R. Brancato, F. Bandello, R. Lattanzio

Atlas of Iris Fluorescein Angiography

Atlas of
IRIS FLUORESCEIN ANGIOGRAPHY

with 1303 pitcures

R. Brancato F. Bandello
R. Lattanzio

kugler & ghedini

R.Brancato
F. Bandello
R. Lattanzio

Department of Ophthalmology and Visual Sciences
Scientific Institute H S. Raffaele
University of Milano
Milano (Italy)

Atlas of Iris Fluorescein Angiography

R. Brancato, F. Bandello, R. Lattanzio

Via G. Pezzotti, 4 - 20141 Milano (Italy)
Tel. (39+2) 89.400.414
Telefax (39+2) 83.23.710
ISBN 88-7780-258-8

P.O. Box 11188 - 1001 GD Amsterdam
The Netherlands
ISBN 90-6299-109-2

P.O. Box 1498 New York, NY 10009-9998
U.S.A.

Cover by:
Yuri De Martin

Phototypesetted and lithos by:
Ghedini Editore - Milano (Italy)

Printed in Italy by:
Centro Poligrafico Milanese
Ponte Sesto di Rozzano - Milano (Italy)

Bounded by:
Nuova Legatoria Liccione Armando s.a.s.
Monza - Milano (Italy)

R. Brancato, F. Bandello, R. Lattanzio
Atlas of Iris
Fluorescein Angiography
Kugler & Ghedini Publications 1995

Table of contents

R. Brancato, F. Bandello, R. Lattanzio
Atlas of Iris
Fluorescein Angiography
Kugler & Ghedini Publications 1995

Preface

It was thirtyfive years ago that MacLean, Maumenee and Norton first sensed the potential importance of fluorescein in ophthalmological diagnosis. A year late Harold Novotny and David Alvis developed the method of retinal fluorescein angiography. These early researchers were too far-sighted for most ophthalmologists of their time, and it was only several years later, as scepticism gave way to clinical testing, that it started to become clear how enormously important this new diagnostic tool could be, in routine clinical practice and for investigative uses. Routine fluorescein angiography was in fact what led to the correct pathogenic interpretation of many chorioretinal pathologies, and provided the basis for the most appropriate treatment. Fluorescein angiography was invaluable in clarifying the cause-effect relationship between retinal ischemic diseases and retinal, papillary and iris neovascularization.

Fluorescein angiography of the iris uses the same principles as angiography of the ocular fundus to examine the anterior segment of the eye. Iris fluorescein angiography, as it is sometimes known, had a harder time getting accepted. We are convinced that this technique is less widely employed because most ophthalmologists are not fully acquainted with its possibilities. In our opinion the lack of enthusiasm for this diagnostic technique in clinical practice is mainly due to the fact that the equipment is not widely available, and not because it provides limited information for diagnosis. We need only look at how useful it is to see the fluorescein angiographic pictures of the iris when cataract surgery is indicated in diabetic patients, at how fluoroiridographic pictures can indicate immediate retinal photocogulation in branch or retinal vein occlusion and at the possibility of detailed monitoring of the evolution of iris tumors.

These are clear examples of how iris fluorescein angiography supplies concrete information useful in diagnosis and treatment, despite its apparent unpopolarity. We believe furthermore, that when the angiographic appearance of the eye is unusual, it can serve to broaden our knowledge of ophthalmology.

We felt this atlas would be useful in extending the use of iris fluorescein angiography, and that in fact was our primary aim.

The illustrations are the fruit of our own work with this method, started 25 years ago and continuing regularly today.

The book starts out with some notes on the history of the method, and describes methodological and technical details. It then proceeds to discuss the various ocular pathologies in which iris fluorescein angiography is most appropriately indicated. Each chapter provides a short introduction, outlining the main pathogenic and clinical points of the diseases which are then amply illustrated in the second iconographic part. To make iconographic consultation easier we thought it convenient to insert an analytical index of the figures.

Clearly the text does not claim to be exhaustive, and we take this early opportunity of apologising for the brevity of the information. However, so that readers can flesh out their knowledge where needed, we have provided a list of bibliographic references with each chapter, besides those mentioned in the brief introductory texts.

Writing a book is always a team job, in which the authors are fortunate when they can rely on numerous helpers. In this case we cannot list all our Department members who have helped put together the caselists on which the book is based, but we must acknowledge the help of two colleagues in particular, whose daily efforts have made a major contribution: Professor Ugo Menchini and Doctor Alfonso Carnevalini.

We are also grateful to Mrs Judy Baggott for her skill and care in translating and editing the text. Mrs Agata Bruno, our secretary, showed unending patience and willingness in organising the various sections. We must also thank our friends and colleagues, for encouraging us on more than one occasion to put this book togheter.

We hope this atlas, with its collection of clinical cases illustrating the use of iris fluorescein angiography, will be useful as a practical tool, and that the layout will permit easy consultation.

Rosario Brancato, Francesco Bandello, Rosangela Lattanzio

Milano, October 1994

R. Brancato, F. Bandello, R. Lattanzio
Atlas of Iris
Fluorescein Angiography
Kugler & Ghedini Publications 1995

Introduction

The year 1990 marked the thirtieth "anniversary" of the introduction of fluorescein angiography as an investigational method in clinical Ophthalmology. Today's fluorangiographic technique has a long history, dating back about 140 years.

In 1850 Hershell and Brewster first described the phenomenon of fluorescence which was studied further by Stokes, two years later. Stokes' law states, in fact, that light emitted from a substance excited by a light source, usually at shorter wavelength, is "fluorescent".[(70)]

Ehrlich was the first to use fluorescein in Ophthalmology. In 1882 he described the appearance of a vertical yellow-green line (Ehrlich's line) in the anterior chamber of a rabbit's eye after injection of a dye into bloodstream.[(33)] Ehrlich went on to use fluorescein to investigate the circulation of aqueous humor and its relation to intraocular pressure. His research was followed by experimental studies by Seidel,[(69)] whose test is still used in clinical practice, by Franceschetti,[(36)] who introduced the concept of the blood-aqueous barrier, and by Goldmann[(44)] whose intuitions on fluorimetry form in fact the groundstones of today's fluorophotometric methods.

Fluorescence was first used in human medicine in 1954, when Mac Lean and Maumenee employed it for diagnostic purposes in a patient with an uveal neoformation, as a basis for deciding whether to enucleate. Their work was later published in 1959.[(51)] Subsequent years witnessed attempts by Maumenee and other researchers such as Flocks and Chao to fix what they saw in the biomicroscope on film, using a cobalt blue filter. In 1958 Chao and Flocks tried out their method in cats and recorded retinal circulation first with serial photographs, using a cine camera to provide a continuous record of fluorescein's passage through the blood vessels.[(21)]

In 1959 two young scientists from Indianapolis, David Alvis and Harold Novotny, achieved good photographic results in human patients; their fluorangiograms are now on display in the American Academy of Ophthalmology's museum in San Francisco. Novotny and Alvis foresaw the clinical importance of this method which made it possible to photograph fluorescence in circulating blood in the human retina, and started to apply it in diabetic and hypertensive patients. They submitted a paper entitled: "A method of photographing fluorescence in circulating blood in the human retina", to the American Journal of Ophthalmology in 1960, but it was rejected as not being original, in the light of the studies by Chao and Flocks. Their clinical experience was eventually published in 1961 in Circulation, and Alvis and Novotny today are recognised as the first to have worked with retinal fluorescein angiography.[(62)]

Their studies opened the way to clinical research by Dollery, Norton, Amalric and Gass who exploited fluorescein angiography to provide a tentative pathogenic interpretation of most ocular vascular disorders.[(1,29,30,38-43,61)] This led to radical changes in the therapeutic approaches to these pathologies.

Fluorescein angiography of the fundus of the eye has been vastly improved since its early stages, and nowadays it is a routine examination for patients with chorioretinal pathology.

In the late Sixties fluorescein angiography started to be used in the anterior segment, particularly the iris. Basing themselves on the principles of retinal fluorescein angiography, Brancato and Frosini used a modified photographic slit-lamp with selected filters, and in 1968 they were among the first to propose this new method for investigating anterior segment of the eye and what they called the surface microcirculation of the eye.[11-18]

Compared to biomicroscopy, this procedure gave an objective assessment of the morphology and the vascular dynamics of conjunctival and ciliary anterior vessels. For the first time, therefore, the physiology and pathology of local vascular systems could be studied in vivo, and the rate of forearm-brain circulation could be measured, particularly in patients with ocular opacities that made it impossible to explore the fundus.

Improvements followed on rapidly and the new technique aroused widespread interest. Some of the first to publish results with this method were Jensen & Lundbaek,[48,49] Cobb,[22,23] Amalric,[2-6] Raitta & Vannas,[64,65] Baggesen,[7] Vannas,[72-73] Mitsui & Matsubara,[59] Rosen,[66,67] Bruun-Jensen,[20] Crandijk & Aan de Kerk,[24] Bron & Easty,[19] Deodati,[25-27] Diversi,[28] Gallenga,[37] Bouchat[10] and Bec.[8,9]

Early studies aimed mainly at establishing fluorangiographic patterns in the normal iris, and the findings extended our knowledge of the vascular anatomy of the iris and - in general - of the anterior segment of the eye. It became increasingly clear that the new method had far-reaching clinical implications.

Fluorescein angiography of the anterior segment was used by many investigators to clarify the vascular anomalies induced by systemic and local pathogenic noxae. Various pathologies of the cornea, episclera and conjunctiva could be analyzed.

Investigation of the iris has remained the most interesting aspect of fluorescein angiography of the anterior segment of the eye but in its twentyfive years of use this method has not received the recognition it deserves, and for a long time it tended to be regarded as a technique mainly useful for researchers. Now, however, it has attracted practical interest for the objective clinical assessment of vascular alterations to the iris. Today it is considered a valid semeiological - hence diagnostic - technique for qualitative and quantitative assessment of pathological damage to the various anatomical structures of the iris.

This method offers the additional advantage, in clinical use, of providing indirect but reliable information on the retinal circulation in situations in which this cannot be examined directly. In many pathologies there is in fact a close relationship between vascular anomalies of the fundus and of the anterior segment. Consequently it is often possible to establish the characteristics of the retinal lesions from a careful analysis of the alterations detected by iris fluorescein angiography.

References

1 Amalric P, Bessou P, Aubry JP: Quelques resultats de retinographie par la fluorescein. Bull Soc Ophtalmol Fr 67: 290, 1967.

2 Amalric P, Bonnin P: L'angiographie fluorescéinique. Bull Soc Ophtalmol Fr, Rapport annuel: 69, 1969.

3 Amalric P, Rebière P, Jourdes JC: Nouvelles indications de l'angiographie fluoresceinique du segment an-

terieur de l'oeil. Ann Ocul 204: 455, 1971.

4 Amalric P, Rebière P, Jourdes JC: Nouvelles indications de l'angiographie fluoresceinique du segment anterieur de l'oeil: Les veines aqueuses. Ann Ocul 204: 469, 1971.

5 Amalric P, Rebière P, Jourdes JC: Nouvelles indications de l'angiographie fluoresceinique du segment anterieur de l'oeil. III Chapitre: Altérations des vaissaux conjonctivaux. Ann Ocul 204: 595, 1971.

6 Amalric P, Rebière P, Jourdes JC: Nouvelles indications de l'angiographie fluoresceinique du segment anterieur de l'oeil. Ann Ocul 204: 731, 1971.

7 Baggesen LH: Fluorescence angiography of the iris in diabetics and non-diabetics. Acta Ophthalmol 47: 449, 1969.

8 Bec P: Discussion des comminication de P. Amalric. Bull Mem Soc Fr Ophtalmol 84: 388, 1971.

9 Bec P, Labro JB: L'angiographie fluorescéinique du segment anterieur. Ann Ther Clin Ophtalmol 33: 257, 1971.

10 Bouchat J: Discussion des comminication de P. Amalric. Bull Mem Soc Fr Ophtalmol 84: 390, 1971.

11 Brancato R: Symposium international sur l'angiographie fluorescéinique. Dynamique circulatoire. Discussion. In Amalric P: Fluorescein angiography. Proc International Symposium on Fluorescein Angiography, Albi, 1969. S Karger, Basel, 1971.

12 Brancato R, Frosini R: Fluorescein microangiography of the anterior segment of the eye. Ann Ottalmol Clin Ocul 96: 543, 1970.

13 Brancato R, Frosini R: Premiers resultats de l'angiographie fluoresceinique superficielle du globe oculaire. Proc 21th International Congress, Mexico 1970. Excerpta Medica International Congress Series 222: 968, 1970.

14 Brancato R, Frosini R: Aspetti fluoroiridografici della ciclite eterocromica. Ann Ottalmol Clin Ocul 97: 107, 1971.

15 Brancato R, Frosini R: La micro-angiographie fluorescéinique du segment antérieur de l'oeil. Bull Mem Soc Franc Ophtalmol 84: 382, 1971.

16 Brancato R, Frosini R: L'angiographie fluorescéinique superficielle du bulbe oculaire. Nouvelle méthode d'exploration. In Amalric P: Fluorescein angiography. Proc International Symposium on Fluorescein Angiography. Albi, 1969. S Karger, Basel, 1971.

17 Brancato R, Frosini R, Boschi MC: L'angiografia superficiale a fluorescenza del bulbo oculare. Ann Ottalmol Clin Ocul 95: 433, 1969.

18 Brancato R, Menchini U: Studio fluorangiografico nelle neovascolarizzazioni corneali. Ann Ottalmol Clin Ocul 98: 531, 1972.

19 Bron AJ, Easty DL: Fluorescein angiography of the globe and anterior segment. Trans Ophthalmol Soc UK 90: 339, 1970.

20 Brunn-Jensen J: Fluorescein angiography of the anterior segment. Am J Ophthalmol 67: 842, 1969.

21 Chao P, Flocks M: The retinal circulation time. Am J Ophthalmol 46: 8, 1958.

22 Cobb B: Vascular tufts at the pupillary margin. Trans Ophthalmol Soc UK 88: 211, 1968.

23 Cobb B, Shilling JS, Chisholm IH: Vascular tufts at the pupillary margin in myotonic dystrophy. Am J Ophthalmol 69: 573, 1970.

24 Craandijk A, Aan de Kerk AL: Fluorescence angiography of the iris. Br J Ophthalmol 54: 229, 1970.

25 Deodati F, Bec P, Labro JB et al.: Angiographie fluorescéinique du segment antérieur. Premiers résultats cliniques. Bull Soc Ophtalmol Fr 69: 1099, 1969.

26 Deodati F, Bec P, Labro JB et al.: L'angiographie fluorescéinique du segment antérieur: son intéret, ses possibilitiés. Bull Soc Ophtalmol Fr 70: 33, 1970.

27 Deodati F, Bec P, Labro JB et al.: Angiographie fluorescéinique du segment antérieur dans les hypertensions oculaires. Bull Soc Ophtalmol Fr 83: 561, 1970.

28 Diversi A: L'iridopathie diabétique étudiée par la fluorescence. In Amalric P: Fluorescein angiography. Proc International Symposium on Fluorescein Angiography Albi, 1969. S Karger, Basel, 1971.

29 Dollery CT, Hodge JV, Engel M: Studies of the retinal circulation with fluorescein. Br Med J 2: 1210, 1969.

30 Dollery CT, Hodge JV, Scott DJ: Studies in fluorescence retinal photography. Trans Ophthalmol Soc UK 83: 429, 1963.

31 Drachenko KG, Shaer EG, Starodubtseva EI: Fluorescence angiography of the anterior segment of the eye. J Audiov Media Med 2: 49, 1979.

32 Editorial: Fluorescein angiography of the iris. Br J Ophthalmol 63: 143, 1979.

33 Ehrlich P: Uber provocirte Fluorescenzerscheinungen am Auge. Dtsch Med Wochenschr 8: 21, 1882.

34 Faggioni R, Grounauer PA, Gailloud C: Angiographie du segment anterieur. Klin Monatsbl Augenheilkd 168: 94, 1976.

35 Flocks M, Miller J, Chao P: Retinal circulation time with the aid of fundus cinephotography. Am J Ophthalmol 48: 3, 1959.

36 Franceschetti A: Uber pharmakologische Beeinflussung der intraocularen Flussigkeiten. Schweiz Med Wochenschr 57: 1089, 1927.

37 Gallenga R: La biofluoroscopie des tumeurs de l'iris. In Amalric P: Fluorescein angiography. Proc International Symposium on Fluorescein Angiography. Albi, 1969. S Karger, Basel, 1971.

38 Gass JDM: A fluorescein angiographic study of macular disfunction secondary to retinal vascular disease: I. Embolic retinal artery obstruction. Arch Ophthalmol 80: 535, 1968.

39 Gass JDM: A fluorescein angiographic study of macular disfunction secondary to retinal vascular disease: II. Retinal vein obstruction. Arch Ophthalmol 80: 550, 1968.

40 Gass JDM: A fluorescein angiographic study of macular disfunction secondary to retinal vascular disease: III. Hypertensive retinopathy. Arch Ophthalmol 80: 569, 1968.

41 Gass JDM: A fluorescein angiographic study of macular disfunction secondary to retinal vascular disease: IV. Diabetic retinal angiopathy. Arch Ophthalmol 80: 583, 1968.

42 Gass JDM: A fluorescein angiographic study of macular disfunction secondary to retinal vascular disease: V. Retinal telengiectasis. Arch Ophthalmol 80: 592, 1968.

43 Gass JDM: A fluorescein angiographic study of macular disfunction secondary to retinal vascular disease: VI. X-ray irradiation, carotid artery occlusion, collagen vascular disease, and vitritis. Arch Ophthalmol 80: 606, 1968.

44 Goldmann H: Uber Fluorescein in der menschlichen Vordekammer. Ophthalmologica 119: 65, 1950.

45 Harris LS, Toyofuku H, Shimmyo M: Fluorescein iris angiography in the albino rabbit. Arch Ophthalmol 88: 193, 1972.

46 Helve J, Nieminen H: Simultaneous bilateral fluorescein angiography of the anterior eye. Acta Ophthalmol 10: 134, 1973.

47 Ikegami M: Fluorescein angiography of the anterior ocular segment. Nippon Ganka Gakkai Zasshi 78: 371, 1974.

48 Jensen VA, Lundbaek K: Fluorescence angiography of the iris in recent and long-term diabetes. Acta Ophthalmol (Kbh) 46: 584, 1968.

49 Jensen VA, Lundbaek K: Fluorescence angiography of the iris in recent and long-term diabetes: preliminary communications. Diabetologica 4: 161, 1968.

50 Koh K: Studies on the fluorescence photography of the bulbar conjunctival vessels, on the techniques of photography. Nich Igaku Zash 27: 386, 1969.

51 MacLean AL, Maumenee AE: Hemangioma of the choroid. Trans Am Ophthalmol Soc 57: 171, 1959.

52 Mapstone R: Fluorescein iridography. Br J Ophthalmol 55: 400, 1971.

53 Matsui M, Asai Y, Sato M 0et al.: Studies on anterior segment fluorescein angiography: II. Improvement of the apparatus. Jpn J Clin Ophthalmol 28: 1347, 1974.

54 Matsui M, Justice J Jr: Anterior segment fluorescein angiography. Int Ophthalmol Clin 16: 189, 1976.

55 Matsui M, Parel JM, Weder H et al.: Some improved methods of anterior segment fluorescein angiography: I. Basic system. Am J Ophthalmol 74: 1075, 1972.

56 Maumenee AE: Clinical manifestations. Ophthalmology 69: 605, 1965.

57 Maumenee AE: Fluorescein angiography in the diagnosis and treatment of lesions of the ocular fundus. Trans Ophthalmol Soc UK 88: 529, 1968.

58 Maurice DM: The use of fluorescein in ophthalmological research. Inv Ophthalmol 6: 464, 1967.

59 Mitsui Y, Matsubara M, Kanagawa M et al.: Fluorescence iridocorneal photography. Br J Ophthalmol 53: 503, 1969.

60 Norton EWD, Smith JL, Curtin VT et al: Fluorescein fundus photography: an aid in the differential diagnosis of posterior ocular lesion. Ophthalmology 68: 755, 1964.

61 Norton EWD, Gass JDM, Smith JL et al: Diagnosis: Fluorescein in the study of macular disease. Ophthalmology 69: 631, 1965.

62 Novotny HR, Alvis DL: A method of photographing fluorescence in circulating blood in the human retina. Circulation 24: 82, 1961.

63 Novotny HR, Alvis DL: A method of photographing fluorescence in circulating blood of the human eye. Aero Med 60: 82, 1962.

64 Raitta C, Vannas S: Fluoresceinangiographie der Irisgefasse nach Zentralvenenverschluss. Albrecht von Graefes Arch Klin Exp Ophthalmol 177: 33, 1969.

65 Raitta C, Vannas S: Fluorescein angiographic features of the limbus and perilimbal vessels. Ear Nose Throat J 50: 58, 1971.

66 Rosen E: Photographie du segment antérieur de l'oeil avec fluorescence. In Amalric P: Fluorescein angiography. Proc International Symposium on Fluorescein Angiography. Albi, 1969. S. Karger, Basel, 1971.

67 Rosen E, Lyons D: Microhemangiomas at the pupillary border demonstrated by fluorescein photography. Am J Ophthalmol 67: 846, 1969.

68 Rumelt MB: A simple technique for anterior segment fluorescein angiography. Am J Ophthalmol 78: 1029, 1974.

69 Seidel E: Weitere experimentale Untersuchungen uber die Quelle und den Verlauf der intraokularen Safstromung: III. Uber den Vorgang der physiologischen Kammerwasserabsonderung und seine pharmakologische Beeinflussung. Graefe's Arch Clin Exp Ophthalmol 102: 372, 1920.

70 Stokes GG, cited by Duke-Elder S: Text-Book of Ophthalmology. CV Mosby, St Louis, 1942.

71 Szalay J, Nunziata B, Henkind P: Permeability od iridial blood vessels. Exp Eye Res 21: 531, 1975.

72 Vannas A: Nouvelle méthode d'angiographie de l'iris. In Amalric P: Fluorescein angiography. Proc International Symposium on Fluorescein Angiography. Albi, 1969. S Karger, Basel, 1971.

73 Vannas A: Fluorescein angiography of the vessels of the iris in pseudoexfoliation of the lens capsule, capsular glaucoma and some other forms of glaucoma. Acta Ophthalmol 105 (Suppl): 75, 1969.

74 Wong IG, Frazier O: Clinical use of iris fluorescein angiography. In Blodi FC: Current concepts in Ophthalmology. CV Mosby, St Louis, 1972.

R. Brancato, F. Bandello, R. Lattanzio
Atlas of Iris
Fluorescein Angiography
Kugler & Ghedini Publications 1995

Section one

Technical Equipment

- Equipment

- Other instruments and new ideas for iris angiography

R. Brancato, F. Bandello, R. Lattanzio
Atlas of Iris
Fluorescein Angiography
Kugler & Ghedini Publications 1995

Chapter 1.1

Equipment

The instrumentation employed for examining the iris with fluorescein angiography has enormously improved over these twenty-five years. The drawbacks of earlier apparatus have been overcome and the examination can be conducted nowadays with extraordinary technical precision.

A photographic slit-lamp is used, modified as necessary and fitted with the accessories required to photograph the anterior segment of the eye. An incandescent lamp is used for observation, and an electronic flash-lamp is built into the optical path for the photography. The depth of field is adjusted with an aperture stop so as to make sure the cornea, anterior chamber and lens are all in focus in the same photo. The image to be photographed can be enlarged as required with a magnification changer.

The slit-lamp has its own camera connected to the microscope. The photographic equipment with its adapter is applied, using an optical beam splitting system, between the magnification changer and the binocular tube.

The camera can be fitted with a system for printing the patient's data and personal number on the film, and the examination time, starting from the fluorescein injection time.

The photo slit-lamp has its own high-power, variable-angle, high-speed charge flash unit.

Fluorescent light

Fluorescein angiographic photography has developed out of the physical phenomenon of *luminescence*, and a system of filters is employed. Luminescence is light emission by a material in response to various types of excitation. If this emission is the response to excitation by another light it is called *fluorescence*. Fluorescence is actually luminescence maintained by continuous excitation which gives rise to immediate emission, only stopping when the stimulus ceases.

Certain substances, when excited by electromagnetic radiation in the visible spectrum, become fluorescent and give off energy at an optical frequency (Fig. **1.1**,1).

Excitation at higher frequencies may cause the fluorescence to contain other frequencies too. According to Stokes' law, the light emitted always comprises lower frequencies, i.e. longer wavelengths. In fact, energy and wavelength are inversely proportional (**E** = **h/l**, where **h** is Planck's constant).

From the beam of exciting light at frequency v, an atom of the excited substance absorbs a finite amount of energy, **hv**. This absorption causes one electron from the atom to pass out of its orbit into a larger orbit. This shift produces the excitation. This electron, now in its wider orbit, can after a very short time - of the order of magnitude of 1 picosecond - return directly to its previous orbit, emitting the same amount of energy, **hv**, and giving rise to waves of the same frequency, **v**.

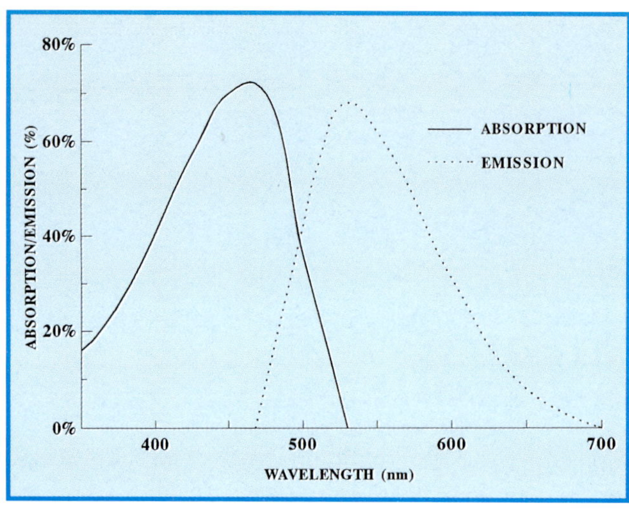

*Fig. **1.1**,1: Curve of absorption and emission of fluorescence.*

Otherwise the electron can return to its initial state not directly but passing through intermediate states, at each of which it emits a certain amount of energy, **hv1**, **hv2**, etc. If this happens the waves emitted may be of different frequencies, but as no new energy reaches the atom between its absorbing the amount of energy hv and emitting the amounts **hv1**, **hv2**, etc., the equation:

hv = **hv1** + **hv2**...must hold; this gives **v** > **v1, v2**, ..., in accordance with Stokes' law.

Fluorescein dye

Fluorescein angiography exploits the chemical and physical features of fluorescein, which in this case is the substance excited. This crystalline molecule has a chemical formula of $C_{20}H_{14}O_5$, and its molecular weight is 376.27 daltons. The molecular structure contains a chinoid ring, which gives it colour. Like other dyes, its main constituent is triphenylmethane. Fluorescein is obtained by reacting phithalic anhydride with resorcin at high temperature, using sulphuric acid as catalyst. Its fluorescence makes it visible even at very low concentrations - down to 10 ng/L (1:100,000,000). As the fluorescence depends on the pH of the solvent and only becomes visible at pH over 6, the characteristic yellow-green colour can only be seen when it is dissolved in alkaline sodium solutions (sodium fluoresceinate).

Fluorescein in solution, excited at wavelengths between 465-490 nm (*absorption spectrum*), emits fluorescence at a wavelength of 520-530 nm (*emission spectrum*). On becoming excited, this dye absorbs light in the visible blue range, and emits light in the yellow-green spectrum.

All the structures and vessels in the body that take up fluorescein show a yellow-green fluorescence. This is because the equipment used has a dual filter system, one known as the *exciter filter* and the other as the *barrier filter*. The ideal exciter filter for fluorescein is blue, which blocks incident light at all wavelengths except between 465 and 490 nm. This filter is placed between the light source (the electronic flash generator) and the eye to be photographed. The ideal barrier filter is yellow-green, which cuts out all wavelengths except those of the fluorescence. This second filter is placed between the patient's eye to be photographed and the film in the camera. This dual filter set-up should allow all light at the desired wavelengths through, and none of the others (Fig. **1.1**,2).

An unwanted effect of in this process is *pseudofluorescence*, caused by non-fluorescent light that does get through the two filters, stimulating the photographic film and creating artefactual fluorescence that reduces the contrast, hence the resolution of the image.

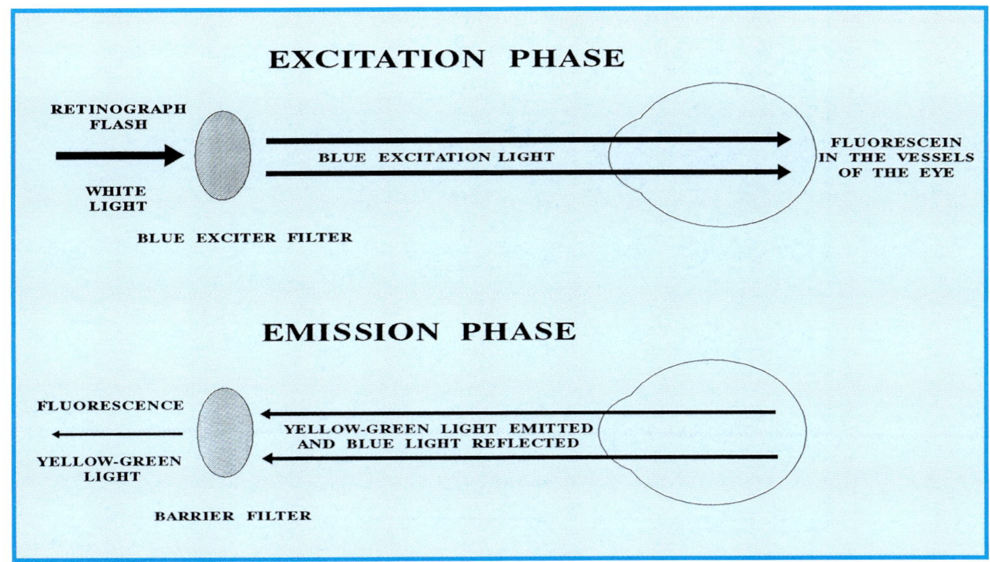

*Fig. **1.1**,2: Fluorescein excitation and emission phases.*

Pseudofluorescence arises where the wavelengths in the two filters overlap (energy cross-over) (Fig. **1.1**,3).

This can be overcome by upairing the filters properly, with clear-cut transmission limits, to minimize the area of overlap of the two curves (Fig. **1.1**,4). *Interferential filters* offer these characteristics (Fig. **1.1**,5).

At the start of the iris angiographic examination, fluorescein is injected intravenously just as for retinal angiography. Generally a 20% solution of fluorescein is employed, and the dose injected is 5 cc (about 14 mg/kg of body weight); this achieves adequate fluorescence.

The concentration of dye used is very important in relation to the intensity of the fluorescence obtained. At a higher concentration of fluorescein the molecules interact, causing loss of energy without any emission of radiation, so without producing any fluorescence. The intensity of the fluorescence does not rise proportionally with the concentration, but remains slightly lower than expected. This self-limiting effect is known as *Excimer quenching*.

Thus a concentration higher than 10^{-2} mg in 100 ml of solution leads to reduced fluorescence. Below 10^{-3}, however, it becomes difficult to distinguish the weak real fluorescence from the tissue autofluorescence.

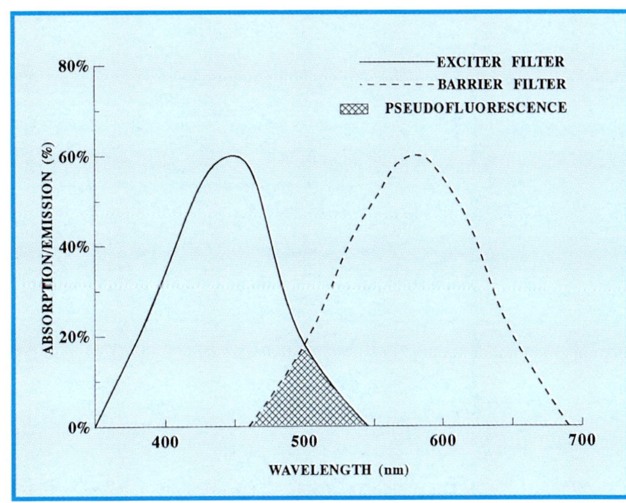

*Fig. **1.1**,3: Pseudofluorescence.*

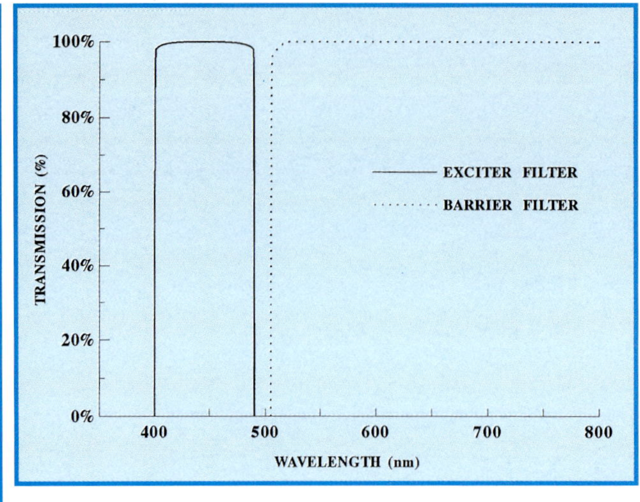

*Fig. **1.1**,4: Ideal combination of filters.*

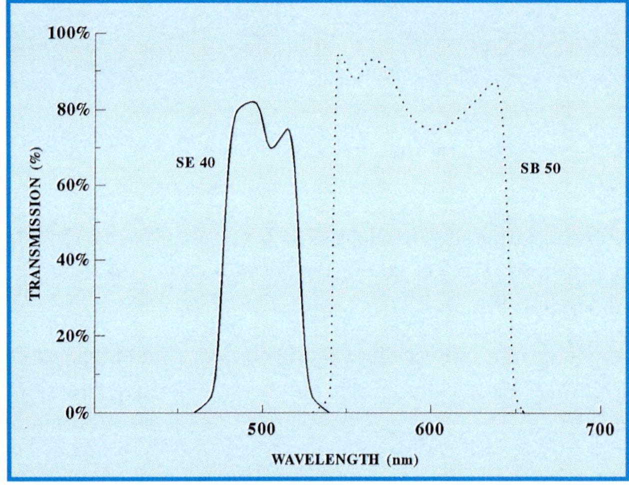

*Fig **1.1**,5: The exciter and barrier filters are separated by approx. 530 nm instead of the usual 500 nm (Interferential filters).*

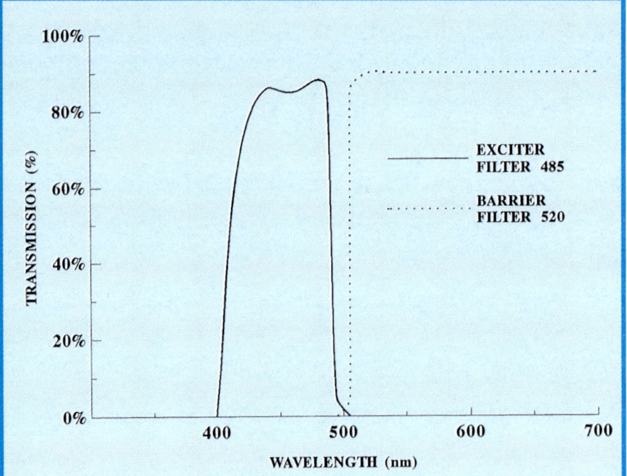

*Fig. **1.1**,6: Combination of exciter and barrier filters in Zeiss photo slit-lamp.*

Once injected, fluorescein largely becomes bound to plasma proteins and to the figured elements in blood. Its molecules remain mainly on the surface of red blood cells, without actually entering them. A large part of the emitted light is absorbed by hemoglobin, thus reducing the intensity of the fluorescence. Binding to proteins in plasma causes alterations in fluorescein's electron structure through the van der Waal reaction, leading to changes in the properties of the fluorescence. The absorption spectra of the fluorescein and plasma proteins overlap, and the whole absorption spectrum shifts. All these factors combined make the fluorescence weaker.

Technique

We have been working with iris fluorescein angiography for twenty-five years. During most of this time we have been using the following equipment:[1]

Zeiss photo slit-lamp with standard optics (lens f.125, binocular tube f. 125, eyepieces 16X), modified to meet our needs with:

a) insertion of a photo adapter in the beam splitter;
b) Contax camera body with Zeiss Dataphot data back;
c) direct connection with a Siemens-Zeiss high-speed charge electronic flash unit, producing 120-720 W/sec.;
d) a Zeiss 485 exciter filter fitted directly on the prism head;
e) a Zeiss P 520 barrier filter mounted between the camera body and the photo adapter (Fig. **1.1**,6).

Since iris fluorescein angiography is a dynamic examination and a timer is employed, the time for each photogram can be recorded on the film, in relation to the fluorescein injection time. This is useful, for example, in assessing changes in the intensity over time, or the extent of pathological hyperfluorescence, or for documenting delays in flow to iris vessels, compared to normal filling times, or rheological differences between the two eyes.

Technical measures

We normally use the enlargement provided by position 16 (factor l in the Galilean system), corresponding to a real enlargement on the photo of 1.76X. When necessary, however, for diagnostic purposes or for documentation, other magnification factors can be used, although these cover either too small or too large a field for routine work.

We currently use a 7° angle for the flash in the pupillary field. This avoids the image of the flash overlapping even a small part of the iris, by saturation, and almost completely reduces the shadow cast by the pupillary border on the lens, which interferes with visualization of the pars pupillaris. It also excludes any interference with the optical path used (set by the side of the camera) and enables one to place the slit prism (with the exciter filter mounted on it) so as to cover the other optical path. A larger flash angle can be useful in some cases to obtain a particular effect of pseudostereopsis.

The flash unit is employed at the maximum power of the instrument we currently have available (position IV), corresponding to 720 W/sec. We use a 50/50 deviator. The photo adapter stop is normally set at f/22. We use black and white film ISO 400/21°, normally Kodak Tri-X or Ilford HP5, developed with D76 at 20°C. The Kodak Tri-X film needs 12 min developing time, and the Ilford HP5 12 min 30 sec. Ilford Hypam fixer is used, needing 5 min for Kodak Tri-X film and 7 min for Ilford HP5. We normally print on Agfa Brovira 312 polythenated paper.

The Zeiss (Oberkochen) is sensitive to the problems of fluorescein angiography of the anterior segment of the eye and has developed an instrument specially for this purpose: the 75 SL slit-lamp. This model has overcome some of the drawbacks of the previous instrumentation and provides the following advantages:

- larger surface illuminated by the flash so as to cover the whole of the iris, up to a maximum of 16 mm;
- a better placing of the exciter filter, directly in the optical path, meaning that the slit illumination prism can be placed coaxially;
- the possibility of continuous lighting for dynamic angiographic examination.

The whole optical pathway for lighting and the corneal microscope suspension unit are above the patient's head so that the investigating physician has ample room for work and manoeuvring, and the patient is not bothered by any of the parts of the instrument. The light source is a high-pressure 75W xenon lamp with provides bright light making it easier to distinguish the finest details. A central control panel permits remote control of all functions: width, height and rotation of the slit, diameter of the light field, movements upwards, zoom enlargement system. A sliding feeder provides electrical power, and the frequency and intensity of the light can be pre-set.

There still remain some problems with hyperfluorescence of the lens which in some cases may attenuate the contrast of the pars pupillaris and with the flashlight, which is not perfectly central.

Several other manufacturers make instruments for iris fluorescein angiography. The tables **1.1**,I-V set out the technical details of the photographic slit-lamps available on the market which can be fitted with units for this examination of the anterior segment of the eye (Figs. **1.1**,7-10).[2]

References

1 Brancato R, Menchini U, Carnevalini A: Atlante di iridografia a fluorescenza. C.I.C. Ed Int Gruppo Ed Medico, Roma, 1981.

2 Martonyi CL: Photographic slit-lamp biomicroscopes. Ophthalmology 96 (Suppl): 6, 1989.

Table 1.1,I: Zeiss Standard Photo Slit-Lamp: technical data (Fig. 1.1,7)

Microscope	
Objective lens focal lenght	125mm
Oculars - Magnifications available – Dioptric range – Range of interpupillary distance	12.5X hi-point (16X and 20X available) ± 8 diopters 49 to 72mm
Magnification settings	6X 10X 16X 25X 40X
Corresponding field of view	32mm 21mm 13mm 8mm 5mm diameter
Observer attachment	available
Slit Lamp	
Slit width	0 to 9.5mm continuous
Slit height	0.3, 3, 4.5, 6, 7.5, 9.5mm
Spot	0.3, 3, 4.5, 6, 7.5, 9.5mm round
Double slit	–
Triple slit	–
Slit illuminator – horizontal arc	90° R&L of center
Slit rotation	90° R&L of center
Slit decentration - horizontal	10° R&L of center
Slit - vertical projection	–
Filters	blue, green
Slit beam diffuser	yes
Light source	6V 30W Tungsten
Instrument Base	
Range of instrument movement – longitudinal – lateral – vertical	26mm 160mm 32mm
Range of control lever	13mm from center
Range of chin rest adjustament (vert.)	43mm
Photography	
Image delivery	beam splitter 50/50 or 7:1 constant
Magnification - linear-mono	0.7, 1.1, 1.8, 2.8, 4.4X or 1.4, 2.2, 3.6, 5.6, 8.8X
Light source – slit illuminator – diffuse illuminator (fill light)	840W/S flash 4 step power supply 60W/S flash 7 step aperture control
Exposure control	manual - power level, aperture
Camera backs available	35mm, Polaroid®
Stereo	full frame simultaneously or split frame simultaneously
Data inprinting	available
Shutter release	control lever button
Anterior segment angiographic capability	available
Endothelial specular microscope attachment	available
Power Supply	
Input	AC 100, 110, 115, 127, 240V, 50-60Hz
Others Accessories available	
	Measuring ocular Pachymeter Video and cine adapters

Table 1.1,II: Zeiss Slit-Lamp 75 SL: technical data (Fig. 1.1,8)

Microscope	
Objective lens focal lenght	125mm
Oculars – Magnifications available – Dioptric range – Range of interpupillary distance	12.5X hi-point (16X) (20X) ± 8 diopters 49 to 72mm
Magnification settings	zoom 6 to 30X (8 to 40X) (10 to 50X)
Corresponding field of view	33 - 7.5mm (26-5.2mm) (20-approx.3.7mm)
Observer attachment	available
Slit Lamp	
Slit width Slit height	0 to 9mm continuous (servo-motor drive) 0 to 9mm continuous (servo-motor drive)
Spot	00 to 9mm continuous
Double slit	–
Triple slit	–
Slit illuminator - horizontal arc	90° R&L of center (servo-motor drive)
Slit rotation	360° continuous (servo-motor drive)
Slit decentration - horizontal	3° R&L of center
Slit - vertical projection	3°
Filters	blue, green, N.D. (10%, 20%, 40%)
Slit beam diffuser	yes
Light source	(14V) 75W high pressure Xenon lamp
Instrument Base	
Range of instrument movement – longitudinal – lateral – vertical	26mm 160mm 32mm
Range of control lever	13mm from center
Range of chin rest adjustament (vert.)	43mm
Photography	
Image delivery	beam splitter 50/50 or 7:1 constant
Magnification - linear-mono	.7 to 3X (.9 to 4.4X) (1 to 5.5X)
Light source – slit illuminator – diffuse illuminator (fill light)	75W high pressure Xenon - 3 step cont. accessory flash unit
Exposure control	manual - power level, aperture and duration
Camera backs available	35mm, Polaroid®
Stereo	full frame simultaneously or split frame simultaneously
Data inprinting	available
Shutter release	control panel button
Anterior segment angiographic capability	yes
Endothelial specular microscope attachment	yes
Power Supply	
Input	AC 100, 110, 120, 127, 220, 240V, 50-60Hz
Others Accessories available	
	Video and cine adapters Measuring ocular Applanation tonometer Pachymeter Hruby lens

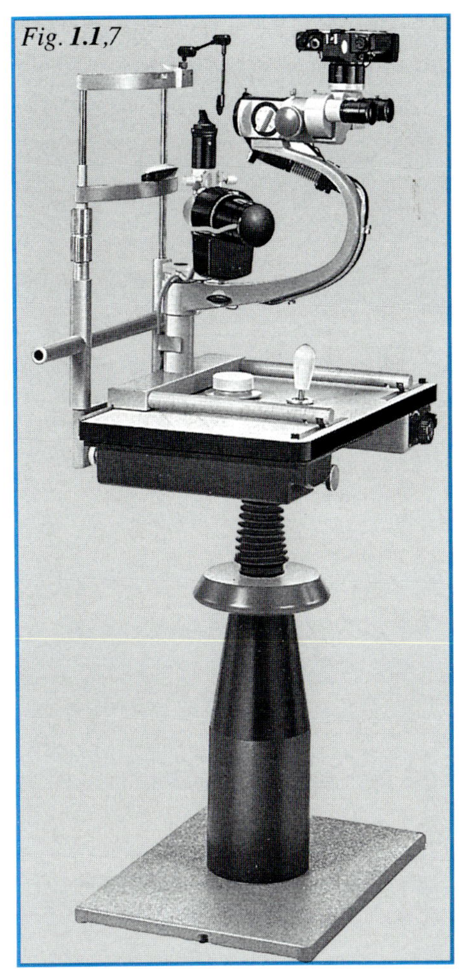
Fig. ***1.1****,7*

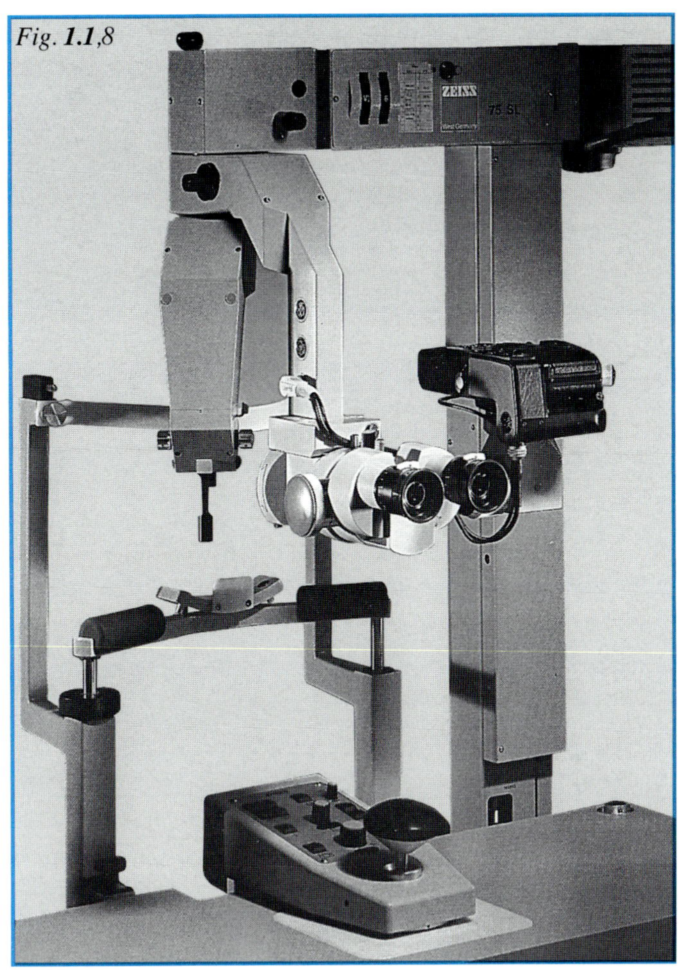

Fig. ***1.1****,8*

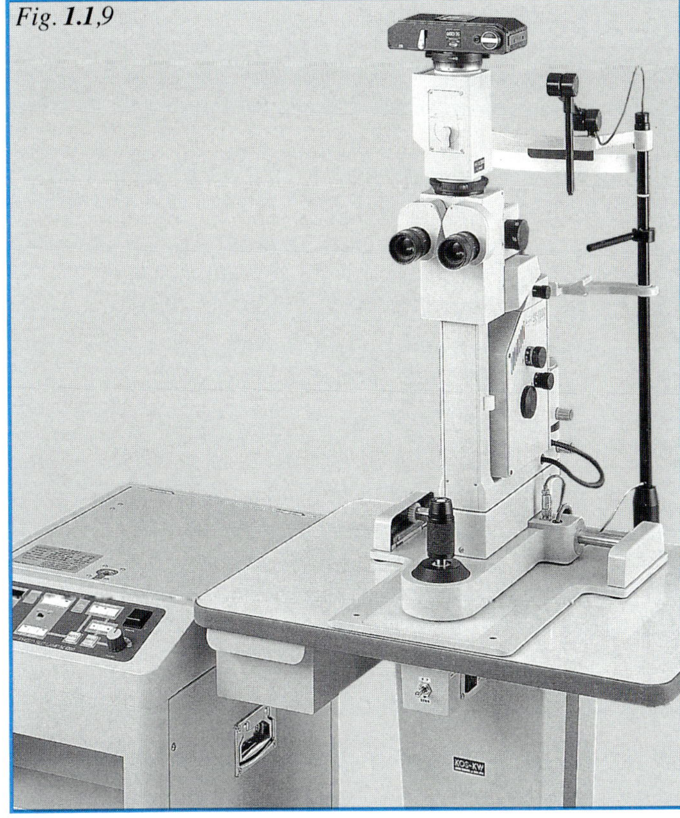
Fig. ***1.1****,9*

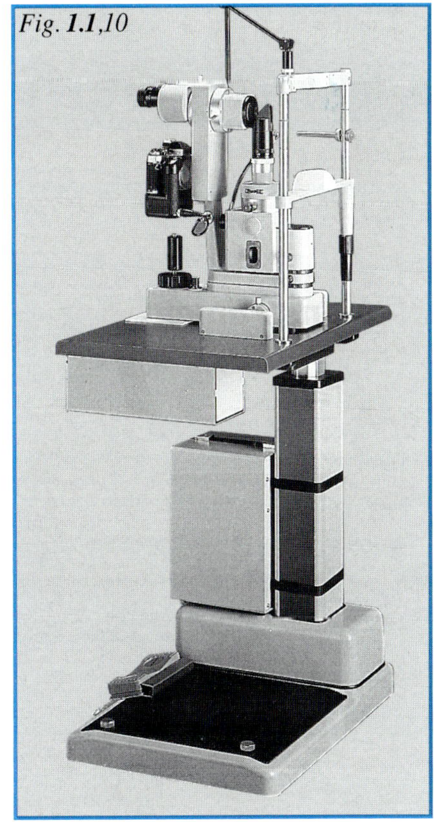
Fig. ***1.1****,10*

Table 1.1,III: Kowa Photo Slit-Lamp SC-1200: technical data (Fig. 1.1,9)

Microscope	
Objective lens focal lenght	120mm
Ocukars – Magnifications available – Dioptric range – Range of interpupillary distance	10X +4 to –8 diopters 55-75mm
Magnification settings	6X 10X 16X 25X 40X
Corresponding field of view	26mm 16.5mm 10mm 6.4mm 4mm diameter
Observer attachment	under development
Slit Lamp	
Slit width Slit height	0 to 11mm continuously adjustable 1, 3, 5, 7, 9, 11 mm in steps
Spot	1, 3, 5, 7, 9, 11 mm in round
Double slit	yes
Triple slit	yes
Slit illuminator - horizontal arc	60° R&L of center
Slit rotation	360°
Slit decentration - horizontal	5° R&L of center
Slit - vertical projection	15°
Filters	blue, green, diffuser on selectable turret
Slit beam diffuser	yes
Light source	6V 30W Halogen lamp
Instrument Base	
Range of instrument movement – longitudinal – lateral – vertical	100mm 120mm 30mm
Range of control lever	6mm from center
Range of chin rest adjustament (vert.)	60mm
Photography	
Magnification - linear-mono	8X 1.3X 2.1X 3.3X 5.2X
Light source	300W/s Xenon -lamp
Exposure control	A7 - step automated flash output is determinated by slit width filters, diaphraghm, ... A5 - step manual control allows the following selections: 300, 200, 100, 50, 25, W/s
Camera backs available	35mm, Polaroid® 600 (ASA 600) interchangeable, cordless contacts
Stereo monocular selection	adjustment lever
Data inprinting	writting data on monocular sqaure picture
Shutter release	control lever button and/or foot switch
Anterior segment angiographic capability	available
Endothelial specular microscope attachment	–
Power Supply	
Input	AC 100, 117, 220, 240V, 50-60Hz
Others Accessories available	
	Tonometer mount (standard equipment) Stereo viewer Video attachment - under development

Table 1.1,IV: Nikon Zoom Photo Slit-Lamp Microscope FS-2: technical data (Fig. 1.1,10)	
Microscope	
Objective lens focal lenght	92mm
Ocukars – Magnifications available – Dioptric range – Range of interpupillary distance	12.5X hi–point (20X hi-point) ±5 diopters 55 to 75mm, adjustable
Magnification settings	zoom 10 to 30X (with click stop at 16X)
Corresponding field of view	22.5 to 7.5mm diameter
Observer attachment	available
Slit Lamp	
Slit width Slit height	0 to 10mm continuous 0 to 10mm continuous
Spot	10mm diameter (smaller sizes are square)
Double slit	–
Triple slit	–
Slit illuminator - horizontal arc	90° R&L of center
Slit rotation	up to 90° on either side of vertical position
Slit decentration - horizontal	10° R&L of center
Slit - vertical projection	0° to 20°
Filters	red-free, cobault, blue, N.D. (28% trasmission)
Slit beam diffuser	yes
Light source	12V 30W Halogen lamp
Instrument Base	
Range of instrument movement – longitudinal – lateral – vertical	100mm 110mm 30mm
Range of control lever	9mm from center
Range of chin rest adjustament (vert.)	50mm
Photography	
Image delivery	beam splitter 70/30, lever controlled
Magnification - linear-mono	1 to 3X (1.4 to 4.2X and 2 to 6X available)
Light source – slit illuminator – diffuse illuminator (fill light)	500W/s Xenon flash, 5 step power supply fiber optic, 3 steps
Exposure control	manual-power level, aperture
Camera backs available	35mm, Polaroid® 600 SX-70
Stereo	split frame simultaneously
Data inprinting	available
Shutter release	control lever button
Anterior segment angiographic capability	under development
Endothelial specular microscope attachment	–
Power Supply	
Input	AC 100, 120, 220, 240V, 50-60Hz
Others Accessories available	
	Stereo photographic attachment El Bayadi-K lens Observation tube Applanation tonometer Pachymeter ITV attachment Observation tube

Table 1.1,V: Mentor Slit-Lamp 22-4600: technical data.

Microscope	
Objective lens focal lenght	102mm
Oculars – Magnifications available – Dioptric range – Range of interpupillary distance	15X hi–point ±8 diopters 54 to 88mm
Magnification settings	5X 7.5X 15X 30X 45X
Corresponding field of view	44mm 20mm 16mm 7mm 4mm diameter
Observer attachment	available
Slit Lamp	
Slit width Slit height	0 to 10mm continuous 0 to 10mm continuous
Spot	.2, 1, 3, 4, 6, 10mm round
Double slit	–
Triple slit	–
Slit illuminator - horizontal arc	90° R&L of center
Slit rotation	90° R&L of center
Slit decentration - horizontal	15° R&L of center
Slit - vertical projection	20° 5 steps
Filters	blue, green, N.D. (50%) (10%)
Slit beam diffuser	yes
Light source	12V 50W Halogen lamp
Instrument Base	
Range of instrument movement – longitudinal – lateral – vertical	76mm 106mm 30mm
Range of control lever	15mm from center
Range of chin rest adjustament (vert.)	88mm
Photography	
Image delivery	separate optical path
Magnification - linear-mono	2.3X (variable)
Light source - slit illuminator – diffuse illuminator (fill light)	200W/s flash, 5 step power supply fiber optics, 4 steps
Exposure control	manual-power level, aperture
Camera backs available	35mm (Polaroid®, available from Tech Enterprises)
Stereo	–
Data inprinting	available
Shutter release	button located just forward of control lever
Anterior segment angiographic capability	may be possible
Endothelial specular microscope attachment	–
Power Supply	
Input	AC 115 or 220V, 50-60Hz
Others Accessories available	
	Applanation tonometer Guyton-Minkowski potential acuity meter

R. Brancato, F. Bandello, R. Lattanzio
Atlas of Iris
Fluorescein Angiography
Kugler & Ghedini Publications 1995

Chapter 1.2

Other instruments and new ideas for iris angiography

A normal retinal fundus camera can be used, with the necessary adaptation, for fluorescein angiography of the anterior segment of the eye. It must be fitted with a compensation lens with a working distance suitable for the required magnification of the iris. Several authors have used a Zeiss fundus camera for the purpose.[25,27,37] In 1978 Fetkenour and Choromokos[9] described another unmodified and not named retinal fundus camera that could be used satisfactorily for this examination. They maintained this method offered several advantages: rapid-sequence exposures, high resolution, time/frame recordings and the dual capability of retinal and anterior segment fluorangiography using the same camera.

The normal limit of fluorangiography using a traditional photographic system, however, lies in its intrinsic features: once the examination is complete time is needed for developing and printing the film before the angiograms can be analysed. Thus a system of angiography independent of the photographic method gets around these problems. The answer is a video-camera that gives real-time fluorescein angiographic images on its monitor. A video-camera also overcomes another limitation that soon becomes apparent in anterior segment angiography: the standard photo slit-lamp does not give a fast enough sequence of photographs during the early phase of fluorescein filling. This is important because in diseased states of the anterior segment, significant changes in the vascular pattern and permeability occur within the first 5 seconds of fluorescein appearing within the eye. In our experience with the Zeiss photo slit-lamp we could obtain at best six consecutive exposures at l-second intervals, after which there was a delay of 13 seconds for recycling.

As early as 1978 Marsh and Ford[28] proposed a technique for cinephotography and video-recording of anterior segment fluorescein angiography. Zeiss has recently designed a system for dynamic documentation of the findings of this iris examination employing a TV system (Fig. **1.2**,1). This instrumentation consists of:

- a Zeiss 20 SL slit-lamp complete with beam splitter and TV adapter (f 74 mm);
- a TV system consisting of:
  a) 1/2" PAL system video camera (single CCD) with linear resolution over 300 lines and automatic gain device to increase the maximum sensitivity up to the threshold of 10 Lux;
  b) monitor with 10" screen and horizontal resolution over 280 lines;
  c) professional video-recorder (U-Matic, 3/4");
  d) exciter filter 483 nm and barrier filter 530 nm.

The selection of a Zeiss slit-lamp 20 SL is based - besides the optical features of the microscope - on the slit width of 12 mm, which means the whole surface of the iris can be illuminated with focused light. The barrier filter with its special mount is positioned by

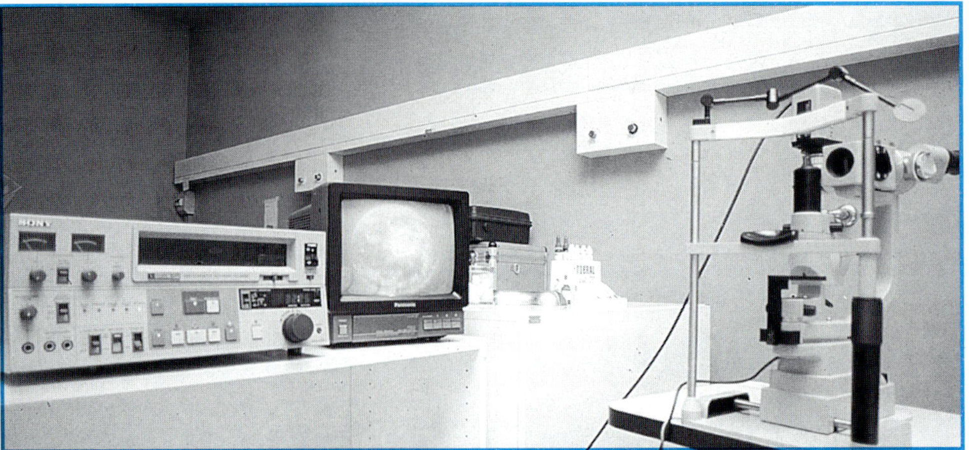

*Fig. **1.2**,1: Zeiss system for cinephotography and video-recording of anterior segment fluorescein angiography.*

dovetailing it onto the illumination prism of the slit lamp, while the barrier filter with special support is introduced between the microscope body and the beam splitter. The splitter can remain permanently in place as it has a special lever to introduce it into the beam path.

For a correct examination the instrument should be set as follows:
- very narrow angle between the slit-lamp illumination and observation system (use the illumination system to cover the beam path not needed for the documentation);
- set the microscope magnification to the required factor;
- set the instrument illumination lamps to maximum brightness;
- activate the automatic gain device on the video-camera;
- take off all colour from the monitor screen and focus the image through the screen itself;
- check that exciter and barrier filters are swung in;
- inject fluorescein and set video-recorder on recording;
- set the stop on the TV adapter in order to achieve correct exposure of the image on the monitor screen.

A personal computer converts the angiograms from the telecamera into digital form and they appear on the monitor in real time. The system comes with the software needed to analyse the images so as to facilitate the interpretation of the angiogram. For example, details can be enlarged as needed, the contrast can be enhanced, and so forth.

Once the examination has been completed, the angiograms can be filed on a high-density optical disk or the whole record can be erased if the results are of no interest. At the end of the examination diagnostic and therapeutic assessments can be drawn from observation of all the images taken. There is no need to wait for the photos to be printed to decide, for example, whether the patient needs retinal photocoagulation. The advantages are evident in the quality of care supplied to out-patients, and the possibility of photocoagulation treatment on the basis of the very latest findings. The patient needs to be kept in hospital less time, with all the advantages this implies for hospital turnover. There is also an appreciable saving in routine photographic material (film, development and printing) and in specialised photographic and laboratory staff.

Over recent years, as advances have been made in electronics and in digital image processing, the high resolution of today's video-camera is closing the gap between the quality of photographic and video images. However, some technical problems persist in current methods for anterior segment fluorescein angiography.

Difficulties with confounding reflexes, off-axis illumination and shallow depth of field have led some investigators[(8)] to develop more complex systems. One uses the

Zeiss 30 fundus camera as the stroboscopic light but powered by a Zeiss FF-4 power pack. A Nikon 2002 camera was chosen as a high-quality, compact, light-weight instrument with its built-in motor drive. The camera was mounted on Nikon PB-6 bellows to provide the variable magnification and the relatively long working distance so that the camera did not obstruct the illumination field of the fundus camera light source. A 75-mm EL-Omegar photographic enlarging lens (Simmon Omega, Woodside, N.Y., USA) was selected to provide a planar image field at high magnification. The lens was relatively inexpensive and fit the bellows without adaptation.

Its designers describe this as a simple method using readily available equipment to provide an inexpensive and optimal photographic system for anterior segment fluorescein angiography.

Another proposal for video fluorescein angiography of the anterior segment employs an angiographic scanning microscope[(32)], which is a modified scanning laser ophthalmolscope. This gives a series of advantages over conventional photographic methods: long focal length, ample visual field, coaxial illumination, low light levels, real-time TV operation and the possibility of video-recording with immediately recall. The video techniques give resolution only slightly below that of photography, and this difference is not felt in clinical practice. Using this instrument a method has been developed that covers the whole anterior episcleral vascular network, facilitating analysis of the vascular dynamics in the sclera and bulbar conjunctiva.

In images obtained with the angiographic scanning microscope the contrast is intensified by creating a uniform black scleral background to the intravascular fluorescence, so that even the smallest vessels become visible. Video images can be filed and employed for digital processing, computerized image analysis and transfer of these electronic data.

Scanning microscope fluorangiography has brought to light a series of principles that can help improve fluorescein angiographic examination of the anterior segment. Some are set out below:

- a fast optical speed is needed in fluorangiography to use as much of the fluorescent light as possible;
- the filling phases must be analysed in real time for studying vascular dynamics;
- coaxial lighting is needed to ensure uniform fluorescence on curved surfaces;
- at useful magnifications, the depth of field must be greater than with traditional photographs or video images;
- "tight" filters must be used to eliminate light reflecting on the bulbar surface;
- improved filter selection will eliminate the loss of contrast sensitivity caused by pseudo-fluorescence.

Indocyanine-green iris angiography

Ophthalmic angiography using indocyanine-green has been re-proposed recently for the study of chorioretinal diseases. This technique was initially developed in the early 1970s,[(6,10-14,26)] but the poor molecular fluorescence of the dye used at that time, inappropriate combinations of excitation and arrest filters, inadequate light sources in the infrared range, poor-quality films and the lack of suitable instruments on the market all prevented the widespread use of this method in clinical practice during these two decades. Nevertheless, there are reports of experience with indocyanine-green choroidal angiography.[(1,2,7,20,22,35,36)]

In recently years the limitations of this technique has been partially overcome by significant advances in infrared imaging technology, such as the development of infrared video cameras (which are really modified retinographs with appropriately treated lenses), improved couples of interferential filters, stronger lighting systems, digital computers systems and the scanning lasers ophthalmoscope.[15,38] This progress has stimulated vigorous interest in the clinical and scientific applications of the method.

Indocyanine-green is an organic substance, a tricarbocyanine dye with peak absorption (805 nm) and peak fluorescence (835 nm) in the near-infrared spectrum. Its actions at these longer wavelengths mean that visibility is better through overlying blood, lipid and pigment that may block fluorescein detection of chorioretinal pathology.[16] In addition, since it binds largely to proteins (98% compared with 60-80% for fluorescein), indocyanine-green diffuses slowly out of fenestrated small choroidal vessels.[2]

The result is that, compared with fluorescein, indocyanine-green gives better visualization of the choroidal circulation and of some membranes that retinal fluorescein angiography only poorly defines because the fluorescein is blocked by overlying substances or structures, or because it rapidly leaks, obscuring neovascular details.[7,17]

Indocyanine-green videoangiography has the additional advantages of providing information on choroidal morphology and dynamics. It is therefore useful for studying and diagnosing inflammatory, neoplastic and ischemic pathologies of the choroid, in vivo. All these disorders offer wide unexplored areas for investigation using indocyanine-green angiography. These various advantages can be put to good use in iris angiography too (Figs. **1.2**,2-12). Initial clinical work with this method has already been described by Podgornaja[34] and by Maruyama.[29]

Although the resolution of this method is still not as good as standard fluorescein angiography and this dye is not likely to replace fluorescein, the information that indocyanine-green investigation can add to fluorescein angiographic findings may possibly improve the detection and subsequent treatment of some poorly defined vascular abnormalities that are currently considered untreatable.[39-41] Indocyanine-green may also possibly provide a dye-enhanced target for infrared laser photocoagulation, to improve the selective closure of neovascular tufts.

References

1 Bischoff PM: Quantitative Untersuchung der normalen Aderhautzirkulation. Fortschr Ophthalmol 86: 107, 1989.

2 Bischoff PM, Flower RW: Ten years experience with choroidal angiography using indocyanine green dye: a new routine examination or an epilogue? Doc Ophthalmol 60: 235, 1985.

3 Brancato R, Menchini U, Carnevalini A: Atlante di iridografia a fluorescenza. C.I.C. Ed Int Gruppo Ed Medico, Roma, 1981.

4 Brown N, Straney R: Infrared fundus angiography. Br J Ophthalmol 57: 797, 1973.

5 Chandler JW, Sewell JH, Kaufman HE: Anterior segment fluorescein angiography: a simple modification of the Zeiss stereo slit lamp camera. Ann Ophthalmol 7: 87, 1975.

6 David NJ: Infra-red absorption fundus angiography. In Amalric P: Fluorescein Angiography. Proc International Symposium on Fluorescein Angiography. Albi, 1969. S Karger, Basel, 1971.

7 Destro M, Puliafito CA: Indocyanine green videoangiography of choroidal neovascularization. Ophthalmology 96: 846, 1989.

8 Fariza E, Ormerod LD, O'Day T et al: Practical anterior segment fluorescein angiography. Graefe's Arch Clin Exp Ophthalmol 229: 105, 1991.

9 Fetkenhour CL, Choromokos E: Anterior segment fluorescein angiography with a retinal fundus camera. Arch Ophthalmol 96: 711, 1978.

10 Flower RW: Infrared absorption angiography of the choroid and some observations on the effects of high intraocular pressures. Am J Ophthalmol 74: 600, 1972.

11 Flower RW: Choroidal fluorescent dye filling patterns: a comparison of high speed indocyanine green and fluorescein angiograms. Int Ophthalmol 2: 143, 1980.

12 Flower RW, Hochheimer BF: Clinical infrared absorption angiography of the choroid (letter). Am J Ophthalmol 73: 458, 1972.

13 Flower RW, Hochheimer BF: A clinical technique and apparatus for simultaneous angiography of the separate retinal and choroidal circulations. Invest Ophthalmol 12: 248, 1973.

14 Flower RW, Hochheimer BF: Infrared fundus angiography (letter). Br J Ophthalmol 58: 635, 1974.

15 Flower RW, Klein GJ: Pulsatile flow in the choroidal circulation: a preliminary investigation. Eye 4: 310, 1990.

16 Geeraets WJ, Berry ER: Ocular spectral characteristics as related to hazards from lasers and other light sources. Am J Ophthalmol 66: 15, 1968.

17 Guyer DR, Puliafito CA, Monés JM et al: Digital indocyanine-green angiography in chorioretinal disorders. Ophthalmology 99: 287, 1992.

18 Hayashi K, deLaey JJ: Indocyanine green angiography of choroidal neovascular membranes. Ophthalmologica 190: 30, 1985.

19 Hayashi K, deLaey JJ: Indocyanine green angiography of submacular choroidal vessels in the human eye. Ophthalmologica 190: 20, 1985.

20 Hayashi K, Hasegawa Y, Tazawa Y et al: Clinical application of indocyanine green angiography to choroidal neovascularization. Jpn J Ophthalmol 33: 57, 1989.

21 Hayashi K, Hasegawa Y, Tokoro T: Indocyanine green angiography of central serous chorioretinopathy. Int Ophthalmol 9: 37, 1986.

22 Hayashi K, Hasegawa Y, Tokoro T et al: Value of indocyanine green angiography in the diagnosis of occult choroidal neovascular membrane. Jpn J Clin Ophthalmol 42: 827, 1988.

23 Hochheimer BF: Angiography of the retina with indocyanine green. Arch Ophthalmol 86: 564, 1971.

24 Hochheimer BF, D'Anna SA: Angiography with the new dye. Exp Eye Res 27: 1, 1978.

25 Jensen VA, Lundbaek K: Fluorescein angiography of the iris in recent and long-term diabetes. Diabetologia 4: 161, 1968.

26 Kogure K, David NJ, Yamanouchi U et al: Infrared absorption angiography of the fundus circulation. Arch Ophthalmol 83: 209, 1970.

27 Mapstone R: Fluorescein iridography. Br J Ophthalmol 55: 400, 1971.

28 Marsh RJ, Ford SM: Cine photography and video recording of anterior segment fluorescein angiography. Br J Ophthalmol 62: 657, 1978.

29 Maruyama Y, Kamei Y, Kishi S et al: ICG iris angiography in exfoliation syndrome. International Symposium of Fluorescence Angiography. Quebec, 1994 (Oral communication).

30 Matsui M, Parel JM, Weder H et al: Some improved methods of anterior segment fluorescein angiography: I. Basic system. Am J Ophthalmol 74: 1075, 1972.

31 Matsui M, Asai Y, Sato M et al: Studies on anterior segment fluorescein angiography. II. Improvement of the apparatus. Jpn J Clin Ophthalmol 28: 1347, 1974.

32 Ormerod LD, Fariza E, Hughes GW et al: Anterior segment fluorescein video-angiography with a scanning angiographic microscope. Ophthalmology 97: 745, 1990.

33 Patz A, Flower RW, Klein ML et al: Clinical applications of indocyanine green angiography. Doc Ophthalmol Proc Ser 9: 245, 1976.

34 Podgornaja NN, Akhmedov AA: Indocyanine green fluorescence iridoangiography in pigmented iris. Vestn Oftalmol 107: 40, 1991.

35 Prunte C, Niesel P: Quantification of choroidal blood-flow parameters using indocyanine green video-fluorescence angiography and statistical picture analysis. Graefe's Arch Clin Exp Ophthalmol 226: 55, 1988.

36 Quentel G, Coscas G: Angiographie en fluorescence infrarouge au vert d'indocyanine. Bull Soc Ophtalmol Fr 84: 559, 1984.

37 Rosen ES: Fluorescence photography of the anterior segment of the eye. In Amalric P: Fluorescein Angiography. Proc International Symposium on Fluorescein Angiography. Albi, 1969. S Karger, Basel, 1971.

38 Scheider A, Schroedel C: High resolution indocyanine green angiography with a scanning laser ophthalmoscope (letter). Am J Ophthalmol 108: 458, 1989.

39 Yannuzzi LA, Slakter JS, Sorenson JA et al: Digital indocyanine green videoangiography and choroidal neovascularization. Retina 12: 191, 1992.

40 Yannuzzi LA, Sorenson JA, Guyer DR et al: Indocyanine-green video-angiography: current status. Eur J Ophthalmol 4: 69, 1994.

41 Yuzawa M, Kawamura A, Matsui M: Clinical evaluation of indocyanine-green video-angiography in the diagnosis of choroidal neovascular membrane associated with age-related macular degeneration. Eur J Ophthalmol 2: 115, 1992.

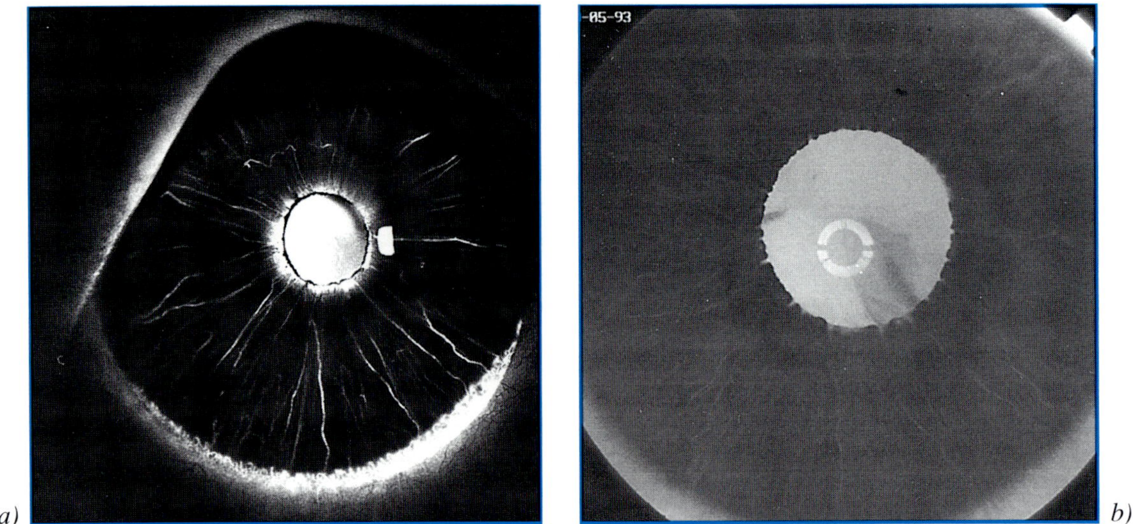

a) *b)*

Fig. ***1.2****,2: Iris fluorescein (a) and indocyanine-green (b) angiographies in a normal 65-year-old subject. The physiological age-related dye leakage observed in the fluorescein image at pupillary margin is probably related to the processes of iris microcirculation aging resulting in the tight-junctions loosening. On the contrary, due to large binding to proteins, indocyanine-green dye diffuses poorly out of capillaries.*

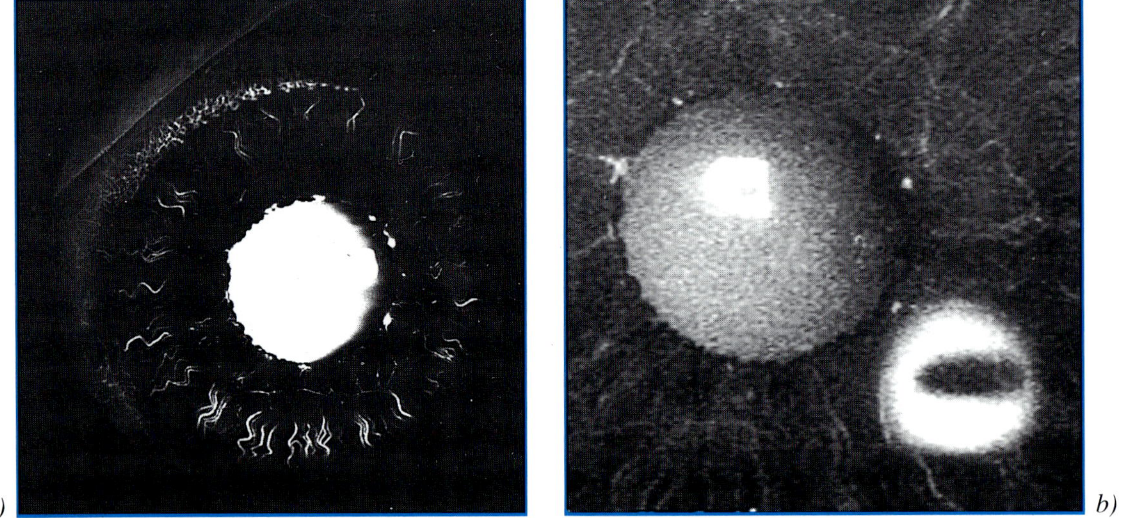

a) *b)*

Fig. ***1.2****,3: Where iris fluorescein angiography shows early neovascular spots at pupillary margin (a), indocyanine-green angiography shows hyperfluorescent rather smaller and not dye-leaking dots (b).*

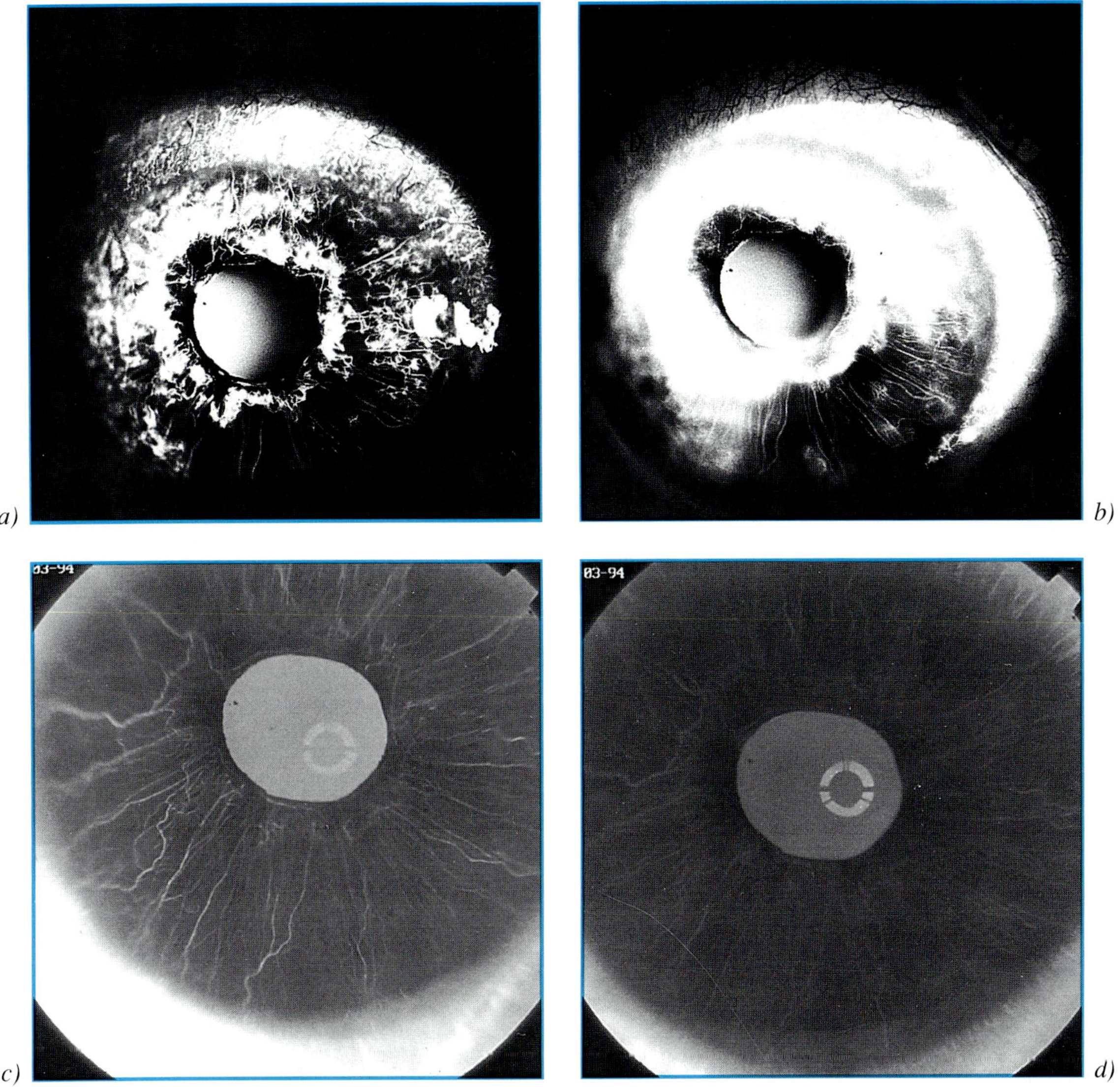

*Fig. **1.2**,4: Iris fluorescein angiography in a diabetic patient with new vessels over the whole iris surface (a,b). Early phase marks the precise site and extent of neovascular growth (a); subsequently, fluorescein leakage from the anomalous vessels covers iris surface (b). In indocyanine-green sequences (c,d) the anarchic morphology and increased permeability of neovascular network are poorly detected.*

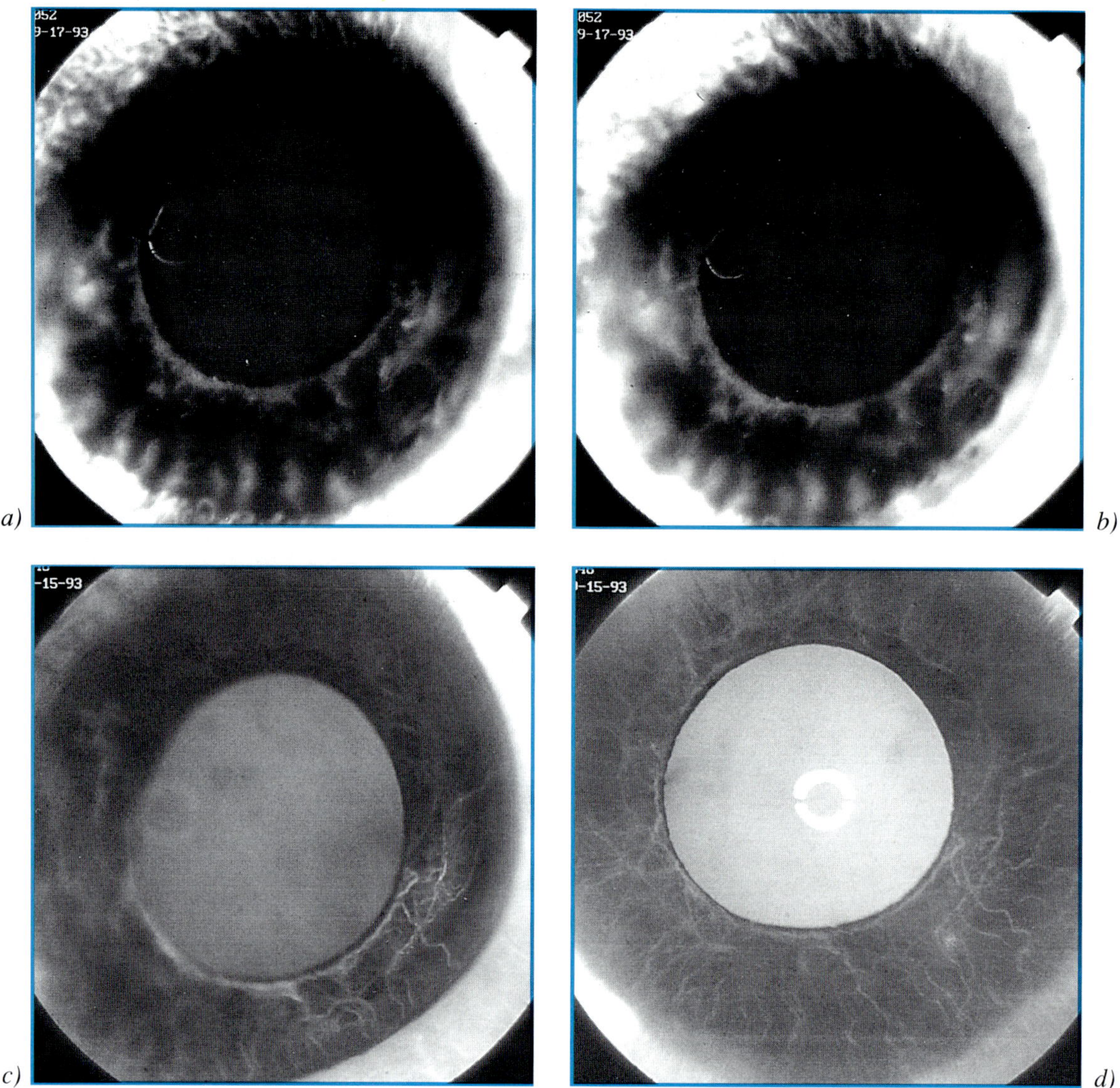

Fig. ***1.2**,5: Neovascular glaucoma in a patient suffering from central retinal vein occlusion. Both fluorescein (a,b) and indocyanine-green (c,d) sequences detect marked filling defects in the superior sectors. Inferiorly, anomalies such as delayed filling, congested iris vessels and neovascular tufts are better visualized by fluorescein (a,b) than by indocyanine-green (c,d).*

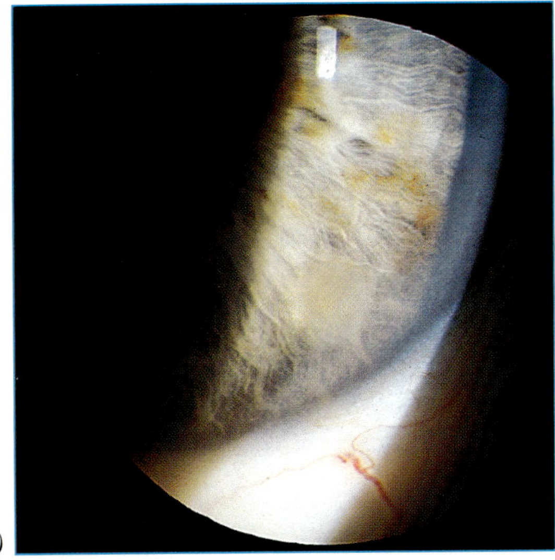

a)

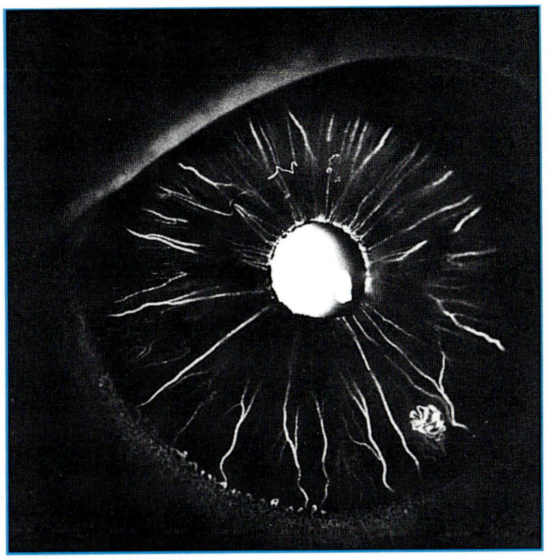

*Fig. **1.2**,6: Biomicroscopy (a) in a 62-year-old patient affected by iris leiomyoma which on fluorescein examination takes up dye early in an intricate vascular network (b) and leaks dye in late phases (c). Dye leakage at the pupillary margin is age-related and increases typically at each phase of examination. On the contrary, indocyanine-green phases show apparently normal iris vessels (d,e).*

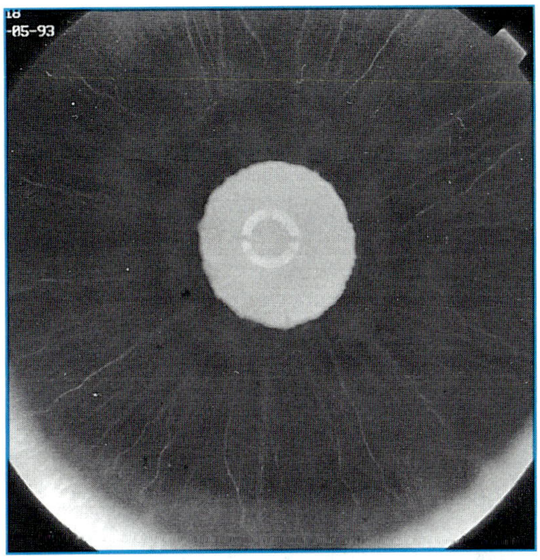

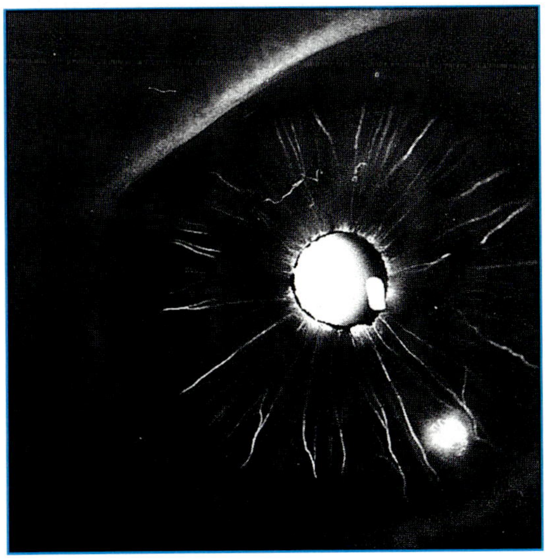

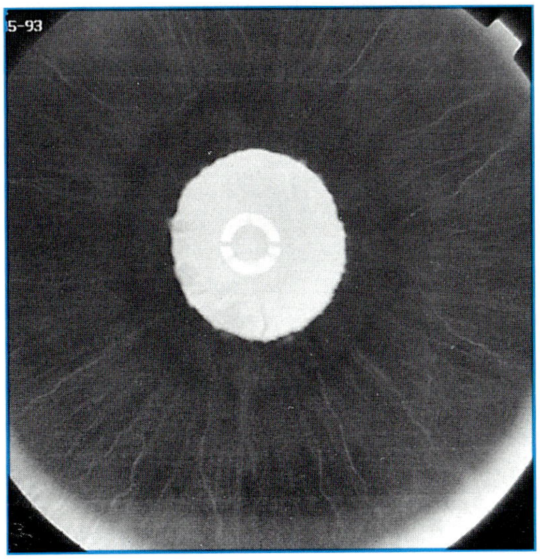

b)

d)

c)

e)

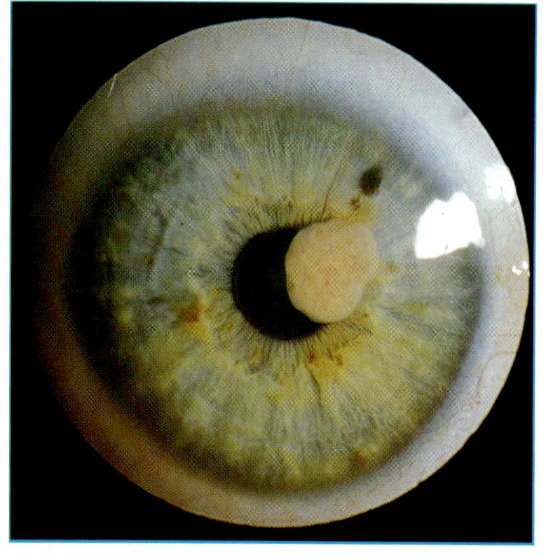

a)

*Fig. **1.2**,7: Biomicroscopy (a) in a case of iris amelanotic melanoma. Because of melanin absence, fluorescein angiography allows a precise picture of tumoral vessels, which perfuse rapidly (b) and leak dye in the later phases (c). Early indocyanine-green injection into the tumor's anarchic vascular network (d) is followed in the later phases (e) by diffuse through the mass but poorly dye-leaking hyperfluorescence. The iris radial vessels at sites remote from the tumor are not properly focused since the angiograms are focused on the mass (b,c,d,e).*

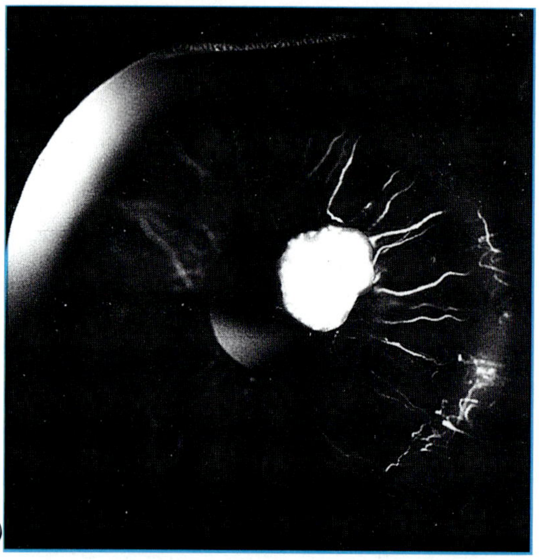

b)

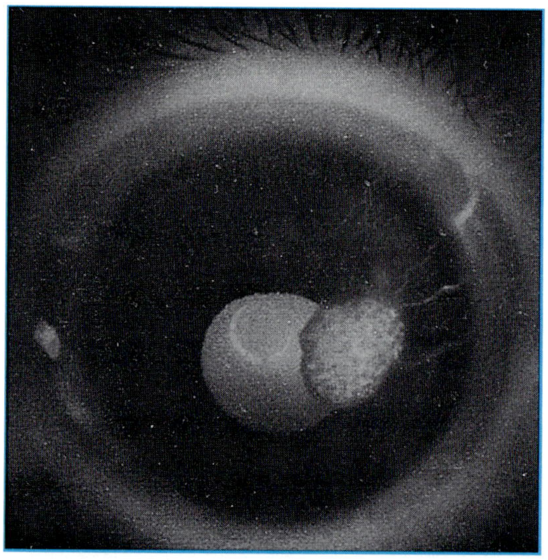

d)

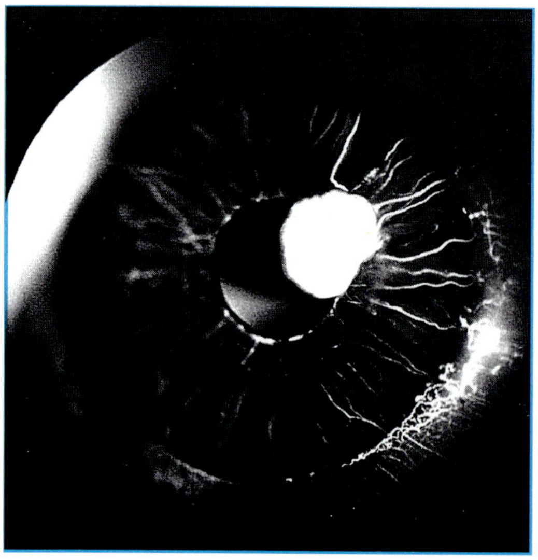

c)

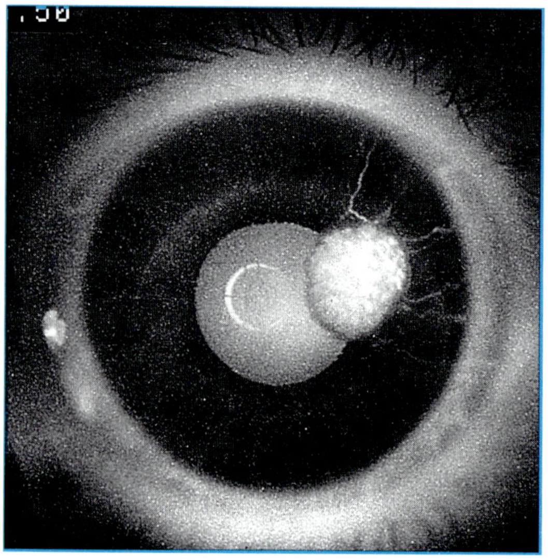

e)

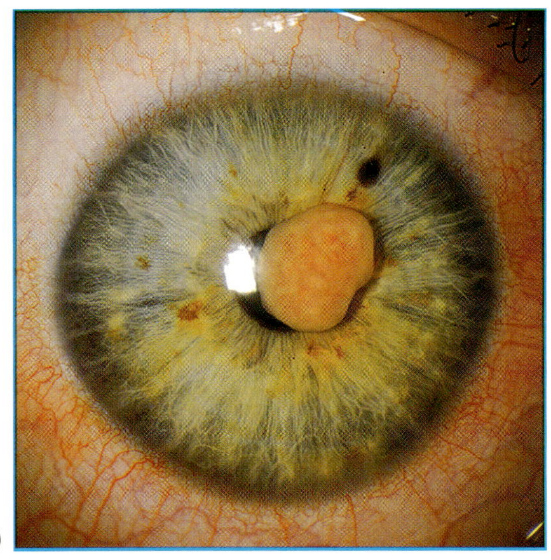

a)

*Fig. **1.2**,8: Same case as in Figure 7 three months later: the mass appears bigger (a) but its fluorescein (b,c) and indocyanine-green (d,e) angiographic characteristics are still the same. A diffuse blood-iris barrier breakdown is only detected by fluorescein (b,c); on the contrary, iris vessels permeability looks normal in indocyanine-green angiograms (d,e).*

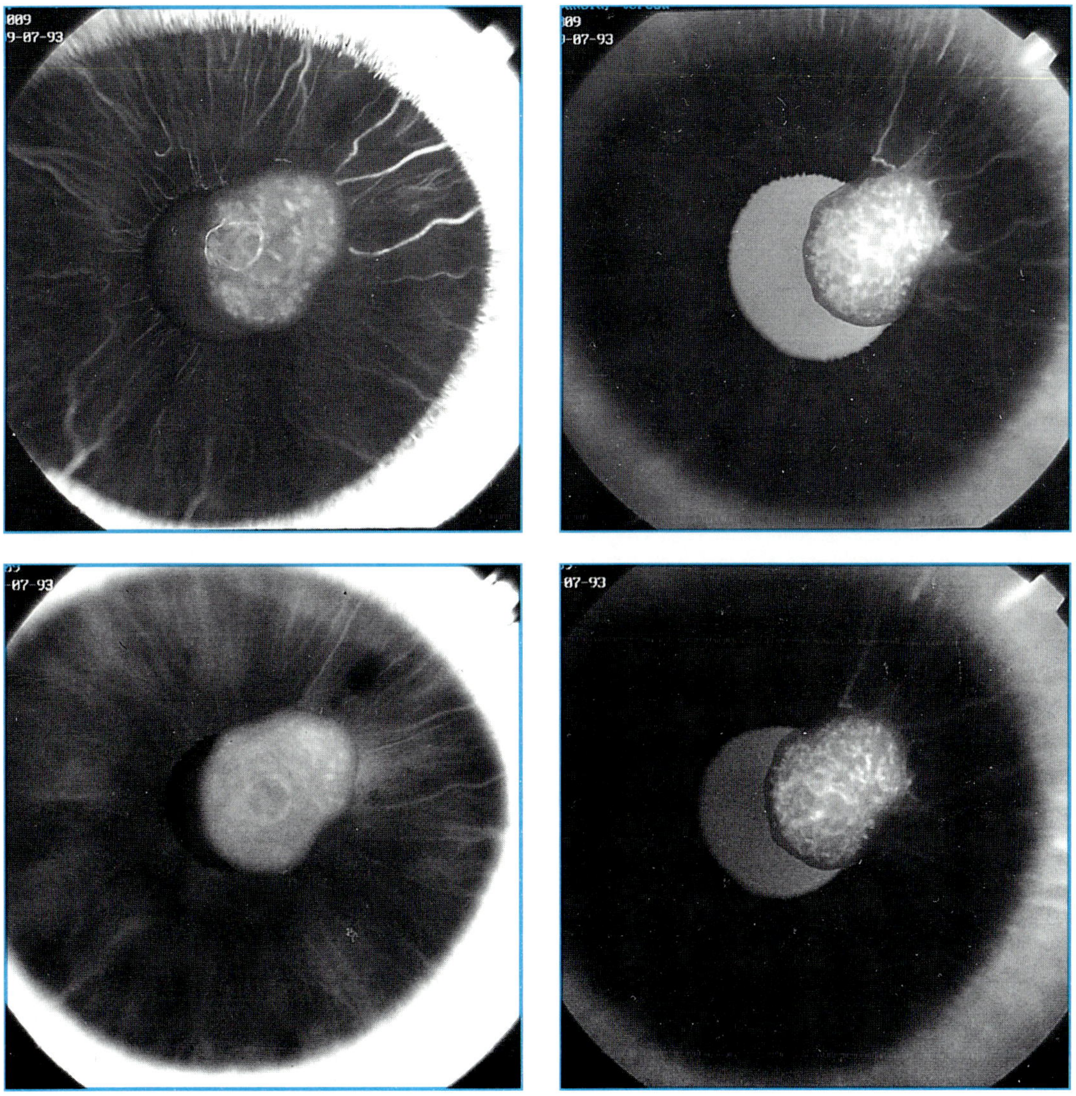

b)

d)

c)

e)

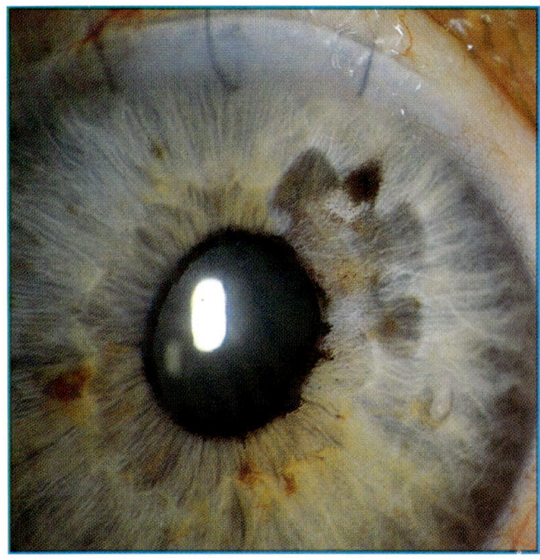

a)

*Fig. **1.2**,9: Colour photo (a), fluorescein (b,c) and indocyanine-green (d,e) angiographies of the same case referred in Figure 7 and 8 after surgical excision. As above, the blood-iris barrier breakdown is not detected by indocyanine-green dye.*

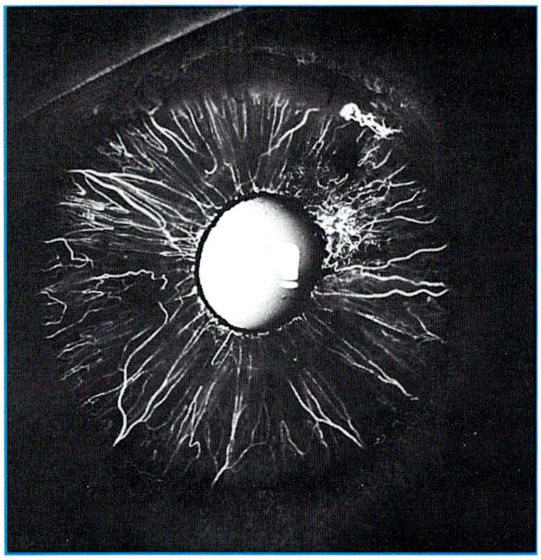

b)

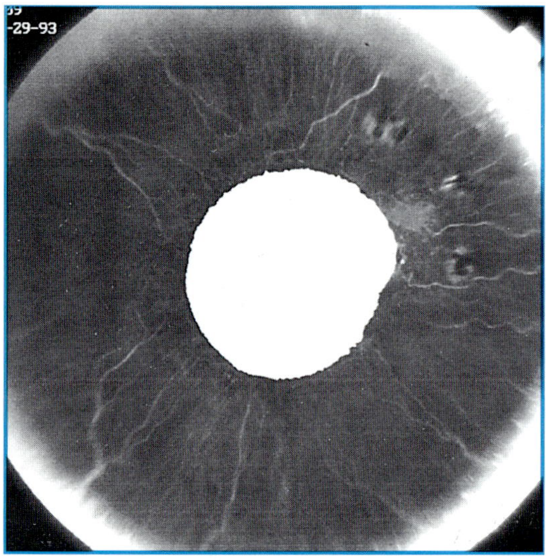

d)

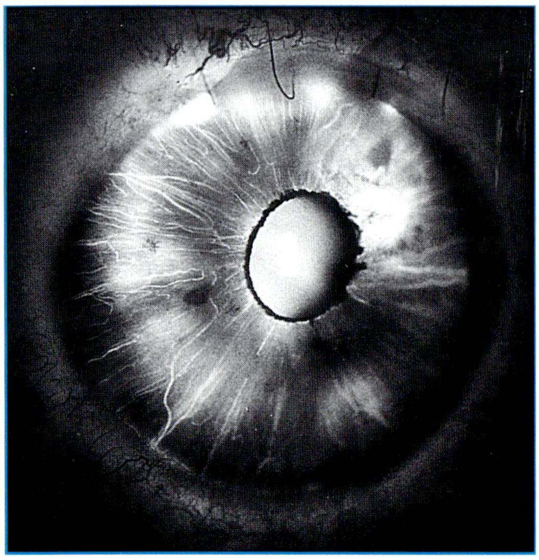

c)

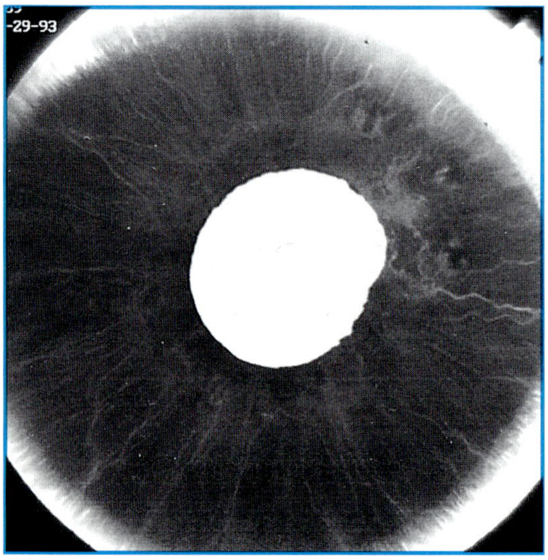

e)

a) 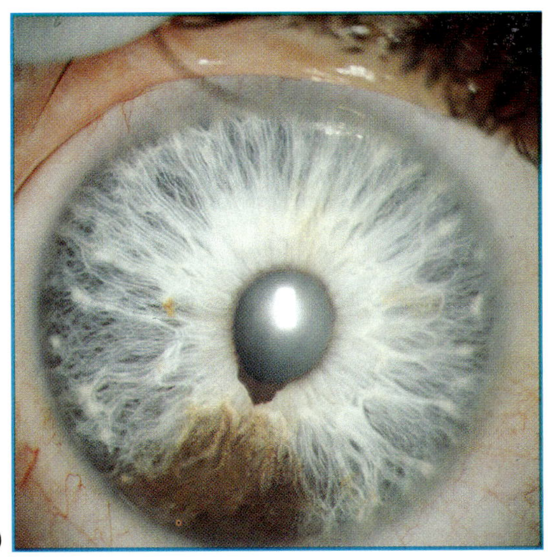

*Fig. **1.2**,10: Biomicroscopy (a) in a case of iris nevus which masks iris neovascularization in the fluorescein angiograms (b,c). The masking effect is less marked on indocyanine-green pictures (d,e).*

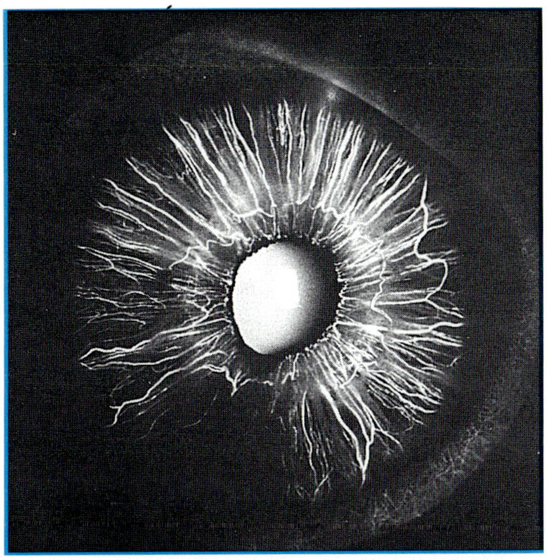

b)

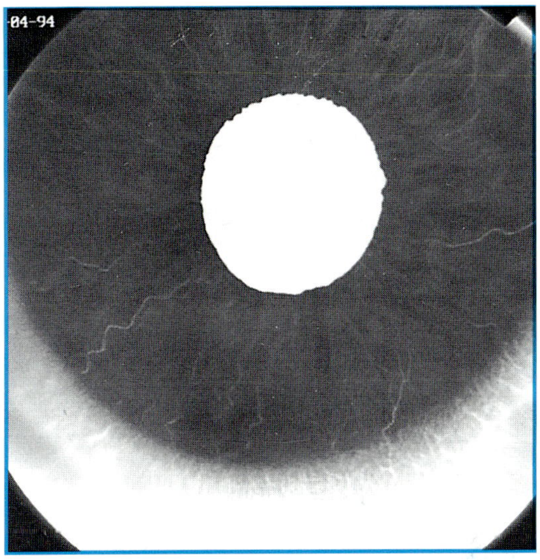

d)

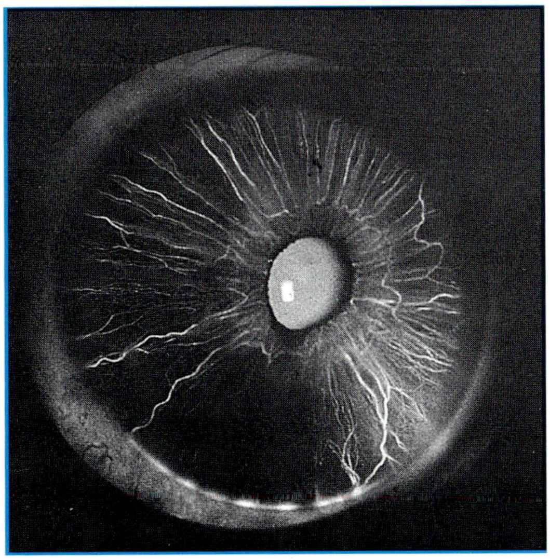

c)

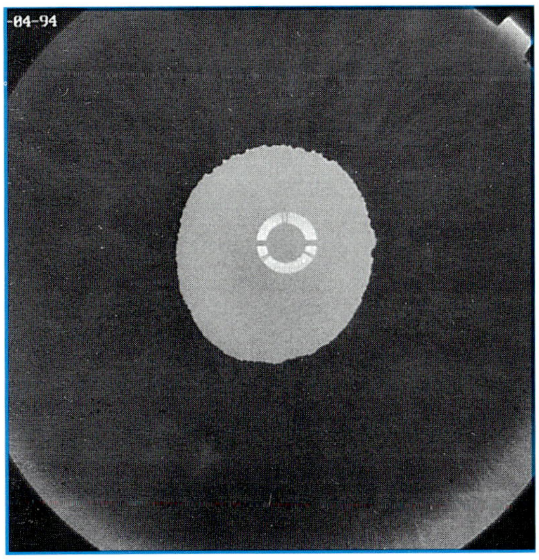

e)

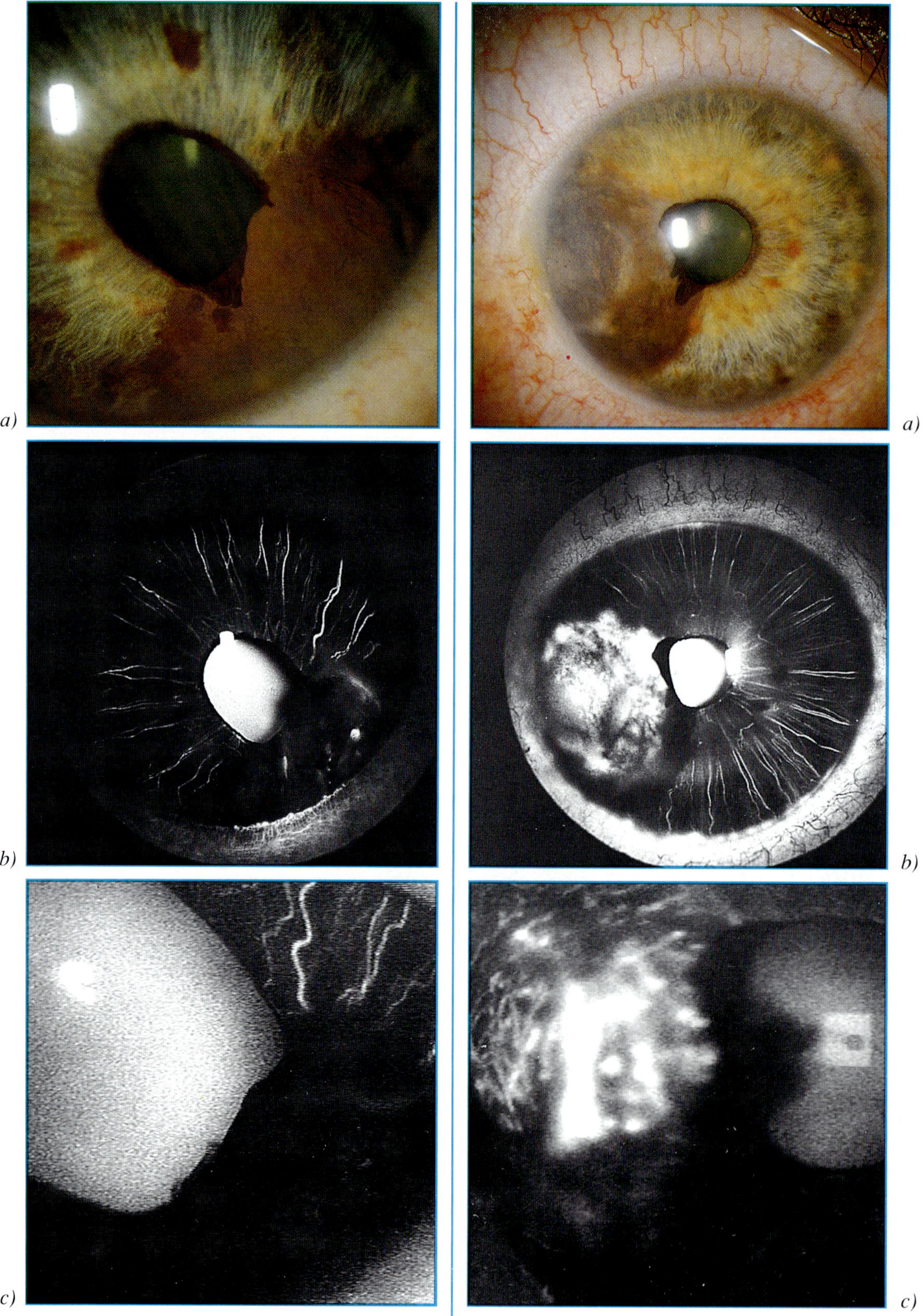

*Fig. **1.2**,11: Colour photo of a pigmented neoformation of the iris which causes deformation of the pupillary margin (a). The excess of pigment in the mass itself masks the tumor vascular network in fluorescein (b) and indocyanine-green (c) images; fluorescein leakage is visible at the tumor periphery (b).*

*Fig. **1.2**,12: When iris melanoma is extensive (a), fluorescein (b) and indocyanine-green (c) angiographic pictures are more complex, with alternating hypo- and hyper-fluorescent areas.*

R. Brancato, F. Bandello, R. Lattanzio
Atlas of Iris
Fluorescein Angiography
Kugler & Ghedini Publications 1995

Section two

The iris: structure and physiology

- Embriology
- Anatomy and histology
- Vascular system
- Nervous system
- Physiology

R. Brancato, F. Bandello, R. Lattanzio
Atlas of Iris
Fluorescein Angiography
Kugler & Ghedini Publications 1995

Chapter 2.1

The iris

The word "iris" comes from the Greek word for a rainbow, and can be traced back to classical times (Rufus of Ephesus). Galen adopted it in his *De uso partium corporis humani* to indicate the ring around which the eye's various membranes converge: he called the iris itself, or the membrane suspended in the front of the eye, the *tunica coerulea.*

The term came to be applied to the anterior surface of what we today know as the iris by Vesalius (*De humani corporis fabrica*, 1543) and by Fallopius (*Observationes Anatomicae Venetiis*, 1561), on account of its brilliant, variegated appearance, while the posterior surface was referred to as the uvea.

In its current usage, referring to the whole membrane, the term iris was first employed by Winslow (Mém. Acad. France, 1711) who was also the first to observe that the nasal part was thinner than the temporal part.

Embryology

Two of the three primitive embryonal leaflets are involved in development of the visual apparatus. The ectoderm gives rise to the optic vesicle and stub of the lens, and the mesoderm provides the adnexa. The iris has a dual embryological origin: the mesoderm gives rise to the iris stroma, and the neuroectoderm gives the posterior pigment epithelium and the pupillary sphincter and dilator muscles.

From the fifth week, for the iris mesoderm mesenchymal cells start to differentiate, giving rise to the formation of the iris-pupillary lamina covering the anterior face of the lens. By the end of the second month the iris-pupillary lamina has further developed in two directions:

a) the peripheral cellular part forms the anterior mesodermal leaflet;
b) the central part, poor in cells, forms the pupillary membrane.

The iris-pupillary mesoderm is rapidly vascularized starting from the anular vessel, leading to the formation of the peripheral and central vascular arcades.

From the seventh month the pupillary membrane is gradually reabsorbed, leaving the pupillary foramen. This involution starts at the centre, taking with it the central vascular arcades. As it extends out to the pupillary border the last anastomotic arcade remains, with the small arterial circle of the iris. The pupillary membrane and its vascular system are not always completely reabsorbed but when regression is complete deep iris crypts form and no residual membrane is left around the collarette of the iris.

From the third month, the iris neuroectoderm extends out from the edge of the optic dome on the front of the lens. It consists of two layers of epithelial cells: the anterior layer, from the third month, starts undergoing myofibrillar differentiation on the inside, the earliest stages of the sphincter muscle. The outer cells of the anterior epithelium differentiate into muscle cells too, which, by the fifth month, form the early dilator muscle. This gradually develops from the periphery towards the sphincter, without ever reaching it. The posterior epithelial cells start to become melanin pigment, from the sixth month. By birth both the posterior epithelial cell layers are pigmented.

Anatomy and histology

The iris differs in colour, appearance and general architecture not only between individuals, but also in the same person with age and with different degrees of dilatation of the pupil. The central aperture of the eye is the pupil, whose size is regulated by movement of the iris; this opening is placed slightly eccentrically, towards the nasal side. This is the equivalent of the diaphragm in a camera, adjusting the amount of light that enters the eye. The iris is the anterior extension of the tunica vasculosa bulbi, known as the uvea, between the tunica fibrosa and the tunica nervosa (Fig. **2.1**,1).

The iris starts about 1 mm from the corneal border and runs transversally in an axial direction, not in contact with the cornea, from which it is separated by the anterior chamber filled with aqueous humor. It is a round disc in front of the lens, with which its central part is in contact. The iris bulges slightly to the front, and resembles the trunk of a cone, with its base at the back. Its total diameter is around 12 mm but this varies with the diameter of the pupil. The iris is not the same thickness throughout, but ranges from 0.3-1.0 mm; it is thickest at the collarette (see below), becoming thinner towards the pupil and even finer at the root where it joins the ciliary body. This explains why this zone is so fragile in cases of trauma.

The iris has two borders:

1) the ciliary or peripheral border, which anteriorly is related to the sclerocorneal angle and proceeds posteriorly to the ciliary body, which the iris joins. This border is held in place by:
   a) the continuity of its stroma and that of the ciliary body;
   b) numerous blood vessels which penetrate the iris from the posterior face of the ciliary muscle, forming the greater arterial circle of the iris;
   c) the lengthening of the pectinate ligament (Hechk's ligament) which runs from the anular ligament (Dollinger's tendinous ring) to the anterior face of the iris. Vessels and nerves pass into the iris through this border.
2) the inner border is the pupillary or free border surrounding the pupillary aperture. It is in contact with the lens, is fine and has a dark brown indented edge where the posterior pigmented epithelial layer curves slightly round to the front. This gives what looks like a brown-black streak which may be 0.06 mm or more wide, but is narrower in the inferior part of the pupil and changes shape with the pupil's movements. The pigmentation tends to diminish with age until in some areas it becomes little more than a fine translucent band.

The iris has an anterior side, towards the anterior chamber and visible through the transparent cornea, and a posterior side facing the posterior chamber of the eye, resting against the lens. The line of contact between the anterior face of the iris and the posterior surface of the cornea is known as the iridocorneal angle, and marks the periphery of the anterior chamber.

The anterior side of the iris is slightly convex, with a grooved, grainy pattern. As the ciliary border of the iris lies slightly behind the pupillary border the anterior surface bulges forward at the centre; it bulges more as the lens becomes more convex for refraction.

About 1 mm from the pupillary border there is a wavy circular line (*collarette*), between the inner third and outer two-thirds on the anterior face of the iris; this marks the zone where the pupillary membrane was reabsorbed and separates two concentric rings

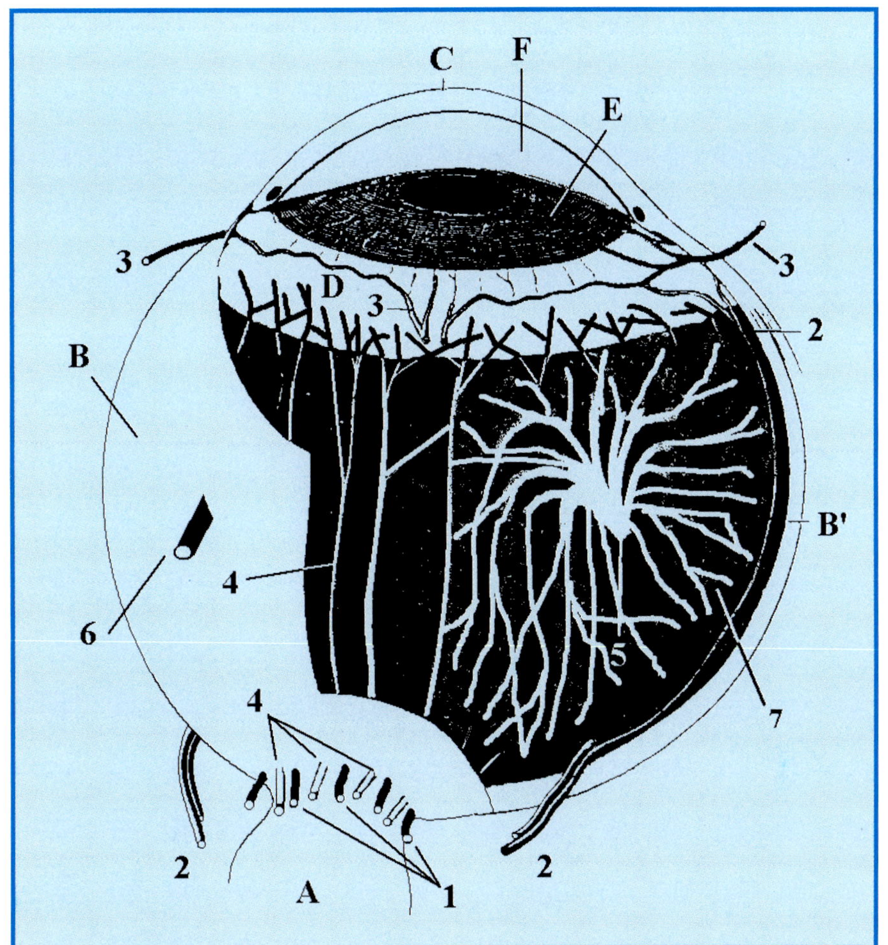

*Fig. **2.1**,1: Section showing schematically the anatomy of the eye.*
A) Optic nerve;
B) sclera;
B')sclera seen in section through the horizontal meridian;
C) section of the cornea;
D) ciliary muscle;
E) iris;
F) anterior chamber of the eye.

1) Short posterior ciliary arteries;
2) long posterior ciliary arteries;
3) anterior ciliary arteries;
4) ciliary nerves;
5) large vein (superolateral vorticose vein) receiving the venae vorticosae from the upper and lateral quarter of the choroid and ciliary processes;
6) superomedial vena vorticosa coming out through the sclera;
7) vena vorticosa in the choroid.

of different colour and thickness:

- a fine inner zone about 1-2 mm wide, the pupillary part or sphincter (the anulus iridis minor of Merkel, 1901);
- a larger peripheral outer zone, 3-4 mm wide, known as the ciliary part (the anulus iridis major of Merkel).

Biomicroscopic examination shows the structures in the two zones are different. In the pupillary zone there are small connecting crests reaching to the pupillary margin. At the collarette deep slits are seen, known as Fuchs crypts or stomates; they are lined at the bottom with a reticulated tissue like the surface of the iris. In the ciliary part there are deep round ruts, mostly incomplete and concentric to the pupillary border; these are known as the *plicae iridis*, or folds of the iris, and are due to the iris contracting. In a lightly pigmented iris one can also see the blood vessels, like pale spokes, straight when the pupil is small, wavy when it is dilated.

The posterior face of the iris is slightly concave, especially when adapting for refraction. With the lens and ciliary bodies it forms the anterior wall of the posterior chamber. In all except albinos the posterior face of the iris is blackish or dark brown on account of the pigment epithelium made up of cells with pigment-filled cytoplasm. This epithelium reflects to varying extents in the pupillary margin so it can be observed in the living being. On the greater circumference, the aboral side of the iris corresponds to the ciliary processes, which leave their mark on it, to varying extents.

Under the biomicroscope, the posterior side of the iris can be seen to have three systems of folds, or plicae:

a) Schwalbe's contraction plicae are fine radial folds in the pupillary region;
b) Schwalbe's structural plicae are also radial, starting about 1.5 mm from the pupillary border and becoming progressively wider towards the periphery. They are related to the blood vessels;
c) the circular plicae are fine concentric circles at the pupil, showing where the thickness of the pigment epithelium differs.

Colour of the iris

Two factors combine to establish the colour of the iris:

1) the large amount of pigment in the deep layer of the iris - from the thickness of the posterior pigment epithelium - which lets no light pass. Light rays hitting the iris are partly reflected and partly diffracted as they pass through the translucent superficial layers. This gives the iris a colour ranging from blue to slate-grey, which is its fundamental colour;
2) the pigmentation of the iris stroma - the more pigment this contains the darker the iris will be. The pigmentation itself derives from several characteristics - the type of pigment, its density and the thickness of the endothelium.

Two types of iris are described depending on their colour:

1) pale irises - generally blue - which have a thin epithelium, limited amounts of pigment and only a few pigment cells in the stroma. In these eyes the vascular network and radial structure are visible;
2) dark irises (brown) which have a thick epithelium and pigmented stroma, giving a velvety look on its front side. The fibrillar structure is only visible between the crypts and collarette, and in many cases may not be visible at all.

Eyes in which the pigment is deposited unevenly may have mottled irises from the spots over the surface. There may thus be a wide variety of colour combinations.

Classification of eyes on the basis of the colour of the iris may have importance in forensic medicine and can be done in different ways, depending on the colour scale employed.[3] Broca proposed a scale comprising twenty shades, most of which do not exist in nature. Bertillon starts out from the fundamental colour, classifying eyes under three headings: blue, intermediate or slate; each of these is then divided into seven categories, depending on the surface pigmentation. Topinard specifies five fundamental shades: black, dark brown, light brown, grey and blue.

The colour of the iris may vary with age: children have paler eyes, as pigmentation is

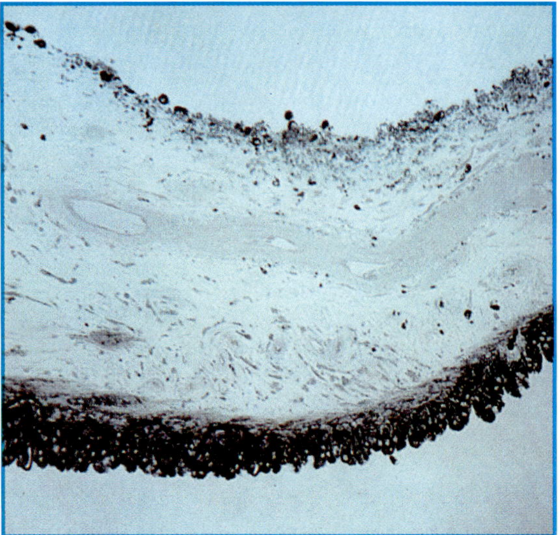

*Fig. **2.1**,2: Light micrograph of iris in normal subject (Methylene blue stain - 400 X).*

only completed at around 15 years, diminishing later as a person grows older. Ethnic differences obviously influence eye colour too.

Structure of the iris

Histological and ultrastructural examination of the iris shows up the following structures, from front to back (Fig. **2.1**,2):

a) an anterior cell layer;

b) the stroma and sphincter muscle;

c) the iris epithelium, comprising:
   - the anterior epithelium and dilator muscle and
   - the posterior pigment epithelium.

Anterior cell layer

The anterior cell layer used to be called the endothelium of the iris. However, ultrastructural studies have shown it is not an endothelial single-cell layer but is actually made up of fibroblasts and melanocytes. The *fibroblasts* do form a single-cell layer covering the whole anterior face of the iris but there are no cell junctions. These appear to be striated cells with a long nucleus. Some have ciliate formations protruding into the aqueous humor. The *melanocytes* are arrayed in one or more layers parallel to the iris surface. Here too, there appear to be no cell junctions. Both cell types have numerous cytoplasmic expansions. In different zones one type or the other may predominate. There seem to be more melanocytes in the thicker parts of the iris, especially near the pupil. They sometimes cluster in freckles.

This layer, often incomplete, forms a totally permeable anterior "barrier", and through the numerous gaps the aqueous humor in the anterior chamber comes into contact with the iris stroma, forming two types of crypts: uncovered ones, with no cells lining their surface, and covered ones, lined with a fine layer of fibroblasts.

Iris stroma

The iris stroma is made up of loose connective tissue and various types of cells - fibroblasts, melanocytes, clump cells and mast cells - blood vessels and nerves.

Fibroblasts aggregate around blood vessels, nerves and muscle elements. Like the fibroblasts in the anterior cell layer they have a flat cell body, an oval nucleus and the usual cytoplasmic organelles. In rare cases mitosis may be observed; they often present ciliate formations.

Melanocytes are rounded with a bulging nucleus. They contain all the usual organelles, but their main content is round or oval melanin granules, from 0.5 micron in diameter, in their various stages of maturation (premelanosomes, melanosomes, melanin granules).

Koganey's *clump cells* cover the surface of the iris stroma (anterior and posterior layers), but tend to congregate around the sphincter muscle. These large globe-like cells measure 100 micron in diameter, and their cytoplasmic expansions may be 1-2 micron long and 1 micron thick. There are numerous granules that may sometimes mask the nucleus. These granules, often containing melanin, are surrounded by a continuous membrane, vary in size, and are structurally similar to the melanin granules in the iris pigment epithelium. Paler granules may be seen, apparently containing lipids, probably with lysosomal residues. These cells used to be considered of epithelial origin on account of their resemblance to melanin granules, but are now believed to be macrophages which have ingested a large number of melanin granules. The only difference between these clump cells and macrophages is that the macrophage cytoplasm is smaller, longer and has various inclusions besides the melanin granules - lipids, blood cells, etc.

Mast cells are often found in the central part of the iris stroma, preferentially around blood vessels. They are characteristically eosinophilic in routine histological preparations. The cytoplasm contains typical crystalline formations, visible under the electron microscope.

The intercellular *connective tissue* of the iris is made of collagen fibres (with no elastic fibres) arrayed obliquely from back to front and from the periphery to the centre. The fibrillar structure is loose so that aqueous humor can circulate freely. Histochemical staining methods show up the following:

- an anterior layer close to the anterior cell layer;
- a deeper, loose intermediate layer;
- a posterior layer in contact with the sphincter and dilator muscles and with the margin of the iris vessels.

Ultrastructure: there are not many fibroblasts. The collagen structure has a periodicity of 600 Å, and a mean fibrillar diameter of 500-600 Å.

Sphincter muscle of the iris

The sphincter muscle of the iris (*musculus sphincter pupillae*) originates from the neuroectoderm and is a flat ring-like muscle lying radially in the posterior, internal part of the iris. It is 0.15 mm thick and 0.8 mm wide, varying in relation to the contraction of the iris - 1.06 mm in myosis, 0.4 mm in midriasis. The muscle is surrounded by collagen tissue, which is thicker towards the pupillary margin. This collagen connects the sphincter to blood vessels, nerves and to the iris connective tissue itself. These connections explain why the pupillary sphincter still works after iridectomy. The back of the sphincter muscle is in contact with the internal part of the iris epithelium.

Ultrastructure: the sphincter muscle of the pupil is made up of fasciae of 5-8 smooth muscle cells, concentric to the pupillary margin, joined by tight cell junctions. Cytoplasmic organelles lie mainly around the nucleus (Golgi apparatus, small mitochondria, some pigment granules, some cisternae of rough endoplasmic reticulum). The cells contain numerous myofilaments lying parallel to the main cell axis, with darker electron-dense zones in them. Pinocytotic vesicles are frequent along the cell membrane. Each smooth muscle cell has its own basement membrane. Melanocytes are often found around these cells. Nerves are visible in the connective tissue separating the muscle units; the fibres are often myelinized.

Iris epithelium

Two layers make up the iris epithelium:

1) a myoepithelial anterior layer, constituting Grynfelt's dilator muscle;
2) a highly pigmented posterior single-cell layer.

Anterior epithelium

The anterior epithelium is 12.5 micron thick. The *dilator muscle* runs from the periphery of the iris to the pupillary sphincter but does not touch the pupillary margin. Its outer edge reaches the root of the iris.

The anterior epithelium of the iris continues on into the pigment cells of the ciliary epithelium. It is made up of *myoepithelial cells*, which are epithelial cells with cytoplasmic expansions. Each one has:

- an apical epithelial portion;

- a basal muscle portion, 4 micron thick, which prolongs the cells radially towards the pupillary sphincter, for about 60 micron, about 7 micron wide per cell;
- a cell nucleus in the epithelial portion;
- pigment granules and the usual intracellular organelles in the cytoplasm.

Ultrastructure: like all other smooth muscle cells, these have a basement membrane. The cytoplasm often contains myofilaments 30 Å in diameter, grouped in radial fasciae. The myofibrils, made of actin, myosin and desmin, are anchored to the dense bodies. Zones of dense cytoplasm, typical of smooth muscle cells, and pinocytotic vesicles are visible along the cell membrane. An intercellular space separates the apical or epithelial portion from the pigment epithelial cells, surrounded by numerous 200 Å microvillosities. Between these cells and the cells of the pigment epithelium there are numerous desmosomes and tight junctions. Muscle cells too are connected by numerous interdigitations, tight junctions and desmosomes. Synergistic contraction of the myoepithelial cells is achieved by amyelinic nervous fibres.

Posterior pigment epithelium

The posterior pigment epithelium covers the whole posterior face of the iris and folds around at the pupillary margin to form the pigmented border of the pupil. It comprises a single layer of highly pigmented cells which must be depigmented for electron the root of the iris where they flow into the ciliary body epithelium. These are polyhedric, cubic or cylinder cells, from 36-55 micron high and 16-25 micron wide.

Ultrastructure: the basal part of the cell membrane presents numerous digitations, and a basement membrane surrounds each cell; they are connected by interdigitations on the cell sides - *maculae adherentes* and *occludentes*. The apical portion is similar to that of the anterior epithelial cells. The nucleus is small, round or oval. The cytoplasm contains round or oval pigment granules, 0.8 micron in diameter and 2.5 micron wide, glycogen and the usual cytoplasmic organelles.

Vascular system

The ophthalmic artery, a branch of the internal carotid artery, supplies the retinal and ciliary vascular systems of the eye. These independent networks provide the eye's whole vascular coverage (Fig. **2.1**,3).

Ciliary system

The ciliary system nourishes the whole eye except for the innermost layers of the retina and part of the optic nerve, whose blood supply comes from the retinal system. The ciliary system comprises the anterior and posterior ciliary arteries.

Posterior ciliary arteries

The main posterior ciliary arteries break up into numerous branches perforating the sclera around the optic nerve (short posterior ciliary arteries), and run to the choroid, the macular region, the pigment epithelium, retinal neuroepithelium and part of the optic nerve itself.

Two long posterior ciliary arteries originate from the posterior ciliary arteries, the medial or nasal, and lateral or temporal. These perforate the sclera nasally and temporally in the horizontal meridian, then run from back to front, together with the ciliary nerves,

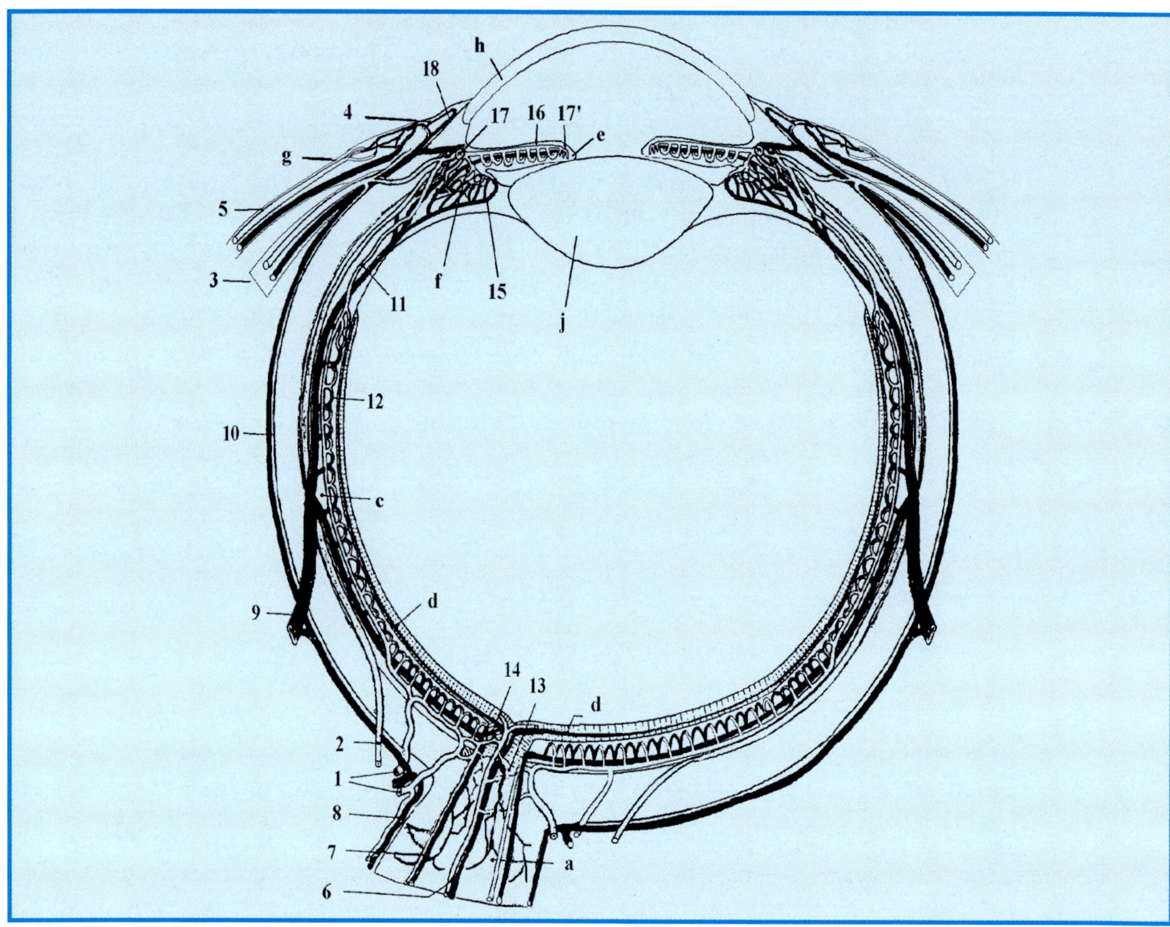

*Fig. **2.1**,3: Horizontal section showing schematically the circulation of the eye.*

1) Short posterior ciliary arteries;
2) long posterior ciliary arteries;
3) anterior ciliary veins and arteries;
4) anterior vessels of the bulbar conjunctiva;
5) posterior vessels of the bulbar conjunctiva;
6) central retinal artery and vein;
7) subdural vessels of the optic nerve;
8) dural vessels of the optic nerve;
9) vasa vorticosa;
10) episcleral artery and vein;
11) recurrent choroid artery;
12) choroid capillaries;
13) anastomosis of the short ciliary arteries with the central retinal artery;
14) anastomosis of the choroid and retinal vessels;
15) vessels of the ciliary processes;
16) iris vessels;
17) greater arterial circle of the iris;
'17) lesser arterial circle of the iris;
18) Schlemm's canal.
a) Optic nerve and its sheath;
b) sclera;
c) choroid;
d) retina;
e) iris;
f) ciliary processes;
g) conjunctiva;
h) cornea;
i) crystalline lens.

in the suprachoroidal space. These arteries have no side branches until the posterior part of the ciliary body, where they divide into an ascending and a descending branch, from which other, smaller branches arise, joining up at many points with branches of the anterior ciliary arteries, to constitute the greater arterial circle of the iris.

Two or three branches of the two main long posterior ciliary arteries, known as recurrent arteries, turn back in the anterior choroid, through the ciliary body.

Anterior ciliary arteries

The anterior ciliary arteries vary in number, and derive from the *arteriae propriae* of the straight muscles which, in turn, originate from the ophthalmic artery. The anterior ciliary arteries run forwards along the tendons and divide into numerous branches when they reach the scleral surface. These are the episcleral, intrascleral and perforating branches. They run perpendicularly down the sclera a few millimeters from the limbus, passing the suprachoroidal space after crossing the ciliary muscle at the height of the anterior part of the ciliary body, then anastomose with the branches of the long posterior ciliary arteries in the greater arterial circle of the iris (Fig. **2.1**,4).

The *greater arterial circle* of the iris is, as its name implies, a circular network parallel to the equator of the eye, running round the anterior part of the ciliary body close to the ciliary margin of the iris, at the height of the root. Sometimes the circle is not complete. According to Marsh[6] it does not consist of a single canal but of several small branches deriving from the vessels mentioned above, all connected by anastomoses. Marsh also sustains that the nasal part of the iris is largely supplied by the lateral posterior ciliary artery, and that the medial anterior ciliary artery plays only a minor role. In the upper, lower and temporal parts of the iris the blood supply is mainly from the superior and inferior anterior ciliary arteries, while the lateral posterior and anterior ciliary arteries are the ones that are less involved.

Vuillemey[16] reported findings partially in agreement with this picture, in that the anterior ciliary arteries did not appear to supply important branches to the greater circle, but more to the ciliary bodies.

Four orders of collateral arteries branch out from the greater arterial circle of the iris:

1) ciliary branches distribute to the ciliary processes;
2) muscle branches go to the ciliary muscle;
3) recurrent choroid branches run back to the anterior part of the choroid;
4) iris branches run radially in the iris stroma.

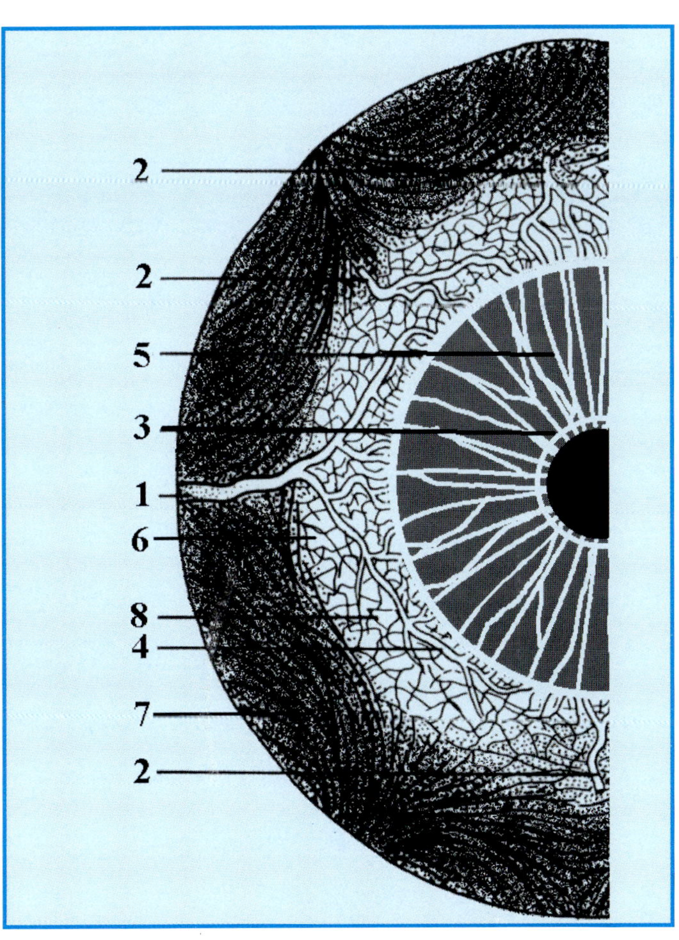

*Fig. **2.1**,4: Blood vessels of the iris and contiguous zones of the vascular tunic (schematic, enlarged drawing). The dark peripheral border corresponds to the choroid, the middle, paler circle to the ciliary muscle, and the innermost ring to the iris.*
1) Long posterior ciliary arteries;
2) five anterior ciliary arteries;
3) lesser arterial circle of the iris;
4) greater arterial circle of the iris (posterior long and anterior ciliary arteries joined);
5) iris arterial branches arrayed radially;
6) ciliary capillaries;
7) choroid capillaries;
8) ciliary capillaries.

Most of these iris branches run to the pupillary margin; others divide dendritically to form the second arterial loop, known as the *lesser arterial circle* of the iris, which runs around the collarette. Vessels in this network are often partially obliterated, so the lesser circle may be incomplete. From the lesser arterial circle, fine arterioles depart radially, running as far as the pupillary margin, and carrying on from there into the capillary plexus.

Capillaries

The capillaries are found mainly around the pupillary margin, closely related to the constrictor muscle. The dilator muscle has another extremely fine capillary network. Capillaries run radially in the rest of the iris.

Veins

The veins run mainly from the peripupillary capillary plexus and follow the path of the arteries, in the opposite direction. The branches grow bigger as they get closer to the periphery of the iris. From the periphery they continue to the ciliary bodies, joining up with the veins from the ciliary processes; together they run through the suprachoroid, flowing into the *venae vorticosae* (one per quadrant) which ultimately empty into the ophthalmic veins (superior and inferior). Anastomoses are frequent between the iris veins, which are more numerous than the arteries, and run deeper in the iris stroma.

Stereomicrodissection techniques have provided the means of confirming these findings and a precise picture can be obtained of the afferent and efferent parts of the iris vascular system.[7] Arteries coming off the greater arterial circle carry blood towards the pupillary margin, running on a superficial plane *(vasa advehentes)*. The venous system carrying blood back towards the ciliary body runs more deeply *(vasa revehentes)* (Fig. **2.1**,5).

The iris vascular system can be divided longitudinally into the *pars ciliaris* and the *pars pupillaris*, separated by the lesser arterial circle of the iris. The ratio between the two sectors is usually around 6:1. Both parts are supplied superficially by the *vasa advehentes*. The first is supplied by the short *vasa advehentes* which stop when they reach

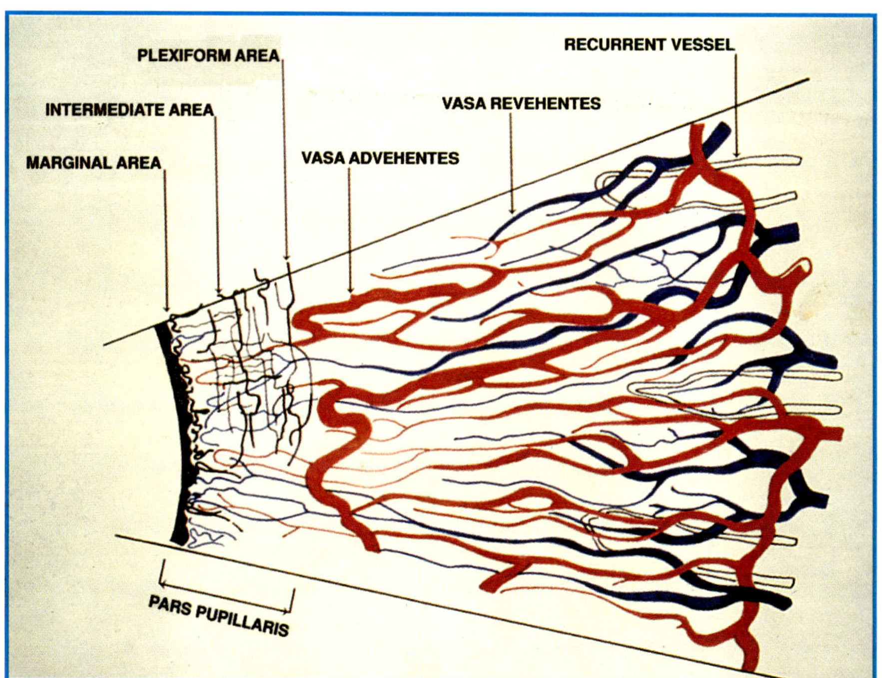

*Fig. **2.1**,5: Scheme of vascular system of the iris.*

the lesser circle and form a capillary arcade that connects with the underlying part of the *revehente* system running the other way. The pars pupillaris, on the other hand, is supplied by long *advehentes* vessels which cross the line between the ciliary and pupillary parts, ending up directly in the pars pupillaris where they break down into the fine capillary mesh that marks this area.

Three areas of fine capillary mesh mark the pars pupillaris (Figs. **2.1**,6,7):
1) the marginal zone, corresponding to the pupillary border;
2) the intermediate zone;
3) the plexiform zone, close to the lesser arterial circle.

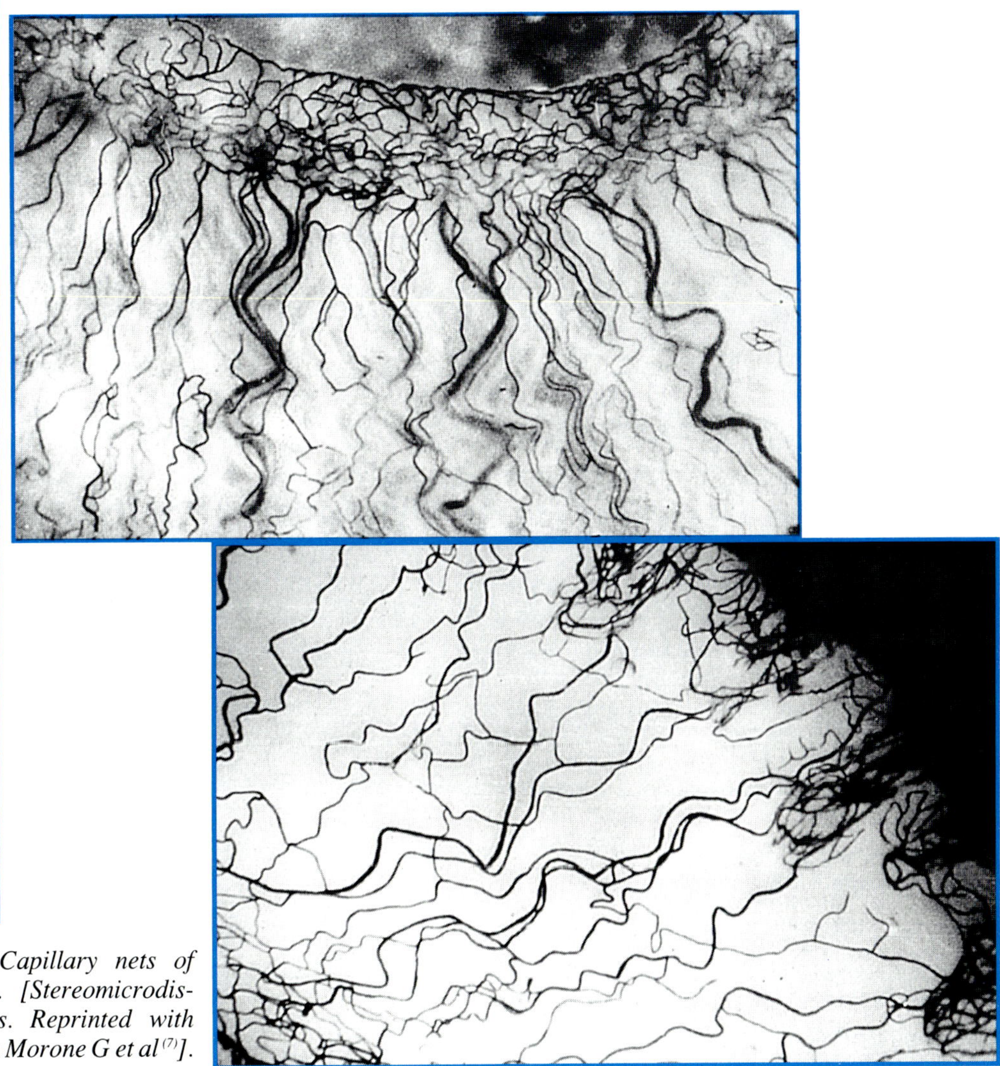

*Figs. **2.1**,6,7: Capillary nets of pars pupillaris. [Stereomicrodissection pictures. Reprinted with permission from Morone G et al[7]].*

The vascular system around the pupillary margin does not always follow the same pattern. At some points there are vessels which seem to run beyond the margin; at others meandering loops follow the curve of the border for a certain distance, then turn away (Fig. **2.1**,8).

The capillary network in this zone is considerably less rich than in the other two areas. The *advehentes* arteries come out to the iris surface with two or three ciliary processes between them (Fig. **2.1**,9). These radial arteries are almost the same caliber and are all the same distance apart. Six or seven veins run deeply between one arterial trunk and the next, draining blood from that district (Fig. **2.1**,10).

From the situation outlined so far and from the figures provided, it is clear that the par-

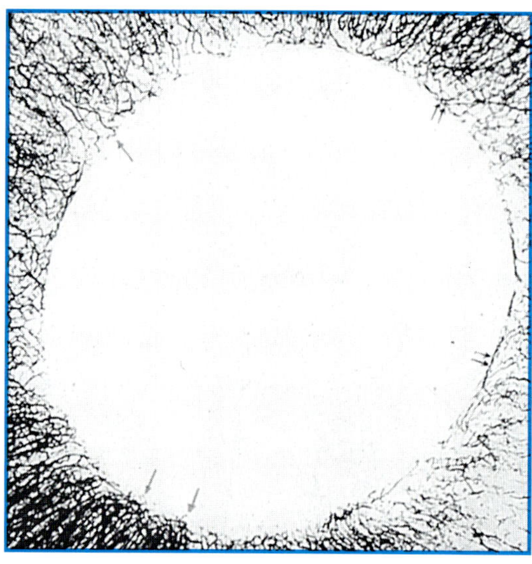

*Fig. **2.1**,8: Vessels at the pupillary border. [Stereomicrodissection picture. Reprinted with permission from Morone G et al [7]].*

ticular segmental vascular arrangement in the iris is one explanation of the sectorial atrophy encountered in a variety of different pathologies. For example, the typical segments of stromal atrophy seen in patients after acute glaucoma attacks are the result of compression of functionally fragile vascular sections of the iris as a consequence of the acute intraocular hypertension, leaving in their wake an ischemic sector where stromal tissue becomes dystrophic.

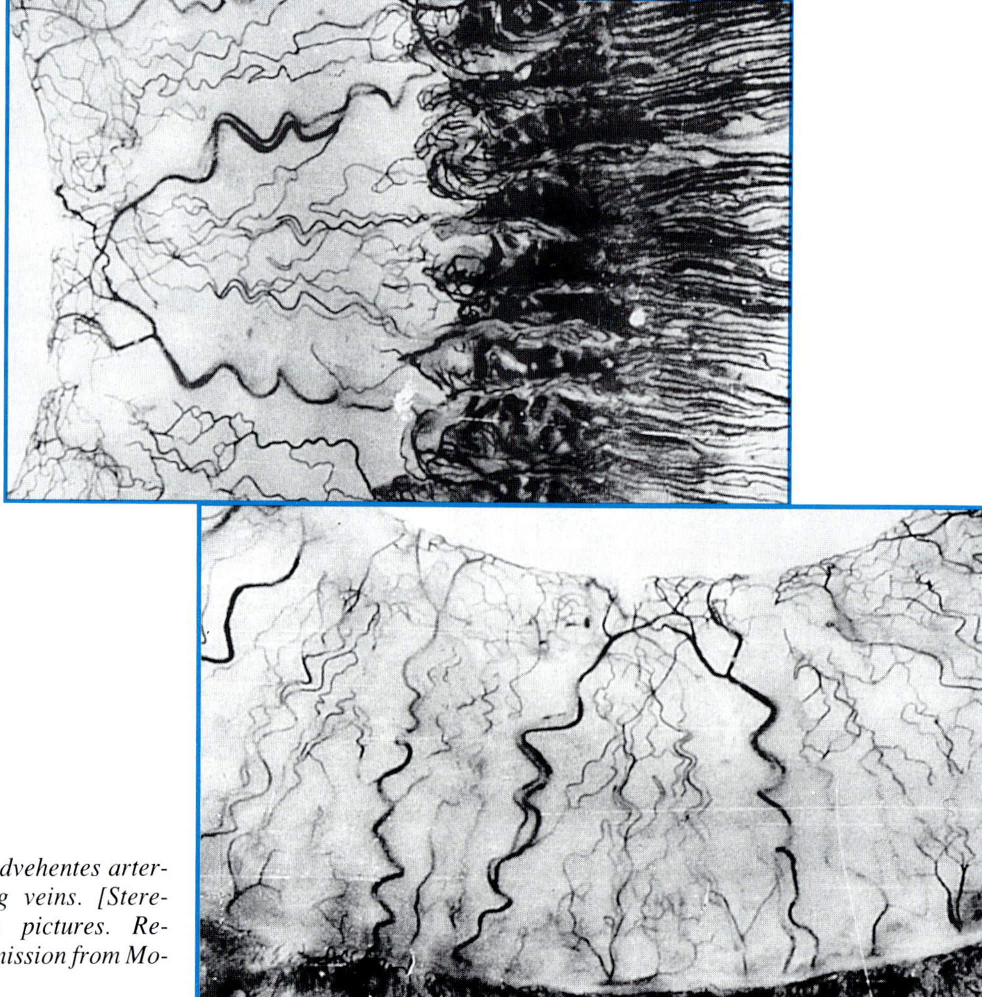

*Figs. **2.1**,9,10: Advehentes arteries and draining veins. [Stereomicrodissection pictures. Reprinted with permission from Morone G et al [7]].*

These angiogenic segmental atrophies can be compared to those seen after Herpes zoster uveal infection, where the stromal lesion however is presumably neurogenic as it reflects the effects of the infection on intrastromal trigeminal nerve endings, which are also laid out in a segmental pattern.

A well-known complication, the string syndrome, is very likely the result of sectorial necrotic ischemia of one metamere of the ciliary body or iris, secondary to circling, occluding some sectors of the venous outflow system from the anterior or intermediate uvea that anatomically are most exposed or rheologically most fragile.

It is also a possibility that senile dystrophy of the iris collarette - a frequent biomicroscopic finding - might be caused by atherogenic atresia of the capillary plexi in the marginal part of the pars pupillaris, whose networks are not only less dense but are also hydrodynamically more impeded.

Ultrastructure

The anatomical structure of the iris vessels is extremely important in the light of the comments that follow on iris neovascularization in ocular or systemic diseases. The arteries have only one muscle layer, with no internal elastic lamina, their adventitia is very thick[4] and rich in collagen and their connective fibres run circularly. The outer layer of the adventitia is continuous with the iris stroma, and is basically a part of it. The adventitia is separated from the muscle layer and endothelium by a virtual space containing a few loose fibres and copious fundamental substance.

The iris vessels are thus made up of two unconnected concentric tubes, the outer one anchored to the stroma and the inner one free. This structure is not found in the choroid or ciliary body and it has been suggested that it is necessary to ensure patency of the iris vessels at all times during pupillary dilatation and contraction.

The vascular endothelial cells are not fenestrated and are joined by tight junctions. Raviola[12] reported that the greater arterial circle sent fenestrated capillaries to the ciliary body, where they are important for filtering the aqueous, and unfenestrated capillaries to the iris. These capillaries have a thick, continuous basement membrane and few pericytes. Like the arterioles, they have tight junctions, making for an efficient blood-iris barrier.

The veins are distinguishable from the arteries on account of the lack of elastic fibres and smooth muscle in the venous wall.

The iris, like the choroid and ciliary body, has no *lymph vessels* as such but merely lymphatic lacunae.[1]

Nervous system

The trigeminus and sympathetic nerves innervate the iris. Nerve branches in the vascular tunic of the eyes derive from the long and short ciliary nerves, the larger originating from the ophthalmic ganglia; only two or three are directly detached from the nasal nerve. The ciliary nerves run through the suprachoroid and form a plexus at the ciliary body. From here amyelinic fibres in Schwann sheaths run out, dividing subsequently into plexi. The anterior plexus leads to the surface layer of the stroma and is mainly sensitive; the vasomotor plexus follows the iris vessels and the motor plexus innervates the smooth muscle fibres.

The pupillary sphincter muscle is innervated by post-ganglial parasympathetic fibres arising in the ciliary plexus which, in turn, receives preganglial fibres from the visceral oculomotor nucleus. The pupillary dilator muscle is innervated by post-ganglial orthosympathetic fibres originating in the superior cervical ganglion. Preganglial fibres arrive here from the spinal cord cilio-spinal centre, at C8-T1 level.

Physiology

The iris has a dual physiological role: it is part of the blood-aqueous barrier, and it also acts as a diaphragm.

To equip it for its first role, the vascular endothelium of the iris has tight intercellular junctions which make it impermeable to high-molecular-weight molecules injected intravenously. In contrast, injection of peroxidase into the anterior chamber is followed by prompt entry into iris vessels. This one-way transport of peroxidases through the vessel wall is a result of endocytosis that carries molecules into the cell from outside. Transcellular transport is ensured by specialized vesicles and this mechanism may be involved in uveo-scleral reabsorption and elimination of aqueous humor. There are still doubts about the type and importance of certain outflow pathways of aqueous humor in man.

The iris is equipped to act as a diaphragm by contraction of the smooth muscle cells in the pupillary sphincter and the myoepithelial cells in the dilator muscle. Dense bodies and desmin microfilaments in the sphincter form an intracellular skeleton for cell contraction. Actin myofilaments are attached to the dense bodies and cause cell shortening by contracting together with the myosin filaments. Their interaction is transmitted through the intermediate desmin microfilaments, and the dense bodies in the cells are shifted. Smooth muscle cells shorten and their borders become festooned. Unlike the faster-twitching striated skeletal muscle, smooth muscle contracts slowly and the cells can hold the contraction for longer without fatigue. Smooth muscle activity is spontaneous even in the absence of nerve stimulation, and innervation serves mainly to modify the contractions.

The myoepithelial cells of the pupillary dilator muscle also contract - like smooth muscle cells - through contraction of the actin and myosin filaments on the dense bodies in the cytoplasm.

References

1 Balboni GC, Bastianini A, Brizzi E et al: Anatomia Umana. Edi Ermes, Milano, 1982.

2 Carella G, Manuelli GF, Ghisolfi A: Ultrastructure, hystoenzymologie et micro-angiotectonique de l'iris humain. Arch Ophtalmol (Paris) 32: 633, 1972.

3 Duke-Elder S: System of Ophthalmology. II. The anatomy of the visual system. CV Mosby, St Louis, 1961.

4 Hogan MJ, Alvarado JA, Weddel JE: Histology of the human eye. WB Saunders, Philadelphia, 1971.

5 Krstic RV: Atlas d'histologie générale. Masson, Paris, 1988.

6 Marsh RJ, Ford SM: Blood flow in the anterior segment of the eye. Trans Ophthalmol Soc UK 100: 388, 1980.

7 Morone G, Tazzi A, Carella G: The vascular system of the eye. La Goliardica Pavese, Pavia, 1981.

8 Mouillon M, Romanet JP: Anatomie de l'uvée. Encycl Méd Chir Ophtalmol, 21003 C10, 4-12-03: 16, 1988.

9 Offret H: Embryologie de l'oeil et de ses annexes. Encycl Méd Chir Ophtalmol, 21080 A10 10: 14, 1988.

10 Offret G, Dhermy P, Offret H: Embryologie et tératologie de l'oeil. Masson, Paris, 1986.

11 Pavan P, Folk J: Diabetic rubeosis and panretinal photocoagulation. A prospective, controlled, masked trial using fluorescein angiography. Arch Ophthalmol 101: 882, 1983.

12 Raviola G: The structural basis of the blood-ocular barriers. J Exp Res (Suppl): 27, 1977.

13 Ropert A, Lapresle J: Physiologie de l'iris. Encycl Méd Chir Ophtalmol, 21024 A10 10: 6, 1990.

14 Saraux H, Biais B: Physiologie oculaire. Masson, Paris, 1983.

15 Sole P, Dalens H, Gentou C: Espaces endoculaires de l'humeur acqueuse. Function motrice irido-ciliaire. In: Biophtalmologie. Société Francaise Ophtalmologie. Masson, Paris, 1992.

16 Vuillemey E, Montard M: Vascularisation iridociliaire. Etude par injection intravasculaire de rèsine polymere. J Fr Ophtalmol 7: 179, 1984.

R. Brancato, F. Bandello, R. Lattanzio
Atlas of Iris
Fluorescein Angiography
Kugler & Ghedini Publications 1995

Section three

The normal iris fluorescein angiography

- Basic procedures

- Nomal patterns

R. Brancato, F. Bandello, R. Lattanzio
Atlas of Iris
Fluorescein Angiography
Kugler & Ghedini Publications 1995

Chapter 3.1

Basic procedures

Before making any analysis of the iris fluorescein angiographic findings in normal situations and in patients with iris pathologies, it is advisable to review some of the basic procedures that must be respected if this investigation is to give worth-while results. These measures are virtually the same as for retinal fluorescein angiography, and can be summarized as follows:

1) the patient must always be informed in advance of the clinical reasons for doing the examination and how it will be done. An informed contest is advisable.[9] Often poor quality angiograms are in fact due to a lack of cooperation from the patient who does not understand what is happening;
2) the physician must question the patient very thoroughly about the possibility of allergies or actual allergic reactions in the past to fluorescein. The tools for emergency reanimation must always be at hand on the premises where the angiography is done;
3) before starting, the investigator should be thoroughly documented on the pathology so that he can assess which sectors to examine and in what order to do the angiograms on the two eyes.

Should a patient present the clinical indication for repeated iris fluorescein angiography, or for retinal fluorescein angiography just after the iris examination, an interval of at least 48 h should be left between the two. This is the time needed for the body to eliminate the fluorescein employed in the first test completely, so that it does not interfere with the results of the second test. Fluorescein is eliminated unchanged through the kidneys and liver, so that in patients with renal failure the dye may remain in the body for several days. In patients requiring dialysis it is therefore preferable to carry out the test shortly before dialysis so that the fluorescein does not remain longer than necessary in the body.

In contrast with retinal fluorescein angiography, an undilated pupil is required to ensure a good-quality iris fluorescein angiogram. This makes it difficult, in cases where this may be necessary, to do fundus and iris fluorescein angiography simultaneously, using a single injection of dye and a standard retinal fundus camera. Nevertheless, Sanborn et al.[11] have shown that the two tests can be done at the same time with good results; in their hands this technique gave better results than simple slit-lamp biomicroscopy in patients with a dilated pupil for detecting rubeosis iridis (sensitivity 97.2%; specificity 98.8%). Iris fluorescein angiography, however, should always be done with an undilated pupil if a clear picture of the morphology and dynamics of the vascular structures of the iris is to be gained.

Using a gonioscopic contact lens during the examination makes it possible to analyse the structures of the iris-corneal angle. This may be particularly useful for early detection of neovascularization at the angle with a view to prevention of neovascular glaucoma. Using the gonioscopic lens also makes iris fluorescein angiography easier for neoformations in the angle. In certain clinical conditions, though, for instance cysts and retro-iris neoformations, the gonioscopic lens is best used with a dilated pupil.

Before starting an iris fluorescein angiographic investigation, colour photographs should be taken as in a large proportion of cases these are essential for correct interpretation of the angiograms. When colour photos cannot be taken, it may be useful to take photographs using a green monochrome filter before angiography since this gives good information for clarifying the biomicroscopic picture. Angiography can then be done on the basis of the colour or green-filter photos.

The dye should be injected fairly fast into an arm vein (in 3-4 sec.) so as to obtain good contrast in the iris. Generally an injection of 5 cc of 20% fluorescein is used (about 14 mg/kg body weight).

Adverse reactions to fluorescein

Sodium fluoresceinate is chemically inert and therefore substantially non-toxic but 3-10% of patients may complain of headache, dizziness, nausea, vomiting and faintness during the examination. These complaints are often psychological in an anxious patient, though some are due to the presence of impurities in the solution, such as mercury or pyrogens.

More serious are the immediate hypersensitivity skin reactions (itching, erythema, urticaria) or - rarely - Quincke's edema. These manifestations may be accompanied by hypotension, tachycardia, involuntary urination or defecation, shock and bronchospasm.

Even more rare are serious cardiovascular or respiratory complications (cardiovascular or acute respiratory arrest). Their frequency is estimated at about 1 per 1900 examinations, and fatal cases amount to 1/222,000.[14]

Usually these symptoms of intolerance arise suddenly, often actually during the injection or immediately after it, more rarely 20-30 minutes after it. They may become rapidly worse or clear up on their own. They may come on in gradually increasing order of severity or else cardiovascular and/or respiratory arrest may occur directly without any warning signs. In any event it is clearly essential to have all the equipment necessary to deal with emergencies at hand (oxygen, cortisone, etc.).

Pathogenic mechanism of adverse reactions to fluorescein injection

If a patient who is already sensitized to the sodium fluoresceinate solution comes into contact again with the allergen, histamine release is rapid and massive. Antigens and antibodies form immune complexes on the surface of mast cells in tissue and blood. As the intraplasmic granules from these cells degranulate they release preformed histamine, large amounts entering the blood. This causes marked hypotonus of the arterioles, leading to vasodilation and vascular collapse. The increased capillary permeability results in tissue infiltration by a protein-rich exudate, inducing edema and hypovolemia. Histamine can also cause bronchostenosis, headache, tachycardia, vomiting and diarrhea.

Anaphylactic reactions of this type are not dose-related - a few micrograms of antigen are enough to trigger them.

References

1 Amalric P, Biau C, Féniès MT: Incidents et accidents au cours de l'angiographie fluoresceinique. Bull Soc Ophtalmol Fr 68: 968, 1968.

2 Bloome MA: Fluorescein angiography: Risks. Vision Res 20: 1083, 1980.

3 Chazan BI, Balodimos MC, Koncz L: Untoward effects of fluorescein retinal angiography in diabetic patients. Ann Ophthalmol 3: 42, 1971.

4 Enzmann V, Ruprecht KW: Zwischenfälle bei der fluoreszenzangiographie der retina. Symptomatik, prophilaxe und therapie. Klin Monatsbl Augenheilkd 181: 235, 1982.

5 Hess JB, Pacurariu RI: Acute pulmonary edema following intravenous fluorescein angiography. Am J Ophthalmol 82: 567, 1976.

6 Ingelstedt S, Ivstam B: Hypersensitivity to fluorescein: a case of anaphylactic reaction to the injection of fluorescein sodium. Int Arch Allergy Appl Immunol 1: 157, 1950.

7 La Piana FG, Penner R: Anaphylactoid reaction to intravenously administered fluorescein. Arch Ophthalmol 79: 161, 1968.

8 Lipson BK, Yannuzzi LA: Complications of intravenous fluorescein injection. Int Ophthalmol Clin 29: 200, 1989.

9 Lee PP, Yang JC, Schachat AP: Is informed consent needed for fluorescein angiography? Arch Ophthalmol 111: 327,1993.

10 Levacy RA, Justice J Jr: Adverse reactions to intravenous fluorescein. Int Ophthalmol Clin 16: 53, 1976.

11 Sanborn GE, Symes DJ, Magargal LE: Fundus-iris fluorescein angiography: evaluation of its use in the diagnosis of rubeosis iridis. Ann Ophthalmol 18: 52, 1986.

12 Stein MR, Parker CW: Reactions following intravenous fluorescein. Am J Ophthalmol 72: 861, 1971.

13 Yannuzzi LA, Justice J Jr, Baldwin HA: Effective differences in the formulation of intravenous fluorescein and related side effects. Am J Ophthalmol 78: 217, 1974.

14 Yannuzzi LA, Rohrer KT, Tindel LJ: Fluorescein angiography complications survey. Ophthalmology 93: 611, 1986.

15 Yokoyama Y, Funahashi T, Horiuchi T et al: Correlation of the fluorescein angiogram with the dye content in the blood. In Shimizu K: Fluorescein angiography. Proc International Symposium on Fluorescein Angiography, Tokyo, 1972. Igaku Shoin Ltd, Tokyo, 1974.

16 Zografos L: Enquète internationale sur l'incidence des accidents graves ou fatals pouvant survenir lors d'une angiographie fluorescéinique. J Fr Ophtalmol 6: 495, 1983.

R. Brancato, F. Bandello, R. Lattanzio
Atlas of Iris
Fluorescein Angiography
Kugler & Ghedini Publications 1995

Chapter 3.2

Normal patterns

Before starting the iris fluorescein angiographic examination, a colour photograph should always be taken, as we mentioned earlier. This not only serves as objective documentation of the state of the iris but may prove useful when the angiogram is being interpreted in assessing the masking effect of any structures such as pigment masses, cysts, nevi or melanomas, metastases, blood or other fluids, etc. A colour photograph also serves to assess the extent to which the iris pigment hides the underlying vessels, in physiological conditions (Figs **3.2**,1-3).

In a highly pigmented iris, fluorangiography only shows up the surface vessels, the deeper ones being completely masked by pigment. Nevertheless, even in these cases fluorescein angiography may give useful information. If the eye presents alterations to vascular permeability, or neovascularization, this will produce some degree of hyperfluorescence which can be assessed as it will normally become evident at the surface (Fig.**3.2**,4).

Hyperfluorescence and vascularization are clearly visible in pale green or blue eyes, which have a thinner epithelium and whose stroma contains less pigment or fewer pigmented cells. In a pale iris fluorescein angiography provides an excellent tool for detailed analysis of the circulation in vivo (Figs **3.2**,5,6).

A colour photo also provides information on pathologies involving components of the anterior segment lying in front of the surface of the iris. In such states the transparency of the ocular dioptric system is altered, and this may make fluorangiography difficult or even impossible. Examples are corneal leukoma, or massive corneal edema (Figs **3.2**,7,8). With pterygium or corneal neovascularization, large-scale early fluorescence from the pathological vascular structures makes iris fluorescein angiography difficult or even prevents it (Figs **3.2**,9-21). This may be the case also in conditions involving changes in the aqueous humor, such as hypopion or hyphema (Fig. **3.2**,22).

Iris fluorescein angiogram in the normal subject

Pathological findings detectable by fluorescein angiography can only be correctly interpreted on the basis of the findings in a normal eye. This calls for an analysis of the anatomical structures of the iris, its morphology and the dynamics of circulation in the iris vessels.

Iris fluorescein angiography times

The iris fluorangiogram can be divided into three periods: the arm-iris time, the arterial and the venous phases. Various investigators have analysed the duration of these phases[6,7,9,10,11,13,37,38] and how they change in relation to age.[16,38,54]

The arm-iris time is the interval between injection of the dye and its appearance in the radial arteries of the limbus of the iris, the part that fills first. Mean times are reported as ranging from 12.5-27.4 sec.,[54] or from 11-22 sec.[38]

The arterial time is the time needed for the dye to reach the pupillary edge from the limbus. It ranges from 3-7 sec. (mean 5 sec.) and appears to remain virtually constant at all ages[13] although some reports give times between 2.9-9.5 sec. (mean 5.5) with a linear tendency to become longer with age, as happens in other parts of the body.

The venous time is the interval needed for the dye to make its way back from the pupillary border to the limbus. Van Nerom found this time ranged between 1.5 and 11.5 sec. (mean 5.4 sec.) (Fig.**3.2**,23).[54]

Circulation in the iris is slower than in the retina, and even slower than in the choroid.[17,32] A state of medium midriasis may influence the iris circulation time, presumably because the tortuosity of the vessels increases the resistance to outflow.[32] This interpretation, however, does not explain the slower circulation time in the iris in miosis, for which no reason is yet known.

Fluorescein patterns

As has been pointed out in many reports[6,9-11,13,32,37] there is no typical fluorescein pattern in the iris since it fills differently in each individual, with a wide variety of times and distribution, all within the limits of normal. Sometimes repeated examinations in the same person give different patterns. It is essential to have a grasp of this physiological variability in order to interpret the findings of iris fluorangiography usefully.

As specified above, about 10-18 sec. after injection, the dye reaches the arteries, filling them first from the root of the iris then spreading radially towards the pupillary region; some arteries, instead, only supply the periphery of the iris.

The arteries and veins are visible only in the first phases of the iris fluorescein angiographic examination. The former are straight, running closer to the surface than the veins, and in a radial direction - out towards the border - growing gradually smaller in caliber. The veins lie on a deeper plane and take up dye at the pupillary border; the caliber becomes larger towards the limbic periphery, and their path is more tortuous (Fig. **3.2**,24).

In the arterial phase filling often shows a segmental pattern, the different sectors of the anterior surface of the iris filling up in no particular order. Fluorescence inside the vessels appears irregular and uneven (Figs. **3.2**,25-29). This is because the iris arteries originate from different parts of the ophthalmic artery, in widely differing ways.

We can confirm - as many others have noticed - that the inferior and superior sectors of the iris fill soonest;[17,38,54] there are some authors, however, who find that the nasal sector is the first to present fluorescence after dye injection.[32]

There is a consensus that the temporal sector is the one that fills slowest, often presenting filling defects. This may be because the anatomical lay-out of the arterial network in this sector is often not complete.[10-11] This finding holds at all ages (Fig. **3.2**,30).[38]

Van Nerom suggests that this sectorial pattern of filling of the iris vessels is explained by the characteristics of the greater arterial circle, which is made up of confluent branches from the anterior and posterior ciliary arteries. They follow quite different paths in the different meridians before meeting up in the greater arterial circle and this might explain the fluorescein patterns described.[54]

Greider and Egberg found that the path of the anterior ciliary arteries was shorter and more direct in the vertical meridian.[31] This might explain why the inferior sector fills before the temporal quadrant, for example, which is fed more by the long posterior ciliary arteries.

The appearance and size of the areas without arteries is generally the same in repeated examinations. Some sectors may not take up dye in the arterial phase, but these filling defects can be considered physiological.

Sectorial filling defects are seen in certain pathologies, however; examples are areas of iris atrophy or after surgical manipulation (Fig. **3.2**,31). Moreover, sometimes the apparently defective filling of the iris or the limbal region may simply be a photographic artefact produced in an area that is not properly focused or is inadequately illuminated (Fig. **3.2**,32).[32]

Occasionally arteries can be seen whose path is not perfectly radial, with small branches running out towards the border. The arteries may also put out collateral branches at acute angles, which then anastomose with other radial arteries or break up into terminal branchlets.[36]

At the end of the arterial phase small arteries are often visible in the pars ciliaris, running a short way then turning towards the ciliary body. These recurrent arteries may also arise from large arterial trunks. Other vessels may be seen with a transverse path (Figs **3.2**,33,34). Often the lesser arterial circle of the iris can also be seen in the collarette, at varying distances from the border. It may be fragmented or incomplete, with even large parts missing. Its branches set out at right angles from the radial arteries and tend to anastomose (Fig. **3.2**,35,36). When the lesser circle is not clearly visible, more recurrent arteries can be seen, with longer paths.

After a few seconds the dye reaches the area between the collarette and the pupillary border; this area varies in diameter and is filled with a dense network of small vessels, many of them have the size of capillaries. At the pupillary border the capillaries join up in hairpin loops (Fig.**3.2**,37).

In the peripupillary region the circulation is normally slower than in the iris periphery. Hayreh concluded that iris fluorescein angiography often indicates sharper edges to the vessels in the zone between the pupilary margin and the collarette than in other parts of the iris. This is because of the anatomical features of this area where the overlying iris tissue is finer.[32]

At the end of the arterial phase, dye appears in the vessels of the pars pupillaris, starting from the margins, then filling in the intermediate and plexiform areas.

As this capillary phase nears completion the venous phase starts. The veins can be seen as more numerous, finer and smaller than the arteries. They lie on a deeper plane, their paths are more tortuous, and they give a less sharp image. Venous filling is not uniform though it is directly related to arterial filling. All the sectors of the iris show dye in the venous phase, even those which had shown filling defects in the arterial phase. This is seen even more clearly with colour computerized equidensitometry of the iris fluorescein angiographic phases (Figs **3.2**,38,39).[14]

Analysis of the density of iris vessels by fluorescein angiography shows, according to Amalric,[1] that the superior nasal sectors present maximal vascularization. Hayreh, on the other hand, sustains the density is virtually the same in all sectors, though possibly greater in the nasal quadrant.[32]

The zone between the collarette and the pupillary margin, at any rate, has the best blood supply, and this might explain why the pathological processes of neovascularization discussed further on originate mainly in this area (Fig. **3.2**,40).

Blood-iris barrier and dye diffusion

The angiogram of a normal adult aged under 40 years shows no appreciable areas of dye leakage.

Kottow[36] conducted experimental histological studies using the optical microscope to clarify the distribution of fluorescein in the eye. The electron microscope has also been used to investigate capillary permeability, using peroxidase as label.[34,55] This enzymatic catalyst has a smaller molecular diameter than fluorescein itself. These studies confirm that retinal and iris vessels do not let the peroxidase pass, whereas choroidal, conjunctival, episcleral and limbal vessels do. Obviously, therefore, these structures act as a barrier to fluorescein with its larger molecular size, and its high degree of albumin binding. However, in the rabbit slight fluorescein "staining" has been described at the root of the iris, where the dye diffuses from the irido-ciliary processes.[30]

Experimental findings agree on the main features of the iris fluorangiogram in the normal subject. The blood-iris barrier in man is not permeable to fluorescein. This barrier, comparable to those of the brain, retina and optic nerve, has also been observed in the mouse, monkey and cat.[44,45,47,48,56]

Thus the anatomical structure of the iris vessels does not theoretically allow intravascular dye through because of the non-fenestrated continuous endothelium with tight junctions like zonulae occludentes between the cell structures.

Marsh and Ford stressed that numerous factors can influence the permeability of the iris vessels, many of them still not understood.[37] In some species permeability increases when the iris is touched or with paracentesis of the anterior chamber, and protein matter comes out.[43,49,50] This effect is prevented by retrobulbar anesthesia, suggesting there a local nerve reflex mediated by prostaglandin release.[58] This appears to be borne out by the finding that salicylic acid reduces this response.[40] The effect has not been proved in man, even though paracentesis ruptures the blood-iris barrier.

High local doses of histamine also enhance iris capillary permeability in patients with ocular hypotension.[3,20-23] Any change in the osmotic equilibrium may lead to rupture of this barrier.[28]

Experimentally deep anesthesia and death lead to dye diffusion, probably on account of the hypoxia resulting from these states.

As discussed further on, the permeability of the iris vessels may be altered in many systemic diseases, or as a result of local vasculopathies and inflammation of the globe. The latter may be a consequence of surgical manipulations. Iris fluorescein angiography is the semeiological method for a qualitative study of the effects of these noxae, and fluorophotometry of the anterior segment can be used for a quantitative assessment. In a normal subject, in fact, iris fluorescein angiographic and fluorophotometric findings are correlated.[38]

Fluorescein leakage has often been reported from the capillaries in the pars pupillaris in physiological conditions, in relation to age. From the fifth decade of life onwards, some leakage in this region is normal, and it is virtually a constant observation from the sixth decade onward.[13]

Van Nerom reported pupillary leakage in nine out of 44 eyes in one study, four only presenting slight staining of iris tissue and five more marked, with dye leakage into the aqueous. Four of these five were older than 40.[54] Similarly, in patients aged 40 or older, Carnevalini found pupillary dye leakage, assessing it as mild in 51.4% of cases,

*Graphic **3.2**,1 - Pupillary margin dye leakage in subjects over 40 years.*[15]

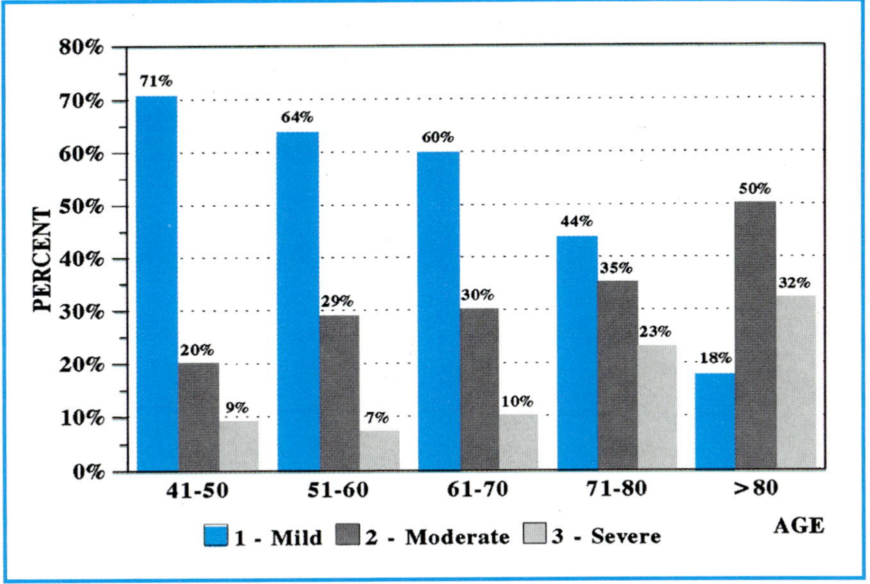

moderate in 30.5% and marked in 18.1% (Graphic **3.2**,1).[15] These findings fully agree with those reported by Chignell and Easty and particularly with Vannas who in 1969 already reported dye spread from the pupillary vessels in 7% of patients younger than 50 but in 31% of those between 50 and 80 years old.[17,52]

This leakage consists of small hyperfluorescent spots appearing around the pupillary border at the end of the arterial phase. Within seconds they start to grow and become brighter, their edges gradually blurring. The dye released into the anterior chamber is carried upward by the convection currents in the aqueous humor[36] and moves towards the supero-temporal part of the anterior chamber, turning in the opposite direction in 50% of cases, after the first minute from dye injection.[38]

This is therefore a physiological form of leakage noted during the entry of the dye and in the first two minutes,[32] but disappears rapidly as the bolus starts to shift (Figs **3.2**,41-46).[54] Conversely, in iris neovascularization the leakage gradually increases with time, and persists even in the late phases.

Physiological pupillary dye leakage in presenile and senile subjects is probably related to the processes of aging of the iris microcirculation, resulting in the tight junctions loosening up somewhat.

However, larger vessels have never been reported to behave the same way in physiological conditions. Thus dye spread from radial vessels should always be considered as an indicator of pathology, even in very old subjects (Fig. **3.2**,47).

Interpretation of the fluorescein angiogram

Just like a retinal fluorescein angiogram, findings in the iris must be read according to a very straightforward principle: the amount of dye in the different zones of different angiograms should ideally be compared with the normal fluorescence. This criterion can then be used to classify all the information in the fluorescein angiogram under the following main headings:

1) a normal amount of dye (*normofluorescence*),
2) more than normal (*hyperfluorescence*),
3) less than normal (*hypofluorescence*).

Hyper- and hypofluorescence may arise for various reasons, summarized in tables **3.2**,I,II. Skill and experience are then needed to interpret the overall information, and draw the appropriate diagnostic conclusions. But the diagnostic path must always follow the basic classification of whether there is more or less fluorescence than in a normal eye, and what might be the causes.

Artefacts in the iris fluorescein angiogram

Just like in retinal fluorescein angiography there are various conditions in the iris which may simulate pathological alterations that in fact do not exist (Fig. **3.2**,48). These possible artefacts must be understood so as to avoid gross errors of interpretation.

There are other aspects of the iris examination which, though not true artefacts, may nevertheless suggest non-existent pathologies:[32]

1) *angiogram not properly focused:* in this case iris vessels seem indistinct, giving the impression of dye spread. This is clearly a technical question, although experience shows that in a single angiogram it is almost impossible for the whole surface of the iris to be perfectly focused, even when the examination has been done correctly;
2) *iris pseudofluorescence:* this phenomenon, mentioned earlier, is linearly related to the thickness of the iris, and is therefore likely to be more marked at the collarette;
3) *lens autofluorescence:* this is the effect produced by the crystalline lens itself during iris fluorescein angiography;
4) *fluorescein staining in the aqueous humor:* since the ciliary body has no blood-ciliary barrier,[43,44,47,48] fluorescein spreads rapidly in the posterior chamber, passing through the pupillary foramen into the anterior chamber. Dye accumulation at the pupillary border may simulate leakage from iris vessels;
5) *capillary loops twisted* at the free edge of the iris may look like fluorescent spots when viewed from the front.

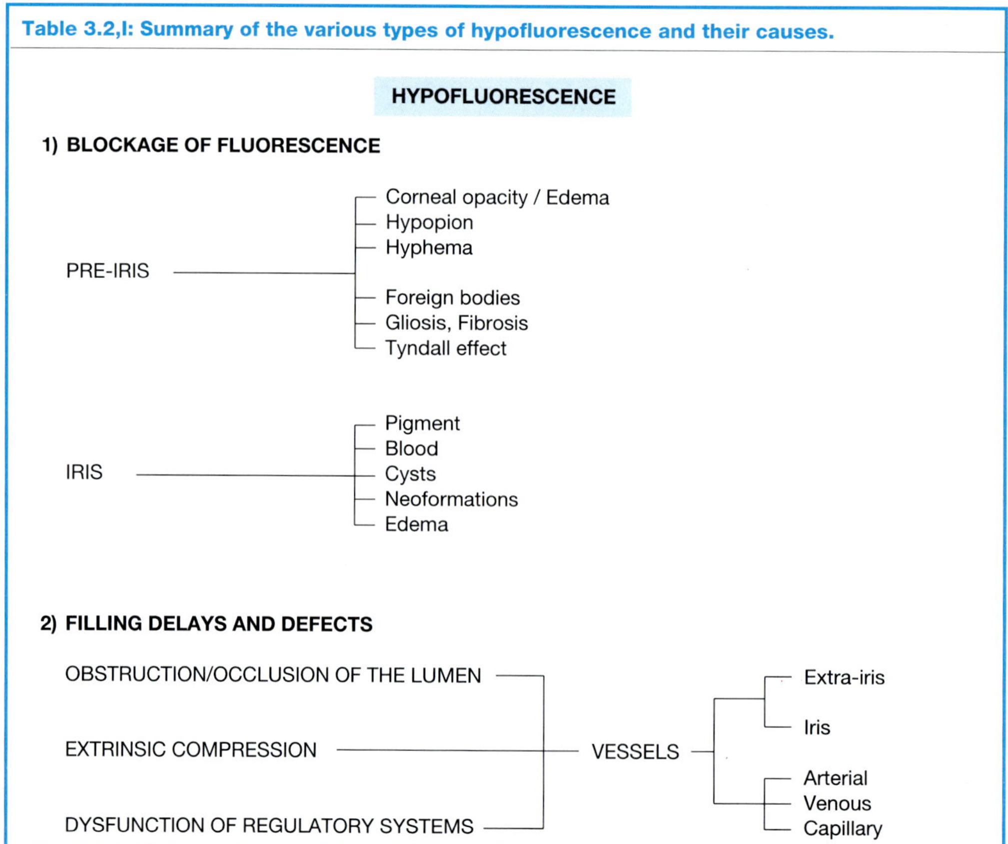

Table 3.2,I: Summary of the various types of hypofluorescence and their causes.

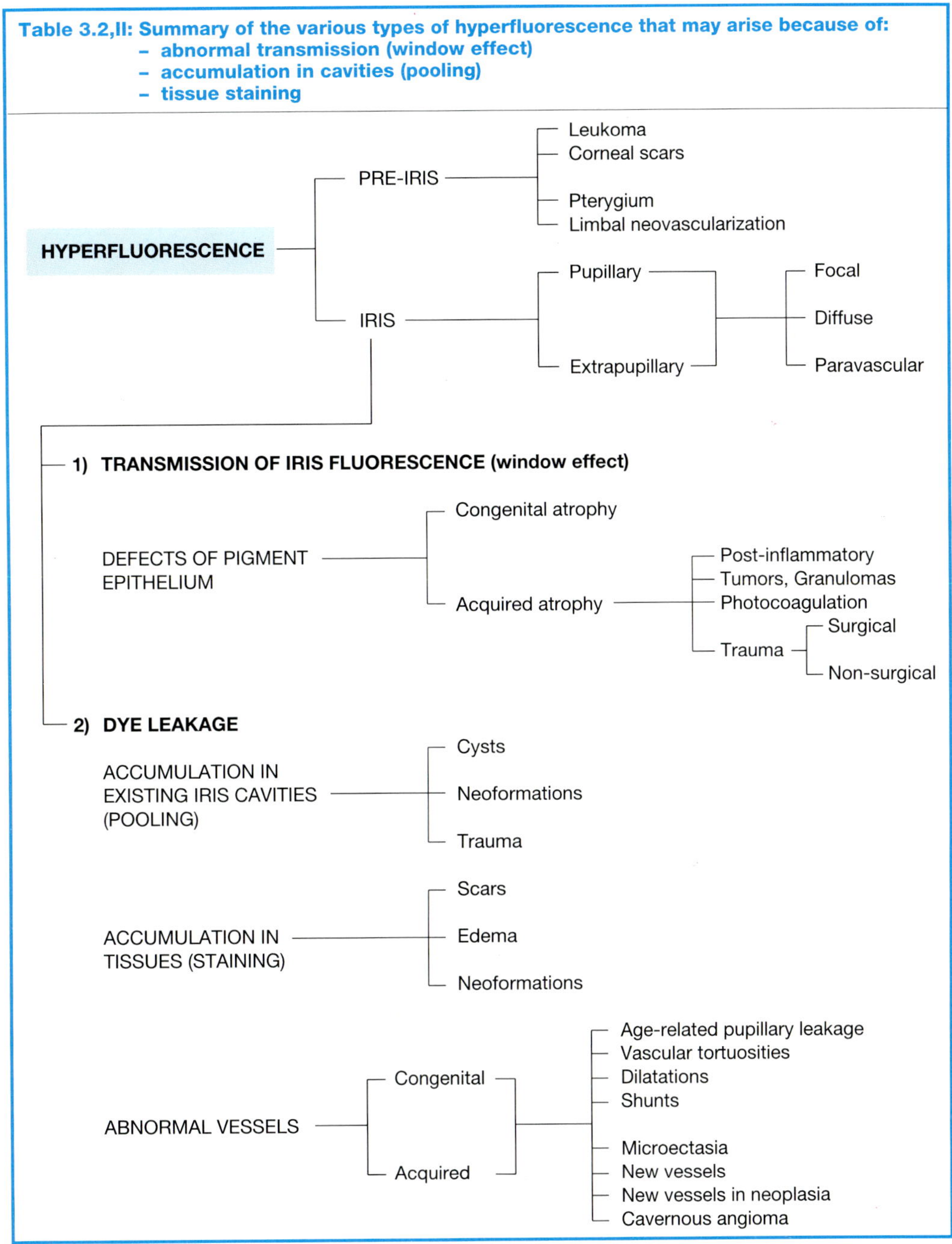

Table 3.2,II: Summary of the various types of hyperfluorescence that may arise because of:
- **abnormal transmission (window effect)**
- **accumulation in cavities (pooling)**
- **tissue staining**

References

1. Amalric P, Rebière P, Jourdes JC: Nouvelles indications de l'angiographie fluoresceinique du segment anterieur de l'oeil. Ann Ocul 204: 455, 1971.
2. Araie M, Sawa M, Nagataki S et al: Aqueous humor dynamics in man as studied by oral fluorescein. Jpn J Ophthalmol 24: 246, 1980.
3. Ashton N, Cunha-Vaz JG: Effect of histamine on the permeability of the ocular vessels. Arch Ophthalmol 73: 211, 1965.
4. Baggesen LH: Fluorescence angiography of the iris in diabetics and non diabetics. In Amalric P: Fluorescein Angiography. Proc International Symposium on Fluorescein Angiography. Albi, 1969. S Karger, Basel, 1971.
5. Brancato R: Sulla natura arteriosa dei vasi ciliari perforanti anteriori. Ann Ottalmol Clin Ocul 98: 501, 1972.

6 Brancato R, Frosini R: L'angiographie fluoresceinique superficielle du bulbe oculaire. Nouvelle methode d'exploration. In Amalric P: Fluorescein Angiography. Proc International Symposium on Fluorescein Angiography. Albi, 1969. S Karger, Basel, 1971.

7 Brancato R, Frosini R: La vascolarizzazione ciliare anteriore studiata mediante l'angiografia a fluorescenza. Atti LII Congresso Società Oftalmologica Italiana, 1969. Cappelli Ed, Bologna, 1969.

8 Brancato R, Frosini R: Possibilità dell'angiografia a fluorescenza nello studio dei vasi congiuntivali. Atti Congresso Società Oftalmologica Meridionale, 1969. Tipografica Publ, Bari, 1969.

9 Brancato R, Frosini R: Premiers resultats de l'angiographie fluoresceinique du globe oculaire. Proc XXI International Congress Ophthalmology, Mexico, 1970. Excerpta Medica Int Congress Series 232: 968, 1970.

10 Brancato R, Frosini R: Fluorescein microangiography of the anterior segment of the eye. Ann Ottalmol Clin Ocul 96: 543, 1970.

11 Brancato R, Frosini R: La microangiographie fluoresceinique du segment anteriour de l'oeil. Bull Mem Soc Fr Ophtalmol 84: 382, 1971.

12 Brancato R, Menchini U: Studio fluorangiografico delle neovascolarizzazioni corneali. Ann Ottalmol Clin Ocul 11 (Suppl): 531, 1972.

13 Brancato R, Menchini U, Carnevalini A: Atlante di iridografia a fluorescenza. C.I.C. Ed Int Gruppo Ed Medico, Roma, 1981.

14 Brancato R, Menchini U, Ravalico G: Computerized colour equidensitometry in fluorescein angiography. Proc VI Congress European Society of Ophthalmology, Brighton, 1980. Grune & Stratton Publ, N.Y. - London, 1980.

15 Carnevalini A, Carassa R, Serini P et al: Fluorophotometric and fluoroiridographic aspects of the blood-iris barrier in normal subjects. In Ocular Fluorophotometry. Proc International Society of Ocular Fluorophotometry, Florence, 1986. Kugler Publications, Ghedini Ed, Milano, 1987.

16 Carnevalini A, Scialdone A, Carassa R et al: Variazione della barriera emato-iridea in rapporto all'età. Atti LX Congresso Società Oftalmologica Italiana, Roma, 1980. Cappelli Ed, Bologna, 1980.

17 Chignell AH, Easty DL: Iris fluorescein photography following retinal detachment and in certain ocular ischaemic disorders. Trans Ophthalmol Soc UK 91: 243, 1971.

18 Cole DF: The site of breakdown of the blood-aqueous barrier under the influence of vaso-dilatator drugs. Exp Eye Res 19: 591, 1974.

19 Cole DF, Rumble R: Effects of catecholamines on circulation in the rabbit iris. Exp Eye Res 9: 219, 1970.

20 Cole DF, Unger WG: Prostaglandins as mediators for the responses of the eye to trauma. Exp Eye Res 17: 357, 1973.

21 Cunha-Vaz JG: The blood-ocular barriers. Surv Ophthalmol 23: 279, 1979.

22 Cunha-Vaz JG, Faria de Abreu JR, Campos AJ et al: Early breakdown of the blood-retinal barrier in diabetes. Br J Ophthalmol 59: 649, 1975.

23 Cunha-Vaz JG, Shakib M, Ashton N: Studies on the permeability of the blood-retinal barrier. I. On the existence, development and site of a blood-retinal barrier. Br J Ophthalmol 50: 441, 1966.

24 D'Anna SA, Hochheimer BF, Joondeph HC et al: Fluorescein angiography of the heavily pigmented iris and new dyes for iris angiography. Arch Ophthalmol 101: 289, 1983.

25 Eakins KE, Whitelocke RAF, Bennett A et al: Prostaglandin-like activity in ocular inflammation. Br Med J 3: 452, 1972.

26 Ehrlich P: Ueber provocirte Fluorescenzerscheinungen am Auge: I. Dtsch Med Wochenschr 8: 21, 1882.

27 Friedburg D, Wigger H, Schultheiss K: Fluoreszenzangiographie der Iris bei diabetikern. Klin Monatsbl Augenheilkd 162: 218, 1973.

28 Goodenough DA, Gilula NB: The splitting of hepatocyte gap junctions and zonulae occludentes with hypertonic disaccharides. J Cell Biol 61: 575, 1974.

29 Grayson MC, Laties AM: Ocular localization of sodium fluorescein: effects of administration in rabbit and monkey. Arch Ophthalmol 85: 600, 1971.

30 Grayson MC, Tsukahara S, Laties AM: Tissue localization in rabbit and monkey eye of intravenously-administered fluorescein. In Shimizu K: Fluorescein Angiography. Proc International Symposium on Fluorescein Angiography, Tokyo, 1972. Igaku Shoin Ltd, Tokyo, 1974.

31 Greider BW, Egbert PR: Anatomy of the major arterial circle of the iris. Inv Ophthalmol Vis Sci 19 (Suppl): 256, 1980.

32 Hayreh SS, Scott WE: Fluorescein iris angiography. I. Normal pattern. Arch Ophthalmol 96: 1383, 1978.

33 Ikegami M: Fluorescein angiography of the anterior ocular segment. I. Hemodynamics in the anterior ciliary vessels. Acta Soc Ophthalmol Jpn 78: 39, 1974.

34 Karnovsky MJ: The ultrastructural basis of capillary permeability studied with peroxidase as a tracer. J Cell Biol 35: 213, 1967.

35 Kluxen G, Bernsmeier H, Weber U: Variabilitat der Irisfluoreszenzangiogramme. Klin Monatsbl Augenheilkd 182: 300, 1983.

36 Kottow MH: Anterior segment fluorescein angiography. Williams & Wilkins, Baltimore, 1978.

37 Marsh RJ, Ford SM: Blood flow in the anterior segment of the eye. Trans Ophthalmol Soc UK 100: 388, 1980.

38 Menchini U, Carnevalini A, Brancato R: I reperti normali della fluoroiridografia. Atti LX Congresso Società Oftalmologica Italiana, Roma, 1980. Cappelli Ed, Bologna, 1980.

39 Miller J, Gravallese E, Bunn HF: Non-enzymatic glycosylation of red cell membrane protein: Relevance to diabetes, abstracted. Clin Res 27: 301, 1979.

40 Miller J, Eakins KE, Atwal M: The release of PGE2-like activity into aqueous humor after paracentesis and its prevention by aspirin. Inv Ophthalmol 12: 939, 1973.

41 Nagataki S: Aqueous humor dynamics of human eyes as studied using fluorescein. Jpn J Ophthalmol 19: 235, 1975.

42 Novack GD, Leopold IH: The blood-aqueous and blood-brain barriers to permeability. Am J Ophthalmol 4: 412, 1988.

43 Raviola G: Effects of paracentesis on the blood-aqueous barrier: an electron microscopic study on Macaca mulatta using horseradish peroxidase as a tracer. Inv Ophthalmol 13: 828, 1974.

44 Raviola G: The structural basis of the blood-ocular barriers. J Exp Res Suppl: 27, 1977.

45 Shabo AL, Maxwell DS: The blood-aqueous barrier to tracer protein. Microvasc Res 4: 142, 1972.

46 Shiose Y: Morphological study on the permeability of the blood-aqueous barrier. Nippon Ganka Gakai Zasshi 74: 1248, 1970.

47 Shiose Y: Electron microscopic studies on blood-retinal and blood-aqueous barriers. Jpn J Ophthalmol 14: 73, 1970.

48 Smith RS: Ultrastructural studies of the blood-aqueous barrier. I. Transport of an electron-dense tracer in the iris and ciliary body of the mouse. Am J Ophthalmol 71: 1066, 1971.

49 Szalay J, Goldberg R, Klug R: The effect of prostaglandin on iridial blood vessel permeability. Acta Ophthalmol (Kbh) 54: 731, 1976.

50 Szalay J, Nunziata B, Henkind P: Permeability of iridial blood vessels. Exp Eye Res 21: 531, 1975.

51 Talusan ED, Schwartz B: Fluorescein angiography. Demonstration of flow pattern of anterior ciliary arteries. Arch Ophthalmol 99: 1074, 1981.

52 Vannas A: Fluorescein angiography of the vessels of the iris in pseudoexfoliation of the lens capsule, capsular glaucoma and some other forms of glaucoma. Acta Ophthalmol 105 (Suppl): 22, 1969.

53 Vannas A: Nouvelle méthode d'angiographie de l'iris. In Amalric P: Fluorescein Angiography. Proc International Symposium on Fluorescein Angiography. Albi, 1969. S Karger, Basel, 1971.

54 Van Nerom PR, Rosenthal AR, Jacobson DR et al: Iris angiography and aqueous photofluorometry in normal subjects. Arch Ophthalmol 99: 489, 1981.

55 Vegge T: An electron microscopic study of the permeability of iris capillaries to horseradish peroxidase in the Vervet monkey (Cercopithecus aethiops). Z Zellforsch 121: 74, 1971.

56 Vegge T, Ringvold A: Ultrastructure of the wall of human iris vessels. Z Zellforsch 94: 19, 1969.

57 Virdi PS, Hayreh SS: Normal fluorescein iris angiographic pattern in subhuman primates. Inv Ophthalmol 24: 790, 1983.

58 Whitelocke RAF, Eakins KE: Vascular changes in the anterior uvea of the rabbit produced by prostaglandins. Arch Ophthalmol 89: 495, 1973.

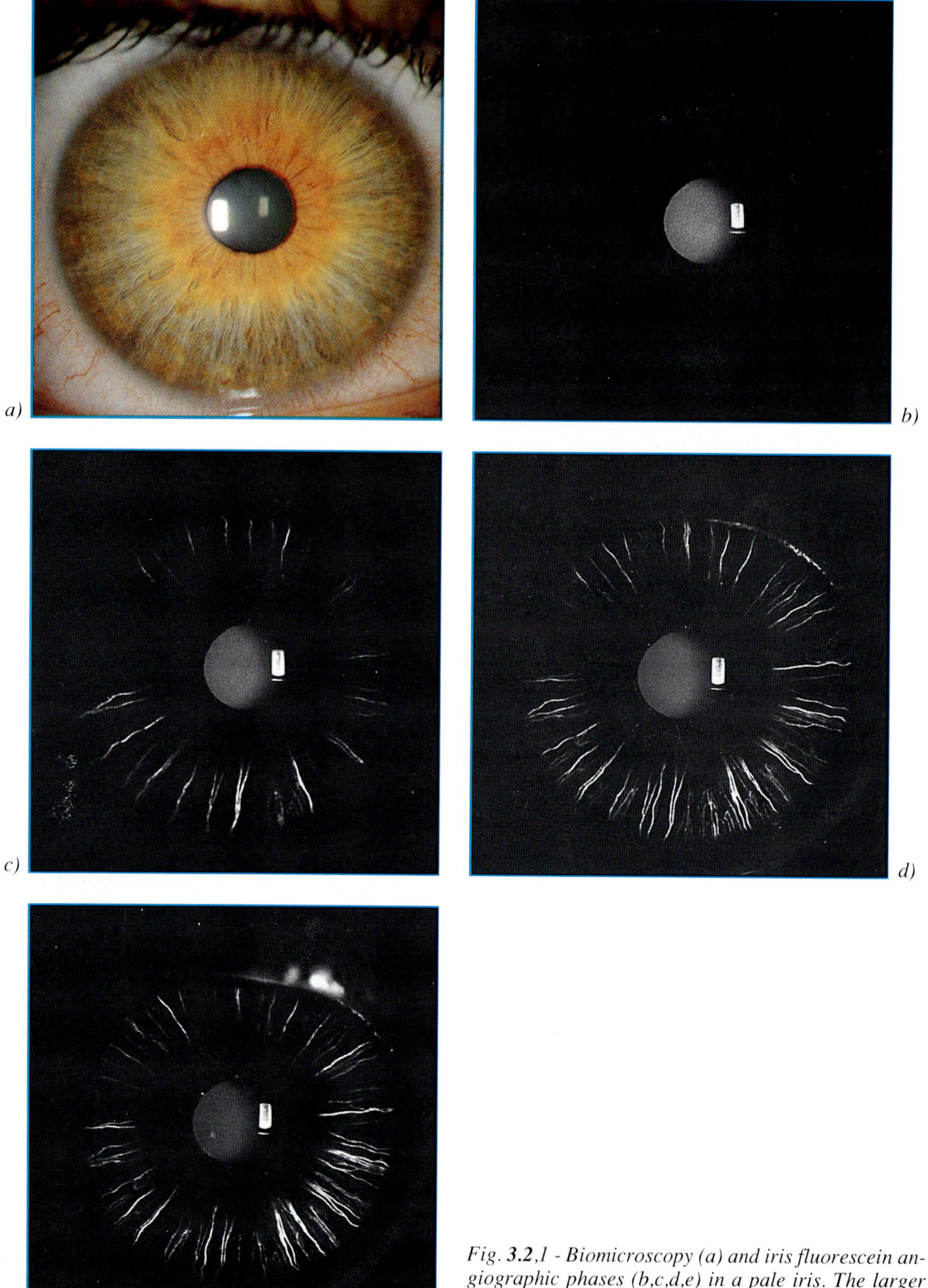

Fig. 3.2,1 - Biomicroscopy (a) and iris fluorescein angiographic phases (b,c,d,e) in a pale iris. The larger amount of pigment in the pupillary part masks the vascular network in this area throughout the examination.

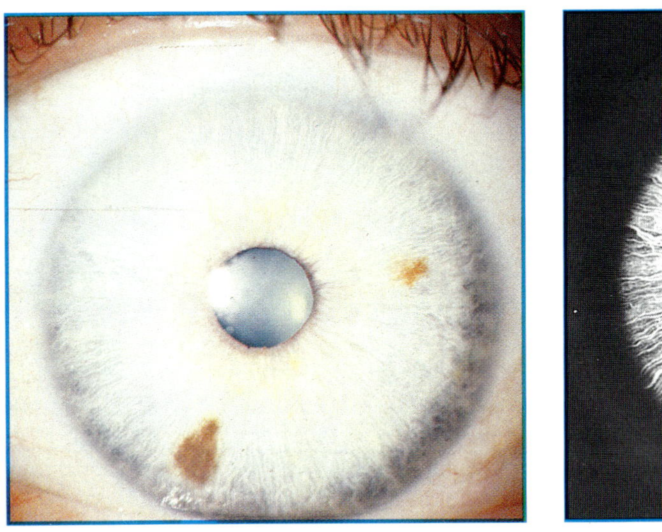

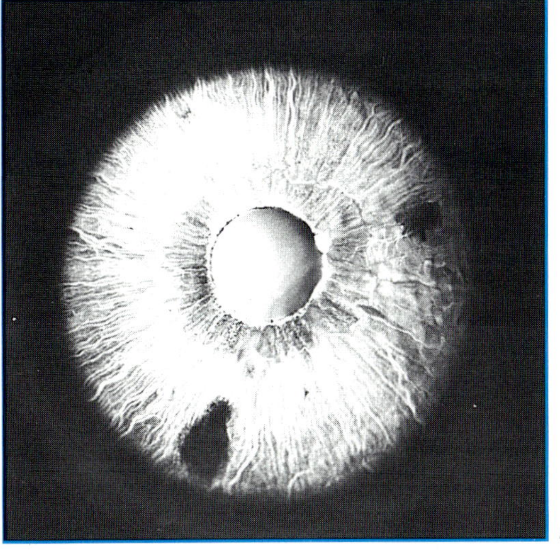

a) b)

Fig. ***3.2****,2 - Biomicroscopy (a) and iris fluorescein angiography (b) of a scantily pigmented iris. Small details of the vascular network are clear. The foci of hyperplasia of the pigment epithelium seen at 3 and 7 o'clock have a masking effect, causing circumscribed areas of hypofluorescence.*

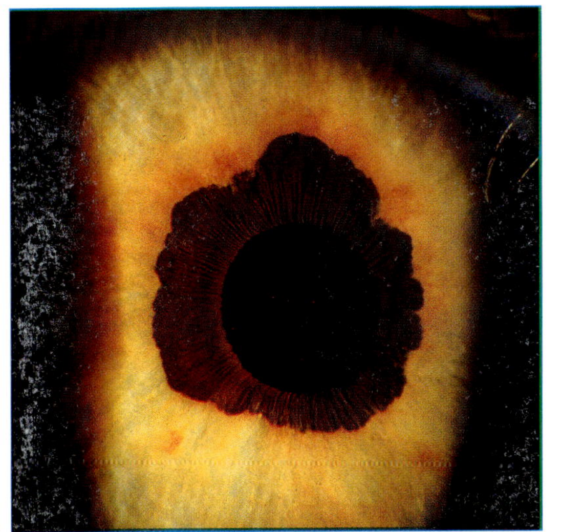

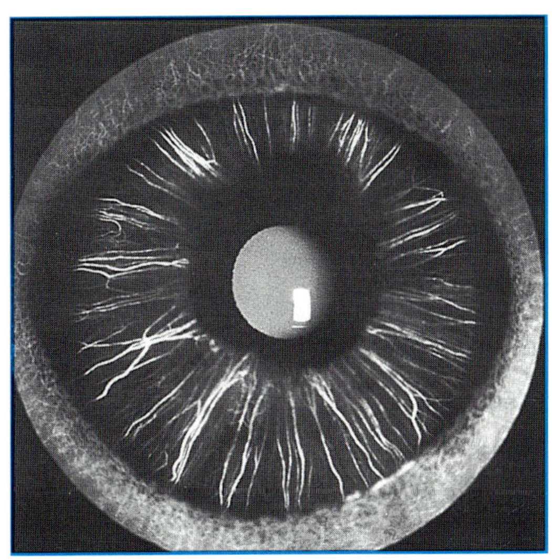

a) b)

Fig. ***3.2****,3 - The ectropion uveae visible by biomicroscopy (a) has a masking effect in iris fluorescein angiography (b).*

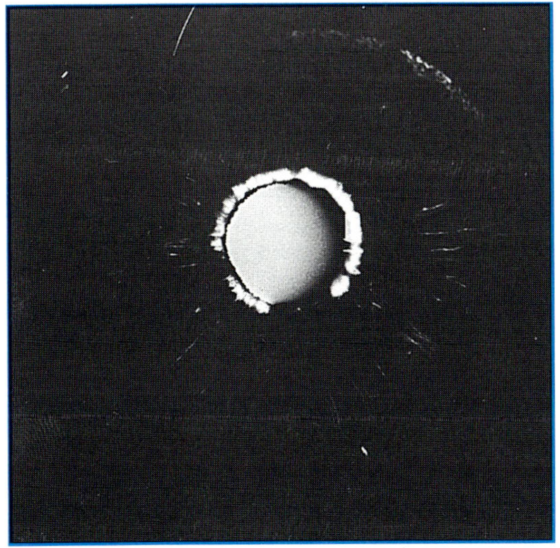

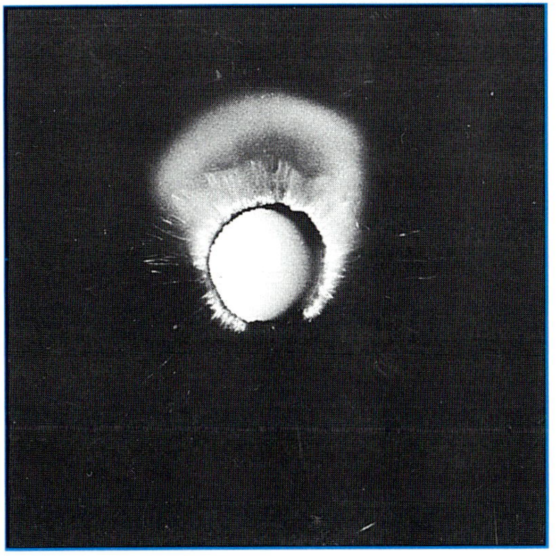

a) b)

Fig. ***3.2****,4 - Early (a) and late (b) iris fluorescein angiographic phases in a highly pigmented iris. The excess of pigment makes it difficult to see even the surface radial vessels. The hyperfluorescence secondary to the vascular anomalies in this case - new vessels in the pupillary margin - is nevertheless clear.*

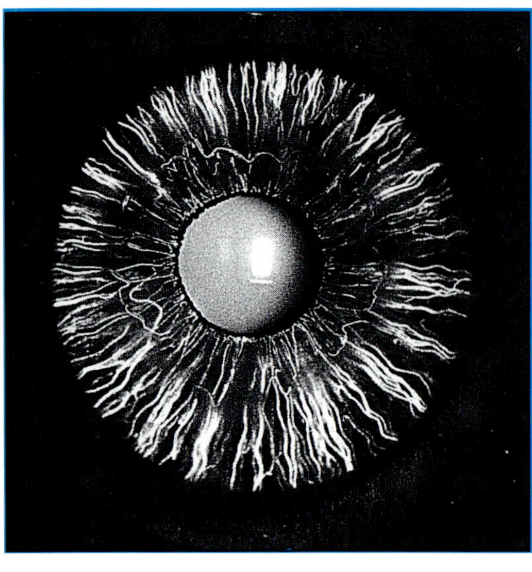

*Fig. **3.2**,5 - Fluorescein angiography of a pale iris in which the scant pigment allows a detailed view of the whole iris circulation.*

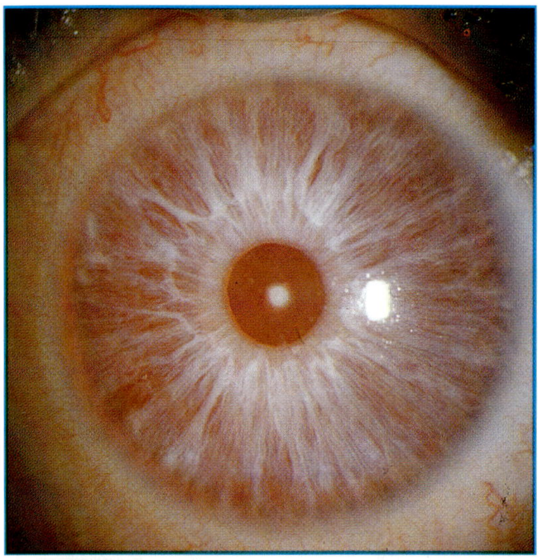

a)

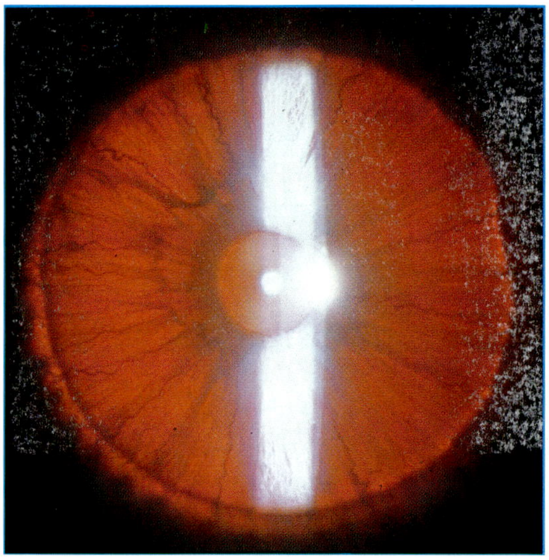

b)

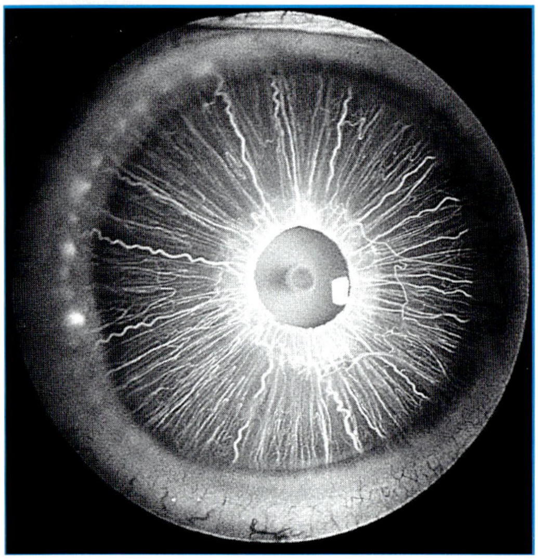

c)

*Fig. **3.2**,6 - Biomicroscopy (a), transillumination (b) and fluorescein angiography (c) of the iris from an albino. The total absence of pigment permits a clear view of the whole vascular network.*

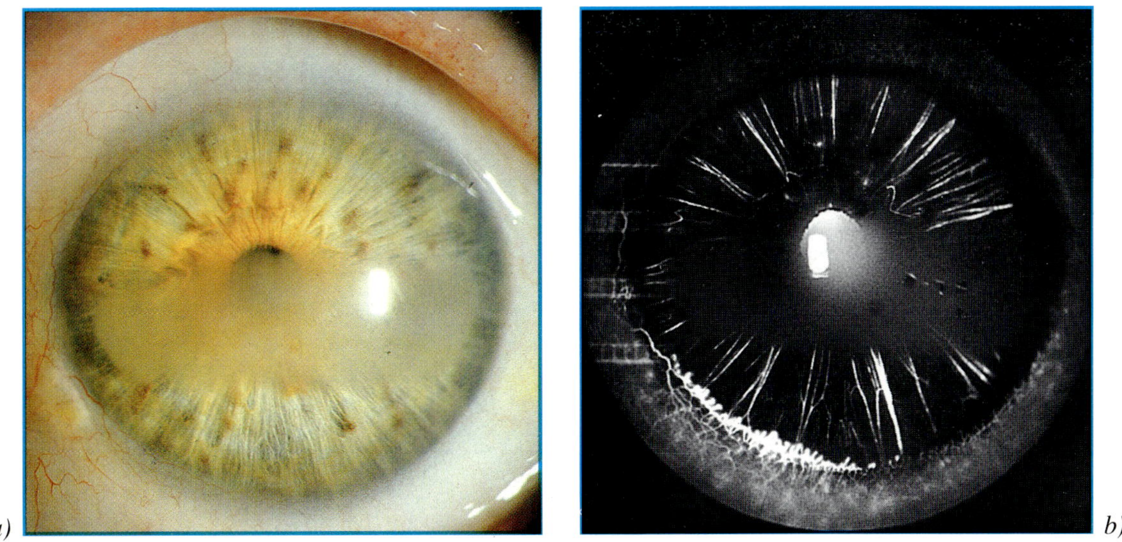

*Fig. **3.2**,7 - Where band keratopathy involves a sector of the cornea, as seen with the biomicroscope (a), fluorescein angiography of the underlying iris structures is impeded (b).*

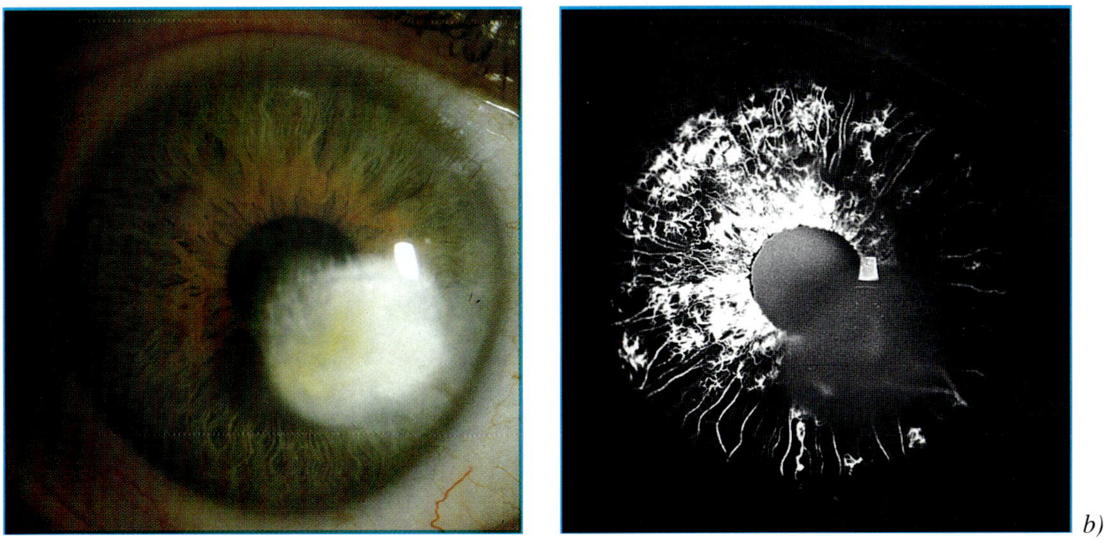

*Fig. **3.2**,8 - Where biomicroscopy shows corneal leukoma (a), fluorescein angiography shows an area of hypofluorescence (b). The hyperfluorescent areas in the sectors of the iris that can be visualized are the result of extensive areas of iris neovascularization.*

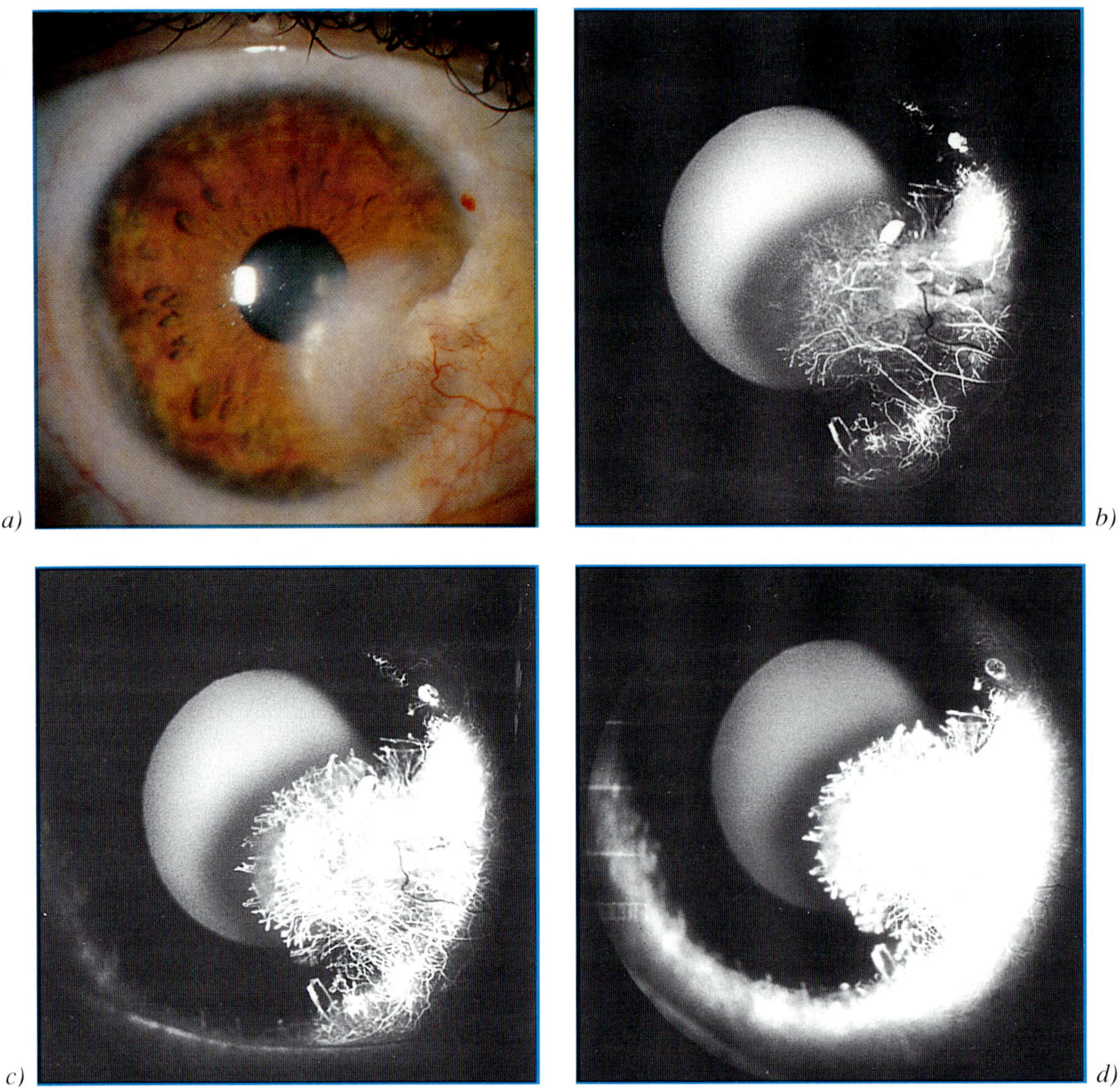

Fig. ***3.2****,9 - Biomicroscopy in a patient operated for pterygium (a). Hyperfluorescence from conjunctival vessels and corneal new vessels dominates the fluorescein angiographic pictures and masks the details of the iris (phases: b,c,d).*

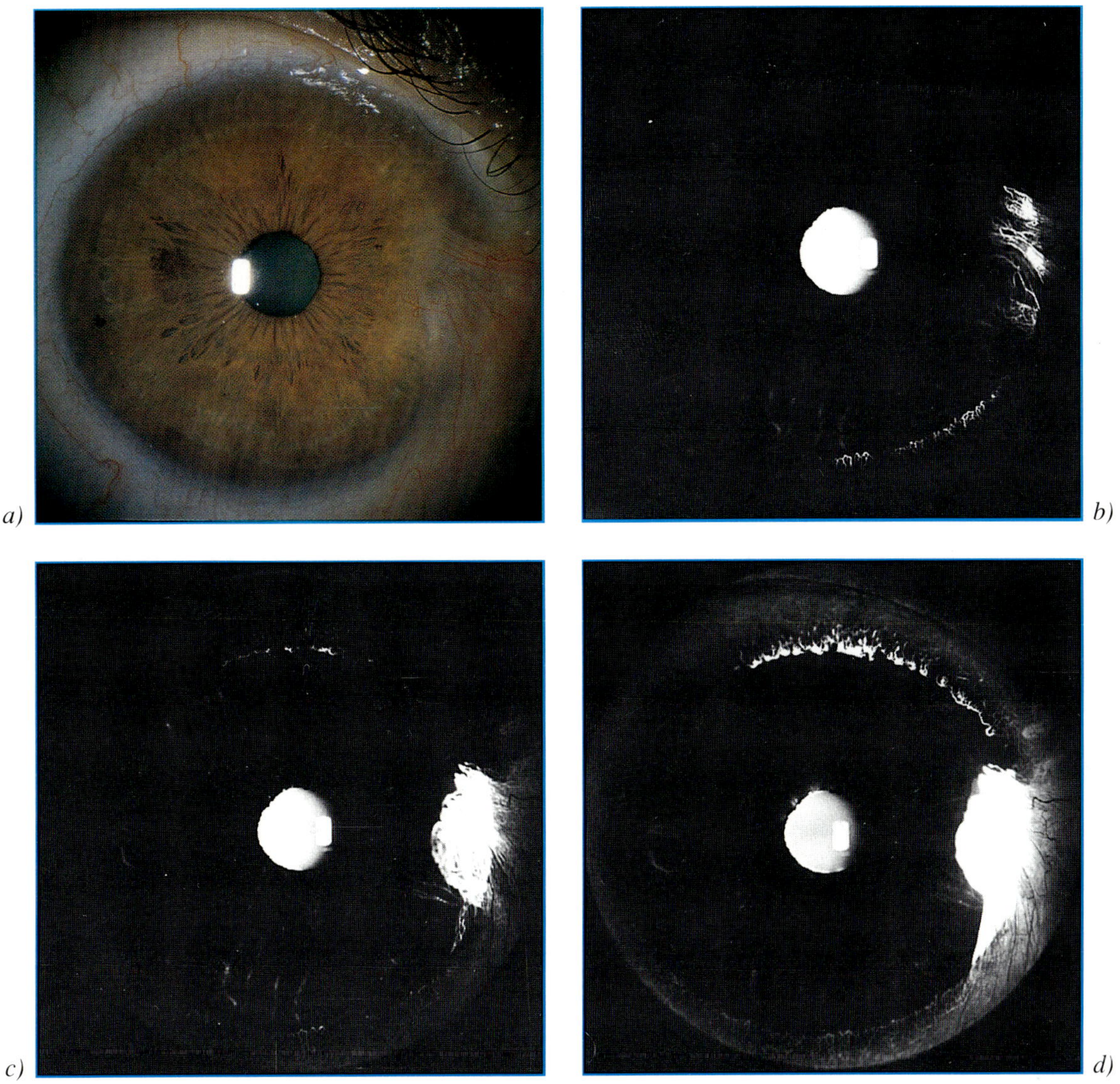

*Fig. **3.2**,10 - Vessels that can be seen inside the pterygium with the biomicroscope (a) fluoresce early on angiographic examination (b) and leak profusely in the later phases (c,d). This iris is too heavily pigmented for the radial vascular network to be visible. However, no hyperfluorescence attributable to vascular anomalies can be seen.*

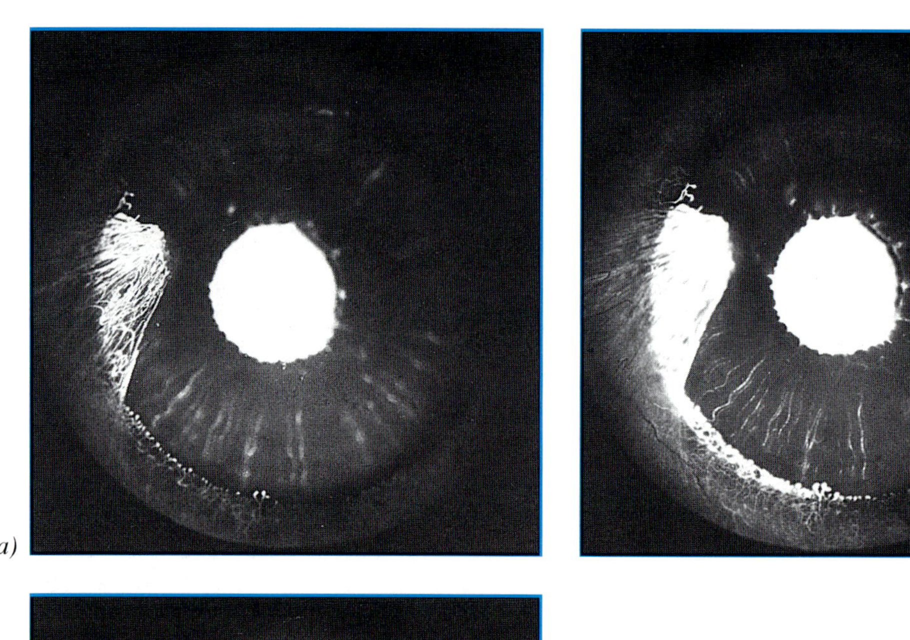

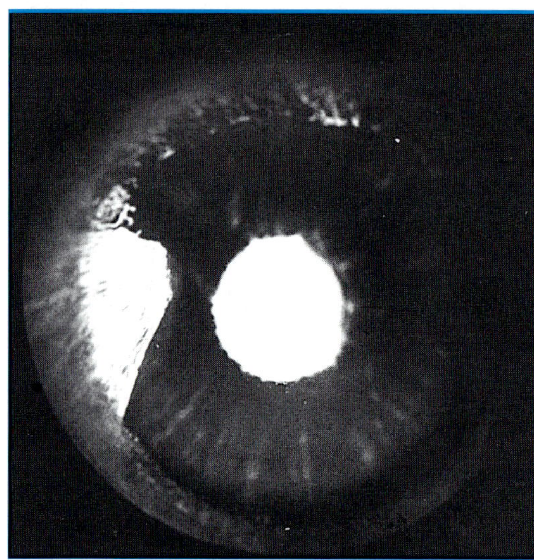

Fig. ***3.2****,11 - Fluorescein angiography in a patient with pterygium at 8-10 o'clock. The instrument was focused on the corneal plane so the iris surface is out of focus. Details of the vascular network of the pterygium can only be seen in the early phases (a); at later angiographic times the dye leaks out through the anomalous vascular walls, leading to increasingly strong hyperfluorescence (b,c).*

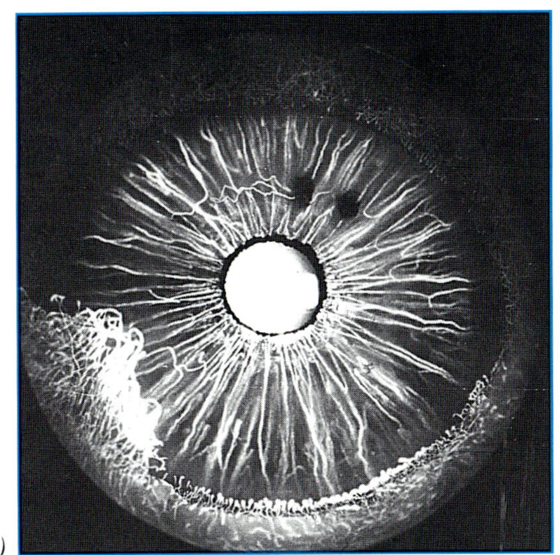

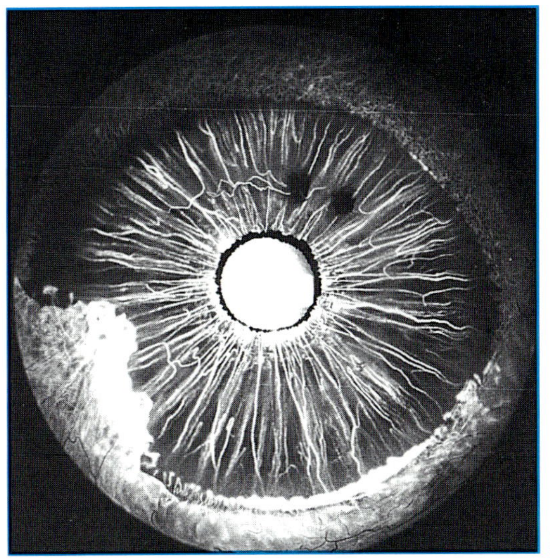

a) *b)*

Fig. ***3.2****,12 - Iris fluorescein angiographic phases (a, early; b, late) in a patient with pterygium (7-9 o'clock) and pale iris. In this case the scant pigmentation permits a detailed view of the iris vessels. The anarchic network of the pterygium results in hyperfluorescence on a plane anterior to the iris surface, becoming brighter in later phases while still keeping within the same margins.*

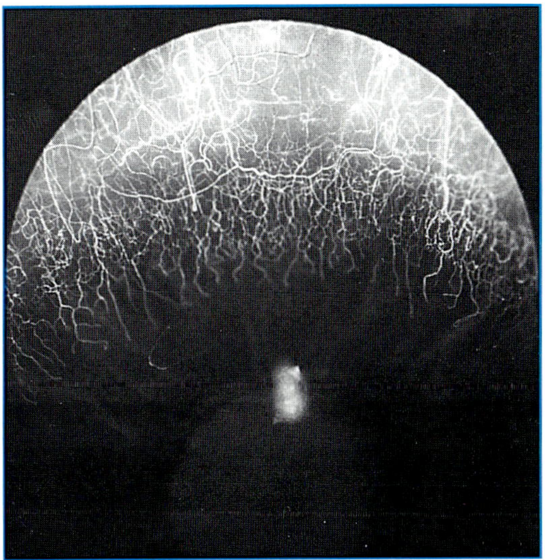

Fig. ***3.2****,13 - Large magnification of an early fluorescein angiographic phase in a patient with long limbal terminal meshes, that pass the limbus and invade the corneal surface. The anomalous vessels fluoresce right down to their tiny end branches, so that details can be seen that are not detectable by biomicroscopy.*

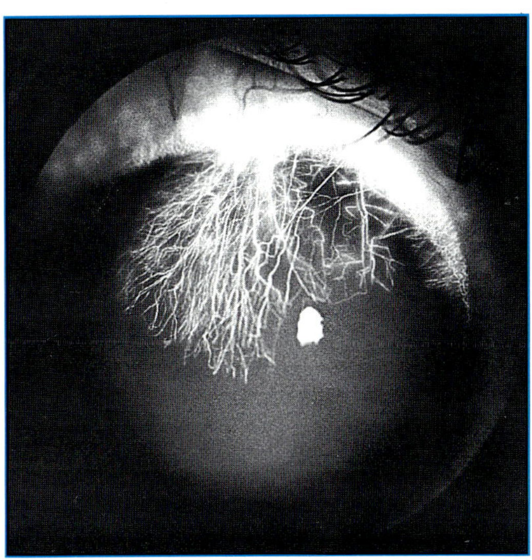

Fig. ***3.2****,14 - The upper corneal sectors are invaded by an arborized mesh of thread-like new vessels originating from the perilimbal conjunctival vascular network (fluorescein angiography). Fluorescein leakage from corneal vessels is only slight.*

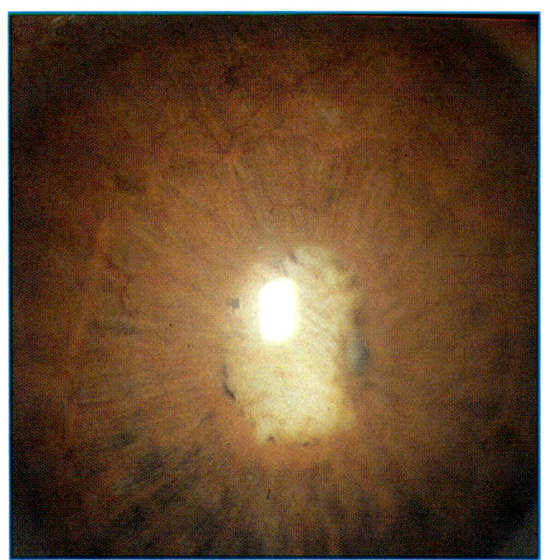

a)

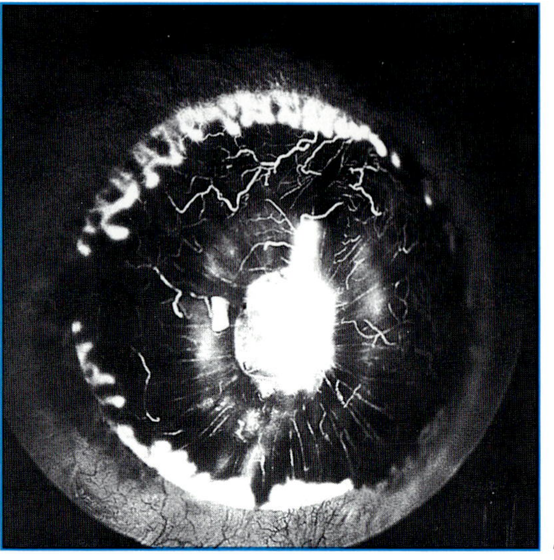

b)

*Fig. **3.2**,15 - Biomicroscopy (a) and fluorescein angiography (b) in a patient who had had anterior uveitis complicated by fibrous pupillary occlusion, corneal new vessels and distortion of the iris vascular structure. The corneal new vessels are mostly on the surface, forming an intricate network of perilimbal branches ending in saccular microaneurysms that fluoresce conspicuously. Biomicroscopy shows the stroma of the iris crossed by anarchic vascular trunks which, on fluorescein angiographic examination, take up dye but only leak it partly through their walls.*

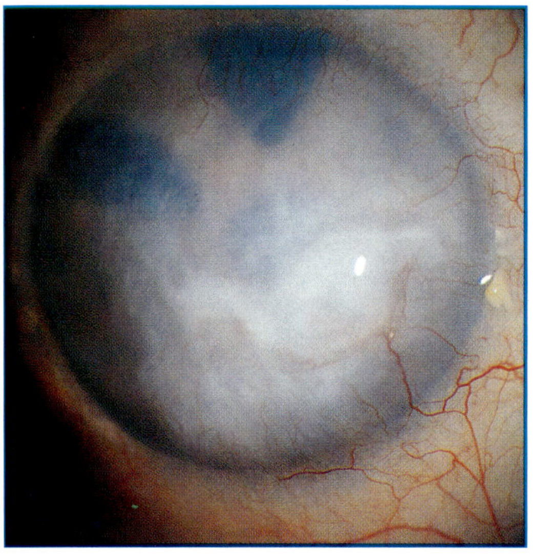

a)

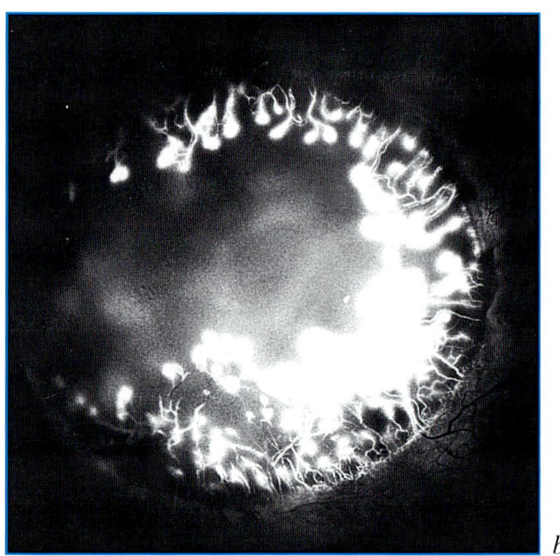

b)

*Fig. **3.2**,16 - Biomicroscopy (a) of an ample vascularized leukoma. Fluorescein angiography (b) shows the sprouts of numerous thread-like vessels, following a serpentine path and ending in microaneurysms that markedly leak fluorescein. Iris dye leakage is seen in the background.*

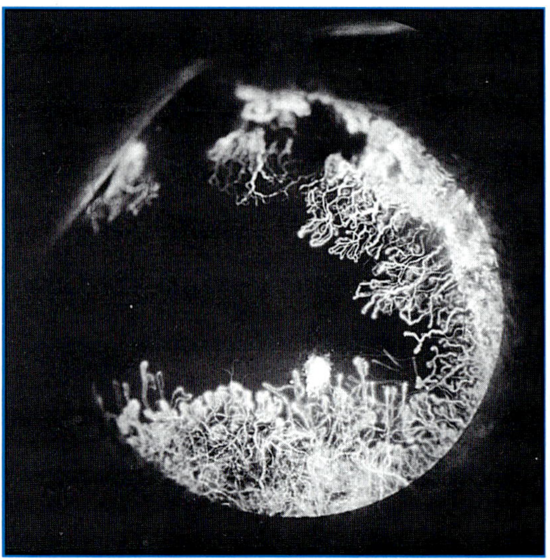

*Fig. **3.2**,17 - Fluorescein angiographic picture of an intricate, complex surface and deeper-lying neovascular network in the cornea whose end branches fan out in an "tree" pattern.*

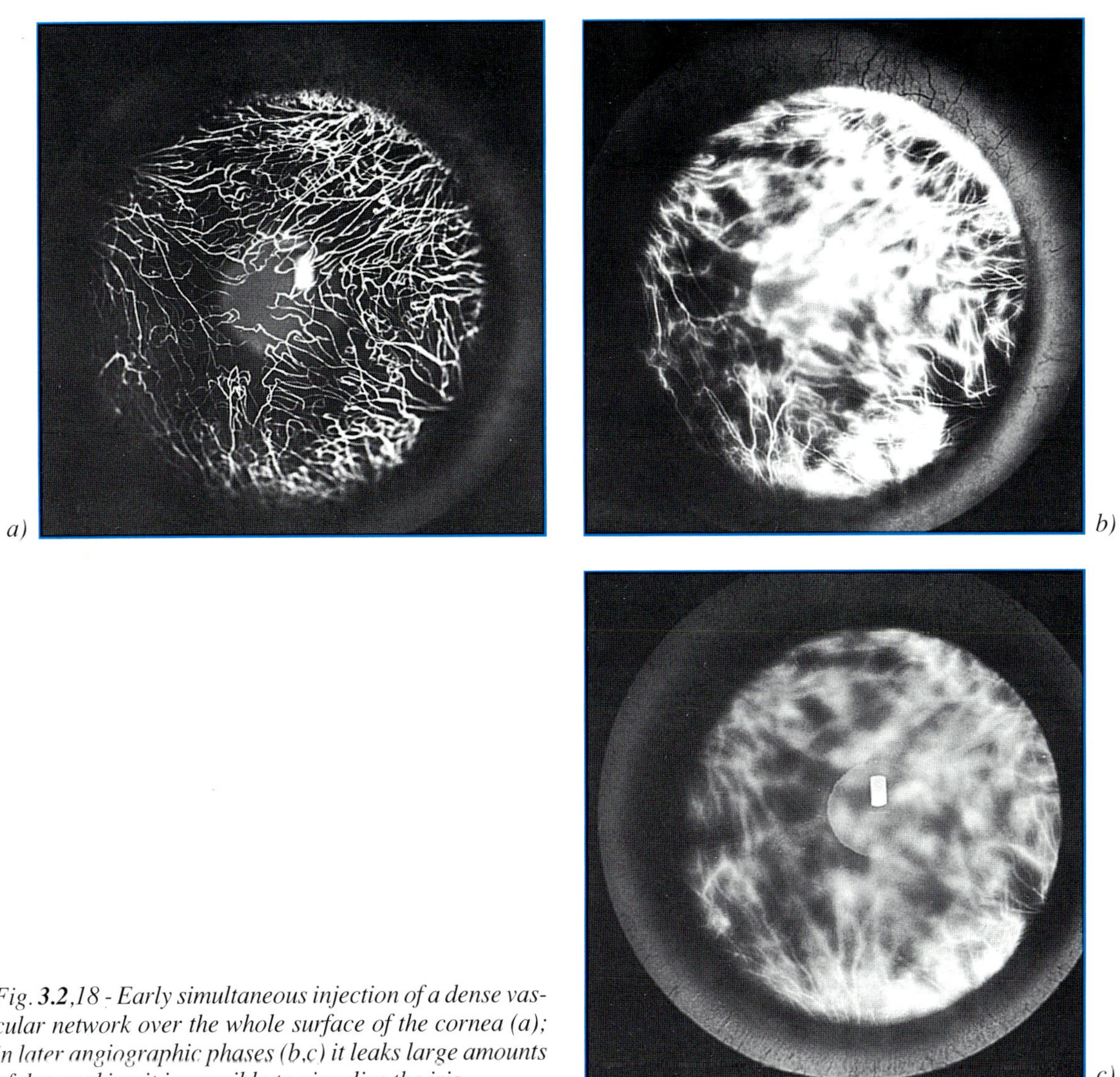

*Fig. **3.2**,18 - Early simultaneous injection of a dense vascular network over the whole surface of the cornea (a); in later angiographic phases (b,c) it leaks large amounts of dye, making it impossible to visualize the iris.*

a) b)

*Fig. **3.2**,19 - Early (a) and late (b) fluorescein angiographic phases showing extensive superficial and deep corneal neovessels. The fluorescein is taken up very fast (a) and dye leakage is massive in later phases (b).*

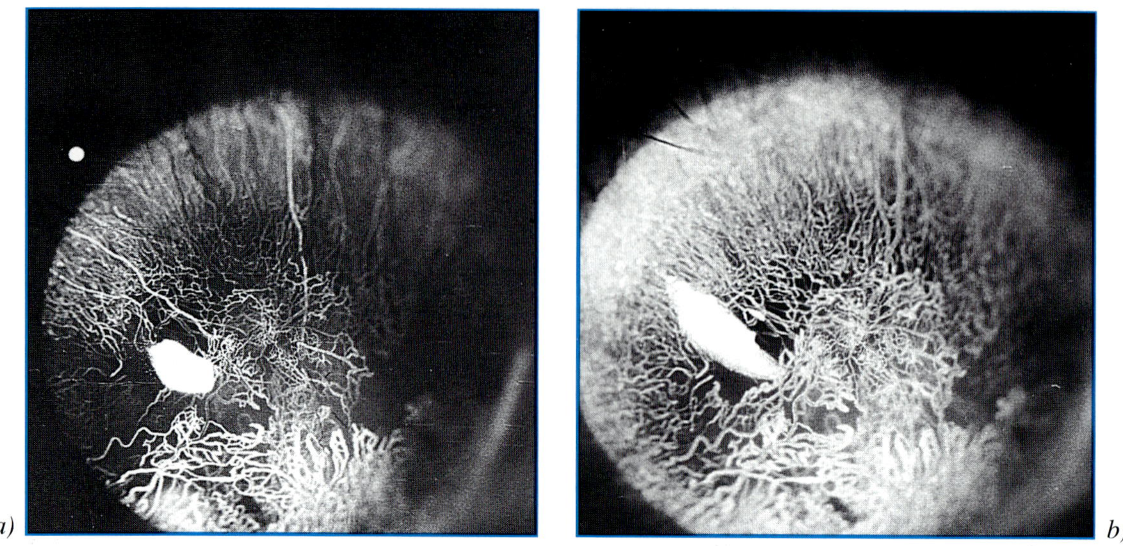

Fig. ***3.2****,20 - Early (a) and late (b) corneal fluorescein angiography of an eye with a vast vascularized leukoma. The neovascular network is extremely complex, lying on several levels, and takes up dye unevenly, at different times in the different zones. The input from branches of perforating ciliary vessels can be seen building up vascular complexes that fan out in a "tree" pattern.*

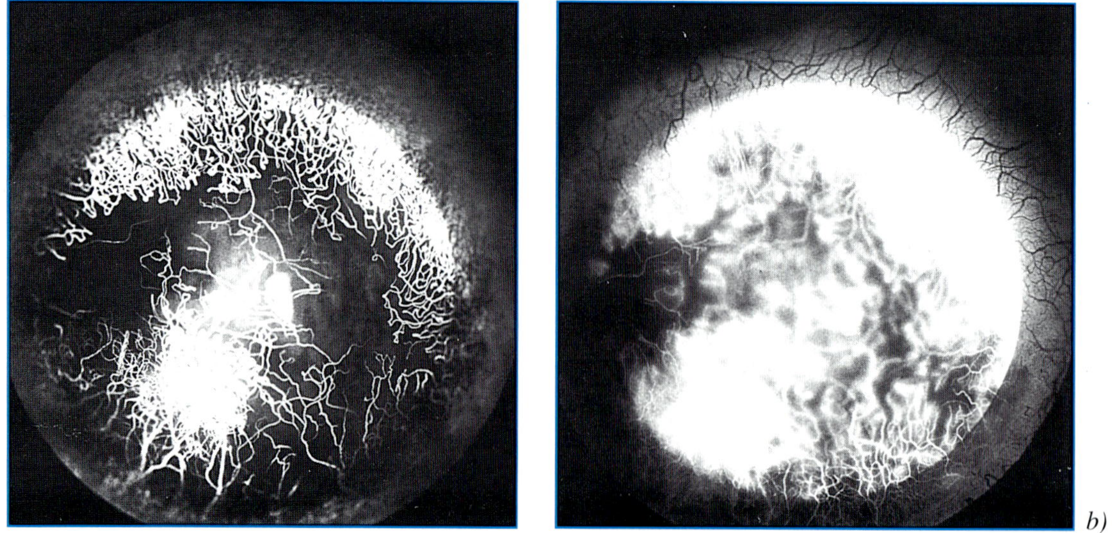

Fig. ***3.2****,21 - Fluorescein angiographic picture of a cicatricial trachomatous pannus. In the early phase (a) the whole neovascular network can be analyzed in detail, with its fine mesh arrayed more regularly in the upper sectors. In the later phase (b) the picture is dominated by diffuse hyperfluorescence, as dye leaks through the walls of the new vessels.*

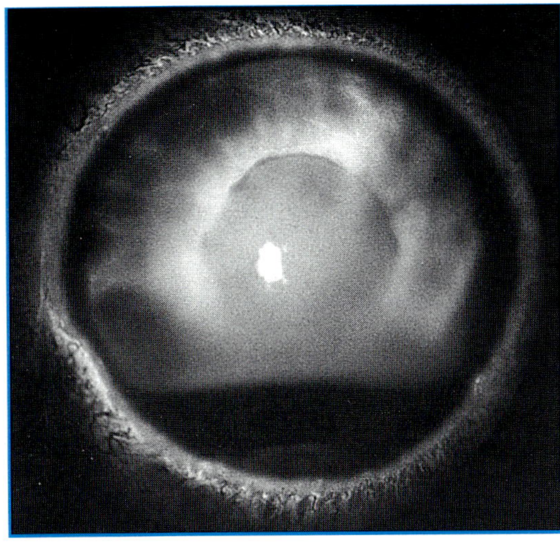

*Fig. **3.2**,22 - Iris fluorescein angiography in a patient with neovascular glaucoma complicated by hyphema. A "level" hypofluorescence resulting from the masking effect of blood covers the lower parts of the iris. Details of the rest of the iris are hard to detect because of the corneal edema though some areas of iris fluorescein leakage can be seen in the background.*

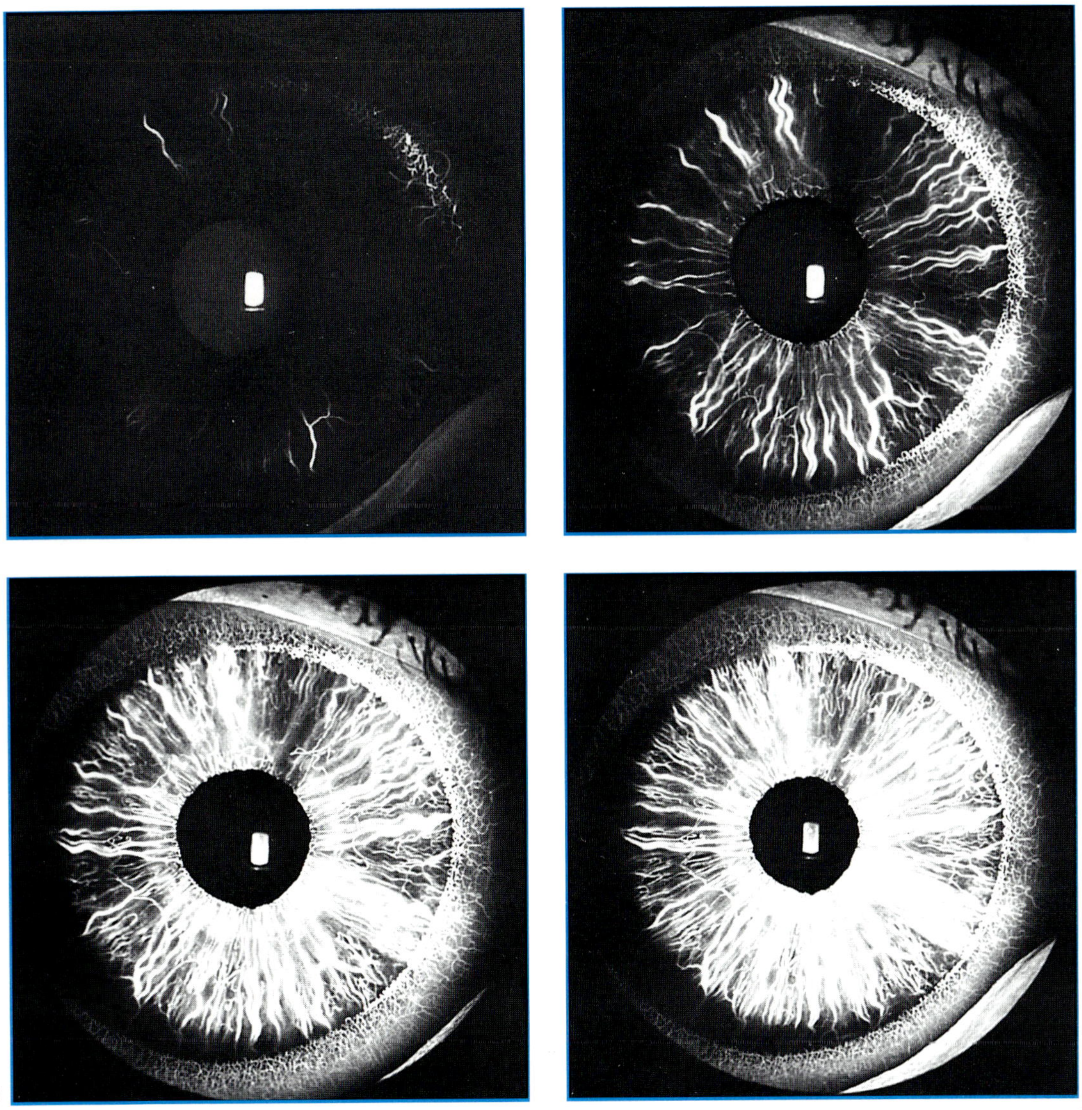

a)

b)

c)

d)

*Fig. **3.2**,23 - Filling phases in a clear iris: the scant pigment means that the morphology and vascular dynamics of the iris vessels can be analyzed in detail by this examination. After injection, the dye appears at the iris root with the same latency as the arm-iris circulation time (a). In the arterial phase (b) the radial arteries gradually fluoresce from the limbus to the pupillary margin. In the venous phase (c) the dye filling the veins flows backwards from the pupillary margin to the limbus. Fluorescence is seen in all the vessels (d) in subsequent angiographic phases.*

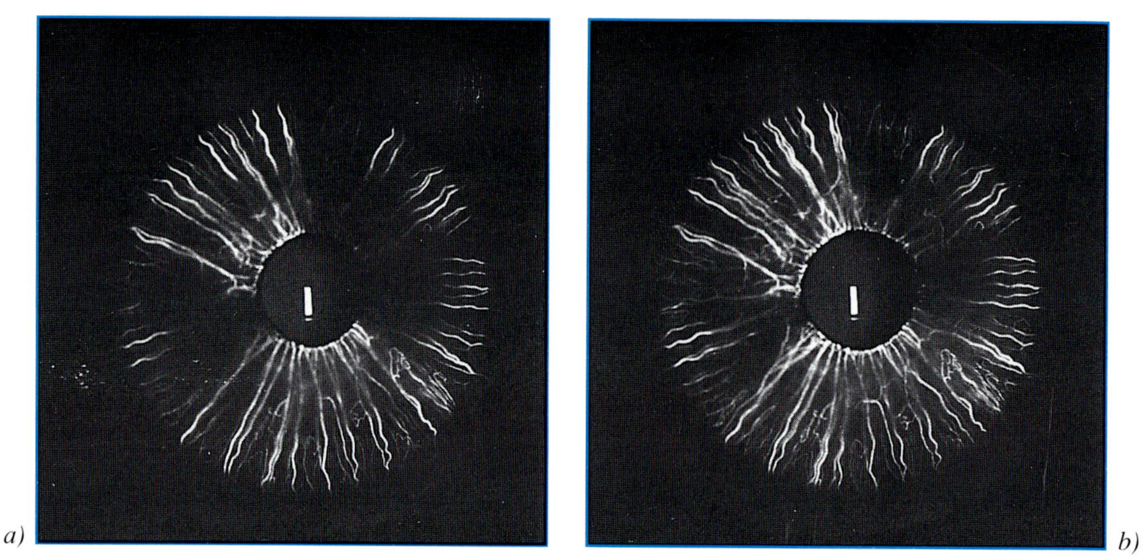

a) b)

Fig. **3.2**,*24 - Iris fluorescein angiographic phases (a: initial arterial phase; b: arteriovenous phase; c: venous phase, d: late venous phase). Arteries fluoresce promptly (a) from the periphery to the pupillary margin, de-* →

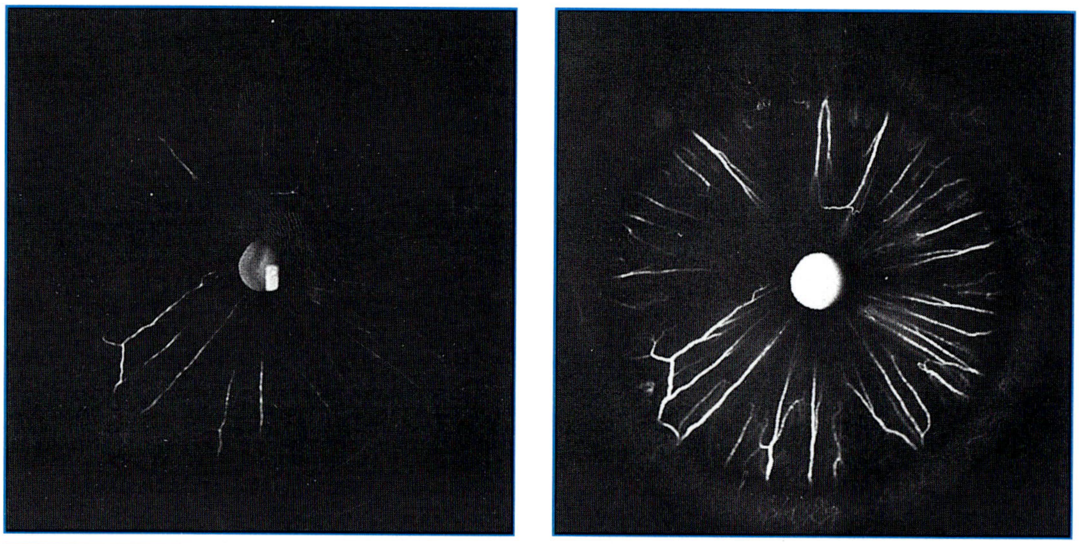

a) b)

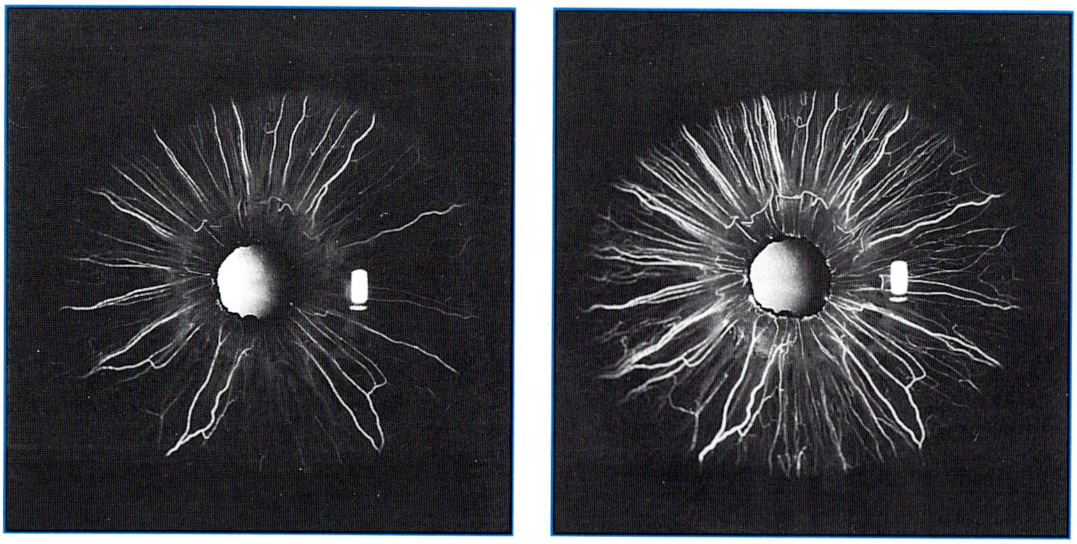

a) b)

Fig. **3.2**,*25-26 - Two iris fluorescein angiographic sequences in normal subjects, illustrating the various phases of iris filling (a,b,c,d). In the early phases (a,b) the arteries in different sectors do not fill in the same* →

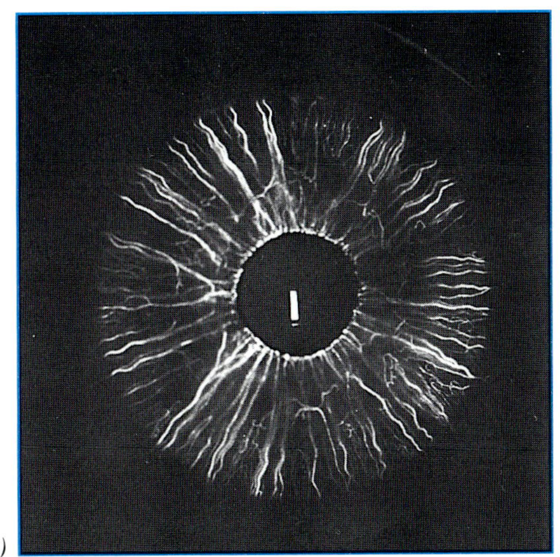
c)

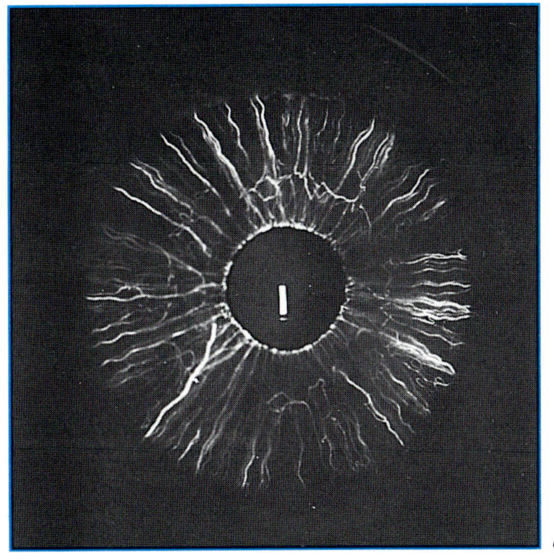
d)

creasing in diameter and running quite straight. The veins become visible later (b,c,d), running deeper and more tortuously; they grow in diameter along the path from the peripupillary capillary plexus to the iris root.

←

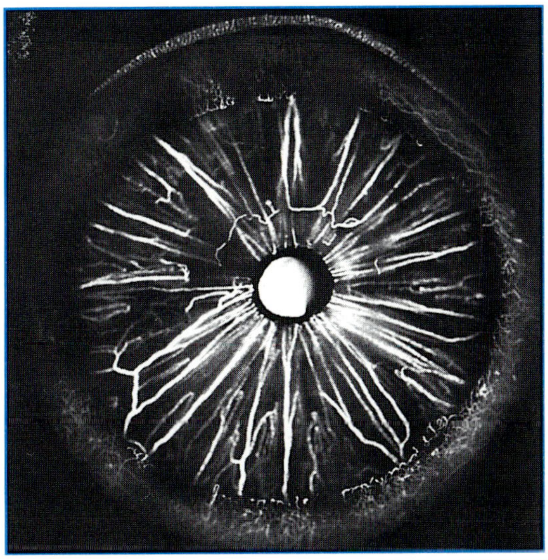

c)

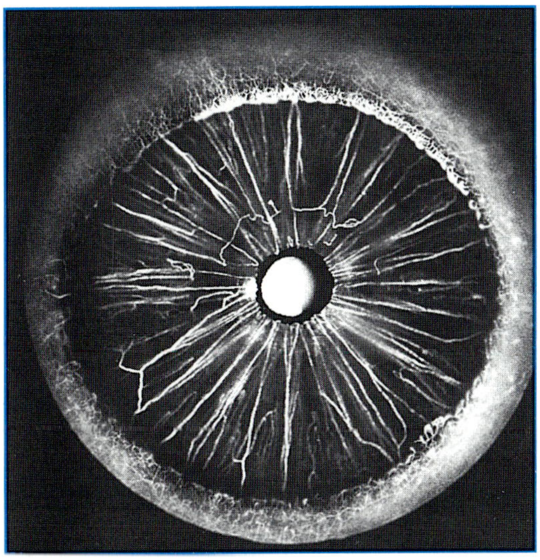

d)

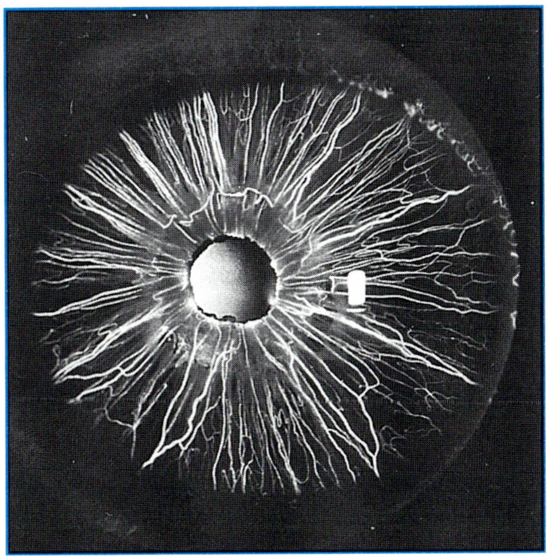

c)

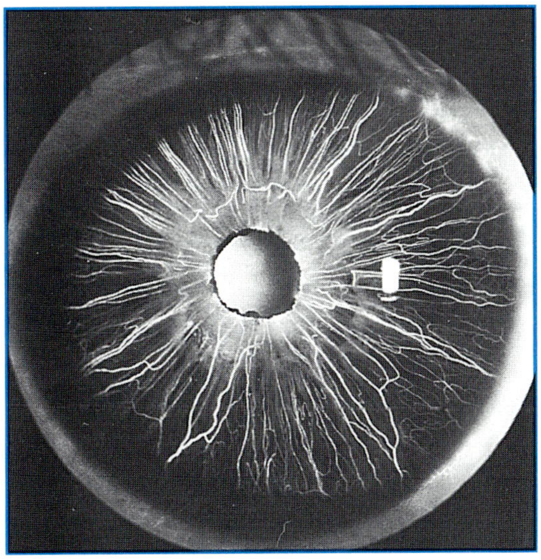

d)

order, but in later phases (c,d) all parts of the iris fluoresce (physiological sectorial delays).

←

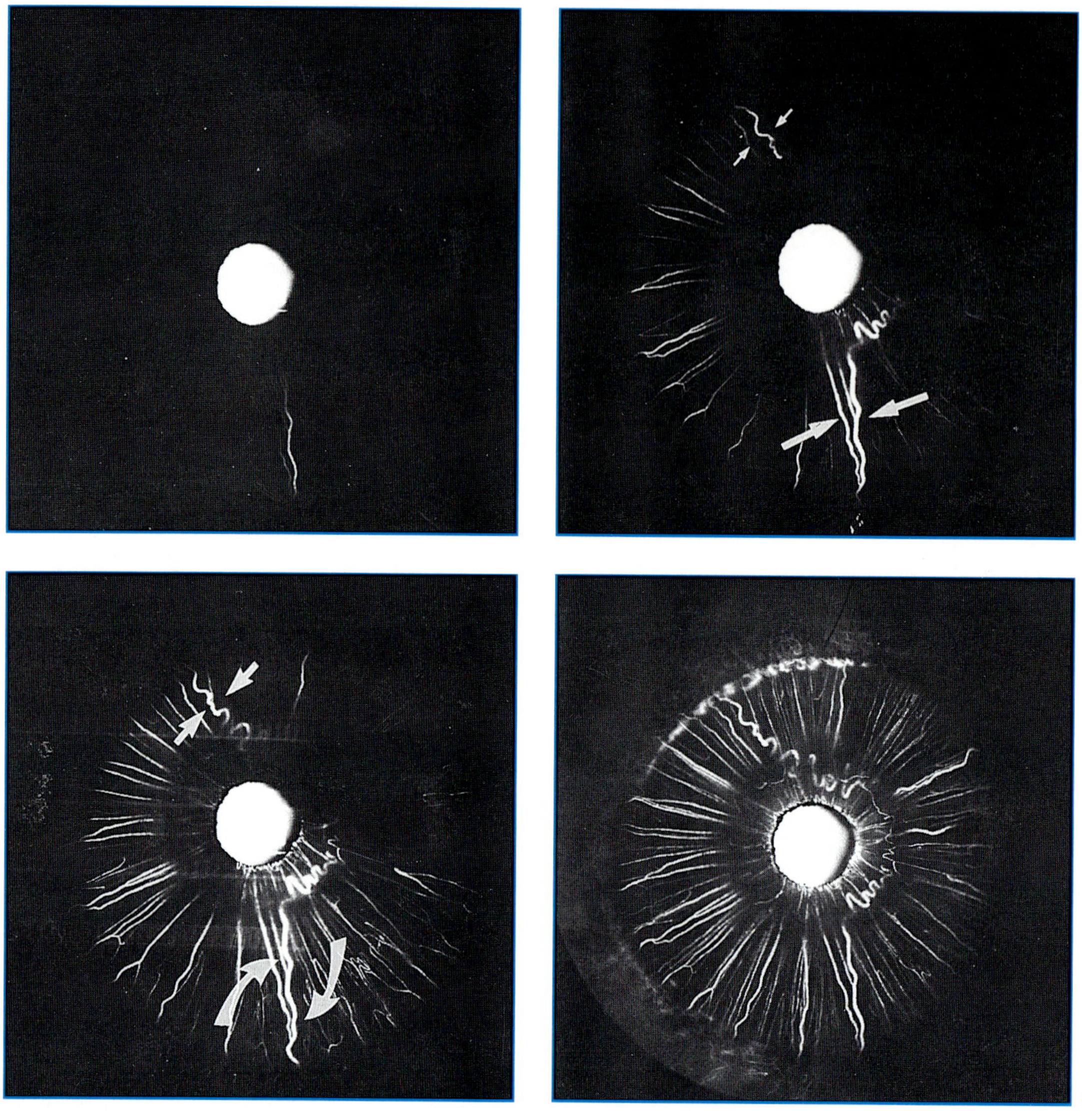

a) b) c) d)

*Fig. **3.2**,27 - Filling phases in an iris with two large arterial trunks (a) following a tortuous path (b,c) (arrows) to reach the pars pupillaris where they form a segment of the minor arterial circle of the iris (d).*

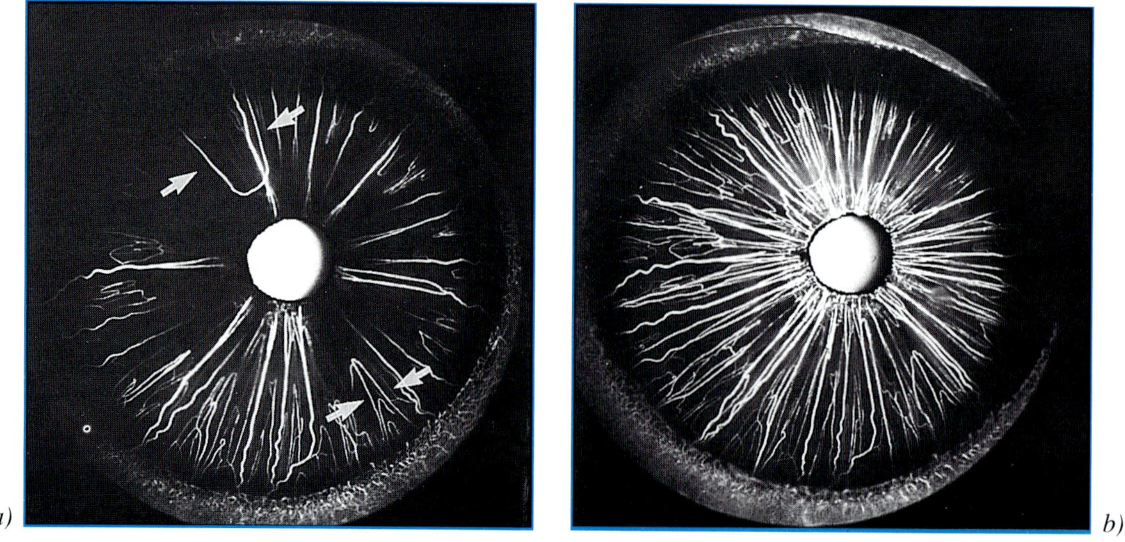

a) b)

*Fig. **3.2**,28 - Iris fluorescein angiography showing recurrent vessels (arrows) (a: arterial filling phase, b: venous phase).*

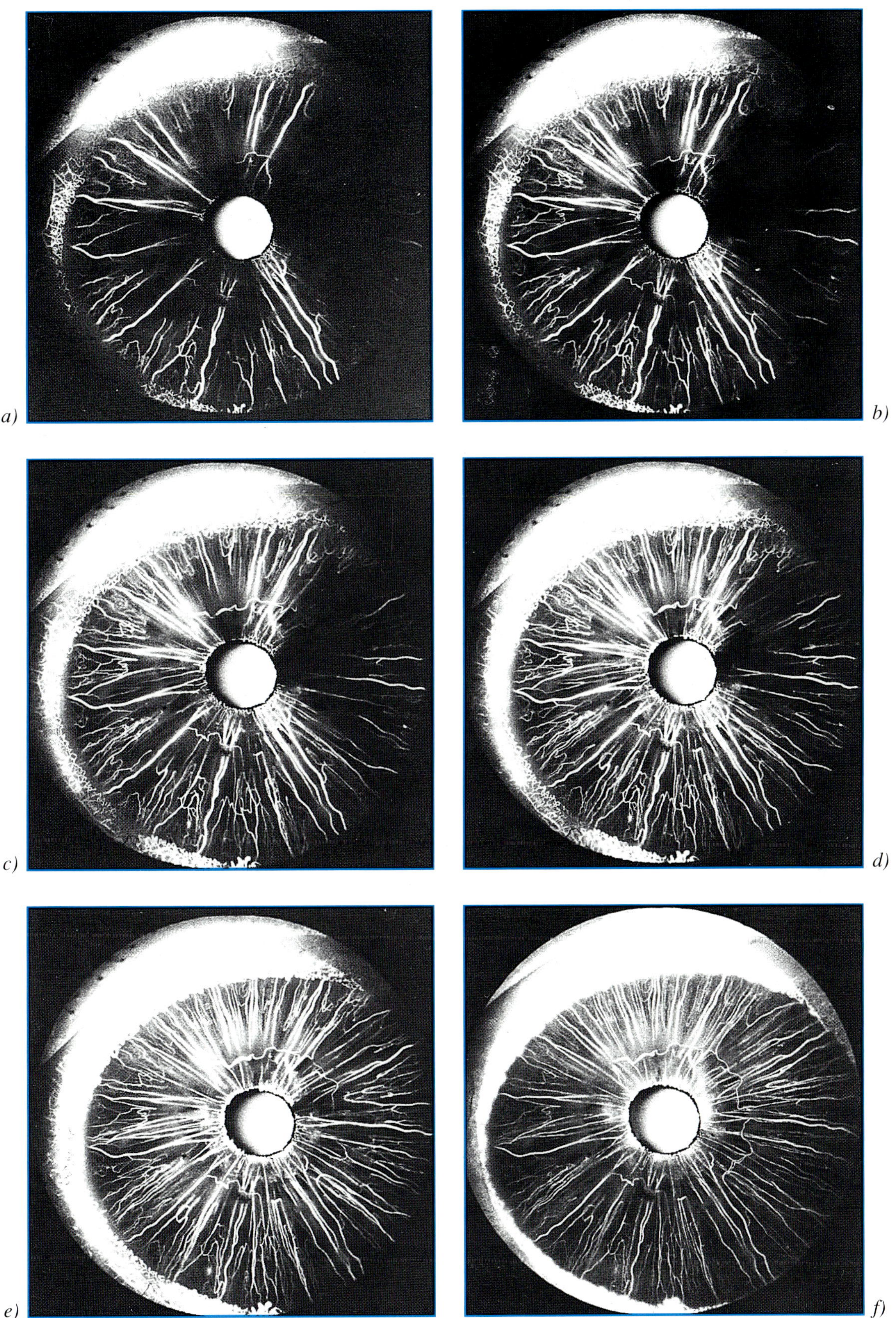

*Fig. **3.2**,29 - Iris fluorescein angiography sequences showing segmental filling (a,b,c,d,e,f). Vascular fluorescence appears in an irregular, uneven pattern in the different sectors, with a definite delay in the temporal hemi-iris (left eye). In the late venous phase (f) all sectors fluoresce well.*

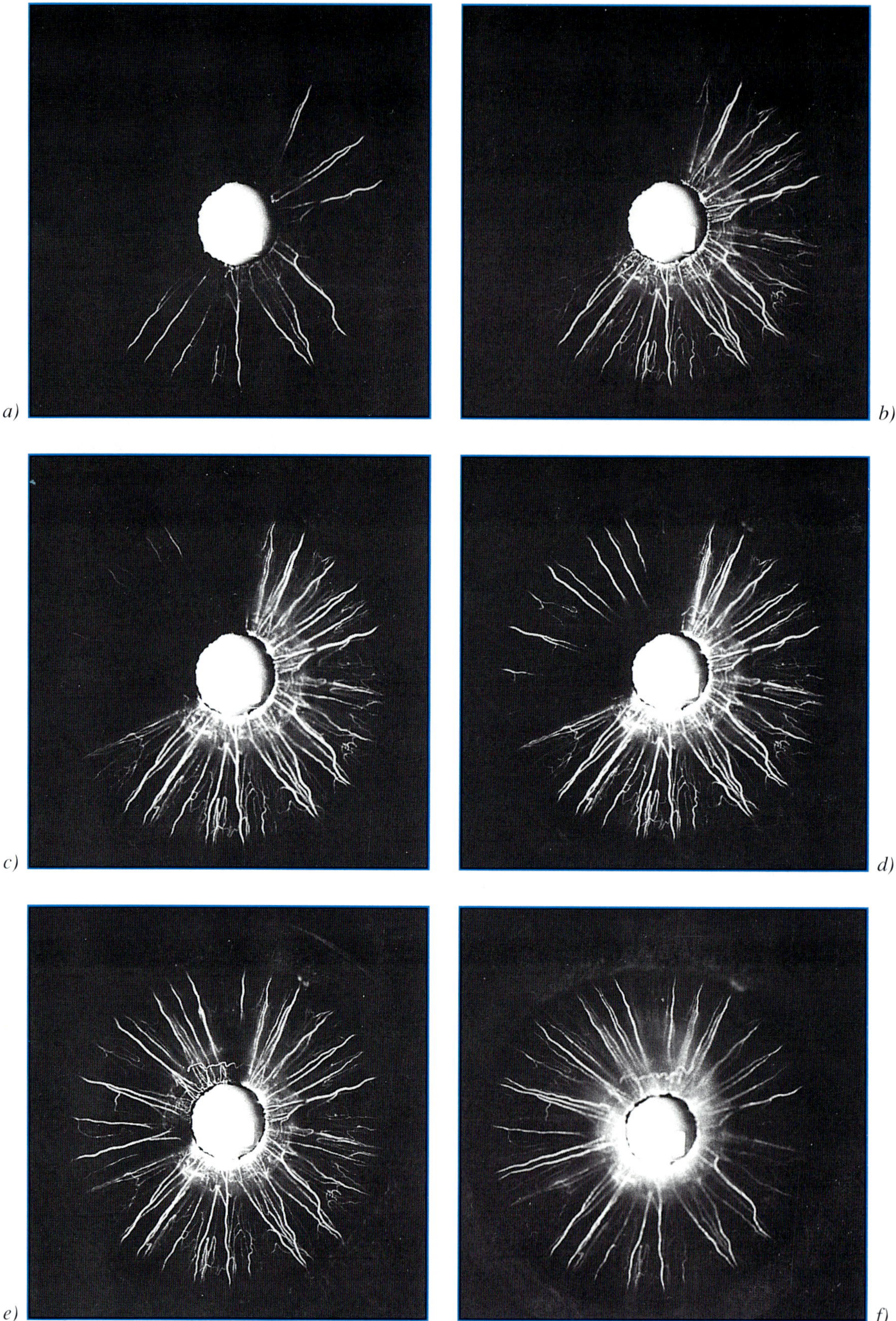

*Fig.**3.2**,30 - Iris fluorescein angiographic phases in a right eye (a,b,c,d,e,f), showing marked filling delays in the temporal sectors.*

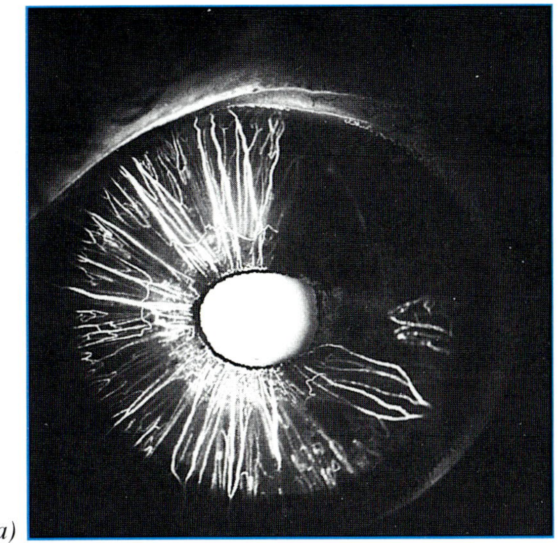

a)

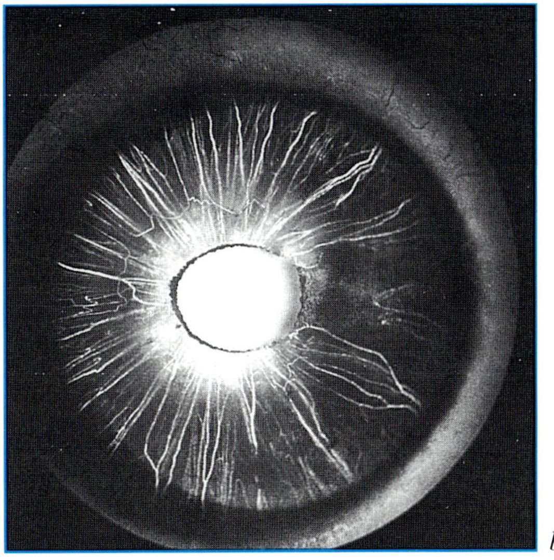

b)

*Fig. **3.2**,31 - Delayed filling in a partially atrophic iris (a). The lack of perfusion in the late venous phase (b) between 2 and 4 o'clock in the iris indicates a pathological filling defect.*

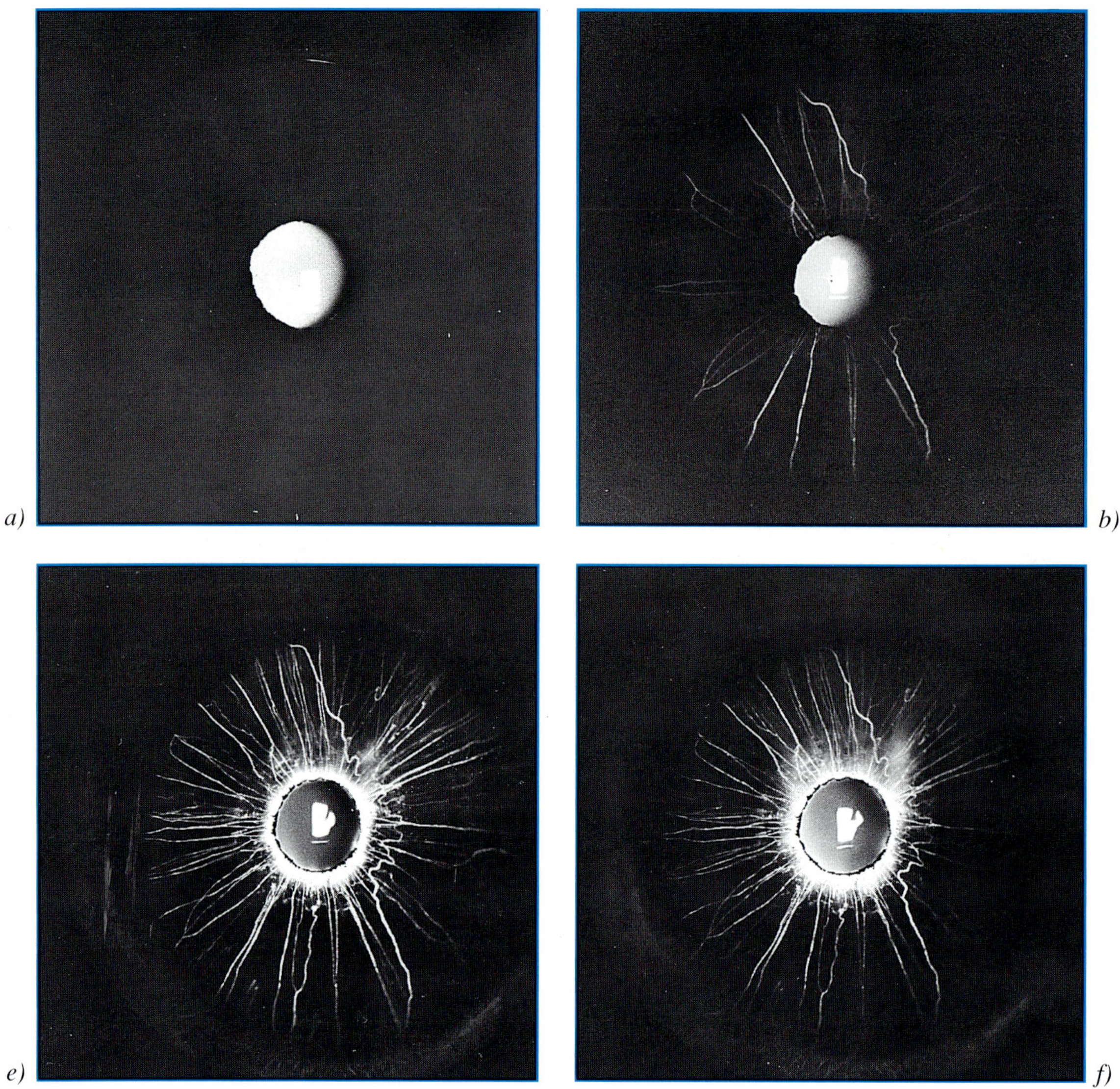

Fig. ***3.2****,32 - Iris fluorescein angiographic sequences (a,b,c,d,e,f,g,h) showing some iris filling defects. Those* →

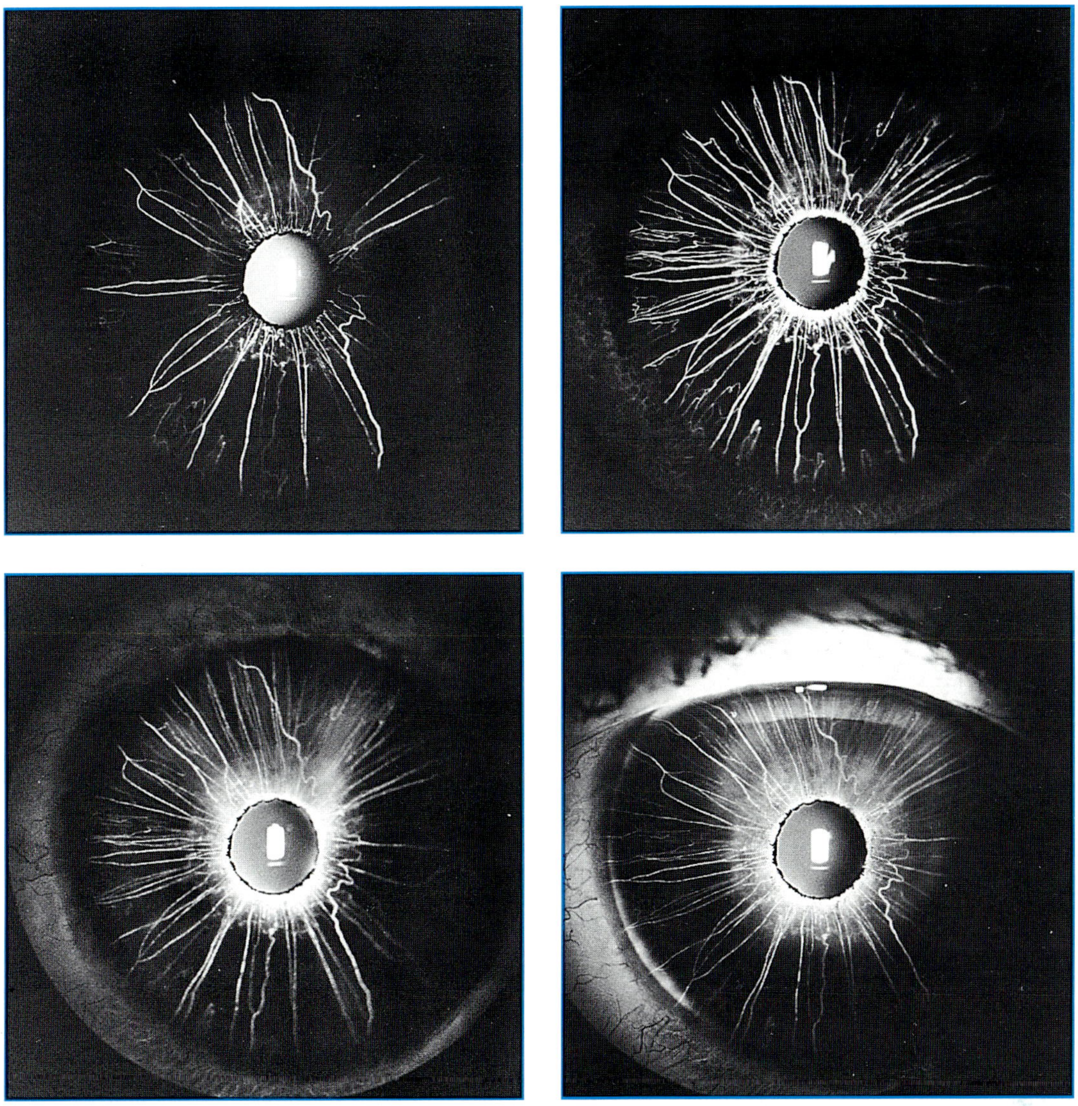

c) d)

g) h)

visible in this example could be photographic artefacts due to an area not being sharply focused or badely lit.
←

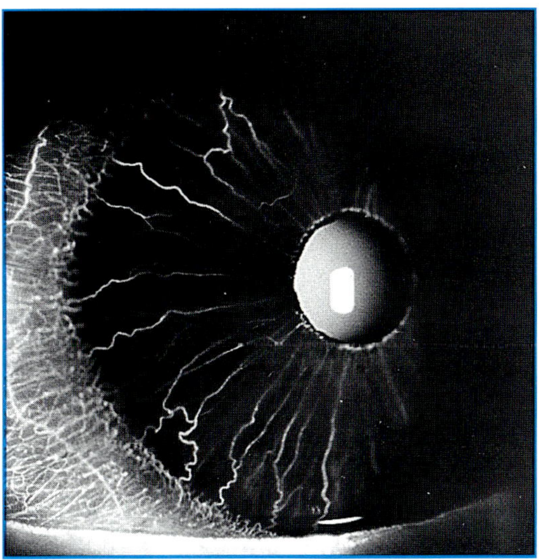

Fig. ***3.2**,33 - Radial arteries may have collateral branches and can anastomose into loops (iris fluorescein angiography).*

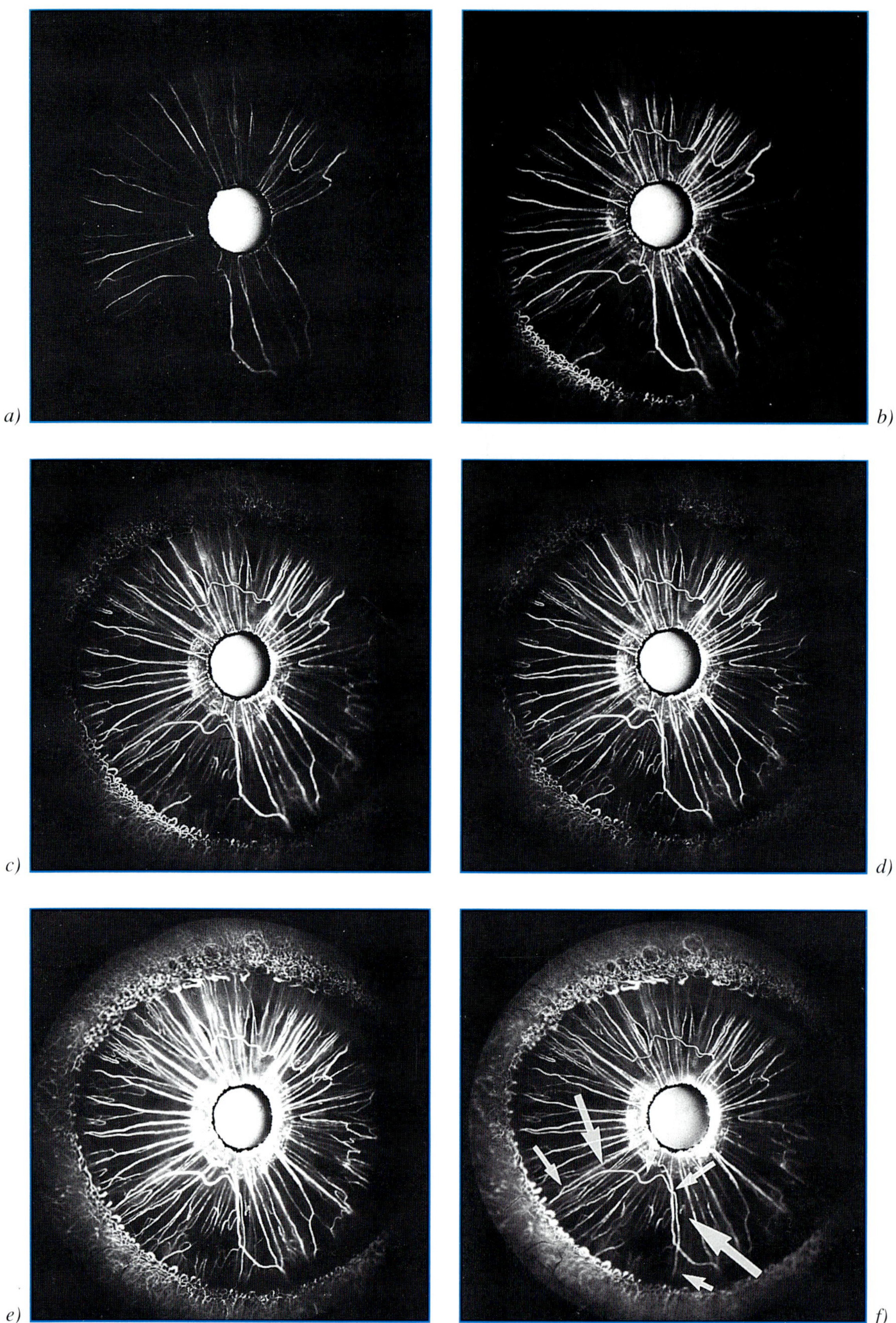

*Fig. **3.2**,34 - The whole sequence of iris fluorescein angiographic phases (a,b,c,d,e,f) provides a good picture of the nature and dynamics of each branch of the iris vascular network. In this example a recurrent vessel can be seen filling in the inferior ciliary portion; after running down to the margin of the pupillary area it turns back round towards the iris root (arrows).*

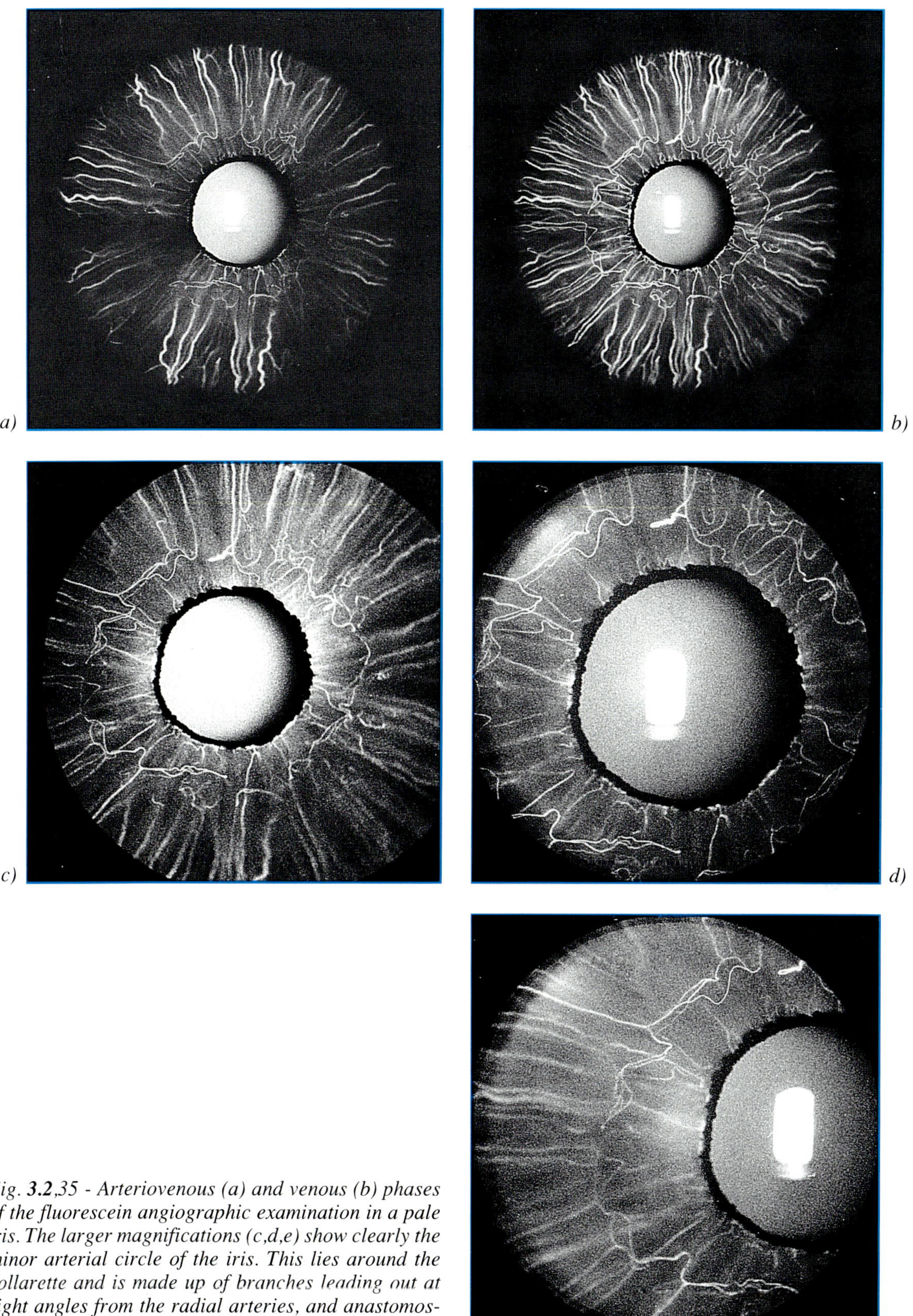

*Fig. **3.2**,35 - Arteriovenous (a) and venous (b) phases of the fluorescein angiographic examination in a pale iris. The larger magnifications (c,d,e) show clearly the minor arterial circle of the iris. This lies around the collarette and is made up of branches leading out at right angles from the radial arteries, and anastomosing in loops.*

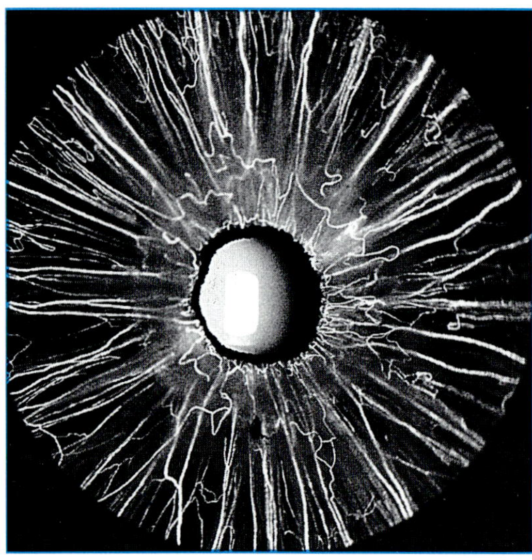

*Fig. **3.2**,36 - The vessels in the minor arterial circle of the iris are often partially obliterated, so the circle is fragmented or incomplete.*

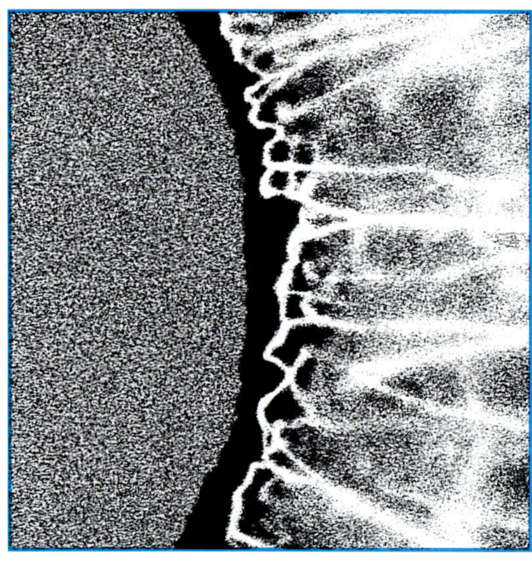

*Fig.**3.2**,37 - Large magnification of the pars pupillaris where the radial arterioles run down to the marginal zone; they continue on into the capillary plexus which is made up of a dense meshwork of small vessels in hairpin loops.*

a)

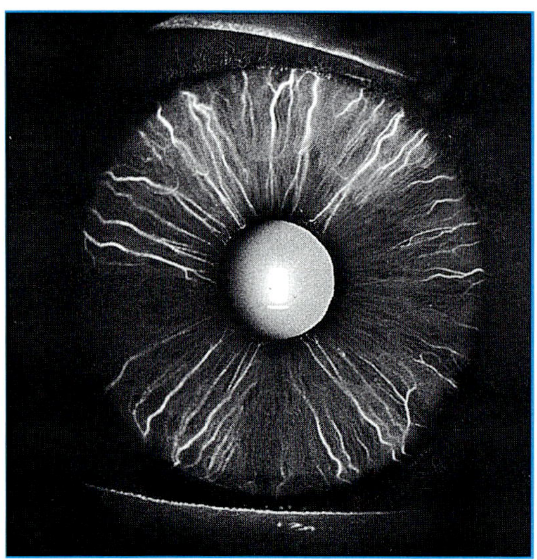

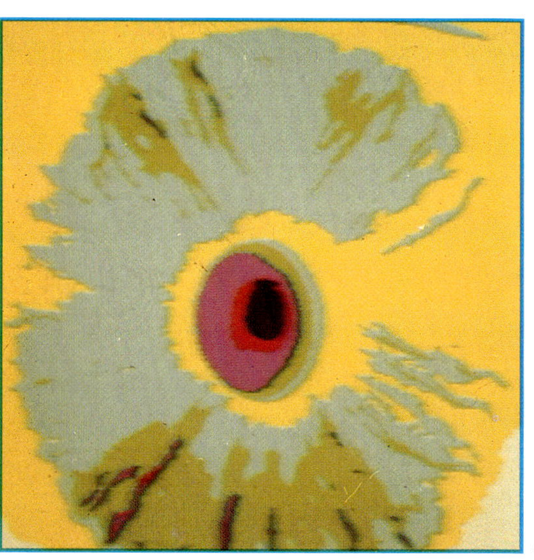

b)

*Fig. **3.2**,38 - Iris fluorescein angiography of a normal eye showing the arterial phase (a), and the corresponding computerized eight-colour equidensitometry (b).*

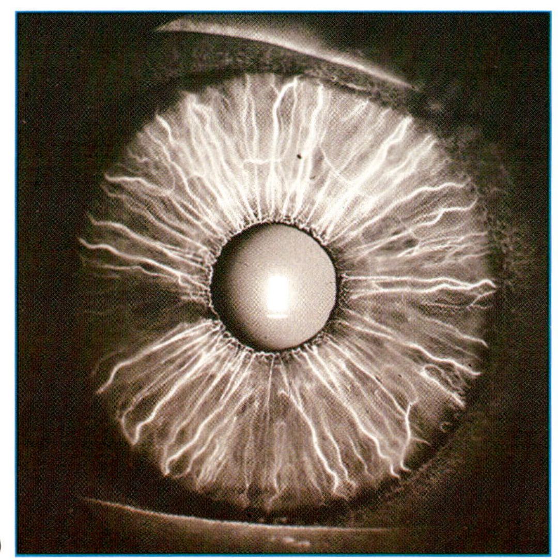

a)

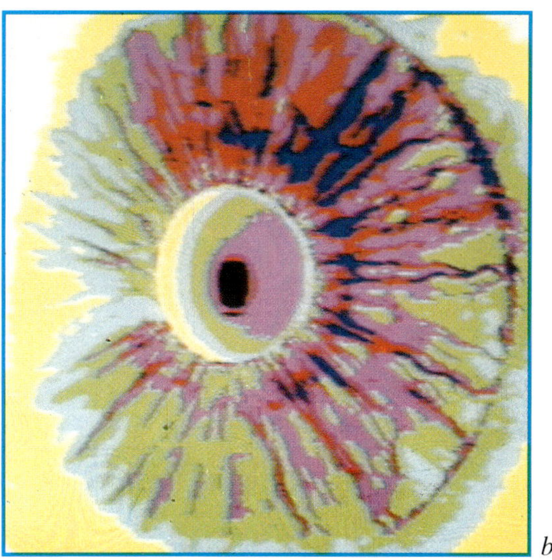

b)

*Fig. **3.2**,39 - Same case as in the previous figure, showing the venous fluorangiographic phase (a), and the corresponding computerized eight-colour equidensitometry (b).*

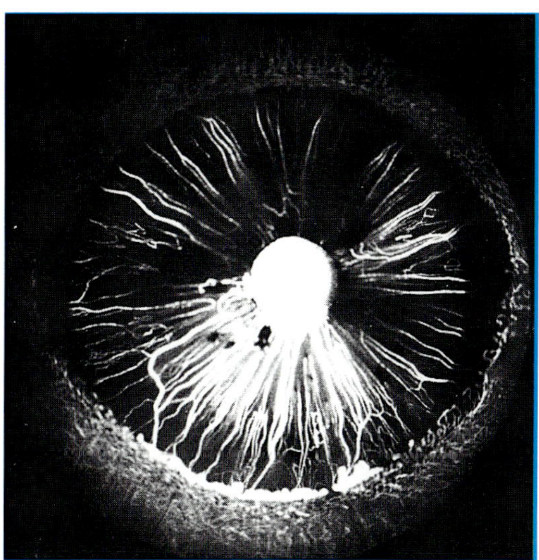

*Fig. **3.2**,40 - In this case fluorescein angiography shows vessels apparently arrayed more densely in the lower sectors of the iris. Correct interpretation of a finding like this calls for a colour photo so as to check whether the iris colouration is uneven, i.e. whether an excess of pigment in the superior sectors is masking the vessels to any extent.*

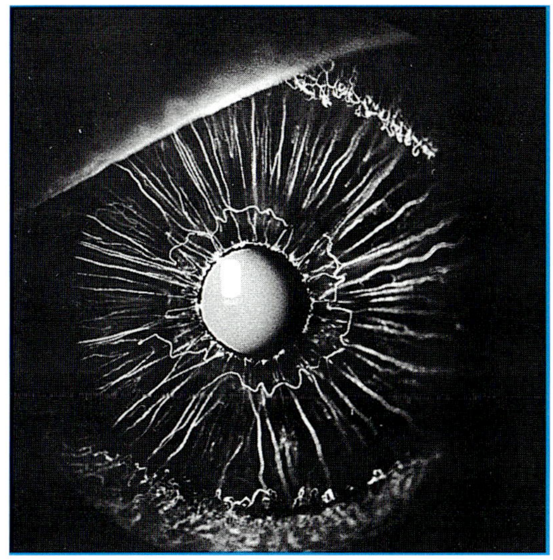

a)

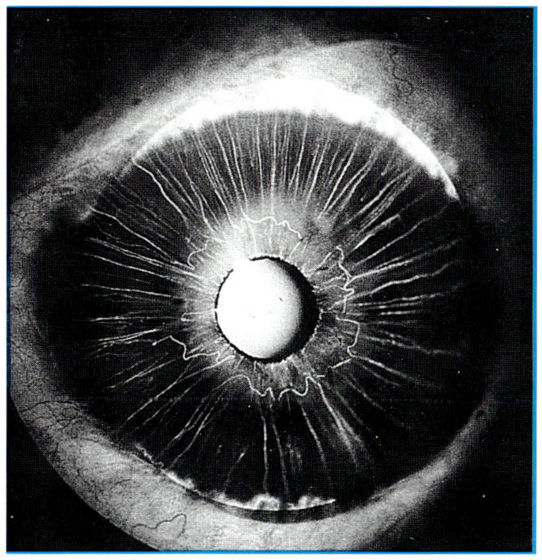

b)

*Fig. **3.2**,41 - Early (a) and late (b) iris fluorescein angiographic phases in a normal 55-year-old subject. Dye leakage from the capillary circulation in the pars pupillaris can be seen.*

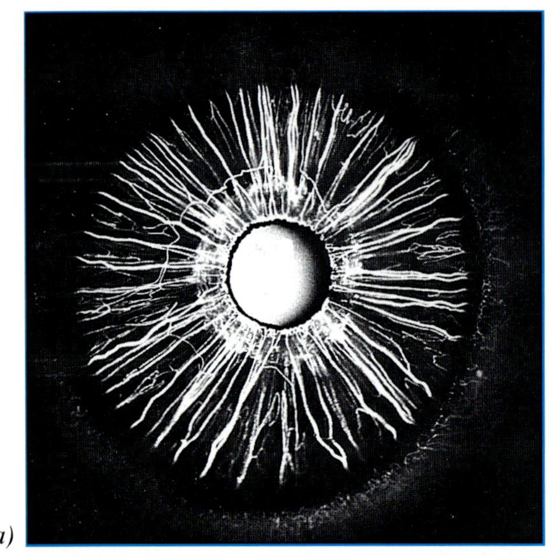

a)

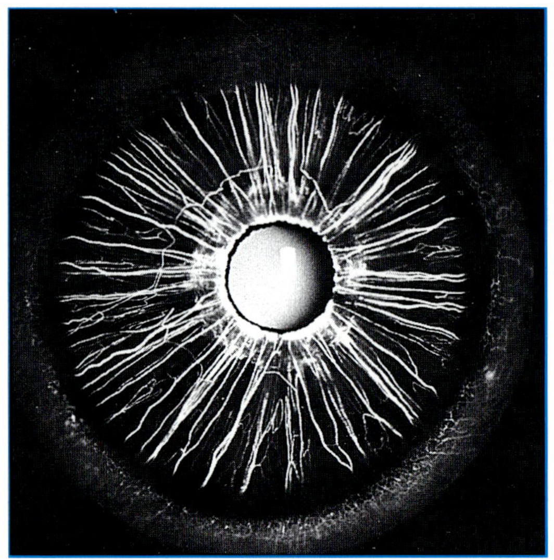

b)

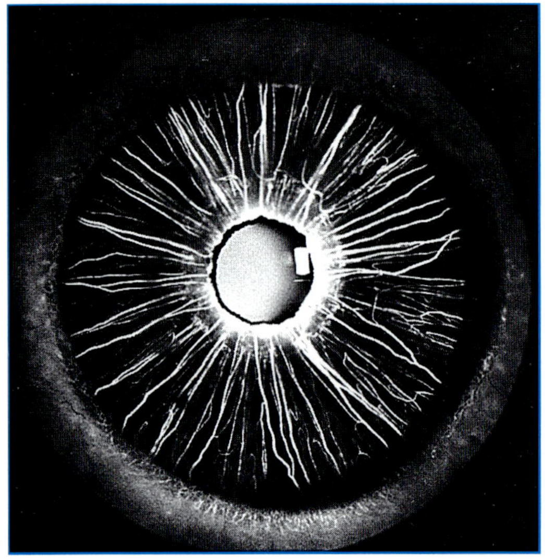

c)

*Fig. **3.2**,42 - Iris fluorescein angiographic sequence (a,b,c) in a normal 60-year-old subject. Vessels in the marginal and plexiform portions are congested and there is dye leakage from the pupillary margin, increasing in subsequent phases of the examination.*

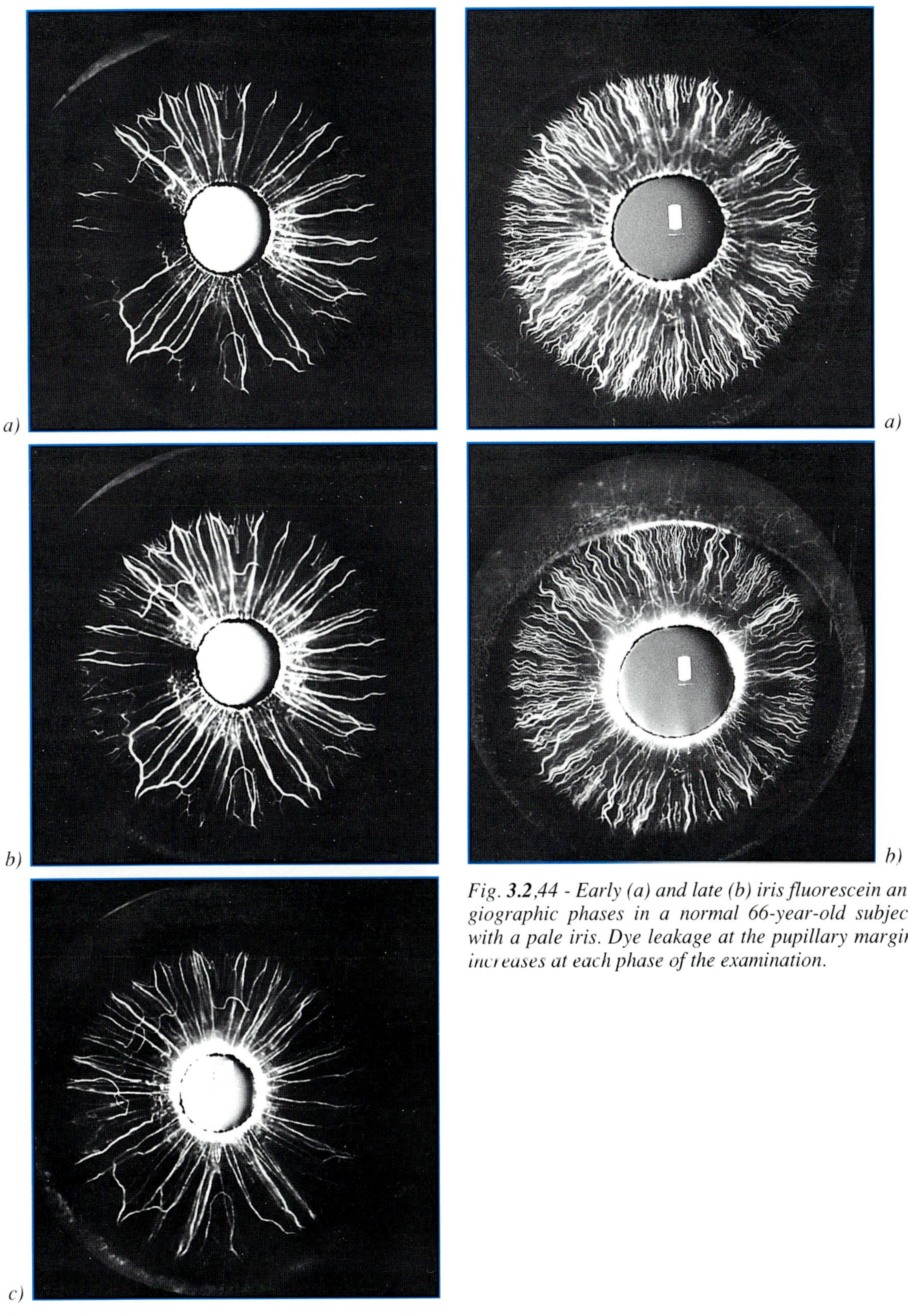

*Fig. **3.2**,43 - Another case of age-related pupillary margin leakage (fluorescein angiographic phases: a,b,c).*

*Fig. **3.2**,44 - Early (a) and late (b) iris fluorescein angiographic phases in a normal 66-year-old subject with a pale iris. Dye leakage at the pupillary margin increases at each phase of the examination.*

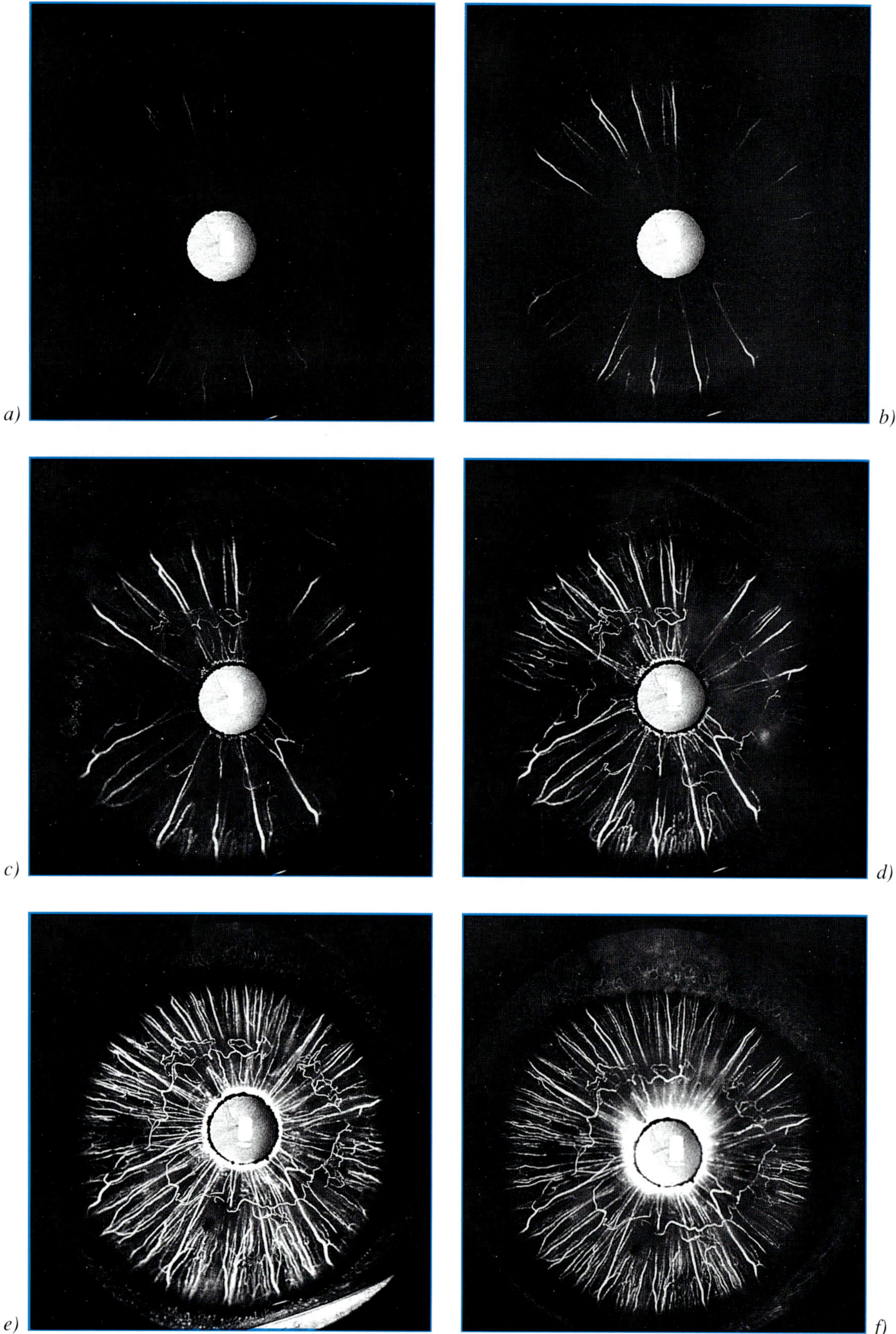

Fig. ***3.2****,45 - Iris fluorescein angiographic sequence (a,b,c,d,e,f) in a normal 70-year-old subject. At the end of the arterial phase (d) small hyperfluorescent spots appear at the pupillary margin; in subsequent phases (e) these grow brighter and bigger and their outlines become blurred. Later hyperfluorescence becomes more marked and dye leaks into the anterior chamber (f). The minor arterial circle of the iris is visible, fragmented and incomplete.*

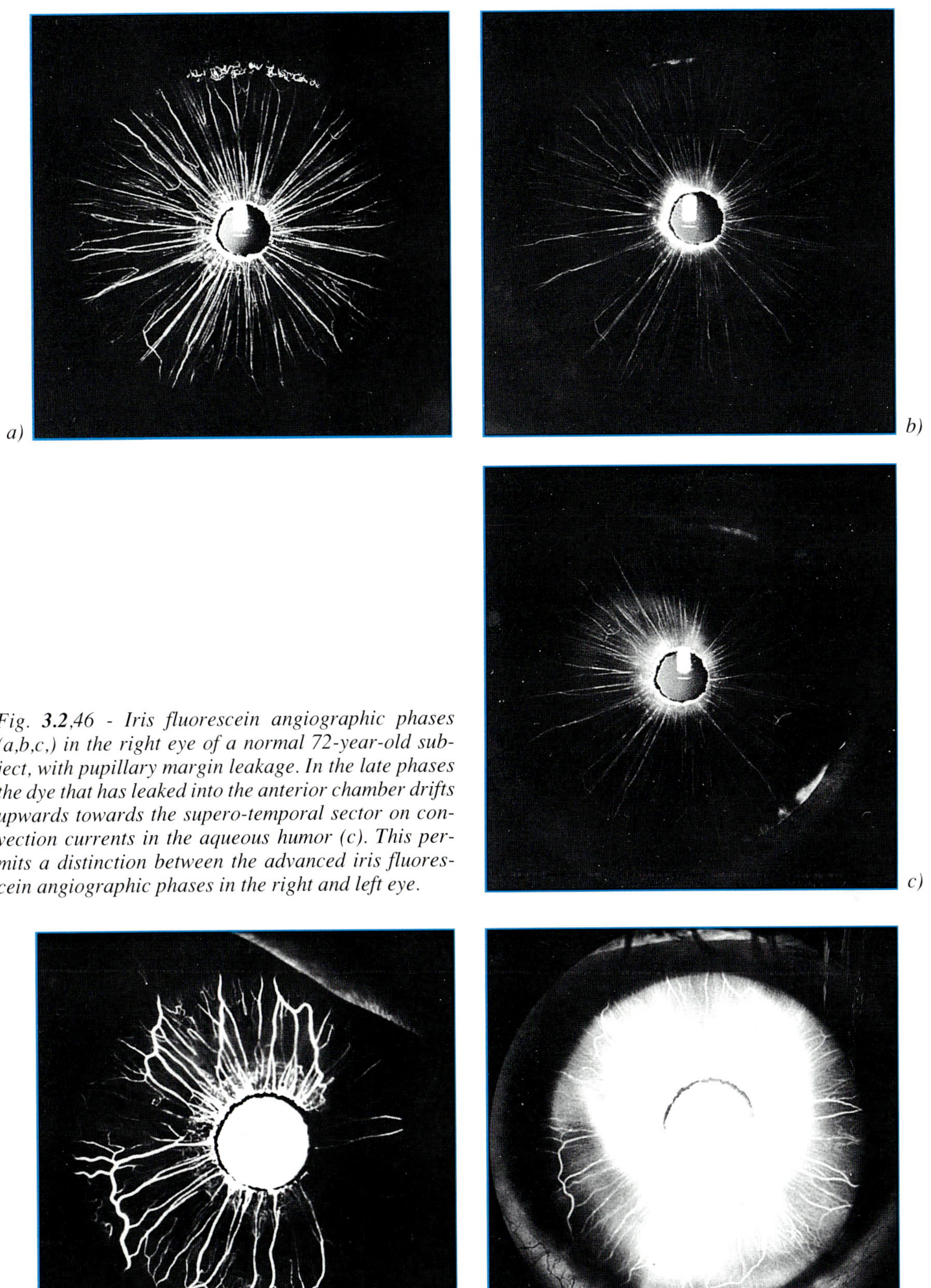

Fig. ***3.2****,46 - Iris fluorescein angiographic phases (a,b,c,) in the right eye of a normal 72-year-old subject, with pupillary margin leakage. In the late phases the dye that has leaked into the anterior chamber drifts upwards towards the supero-temporal sector on convection currents in the aqueous humor (c). This permits a distinction between the advanced iris fluorescein angiographic phases in the right and left eye.*

Fig. ***3.2****,47 - Early (a) and late (b) phases of iris fluorescein angiography in a right eye of a 70-year-old subject. In the early phase filling defects can be seen in the nasal sector, with peripupillary hyperfluorescent spots. In the next phase massive hyperfluorescence makes it impossible to assess any abnormalities. As there are no intermediate phases there is no way of assessing where the blood-iris barrier is ruptured. The intensity of the hyperfluorescence leads one to assume that it is more than just the normal age-related pupillary margin leakage, and that radial vessels are involved too.*

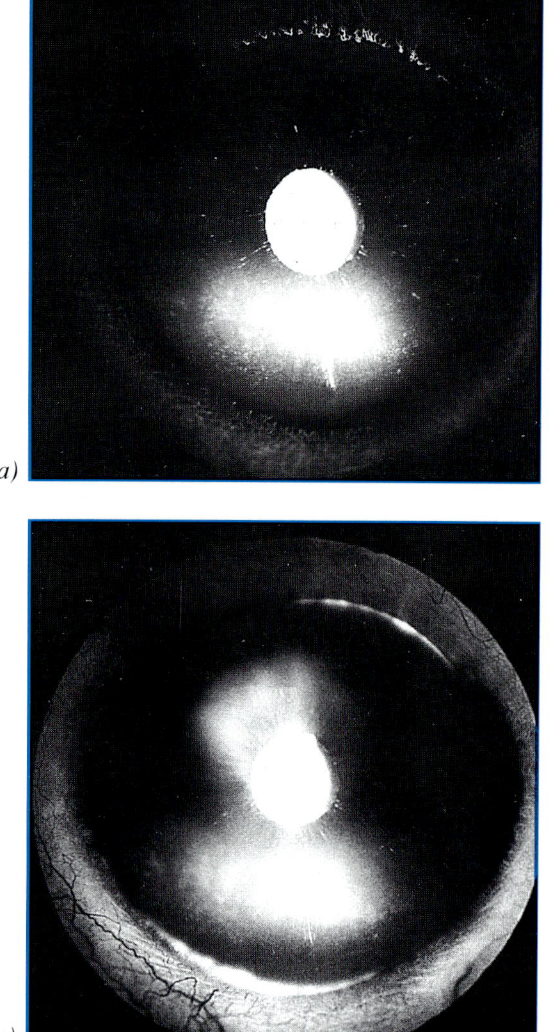

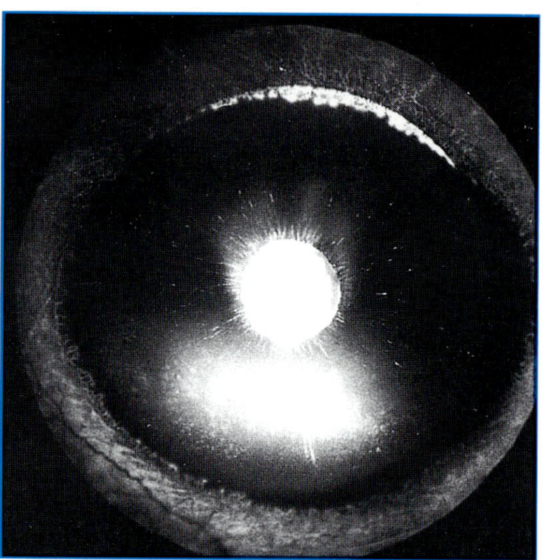

a) b)

c)

*Fig. **3.2**,48 - Iris fluorescein angiographic phases (a,b,c) in a normal 63-year-old subject with a dark iris. Peripupillary fluorescence visible in the intermediate phase (b) and more marked later (c) is the result of physiological age-related dye leakage from the pupillary margin. The hyperfluorescence dominating the lower sectors of the iris from the early phase (a) and right through the later ones (b,c) is a photographic artefact resulting from corneal impregnation with fluorescein after applanation tonometry.*

R. Brancato, F. Bandello, R. Lattanzio
Atlas of Iris
Fluorescein Angiography
Kugler & Ghedini Publications 1995

Section four

The abnormal iris fluorescein angiography

- Developmental diseases
- Degenerative diseases
- Abnormal vessel patterns
- Diabetic microangiopathy
- Retinal vessel occlusions
- Ocular ischemic syndrome
- Uveitis
- Glaucoma
- Surgical diseases
- Iris masses
- Traumas

R. Brancato, F. Bandello, R. Lattanzio
Atlas of Iris
Fluorescein Angiography
Kugler & Ghedini Publications 1995

Chapter 4.1

Developmental diseases

Abnormalities in development of the anterior segment of the eye and the uveal tract may originally affect only one particular structure, or the whole at the same time. Some of these abnormalities are inherited genetically while others are a result of the intrauterine conditions. Some iris abnormalities may be due to tissue hyperplasia or hypoplasia (tissue defects). They present various clinical pictures giving different signs and symptoms, and with different natural history and systemic associations.

Iris abnormalities include albinism, aniridia, coloboma, polycoria, pseudopolycoria, iridodiastasis, iris hypoplasia, microcoria, persistent pupillary membrane, corectopia, dyscoria, heterochromia, hyperplasia of the pigment epithelium, cysts, and Rieger's anomaly. The most frequently encountered forms are summarily described here.

Albinism

This term covers any congenital condition involving the absence of pigmentation in the skin, skin and eyes, or only in the eyes.(27) A clinical distinction is made between oculocutaneous albinism and partial albinism only involving the eyes.(10,18) Biochemically, albinism can be classified in relation to the function of the enzyme tyrosinase.(27)

In the oculocutaneous forms the subject has a subnormal amount of melanin in each melanosomes, and in the ocular forms there is a reduced number of melanosomes and type IV melanosomes are found in the iris.(35) These patients frequently present the following ocular signs and symptoms: foveal hypoplasia, reduced vision, nystagmus, iris transillumination, hypopigmentation of the fundus and photophobia.

The more severe forms of albinism are the result of recessive autosomal transmission, the milder ones are dominant autosomal. There is also an X-linked form(40) in which the mothers of affected males present alterations to the fundus(15) and a striking pigment pattern of the iris stroma.(33)

Albinism may be one of the signs of the Chediak-Higashi syndrome(2) and of the Hermansky-Pudlak syndrome.(48)

Iris fluorescein angiography of an albino iris gives a strikingly clear picture of the radial and peripupillary vascular network. There appear to be numerous radial vessels, especially in the upper portions of the iris (See Fig. **3.2**,6).(29)

Coloboma

Congenital colobomas may involve the iris, ciliary body, choroid and optic nerve, either together or separately. A coloboma is the result of incomplete fusion of the fetal cleft. Some atypical forms may be the consequence of persistence of vascular cords or circumscribed ectodermal defects.

Iris colobomas account for two % of congenital eye abnormalities and are generally bilateral. Typically, they arise in the inferonasal part (Figs. **4.1**,1,2). Histologically, the stroma is rounded and the pigment epithelium folded.[18] The defect may involve the whole section of the iris or only one layer.

Mullaney[38] proposed a classification system for colobomas related to the various associated pathologies (chromosomal defects, systemic abnormalities, phakomatosis, neural tube defects and oculo-renal abnormalities). Bateman[1] classified colobomatous microphthalmia from the genetic viewpoint, with a distinction between conditions inherited by Mendelian law (dominant or recessive autosomal) which only involve the eyes, forms manifesting pleiotropy involving other organs too (dominant autosomal, recessive or X-linked forms) and, third, forms involving chromosomal aberrations.

Uveal colobomas may be one of the abnormalities observed in certain syndromes such as the cat-eye syndrome (Schmid-Fraccaro), the Charge, Meckel-Gruber, Sjögren-Larsson and Lanz syndromes, and Jadassohn's linear sebaceous nevus syndrome.

Iris fluorescein angiography shows no morphological or functional abnormalities in the iris vessels in sectors unaffected by the coloboma (Figs. **4.1**,3-5).[4]

Aniridia

This term comprises a range of conditions involving iris hypoplasia resulting from abnormal growth of the cells of the neural crest.[47] Hereditary and sporadic cases have been reported. Histologically the iris is merely a stump and there is generally no smooth muscle.

Aniridia may be associated with angle, retinal and corneal anomalies, with low visual acuity, glaucoma and cataract.[6,9,12,17,19,22,23,25,31,32,34,39,45,46,50] In a quarter to one third of children with sporadic aniridia a Wilms' tumor appears before the age of three years.[14,17,42] A deletion of chromosome 11 was observed in these patients. Other systemic abnormalities include mental retardation, genito-urinary and craniofacial abnormalities, microcephaly, cerebellar ataxia, ptosis and obesity. Chromosomal deletions have been demonstrated for some of these associations too.[43]

Hittner[22] described the iris fluorescein angiography findings in nine patients from the same family, all with dominant autosomal aniridia. Their iris abnormalities ranged from thinning to full-blown coloboma but they all had sufficient iris tissue for angiographic study. The anomalies found were vascular loops that fluoresced early, and dye leakage from the pupillary margins.

Persistent pupillary membrane

The pupillary membrane may persist when involution of the anterior vascular tunic of the lens is incomplete. When the membrane is extensive there is assumed to have been some damage at the 24th week of gestation. There are reports of dominant autosomal transmission.[36]

The residual membrane is attached to the collarette and strands may float freely or through the pupil, inserting themselves either on the opposite side or on the anterior face of the lens (Figs. **4.1**,6,7). They are sometimes associated with cataract. Generally this malformation is not accompanied by marked visual impairment.

Residual pupillary membranes are normally seen in children and diminish with age, showing that involution of this membrane may happen even after birth.

The membrane residues are generally avascular. Iris fluorescein angiography, however, is essential to detect any vessels present among the strands of residual membrane.[11,28,44] In certain cases hyperfluorescence may even be seen in the later phases as dye spreads from the ectopic vessels.[11] This leakage is not normally profuse, and is only segmental along the vessel's path. It can be assumed from this pattern of leakage that the endothelium is not actually permeable to the dye but that in some cases there is partial loss of its barrier function.[29] Wigger[52] suggested that this might be a consequence of vascular distension because of the attachment to the lens, but in other cases[44] leakage was still found in non-adhering strands.

Idiopathic congenital microcoria

This unilateral abnormality involves marked or total obliteration of the pupil and is probably caused by anomalies in the development of the fetal pupillary membrane. Since the condition involves amblyopia and a high risk of glaucoma surgery is indicated, with prompt occlusive therapy.[30]

Congenital iris cysts

These cysts are the result of fluid accumulating inside iris cavities lined on the inside with stratified squamous epithelium or neuroepithelium. The first type form in the stroma[20] and the second at or behind the pupillary margin. Surgery may be necessary if the cyst is large or sited in such a way as to interfere with vision.

Brushfield spots

These spots around the pupillary margin are frequent in pale irises. They are seen in 85% of patients with trisomy 21.[5] Histologically they appear as hypercellular areas of iris tissue surrounded by stromal hypoplasia.

Iris heterochromia

Heterochromia, meaning irises of different colours in the two eyes, may be congenital or acquired. Congenital forms of heterochromia, with the affected eye darker than the other, may be the result of ocular melanocytosis, oculodermal melanocytosis or sectorial iris hamartoma.[24] Horner's congenital syndrome and Waardenburg's syndrome both involve congenital heterochromia but in these cases the paler eye is the affected one (hypopigmentation).

Acquired heterochromia may be the result of various causes: nevi, tumors, metastasis, siderosis, foreign bodies, long-standing or relapsing hyphema, Fuchs iridocyclitis, juvenile xanthogranuloma, Horner's acquired syndrome, and others.

Rieger's anomaly

This is one of the primary iris developmental abnormalities.[13] It is inherited by dominant autosomal transmission, varying in expression - there may be occasional sporadic forms or new mutations.[21] The anomaly consists of hypoplasia of the anterior iris stroma which makes the iris look flat and featureless (sometimes with coloboma); irido-trabecular bridges to Schwalbe's line, corneal opacity, posterior keratoconus, posterior embryotoxon, pupillary abnormalities, ectropion uveae, lens alterations, anomalies of the optic disc, and high myopia; 60 % of cases present glaucoma.[7,13,21]

When Rieger's anomaly is associated with somatic alterations such as facial and dental abnormalities, hernia and hypospadias, it is known as Rieger's syndrome.

To complete this overview of iris abnormalities, we must mention those arising in the course of primary corneal developmental abnormalities.[13] These may include atrophy of the iris stroma and iridodonesis with megalocornea, mesenchymal dysgenesis of the iris in Peter's anomaly, and bridges of iris tissue crossing the angle to Schwalbe's ring in Axenfeld's anomaly.[51,26]

References

1 Bateman JB: Microphthalmos. Int Ophthalmol Clin 24: 87, 1984.

2 Bedoya V, Grimley PH, Dugue O: Chediak-Higashi syndrome. Arch Pathol 88: 340, 1969.

3 Bernsmeier H, Kluxen G, Weber U: Irisangiographie und Endothelmikroskopie bei Dysgenesis mesodermalis iridis et corneae. Klin Monatsbl Augenheilkd 183: 128, 1983.

4 Brancato R, Menchini U, Carnevalini A: Atlante di Iridografia a fluorescenza. C.I.C. Ed Int Gruppo Ed Medico, Roma, 1981.

5 Brushfield T: Mongolism. Br J Child Dis 21: 241, 1924.

6 Callahan A: Aniridia with ectopia lentis and secondary glaucoma, genetic, pathologic, and surgical consideration. Am J Ophthalmol 32: 28, 1949.

7 Chisholm IA, Chudley AE: Autosomal dominant iridogoniodysgenesis with associated somatic anomalies: four generation family with Rieger's syndrome. Br J Ophthalmol 67: 529, 1983.

8 Cohen SM, Nelson LB: Aniridia with congenital ptosis and glaucoma: a family study. Ann Ophthalmol 20: 53, 1988.

9 David R, MacBeath L, Jenkins T: Aniridia associated with microcornea and subluxated lenses. Br J Ophthalmol 62: 118, 1978.

10 Day S: Uveal tract. In Taylor D: Pediatric Ophthalmology. Blackwell Scientific Publications, London-Boston, 1990.

11 Demeler U: Irisangiographie bei der Membrana pupillaris persistens. Ophthalmologica (Basel) 177: 270, 1978.

12 Elsas TJ, Maumenee IH, Kenyon KR et al: Familial aniridia with preserved ocular function. Am J Ophthalmol 83: 718, 1977.

13 Elston J: Developmental abnormalities of the cornea and iris. In Taylor D: Pediatric Ophthalmology. Blackwell Scientific Publications, London-Boston, 1990.

14 Flanagan JC, DiGeorge AM: Sporadic aniridia and Wilms' tumour. Am J Ophthalmol 67: 558, 1969.

15 Forsius H, Eriksson AW: Ein neues augensyndrom mit x-chromosomaler transmission. Eine sippe mit fundus-albinismus, fovea hypoplasie, nistagmus, myopie, astigmatismus und dyschromatopsie. Klin Monatsbl Augenheilkd 144: 447, 1964.

16 François J, Verschragen-Spae MR, De Sutter E: The aniridia-Wilms' tumour syndrome and other associations of aniridia. Ophthalmol Paediatr Genet 1: 125, 1982.

17 Grant WM, Walton DS: Progressive changes in the angle in congenital aniridia, with development of glaucoma. Am J Ophthalmol 18: 842, 1974.

18 Green WR: Uveal tract. In Spencer WH: Ophthalmic pathology. An atlas and textbook. Saunders WB, Philadelphia, 1986.

19 Grove JH, Shaw MW, Bourgue G: A family study of aniridia. Arch Ophthalmol 65: 81, 1961.

20 Grutzmacher R, Lindquist T, Chittum M et al: Congenital iris cysts. Br J Ophthalmol 71: 227, 1987.

21 Henkind P, Siegel IM, Carr RE: Mesodermal dysgenesis of the anterior segment: Rieger's anomaly. Arch Ophthalmol 73: 810, 1965.

22 Hittner HM, Riccardi VM, Ferrell RE et al: Variable expressivity in autosomal dominant aniridia by clinical electrophysiologic and angiographic criteria. Am J Ophthalmol 89: 531, 1980.

23 Hittner HM, Kretzer FL, Antoszyk JM et al: Variable expressivity of autosomal dominant anterior segment mesenchymal dysgenesis in six generations. Am J Ophthalmol 93: 57, 1982.

24 Jakobiec FA, Howard GM, Devoe AG: Sector hamartoma of the iris. Arch Ophthalmol 93: 614, 1975.

25 Jesberg DO: Aniridia with retinal lipid deposits. Arch Ophthalmol 68: 331, 1962.

26 Kenyon KR: Mesenchymal dysgenesis in Peter's anomaly, sclerocornea and congenital endothelial dystrophy. Exp Eye Res 21: 125, 1975.

27 Kinnear PE, Jay B, Witkop CJ: Albinism. Review. Surv Ophthalmol 30: 75, 1985.

28 Kluxen G: Pupillarmembranfäden in Irisangiographie und Scheimpflug-Photographie. Fortschr Ophthalmol 83: 242, 1986.

29 Kottow MH: Anterior segment fluorescein angiography. Williams & Wilkins, Baltimore, 1978.

30 Lambert SR, Amaya L, Taylor D: Congenital idiopathic microcoria. Am J Ophthalmol 106: 590, 1988.

31 Layman PR, Anderson DR, Flynn JT: Frequent occurrence of hypoplastic optic discs in patients with aniridia. Am J Ophthalmol 77: 573, 1974.

32 Mackman G, Brightbell FS, Opitz JM: Corneal changes in aniridia. Am J Ophthalmol 87: 497, 1979.

33 Maguire AM, Maumenee IH: Iris pigment mosaicism in carriers of X-linked ocular albinism cum pigmento. Am J Ophthalmol 3: 298, 1989.

34 Margo CE: Congenital aniridia: a histopathologic study of the anterior segment in children. J Pediatric Ophthalmol Strabismus 20: 192, 1983.

35 McCartney ACE, Spalton DJ, Bull TB: Type IV melanosomes of the human albino iris. Br J Ophthalmol 69: 537, 1985.

36 Merin S, Crawford JS, Cardarelli J: Hyperplastic persistent pupillary membrane. Am J Ophthalmol 72: 717, 1971.

37 Mullaney J: The anterior chamber cleavage syndrome. Trans Ophthalmol Soc UK 88: 757, 1968.

38 Mullaney J: Curious Colobomata. The Montgomery Lecture 1977. Trans Ophthalmol Soc UK 97: 517, 1977.

39 Nelson LB, Spaeth GL, Nowinski TS et al: Aniridia. A review. Surv Ophthalmol 28: 621, 1984.

40 O'Donnel FE, Green WR, Fleishman JA et al: X-linked ocular albinism in blacks. Ocular albinism cum pigmento. Arch Ophthalmol 96: 1189, 1978.

41 Pearce WG, Kerr CB: Inherited variation in Rieger's malformation. Br J Ophthalmol 49: 503, 1965.

42 Pilling GP: Wilms' tumour in 7 children with congenital aniridia. Pediatr Surg 10: 87, 1975.

43 Riccardi VM, Borges W: Aniridia, cataracts, and Wilms' tumour. Am J Ophthalmol 86: 577, 1978.

44 Rieger G: Zur fluoreszenzangiographischen Darstellung der Gefässe in der Membrana pupillaris persistens. Klin Monatsbl Augenheilkd 165: 483, 1974.

45 Shaffer RN, Cohen JS: Visual reduction in aniridia. J Pediatric Ophthalmol Strabismus 12: 220, 1975.

46 Shaw MW, Falls HF, Neel JV: Congenital aniridia. Am J Hum Genet 12: 389, 1960.

47 Spaeth G, Nelson LB, Beaudoin AR: Ocular teratology. In Jakobiec FA: Ocular Anatomy, Embryology, and Teratology. Harper & Row, Philadelphia, 1982.

48 Summers CG, Knobloch WH, Witkop CJ et al: Hermansky-Pudlak Syndrome: ophthalmic findings. Am J Ophthalmol 95: 545, 1988.

49 Taylor D: Pediatric Ophthalmology. Blackwell Scientific Publications, London-Boston, 1990.

50 Walton DS: Aniridia with glaucoma. In Chandler PA, Grant WM: Glaucoma. Lea & Feiberger, Philadelphia, 1979.

51 Waring GO, Rodrigues MM, Laibson PR: Anterior segment cleavage syndrome: a stepladder classification. Surv Ophthalmol 20: 3, 1975.

52 Wigger H, Friedburg D, Schultheiss A: Irisangiographische Darstellung von Gefässen in der Membrana pupillaris persistens. Klin Monatsbl Augenheilkd 163: 351, 1973.

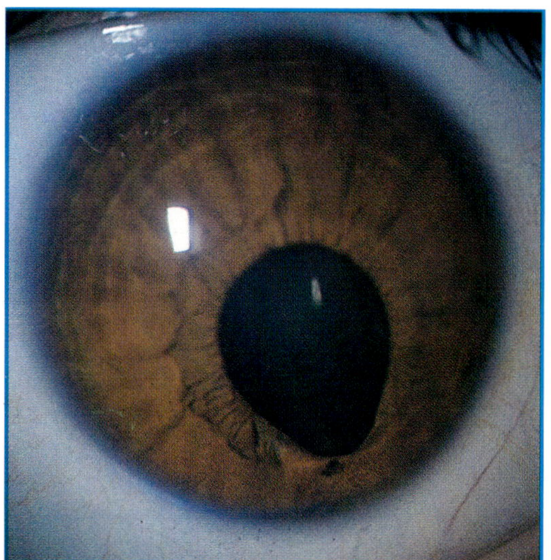

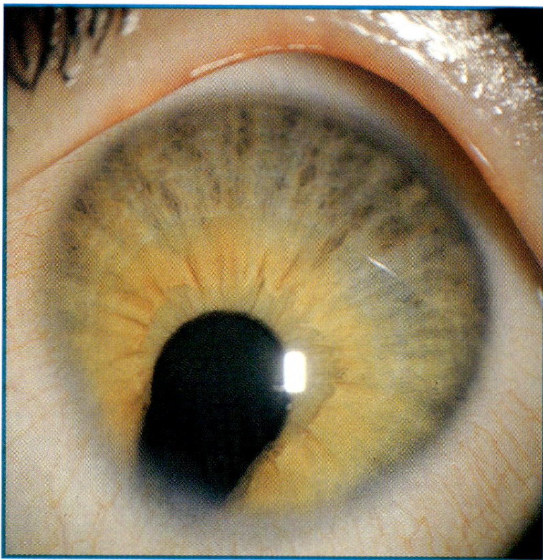

*Figs **4.1**,1,2 - Congenital colobomas of the iris in a right eye (Fig. **4.1**,1) and a left eye (Fig. **4.1**,2): biomicroscopic findings. These defects are typically found in the inferonasal segment.*

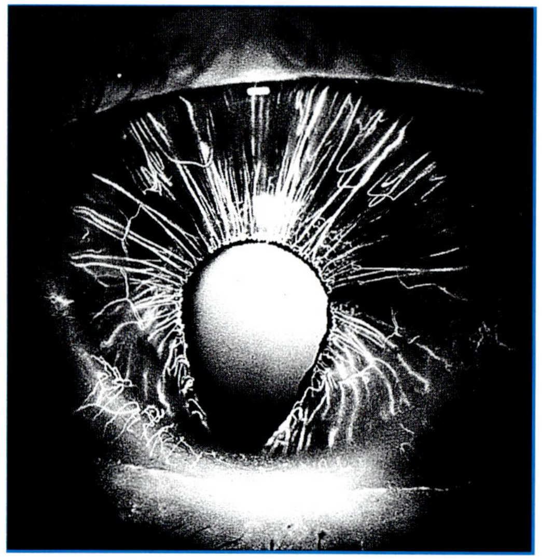

a)

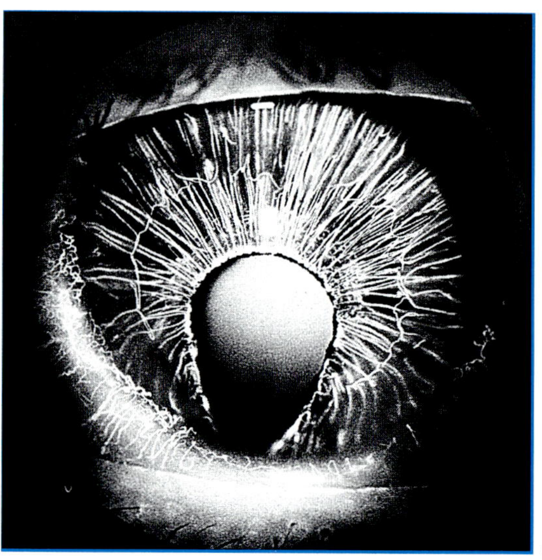

b)

*Fig. **4.1**,3 - Congenital coloboma in a pale iris: early (a) and late (b) iris fluorescein angiographic phases. The radial vascular network in the parts of the iris not affected by the coloboma shows no morphological abnormalities. There is slight dye leakage from the pupillary margin.*

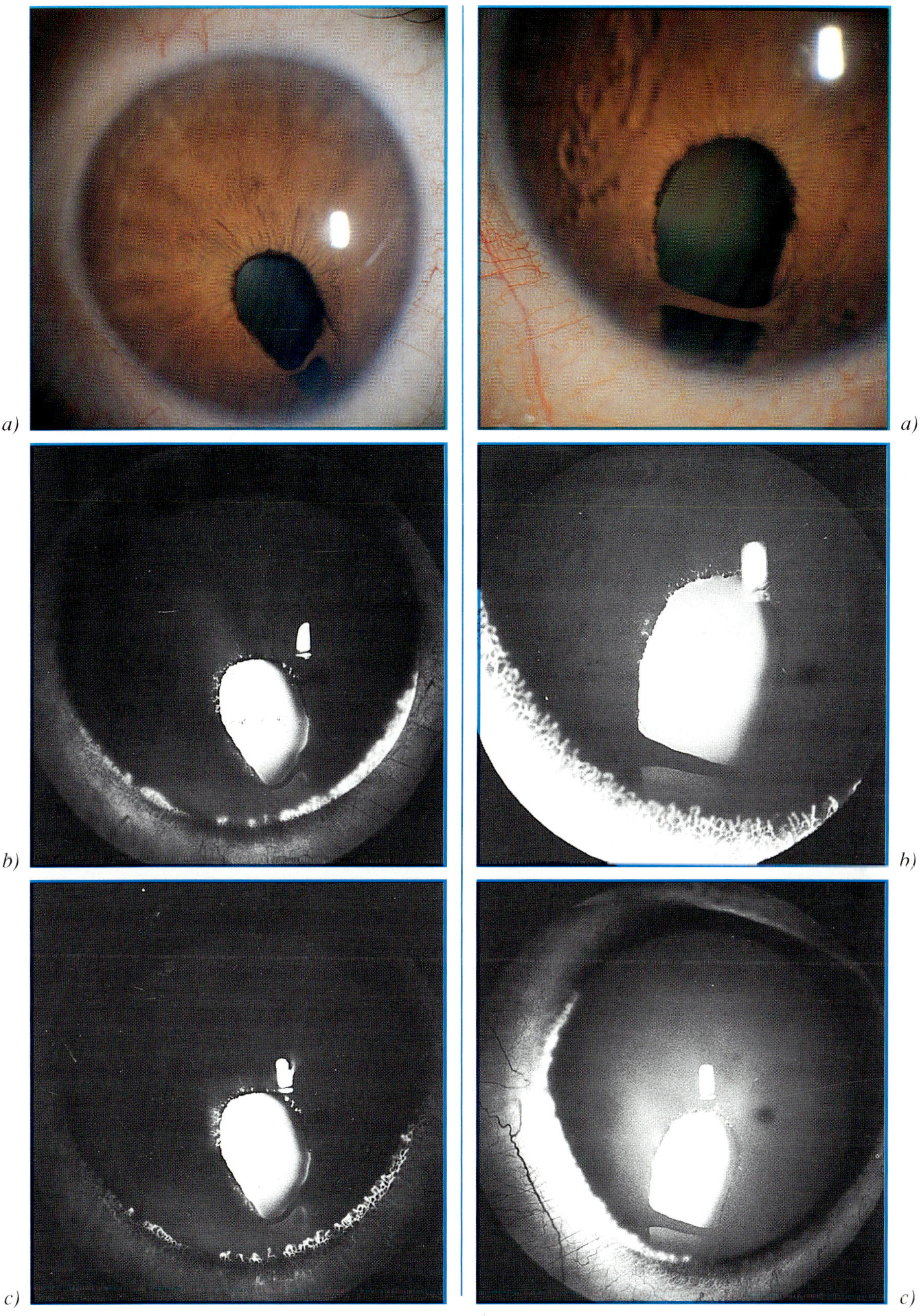

*Figs **4.1**,4,5 - Biomicroscopy (a) and early (b) and late (c) iris fluorescein angiographic phases in a subject with bilateral iris colobomas. The defect is located inferonasally in both eyes (right, Fig. **4.1**,4; left, Fig. **4.1**,5). The pigment of the iris impedes angiographic visualization of the vascular network. The only angiographic abnormality is slight dye leakage from the upper part of the pupillary margin (b), increasing somewhat in the later phase (c).*

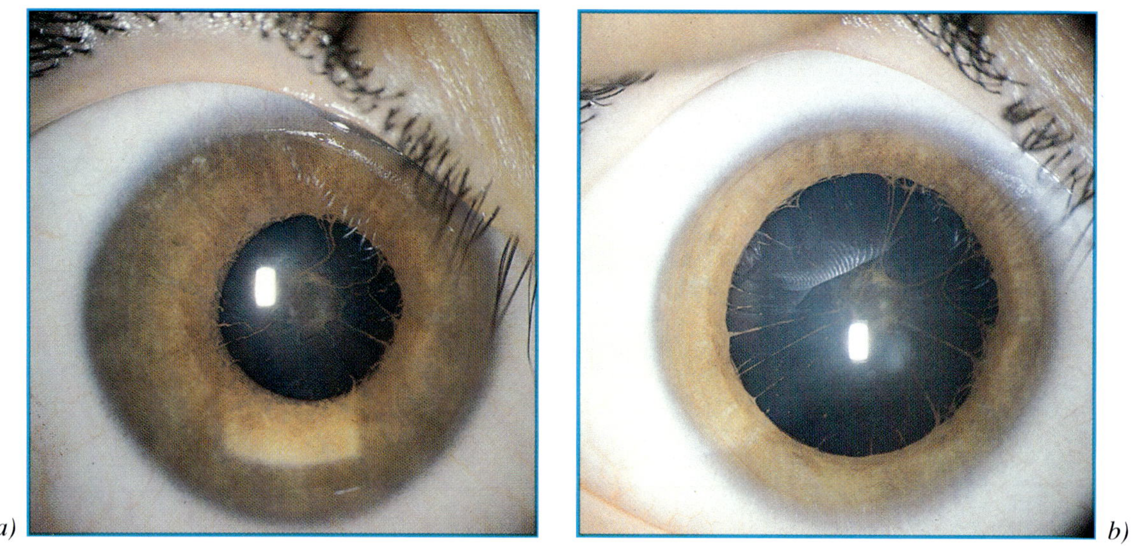

*Fig. **4.1**,6 - Persistent pupillary membrane in miosis (a) and mydriasis (b): biomicroscopic findings. The residues cross the pupillary field and attach on the opposite side of the iris.*

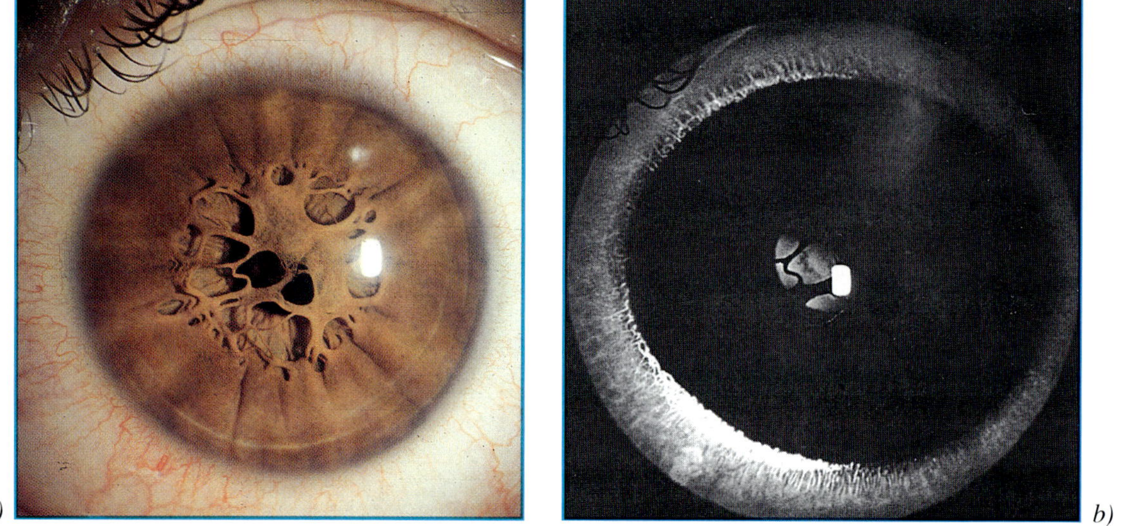

*Fig. **4.1**,7 - Biomicroscopy (a) in a case with heavy residual pupillary membrane covering much of the pupillary foramen. Iris fluorescein angiography (b) shows no vascular strands within the membrane itself.*

R. Brancato, F. Bandello, R. Lattanzio
Atlas of Iris
Fluorescein Angiography
Kugler & Ghedini Publications 1995

Chapter 4.2

Degenerative diseases

These diseases may be *involutive*, such as senile atrophy, or *secondary* to other diseases, such as post-inflammatory or post-traumatic atrophy, or *primary* or idiopathic, like progressive essential atrophy.[28]

Senile atrophy

Senile atrophy is marked by thinning of all the iris tissue as the stroma becomes finer and there is progressive pigment loss. The sphincter becomes almost transparent. Retroillumination shows loss of oval and radial substance in the epithelium.

In some cases atrophy may be due to vascular sclerosis and hyaline degeneration of the connective tissue. The iris then becomes more rigid and pupillary reactions are reduced.[28]

Secondary atrophy

These may be acquired degenerative processes following on the heels of other diseases (Figs. **4.2**,1-5). Post-inflammatory iris atrophy may follow inflammation of the anterior uveal tract alone or other ocular structures too (see chapter on Uveitis).

Post-traumatic atrophy resulting from contusion is probably secondary to transient acute ischemia at the time of the trauma. Generally in these cases atrophy only affects one sector of the iris; it is more marked than other forms, with greater alterations to the pigmentation, following chronic inflammation or iridodialysis. Total aniridia may be the response to perforating trauma or rupture of the globe. Gonioscopic examination in such cases shows no iris residues in front of the ciliary body, and this is the feature that differentiates it from certain forms of congenital aniridia in which portions of the iris can be seen at the angle.

Post-ischemic atrophy may result after surgery (for example on the extrinsic muscles) and is secondary to section of the anterior ciliary arteries (see chapter on Surgical Diseases).

Post-glaucomatous atrophy may follow an acute episode, in which case the pupil remains in mid-mydriasis and no longer reacts to light stimuli (see chapter on Glaucoma).

Neurogenic atrophy of the iris involving the pupillary part may be seen in neurosyphilis on account of lesions to the ciliary ganglion.

The areas of iris atrophy described in sickle-cell anemia[1,9,15] are probably the result of vascular occlusions. Iris fluorescein angiography shows in fact that these atrophic areas are not perfused, the dye leaking at their edges.[1]

A case of progressive iris necrosis of both eyes was described in a patient with retinochoroidal degeneration,[27] and its features were so unusual that nosological classification was difficult.

Primary or idiopathic atrophy

Progressive essential atrophy of the iris was first described in 1903[16] and today it is considered one of the manifestations of the *irido-corneal-endothelial syndrome*. This term, proposed by Yanoff[46] and subsequently employed by others, covers a single pathological process comprising not only essential atrophy of the iris but also Chandler's and Cogan-Reese syndromes.

In clinical practice it may be useful to consider these as three distinct entities but they are in fact the main clinical manifestations of a single disease. A patient may either gradually pass from one form to the other of the irido-corneal-endothelial syndrome, or else the clinical features may all overlap at the same time, making it difficult to distinguish them clearly.

The three clinical characteristics common to the irido-corneal-endothelial syndrome are:
1) anomalies of the posterior aspect of the cornea, leading to corneal edema;
2) peripheral anterior synechia leading to often intractable secondary glaucoma;
3) iris anomalies.[40,41]

The corneal anomalies, characteristic of Chandler's syndrome, are not easy to distinguish clinically in essential atrophy of the iris or in the Cogan-Reese syndrome, but are always visible with the specular microscope.[40,41]

The primary lesion in the irido-corneal-endothelial syndrome is anarchic proliferation of endothelial cells migrating to adjacent structures like the trabecular meshwork or the anterior surface of the iris.[3,21]

Embryogenetically the endothelium, the corneal stroma and the iris stroma all originate from the mesodermal wedge, situated between the edge of the optic cup and the ectodermal surface, along the planes formed by mesostromal membranes. Endothelial colonization of the anterior face of the iris is followed by contraction of these abnormal structures, and deposition of an ectopic Descemet membrane. Peripheral anterior synechiae may then form, closing the angle and leading to secondary glaucoma, with ectropion uveae, distortions or ectopia of the pupil and abnormalities of the iris.

These iris abnormalities may vary widely in type and severity. There is almost always atrophy of the iris stroma, involving a single or several areas, or diffuse. There may also be some slight stretching and thinning of the stroma with enlargement or spindle-shaped deformations of the crypts, sometimes giving rise to real lacunae with the underlying pigment epithelium exposed, and transillumination. In some cases the pigment epithelium may be absent. On microscopic examination the iris atrophic areas show a sudden and striking demarcation from the relatively normal-appearing iris root.[39]

Advanced cases present holes in the iris - referred to variously as perforating holes, through-and-through holes, full-thickness holes or pseudopupillae - generally surrounded by thinned stroma (Fig. **4.2**,6). The atrophy and the holes typically develop in iris sectors on the opposite side from the ectopic pupil.

In some long-standing cases the iris may also contain fine pigmented pedunculated nodules, occasionally associated with flattening and loss of detail of the underlying iris stroma.[40] These nodules become more numerous and darker with time.[6]

These iris abnormalities vary in the different manifestations of the irido-corneal-endothelial syndrome: Chandler's syndrome usually involves only modest atrophy; holes are typical of essential atrophy of the iris[6,45] and are not seen in the Cogan-Reese syndrome. Also known as the Iris Nevus syndrome, this latter is characterized by numerous pigmented iris nodules made up of cells similar to those of nevi, or of true nevi on the anterior surface of the iris. This syndrome also involves ectropion uveae, peripheral anterior synechiae, frequently associated with defects of the adjacent stroma, and secondary glaucoma.

Several signs permit a differential diagnosis of the irido-corneal-endothelial syndrome and other degenerative abnormalities of the iris and cornea[24]:
a) no family history;
b) predominance in females;
c) onset in adult age;
d) unilaterality;
e) iridocorneal synechiae;
f) involvement of the iris stroma;
g) increased intraocular pressure.

Iris fluorescein angiographic examination in the irido-corneal-endothelial syndrome has given conflicting results.[19,20,22,37,38,40,41,45] It must be borne in mind that these patients present introcular hypertension or have already undergone medical or surgical treatment, and that this may affect the angiographic findings.

The following abnormalities have been reported: areas of iris hypoperfusion; peripupillary leakage and capillary dilatation similar to neovascularization.[19] This confirms the existence of hypoxia but does not cast any light on whether these are primary, secondary, concomitant or accidental processes.[22] However, similar abnormalities have been described in uncomplicated cases of glaucoma.[19] Other abnormal findings include sectorial filling defects and leakage from the remaining iris vessels.[37,45] Some investigators, however, report finding a well-preserved vascular system, despite marked iris atrophy, with minimal or no vascular leakage.

Shields[40,41] described two types of holes, giving different iris fluorescein angiographic patterns, in essential atrophy of the iris: "stretching holes" and "melting holes". In the first, iris fluorescein angiography found no associated vascular abnormalities, but around the melting holes ischemic areas were reported, with vessels at their periphery from which dye did leak. The existence of two types of atrophy might explain the different iris fluorescein angiographic findings reported (Fig. **4.2**,7).

Iridoschisis

This is a rare degenerative disease affecting males and females in equal measure, usually after the age of 60. It may be uni- or bilateral and no hereditary factors are known.[28] The term is taken to mean a cleavage of the iris leaflets originating from the mesoderm.[12] The cleavage is localized in the iris stroma which separates into two layers; the posterior layer remains attached to the pigment layer, while the anterior one atrophies or degenerates into disconnected fibers which float in the aqueous humor or stick to the corneal endothelium. The pupil remains central and its reactions are preserved.

Clinically, the alterations usually affect the lower sectors of the iris, subsequently extending to the whole iris. With time the remains of the posterior layer of the stroma become detached and the epithelial layer is exposed, with the sphincter. At the outset, however, in all cases, histological examination shows a thick stromal layer remaining on the epithelium. The chamber angle is normally narrow but only about half the cases present glaucoma, and it is not clear whether this is linked to the degenerative disease.

The pathogenesis of iridoschisis is still not clear, and there are many theories. Some hold that it is related to increases in intraocular pressure, or to the presence of post-inflammatory synechiae, or to mechanical factors secondary to trauma. There is also a vascular theory according to which progressive obliteration of the vessels leads to tissue malnutrition with secondary atrophy.[2,23,26] Vascular occlusion might also explain why no hemorrhages occur in iridoschisis even when there is gross damage to the iris stroma. The vascular hypothesis is borne out by the histological findings of disintegrated, occluded or hyalinized vessels, and the fact that iris fluorescein angiography shows anomalous radial vessels, straightened but with an irregular path, and perfusion defects.

Once again, though, the eyes described in published reports[22,42] were all complicated by glaucoma or anterior synechiae, or had already undergone medical or surgical therapy, so that interpretation of the angiographic findings becomes difficult. There was one study in which iris fluorescein angiography showed no vascular abnormalities in a case of iridoschisis.[8] However, the sole common feature of all cases examined to date is simply that the detachment of the leaflets makes it easier to see the stromal vessels around the cleavage.

References

1 Acheson RW, Ford SM, Maude GH et al: Iris atrophy in sickle cell disease. Br J Ophthalmol 70: 516, 1986.

2 Alber EC, Klien BA: Iridoschisis: a clinical and histopathologic study. Am J Ophthalmol 46: 794, 1958.

3 Alvarado JA, Murphy CG, Maglio M et al: Pathogenesis of Chandler's Syndrome, essential iris atrophy and the Cogan-Reese Syndrome. Invest Ophthalmol Vis Sci 27: 853, 1986.

4 Bouchat J, André J, Conrad J: Étude fluoro-angiographique d'un cas d'atrophie essentielle de l'iris. Bull Soc Ophtalmol Fr 70: 854, 1970.

5 Brancato R, Menchini U, Carnevalini A: Atlante di iridografia a fluorescenzà. C.I.C. Ed Int Gruppo Ed Medico, Roma, 1981.

6 Buxton JN, Lash RS: Results of penetrating keratoplasty in the iridocorneal endothelial syndrome. Am J Ophthalmol 98: 297, 1984.

7 Campbell DG, Shields MB, Smith TR: The corneal endothelium and the spectrum of essential iris atrophy. Am J Ophthalmol 86: 317, 1978.

8 Carnevalini A, Menchini U, Bandello F et al: Aspects fluoroiridographiques de l'iridoschisis. J Fr Ophtalmol 11: 329, 1988.

9 Chambers J, Puglisi J, Kernitsky R et al: Iris atrophy in hemoglobin SC disease. Am J Ophthalmol 77: 247, 1974.

10 Chandler PA: Atrophy of the stroma of the iris: endothelial dystrophy, corneal edema, and glaucoma. Am J Ophthalmol 41: 607, 1956.

11 Dollfus MA: Dégénérescence irienne d'un type particulier. Bull Soc Ophtalmol Fr: 170, 1927.

12 Duke-Elder S: Iridoschisis. In: System of Ophthalmology. IX. Diseases of the uvea. Kimpton Ed, London, 1966.

13 Eagle RC Jr, Font RL, Yanoff M et al: Proliferative endotheliopathy with iris abnormalities. The iridocorneal endothelial syndrome. Arch Ophthalmol 97: 2104, 1979.

14 Feingold M: Essential atrophy of the iris. Am J Ophthalmol 1: 1, 1918.

15 Galinos S, Rabb MF, Goldberg MF et al: Hemoglobin SC disease and iris atrophy. Am J Ophthalmol 75: 421, 1973.

16 Harms C: Eiseitige spontane Lukenbildun ber Iris durch Atrophic ohne mechanische Zerrung. Klin Monatsbl Augenheilkd 41: 522, 1903.

17 Hetherington J: The spectrum of Chandler's syndrome. Trans Am Acad Ophthalmol Otolaryngol 85: 240, 1978.

18 Hirst LW, Quigley HA, Stark WJ et al: Specular microscopy of iridocorneal endothelial syndrome. Am J Ophthalmol 89: 11, 1980.

19 Jampol LM, Rosser MJ, Sears ML: Unusual aspects of essential progressive iris atrophy. Am J Ophthalmol 77: 353, 1974.

20 Kaiser-Kupfer M, Kuwabara T, Kupfer C: Progressive bilateral essential iris atrophy. Am J Ophthalmol 83: 340, 1977.

21 Kidd M, Hetherington J, Magee S: Surgical results in iridocorneal endothelial syndrome. Arch Ophthalmol 106: 199, 1988.

22 Kottow MH: Anterior segment fluorescein angiography. Williams & Wilkins, Baltimore, 1978.

23 Krohn DL, Garret EE: Iridoschisis et keratoconus. Report of a case in a twenty years old man. Arch Ophthalmol 52: 426, 1954.

24 Lefrancois A: Dégénérescences de l'iris et du corps ciliaire. Une variété d'atrophie essentielle de l'iris: le syndrome de Chandler. Encycl Méd Chir Paris Ophtalmol 1-21225 D-10, 9, 1980.

25 Lichter PR: The spectrum of Chandler's syndrome: an often overlooked cause of unilateral glaucoma. Trans Am Acad Ophthalmol Otolaryngol 85: 245, 1978.

26 Loewenstein A, Foster J: Iridoschisis with multiple rupture of the stromal treads. Br J Ophthalmol 29: 277, 1945.

27 Margo CE, Friedman SM, Purdy EP et al: Retinochoroidal degeneration associated with progressive iris necrosis. Arch Ophthalmol 108: 989, 1990.

28 Martenet AC: Dégénérescences de l'iris et du corps ciliaire. Encycl Méd Chir Paris Ophtalmol, 21225 D-10, 12, 1979.

29 Maselli E, Avanza C: Considerazioni su alcuni casi di iridoschisi. Ann Ottalmol Clin Ocul 88: 683, 1962.

30 McCulloch C: Iridoschisis as a cause of glaucoma. Am J Ophthalmol 33: 1398, 1950.

31 Mills PV: Iridoschisis. Br J Ophthalmol 51: 158, 1967.

32 Patel A, Kenyon KR, Hirst LW et al: Clinicopathologic features of Chandler's syndrome. Surv Ophthalmol 27: 327, 1983.

33 Portis JM, Stamper RL, Spencer WH et al: The corneal endothelium and Descemet's membrane in the iridocorneal endothelial syndrome. Trans Am Ophthalmol Soc 83: 316, 1985.

34 Recupero SM, Lesnoni La Parola G, Sampalmieri M et al: Iridoschisi senile. Clin Ocul 6: 486, 1984.

35 Redi F, Ragnetti E: Studio di un caso di iridoschisi con corredo istologico. Ann Ottalmol Clin Ocul 86: 147, 1960.

36 Rodrigues MM, Spaeth GL, Krachmer JH et al: Iridoschisis associated with glaucoma and bullous keratopathy. Am J Ophthalmol 95: 73, 1983.

37 Rodrigues MM, Streeten BW, Spaeth GL: Chandler's syndrome as a variant of essential iris atrophy. Arch Ophthalmol 96: 643, 1978.

38 Sautter H, Demeler U: Ein Beitrag zur Klinik, Fluoreszenzangiographie und Histologie der essentiellen progressiven Irisatrophie. Klin Monatsbl Augenheilkd 170: 592, 1977.

39 Scheie HG, Yanoff M, Kellogg WT: Essential iris atrophy. Report of a case. Arch Ophthalmol 94: 1315, 1976.

40 Shields MB: Progressive essential iris atrophy. Chandler's syndrome, and the iris nevus (Cogan Reese) syndrome: a spectrum of disease. Surv Ophthalmol 24: 3, 1979.

41 Shields MB, Campbell DG, Simmons RJ: The essential iris atrophies. Am J Ophthalmol 85: 749, 1978.

42 Vannas A: Fluorescein angiography of the vessels of the iris in pseudoexfoliation of the lens capsule, capsular glaucoma and some other forms of glaucoma. Acta Ophthalmol 105 (Suppl): 1, 1969.

43 Vogt A: Detached anterior iris plate as a senile change. Klin Monatsbl Augenheilkd 77: 710, 1926.

44 Wistanley J: Iris atrophy in primary glaucoma. Trans Ophthalmol Soc UK 81: 23, 1963.

45 Wittebol-Post D, van Bijsterveld OP: Essential progressive iris atrophy. Report of two cases. Ophthalmologica (Basel) 178: 303, 1979.

46 Yanoff M: Iridocorneal endothelial syndrome. Unification of a disease. Editorial. Surv Ophthalmol 24: 1, 1979.

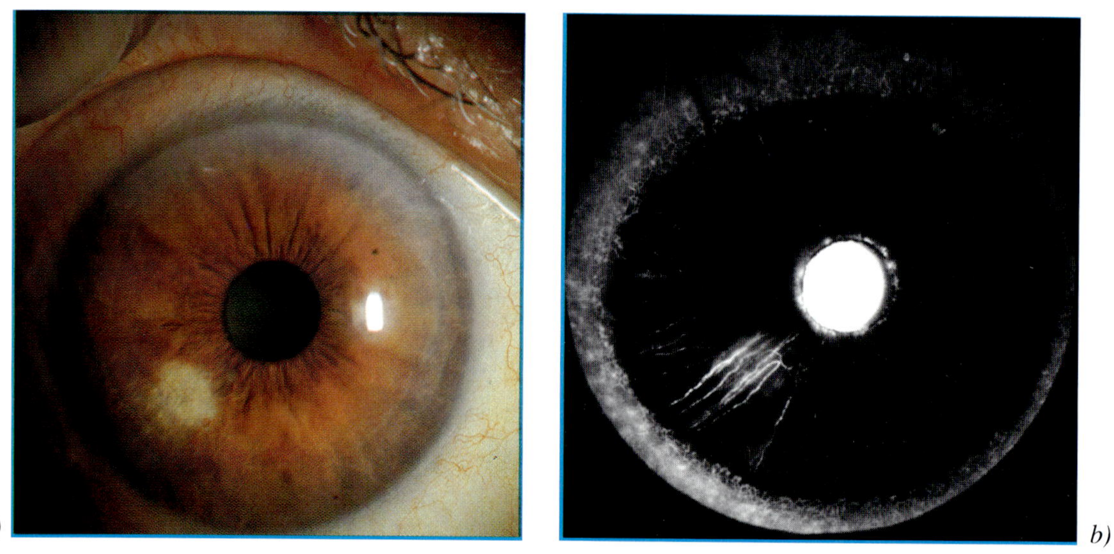

*Fig. **4.2**,1 - Biomicroscopy (a) in a 70-year-old patient with area of atrophy at the 7-8 o' clock position. In the same area there is marked pigment loss permitting fluorescein angiographic visualization of the underlying radial vessels (b). The slight dye leakage from the pupillary margin is age-related (b).*

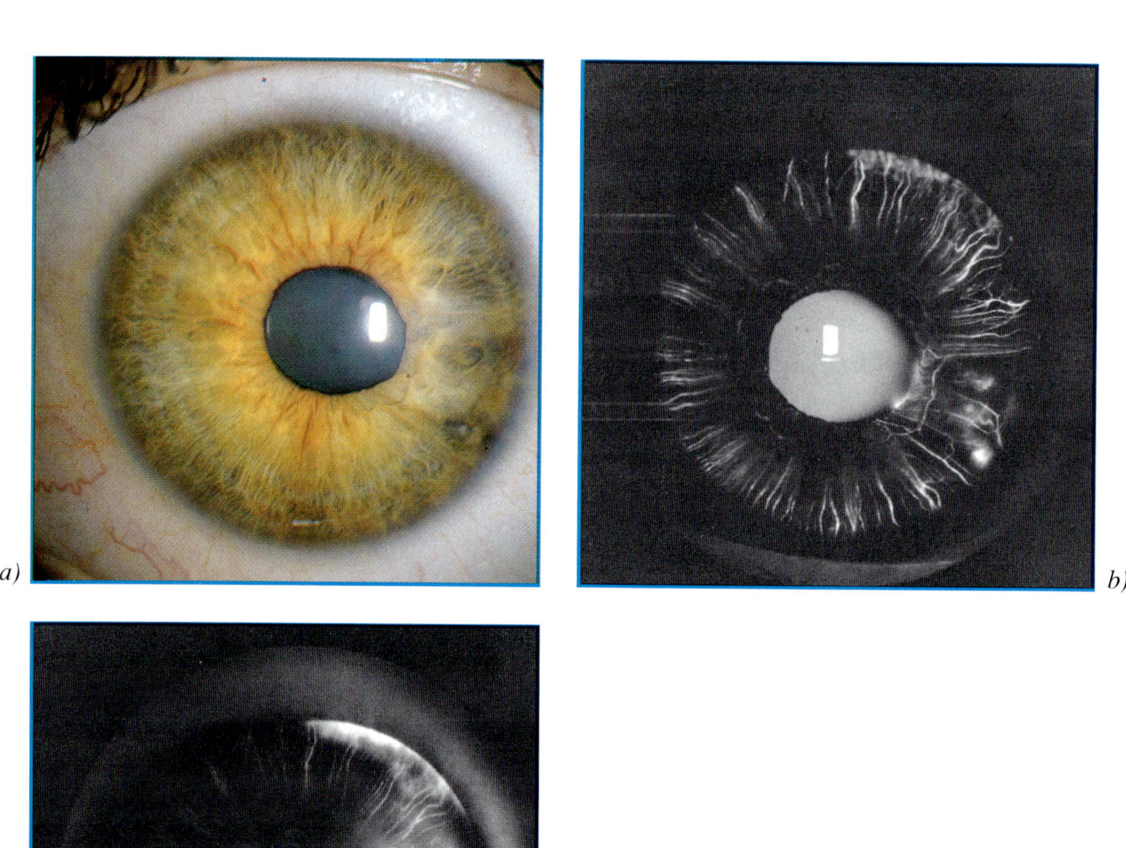

*Fig. **4.2**,2 - Biomicroscopy (a) and iris fluorescein angiographic phases (b,c) in an eye operated for retinal detachment. Corresponding to the area of atrophy at the 3-5 o' clock position, detectable biomicroscopically, iris fluorescein angiography shows a hypofluorescent area where perfusion is inadequate (b), and hyperfluorescent buds indicating neovascularization (b,c).*

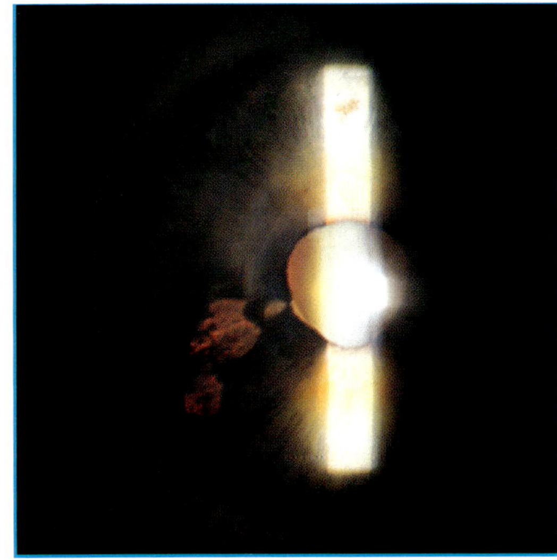

*Fig. **4.2**,3 - Biomicroscopic examination in a patient with necrosis of the anterior segment as a result of an encircling procedure for retinal detachment. There is one segment of the iris with stromal atrophy and loss of the pigment epithelium, so marked that it can be transilluminated at some points.*

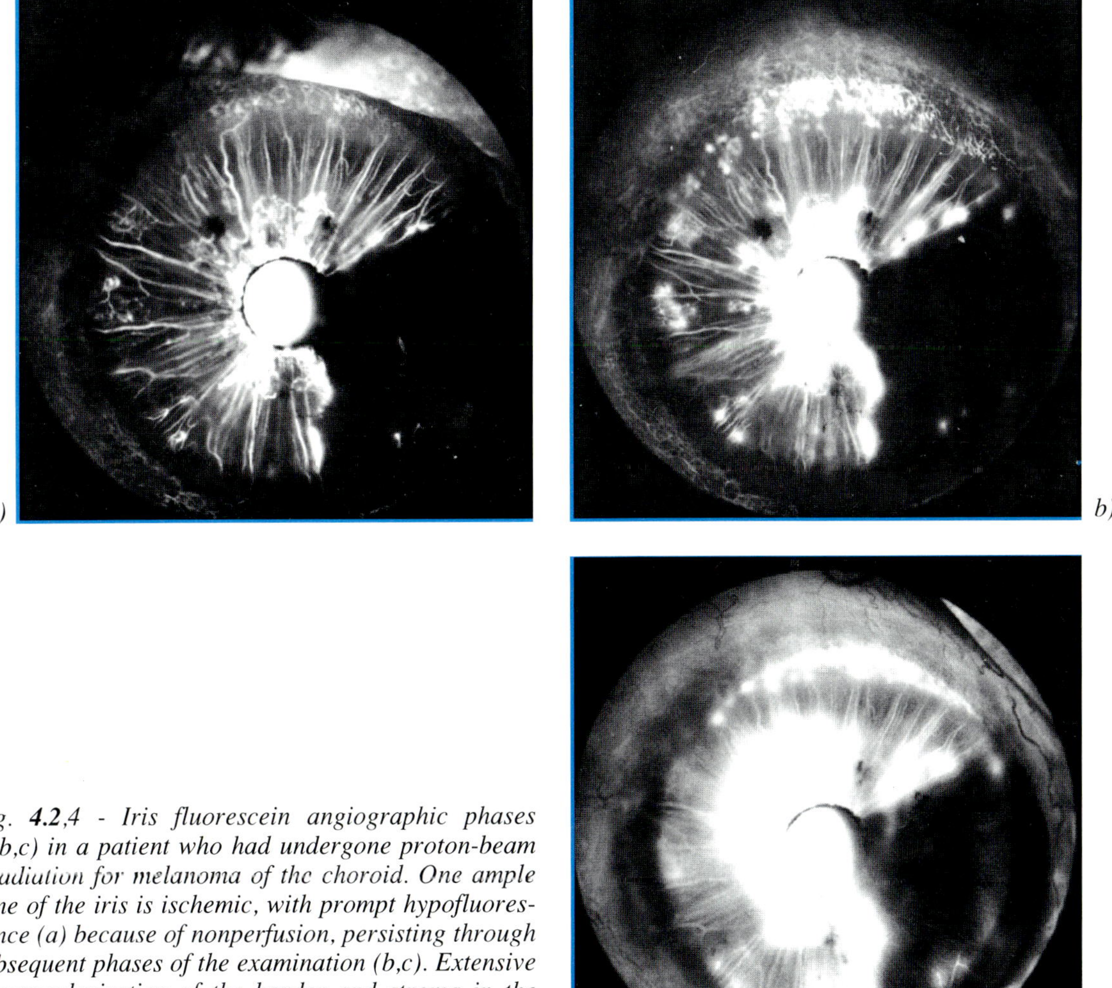

a) *b)* *c)*

*Fig. **4.2**,4 - Iris fluorescein angiographic phases (a,b,c) in a patient who had undergone proton-beam irradiation for melanoma of the choroid. One ample zone of the iris is ischemic, with prompt hypofluorescence (a) because of nonperfusion, persisting through subsequent phases of the examination (b,c). Extensive neovascularization of the border and stroma in the other sectors of the iris cause patches of hyperfluorescence, becoming larger and brighter in subsequent phases of the examination.*

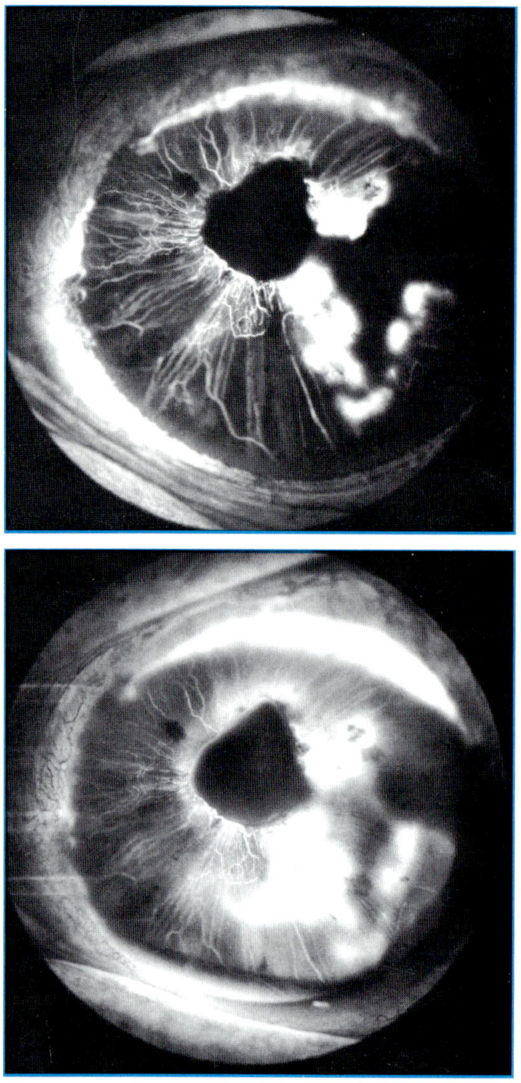

a)

b)

*Fig. **4.2**,5 - Early (a) and late (b) iris fluorescein angiographic phases in the same patient as above, six months later. In the interval the patient had been operated for cataract removal. The area of iris nonperfusion seems smaller. The hyperfluorescence due to new vessels is stronger but limited to the edges of the ischemic area.*

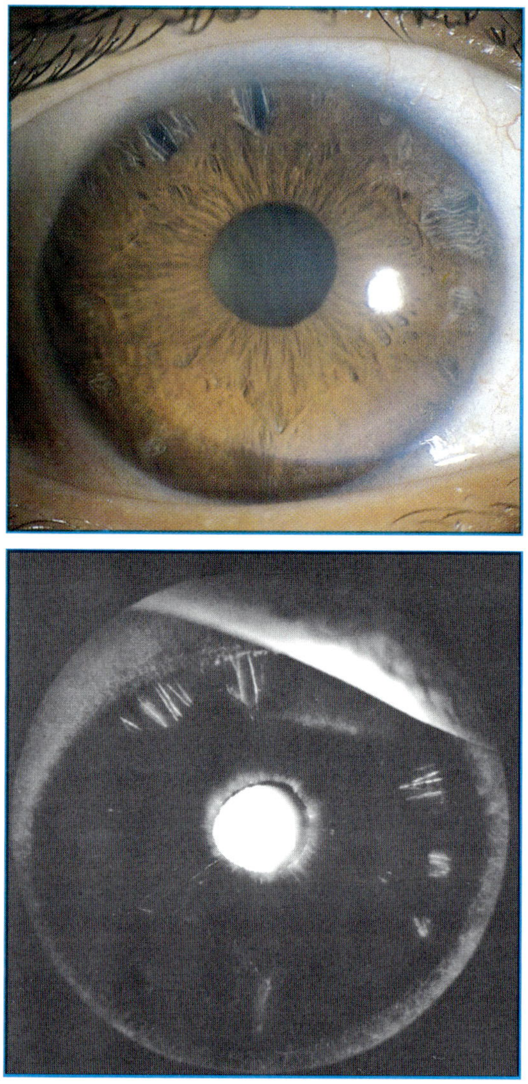

a)

b)

*Fig. **4.2**,7 - Biomicroscopy (a) and iris fluorescein angiography (b) in a patient with the irido-corneal-endothelial syndrome.*

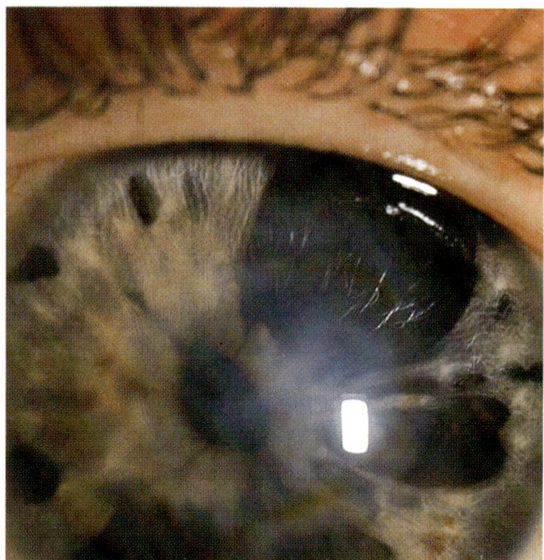

*Fig. **4.2**,6 - Biomicroscopy in a patient with progressive essential atrophy of the iris. The characteristic "through-and-through" holes appear particularly marked in this case .*

R. Brancato, F. Bandello, R. Lattanzio
Atlas of Iris
Fluorescein Angiography
Kugler & Ghedini Publications 1995

Chapter 4.3

Abnormal vessel patterns

The iris may present various types of vascular anomalies, each with its own distinct iris fluorescein angiographic picture. The main headings are:

1) well demarcated vascular arcades;
2) large-caliber arteries;
3) anomalous vessels;
4) vascular tufts;
5) iris new vessels.

Well demarcated vascular arcades

These clearly outlined vascular arcades, that rarely leak fluorescein, lie at the periphery of sectors with filling defects. They are probably shunt systems which dilate and becogme canalized when normal perfusion is impaired.[24]

Large-caliber arteries

Another type of vascular anomaly is the finding of tortuous arteries with a larger than normal diameter, emerging from the iris root and running anomalously (Figs. **4.3**,1-5). They do not always run in a strictly radial direction, tending in fact to circumvent the pupil, running paramarginally then dissolving into capillaries, or else turning back toward the periphery and continuing to the iris base as a vein.[24] In other instances, despite their serpentine, irregular route, these vessels do approximately follow the path of normal iris vessels, and take on the appearance of recurrent vessels, or vessels of the minor arterial circle of the iris. Sometimes the anomalous vessel is continuous with the normal vascular network, being either directly linked or a branch of it.

These are unusually thick serpentine vessels of the surface vascular network of the iris, standing out from the stromal surface; they can be seen with the biomicroscope, especially in pale irises with little pigment (Fig. **4.3**,6).

On iris fluorescein angiography they present as dilated channels; their filling appears in the arterial phase,[34] generally earlier than in normal stromal vasculature, and is synchronous with that of conjunctival vessels.[32] They generally fill completely before normal capillary filling. These anomalous vessels do not normally have permeable walls, so there is no dye leakage.[22,24,32,34] Occasional slight leakage reported may have been at least in part an artefact caused by the iris vessels being slightly out of focus.[37]

Anomalous vessels

Two functional angiographic pictures of anomalous vessels may be observed:[32]

a) vessels with an abnormal diameter and path, approximately following the normal iris vessel arrangement;

b) atypical vessels with wide communicating shunts between artery and vein, without collaterals.

These manifestations can be compared with retinal angioma that has not developed overtly. True iris hemangiomas are in fact extremely rare,[3,17,19,39] as are capillary[1,3,11,19] or cavernous hemangiomas,[3,27,33] and the so-called racemose hemangiomas.[46] These are not true tumors, but are anatomical anomalies of the vessels. They have been defined as abnormal, direct bypassing capillary bed communications between more or less fully developed, dilated and tortuous arteries and veins.[2,6,37] Other terms proposed include arteriovenous communications, arteriovenous anastomoses[6] or arteriovenous malformations.[34] Lesions of this type occur mainly in the retina[6,39] and there are very few reports of arteriovenous communications in the iris.[46]

Such arteriovenous communications appear to be congenital anomalies,[6] whose pathogenesis is not known, but they probably arise from a local defect in the maturation of the primitive mesenchymal cells. In the early stages of development of the vascular system, the primitive mesenchymal cells do in fact differentiate into solid cords of endothelial cells which gradually become canalized to form an early capillary network.[3] As blood starts to flow through these networks the primitive vessels develop into arteries, veins and connecting capillaries, while the primitive capillaries themselves retract and become atrophic. In arteriovenous communications extensive capillary retraction and atrophy may occur, and a single channel develops to shunt blood across this defective capillary zone.

These anomalies are slow in developing and only become evident in the second or third decade of life,[6,46] as conglomerates of greatly dilated and tortuous vessels. Their larger diameter and tortuosity might be a response to the greater blood flow they have to carry, which shifts the vascular path over time.[32]

Fluorescein angiography of the iris permits a distinction between the afferent and efferent vessels in the communication (Figs. **4.3**,7-14).[37] Angiography generally shows reduced perfusion in the iris sector where the lesion is, suggesting there may be some sort of slight "decompensation" in the arteriovenous communication (Fig. **4.3**,15).[37]

Arteriovenous malformations of the iris need to be distinguished mainly from secondary vascular alterations arising in the course of various iris diseases; these include the dilated and tortuous vessels of the iris observed in association with expansive lesions, or local inflammation.[1,24,28,37,39]

Vascular tufts

Vascular tufts of the pupillary margin are another anomaly of the iris; these are coiled, intertwined tight clusters of tiny vessels.[7,12,14,16,20,31,35,36,41,43,44] Often multiple, these microhemangiomas are asymptomatic. Unless trauma arises, they may cause hyphema,[5,7,14,16,20,35,36,41,43,44] sometimes recurrent, which goes and comes of its own accord, with no functional aftermaths. Frequently it is the hyphema that leads to diagnosis.

These microhemangiomas are not anatomically correlated with the minor arterial circle of the iris, but presumably derive from the capillary network at the end of the radial vessels, surrounding the iris sphincter.[41] Their vascular nature has been confirmed histologically[14] and also by iris fluorescein angiography which establishes the site and number with precision.[5,36,41] This latter examination shows them up as bright spots which take up dye early and abundantly; the resulting hyperfluorescence becomes brighter in subsequent angiographic phases[41] and persists late in the examination (Figs. **4.3**,16-17).[7,31]

Some investigators report that vascular tufts are frequently associated with serious heart or lung diseases.[12,13,25,44] They also appear to be associated with myotonic dystrophy in from 22-50% of cases.[10,13,30,45]

The etiology of these tufts, when not associated with systemic disease, is not known. It has been suggested that they are congenital[16,36,41] although the age at diagnosis is late.[41] Savir reported one case of contralateral orbital cavernous hemangioma.[43]

Hyphema, especially when recurrent, is best dealt with by laser photocoagulation to directly obliterate the vascular anomaly (Fig. **4.3**,18).[5,14,36] The main point, however, is differential diagnosis from iris new vessels, excluding all potentially causal local or systemic pathology which might require a different therapeutic approach.

Iris new vessels

Neovascular proliferation of the iris is another form of vascular anomaly. Defined as *rubeosis iridis* since 1928, iris neovascularization is a calamity for the eye since it may lead to intractable glaucoma. It is not a primary disorder of the iris but is always secondary to any of a range of ocular or systemic pathologies (Table **4.3**,I).[18] Rubeosis iridis may arise in different positions, and vary in extent, giving a range of clinical pictures.

Iris fluorescein angiography shows the new-formed vessels behaving in a typical way, with dye leakage from their anomalous walls, causing dots that fluoresce early, getting bigger and brighter in subsequent angiographic phases. This is the examination that gives the best visualization of any new vessels, and is much more sensitive than biomicroscopy alone.[4] However, the fluorescein angiographic finding is non-specific and gives no indication whatsoever of the etiopathogenesis of any new vessels found.

Tab. 4.3,I: Causes of neovascularization of the iris[18]

1. Systemic diseases Diabetes Norrie's disease Sickle cell disease Neurofibromatosis Lupus erythematosus Marfan's syndrome	Glaucoma - Open-angle glaucoma - Closed-angle glaucoma - Secondary glaucoma Retinal detachment Persistent hyperplastic vitreous Coats' disease Eales' disease Pseudoexfoliation of lens capsule Essential iris atrophy
2. Vascular disorders Central retinal vein occlusion Central retinal artery occlusion Branch vein occlusion Carotid occlusive disease Takayasu's disease (Pulseless disease) Giant cell arteritis Carotid artery ligation Carotid-cavernous fistula Leber's ciliary aneurysms Retrolental fibroplasia Sturge-Weber with choroidal hemangioma	**4. Surgery and radiation therapy** Retinal detachment surgery Vitrectomy Laser coreoplasty Cataract extraction Radiation **5. Trauma**
3. Ocular diseases Uveitis - Endophthalmitis - Sympathetic ophthalmia - Vogt-Koyanagi syndrome	**6. Neoplastic diseases** Retinoblastoma Melanoma of choroid Melanoma of iris Metastatic carcinoma Reticulum cell sarcoma of ciliary body

Rubeosis iridis is discussed in detail in the various chapters dealing with the diseases that may cause it (Figs. **4.3**,19-27).

Iris fluorescein angiography sometimes shows up abnormalities in the path and diameter of iris vessels that could suggest impending neovascularization or alterations preceding the formation of true neovascular processes (Fig. **4.3**,28). Kluxen[23] examined patients with diabetes or retinal venous occlusion using iris fluorescein angiography, and described duplications of the anastomoses in the minor arterial circle of the iris (*circular neovascularization*) which gave no dye leakage even in the late phases of the examination. These alterations turned out to be the result of a non-aggressive process and in four years of follow-up none of these cases developed rubeosis (Fig. **4.3**,29).

Other iris fluorescein angiographic findings mentioned in the literature as vascular anomalies include straightening, narrowing, and congestion of the iris vessels.[38,48] Iris fluorescein angiography is a useful method for detecting a series of furtherfocal abnormal vessel patterns, sometimes hard to classify, which may escape biomicroscopic detection and which may be partly masked by the colour of the iris (Figs. **4.3**,30-33).

References

1 Amasio E, Brovarone FV, Musso M: Angioma of the iris. Ophthalmologica 180: 15, 1980.

2 Apple DJ, Rabb MF: Clinicopathologic correlation of ocular disease. CV Mosby, St Louis, 1978.

3 Ashton N: Primary tumours of the iris. Br J Ophthalmol 48: 650, 1964.

4 Bandello F, Brancato R, Lattanzio R et al: Biomicroscopy versus fluorescein angiography of the iris in the detection of diabetic iridopathy. Graefe's Arch Clin Exp Ophthalmol 231: 444, 1993.

5 Bandello F, Brancato R, Lattanzio R et al: Laser treatment of iris vascular tufts. Ophthalmologica (Basel) 206: 187, 1993.

6 Baurmann H, Meyer F, Oberhoff P: Komplikationen bei der arteriovenösen Anastomose der Netzhaut. Klin Monatsbl Augenheilkd 153: 562, 1968.

7 Blanksma LJ, Hooijmans JMM: Vascular tufts of the pupillary border causing a spontaneous hyphaema. Ophthalmologica (Basel) 178: 297, 1979.

8 Brancato R, Menchini U, Carnevalini A: Atlante di iridografia a fluorescenza. C.I.C. Ed Int Gruppo Ed Medico, Roma, 1981.

9 Brown GC, Magargal LA, Schachat A et al: Neovascular glaucoma. Etiologic considerations. Ophthalmology 91: 315, 1984.

10 Burian HM, Burns CA: Ocular changes in myotonic dystrophy. Am J Ophthalmol 63: 222, 1967.

11 Cashell GTW: Angioma of the iris. Br J Ophthalmol 51: 633, 1967.

12 Cobb B: Vascular tufts at the pupillary margin. A preliminary report on 44 patients. Trans Ophthalmol Soc UK 88: 211, 1968.

13 Cobb B, Shilling JS, Chisholm IH: Vascular tufts at the pupillary margin in myotonic dystrophy. Am J Ophthalmol 69: 573, 1970.

14 Coleman ST, Green WR, Patz A: Vascular tufts of pupillary margin of iris. Am J Ophthalmol 83: 881, 1977.

15 Duke Elder S: System of Ophthalmology. 3/II. Congenital Deformities. Kimpton, London, 1966.

16 Fechner PU: Spontaneous hyphema with abnormal iris vessels. Br J Ophthalmol 42: 311, 1958.

17 Ferry AP: Hemangiomas of the iris and ciliary body: Do they exist? A search for a histologically proved case. Int Ophthalmol Clin 12: 177, 1972.

18 Gartner S, Henkind P: Neovascularization of the iris (Rubeosis iridis). Review. Surv Ophthalmol 22: 291, 1978.

19 Goder G, Lommatsch P, Noor MS: Differentialdiagnostische Probleme bei Tumoren der vorderen Uvea. Klin Monatsbl Augenheilkd 166: 340, 1975.

20 Israel MP, Lorenzetti DWC: Bilateral microhemangiomas of the pupillary border with later hyphema. Can J Ophthalmol 9: 138, 1974.

21 Klein S, Zenker HJ: Zum Stellenwert der Irisfluoreszenzangiographie bei der Fruhdiagnostik von Gefässlasionen. Klin Monatsbl Augenheilkd 187: 184, 1985.

22 Kluxen G, Friedburg D: Gefässanomalien der Iris im Fluoreszenzangiogramm. Klin Monatsbl Augenheilkd 175: 211, 1979.

23 Kluxen G, Friedburg D, Ruppert A: Zirkuläre Gefässneubildungen des Circulus arteriosus iridis minor. Klin Monatsbl Augenheilkd 176: 160, 1980.

24 Kottow MH: Anterior segment fluorescein angiography. William & Wilkins, Baltimore, 1978.

25 Krarup JC: Atypical rubeosis iridis in congenital cyanotic heart disease. Report of a case with microhaemangiomas at the pupillary margin causing spontaneous hyphaemas. Acta Ophthalmol 55: 581, 1977.

26 Magauran DM: Unilateral spontaneous hyphema. Br J Ophthalmol 57: 945, 1973.

27 Magrane WG: Cavernous hemangioma of the iris. North Am Veterinarian 35: 516, 1954.

28 Mann I: Developmental abnormalities of the eye. British Medical Association, London, 1957.

29 Manor RS, Sachs W: Spontaneous hyphema. Am J Ophthalmol 74: 293, 1972.

30 Mason GI: Iris neovascular tufts. Relationship to rubeosis, insulin, and hypotony. Arch Ophthalmol 97: 2346, 1979.

31 Mason GI, Ferry AP: Bilateral spontaneous hyphema arising from iridic microhemangiomas. Ann Ophthalmol 11: 87, 1979.

32 Menchini U, Carnevalini A, Meloni P: Anomalies vasculaires iriennes: aspects fluoroiridographiques. J Fr Ophtalmol 13: 177, 1989.

33 Naidoff MA, Kenyon KR, Green WR: Iris hemangioma and abnormal retinal vasculature in a case of diffuse congenital hemangiomatosis. Am J Ophthalmol 72: 633, 1971.

34 Perkins SA, Magargal LE: Arteriovenous malformations of the iris. Ann Ophthalmol 17: 679, 1985.

35 Perry HD, Mallen FJ, Sussman W: Microhaemangiomas of the iris with spontaneous hyphaema and acute glaucoma. Br J Ophthalmol 61: 114, 1977.

36 Podolsky MM, Srinivasan BD: Spontaneous hyphema secondary to vascular tuft of pupillary margin of the iris. Arch Ophthalmol 97: 301, 1979.

37 Prost M: Arteriovenous communication of the iris. Br J Ophthalmol 70: 856, 1986.

38 Raitta C, Vannas S: Fluoresceinangiographie der Irisgefässe nach Zentralvenenverschluss. Albrecht von Graefes Arch Klin Ophthalmol 177: 33, 1969.

39 Reese AB: Tumors of the eye. Harper & Row, New York, 1963.

40 Riffenburgh RS: Recurrent spontaneous iris arterial haemorrhage. Am J Ophthalmol 53: 319, 1965.

41 Rosen E, Lyons D: Microhemangiomas at the pupillary border demonstrated by fluorescein photography. Am J Ophthalmol 67: 846, 1969.

42 Rydberg M: Svenska Ögonläkarföreningens sammanträde. Nord Med 72: 1488, 1964.

43 Savir H, Manor RS: Spontaneous hyphema and vessel anomaly. Arch Ophthalmol 93: 1056, 1975.

44 Sellman A: Hyphaema from microhaemangiomas. Acta Ophthalmol 50: 58, 1972.

45 Stern LZ, Cross HE, Crebo AR: Abnormal iris vasculature in myotonic dystrophy: an anterior segment angiographic study. Arch Neurol 35: 224, 1978.

46 Stur M, Strasser G: Sektorförmige Gefässmissbildung der Iris vom razemösen Typ. Klin Monatsbl Augenheilkd 183: 50, 1983.

47 Troost TB: Glaser aneurysms, arteriovenous communications, and related vascular malformations. In Duane TD: Clinical Ophthalmology. Harper & Row, Hagerstown, 1979.

48 Vannas S, Raitta C, Vannas A: A study of retinal and iris circulation in dystrophia retinae pigmentosa. In Amalric P: Fluorescein Angiography. Proc International Symposium on Fluorescein Angiography. Albi, 1969. S Karger, Basel, 1971.

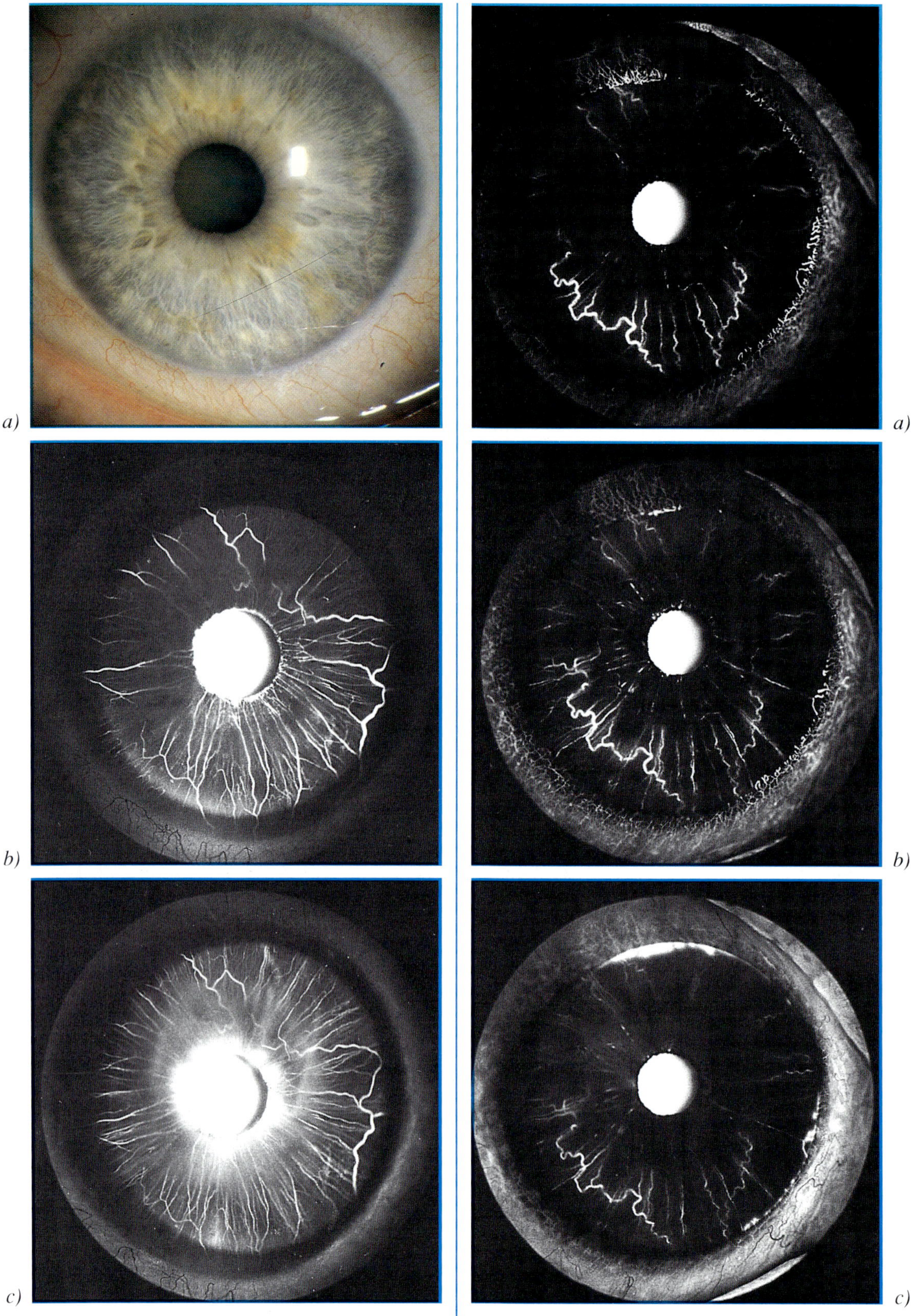

*Fig. **4.3**,1 - Biomicroscopy (a) shows a large-caliber vessel running crosswise close to the iris root at 3-5 o'clock. Iris fluorescein angiographic examination shows the vessel takes up dye in the arterial phase (b), and has radial branches running out towards the pupillary border. Dye leakage is seen at the pupillary margin, causing marked hyperfluorescence in the late phases (c).*

*Fig. **4.3**,2 - Iris fluorescein angiographic phases (a,b,c). The radial arteries of the lower sectors of the iris start out mostly from tortuous arterial trunks running parallel to the base of the iris and becoming hyperfluorescent early.*

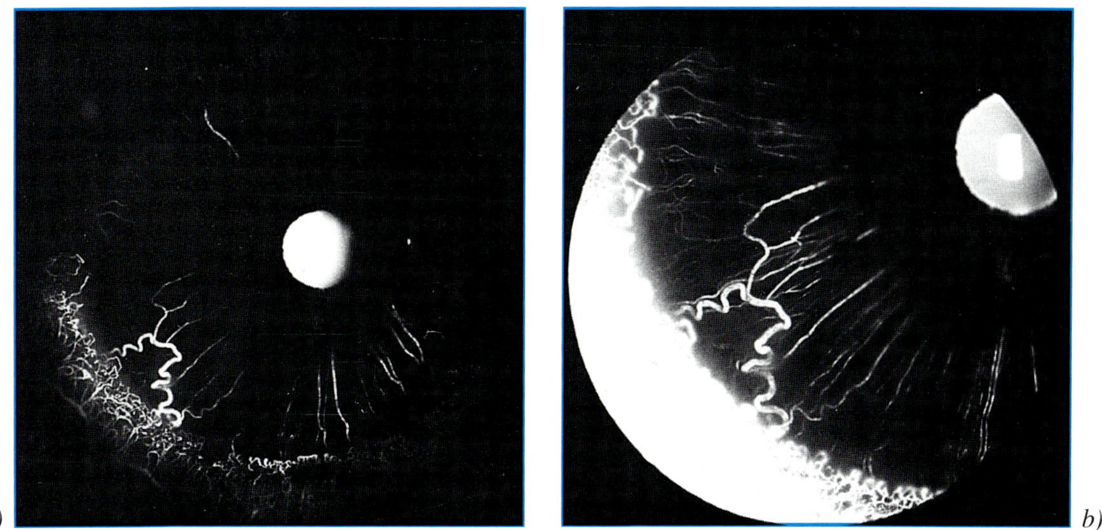

a) b)

*Fig. **4.3**,3 - At 7-8 o'clock there is an anomalous tortuous recurrent vessel that already fluoresces in the arterial phase (a); radial arteries lead off this, running either directly or through collateral branches towards the pupillary border (b: subsequent fluorangiographic phase and greater enlargement).*

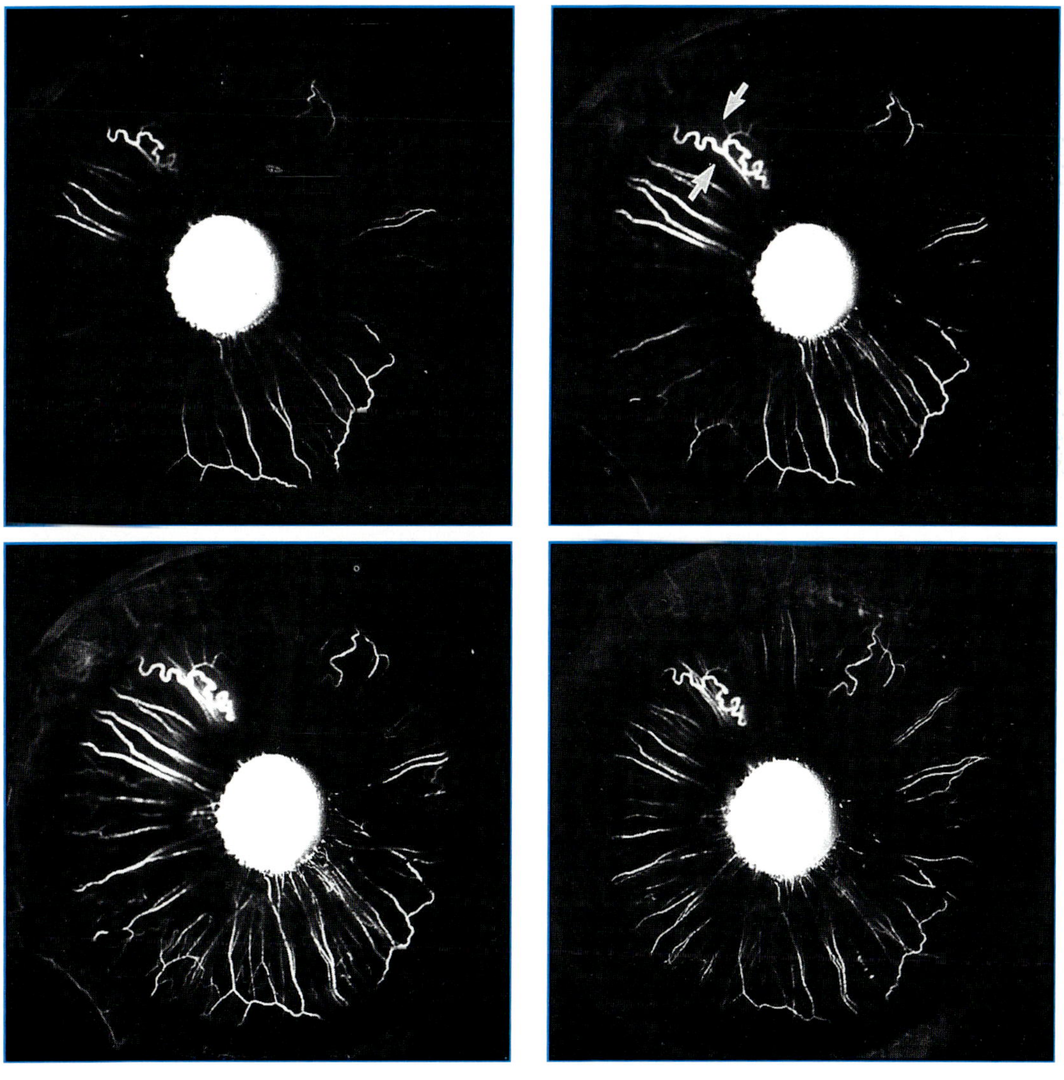

a) b)

c) d)

*Fig. **4.3**,4 - Iris fluorescein angiographic appearance of an anomalous arterial branch (arrows), with its large caliber and tortuous path. There is so much pigment in the upper sectors of the pupillary portion that its path towards the pupillary border cannot be seen (a,b,c,d: subsequent phases of the examination).*

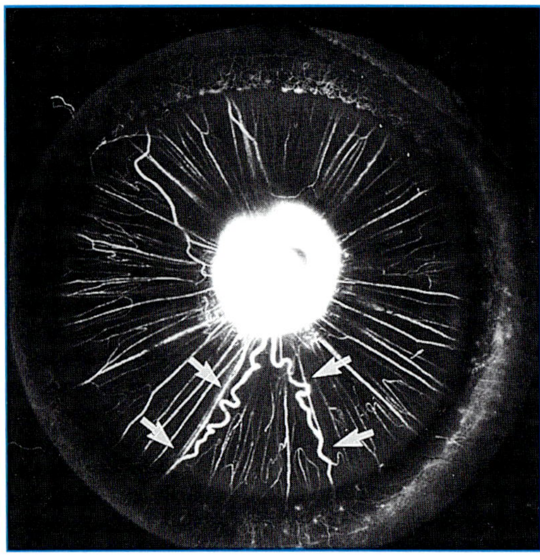

*Fig. **4.3**,5 - Tortuous radial vessels of increased caliber (arrows): iris fluorescein angiography.*

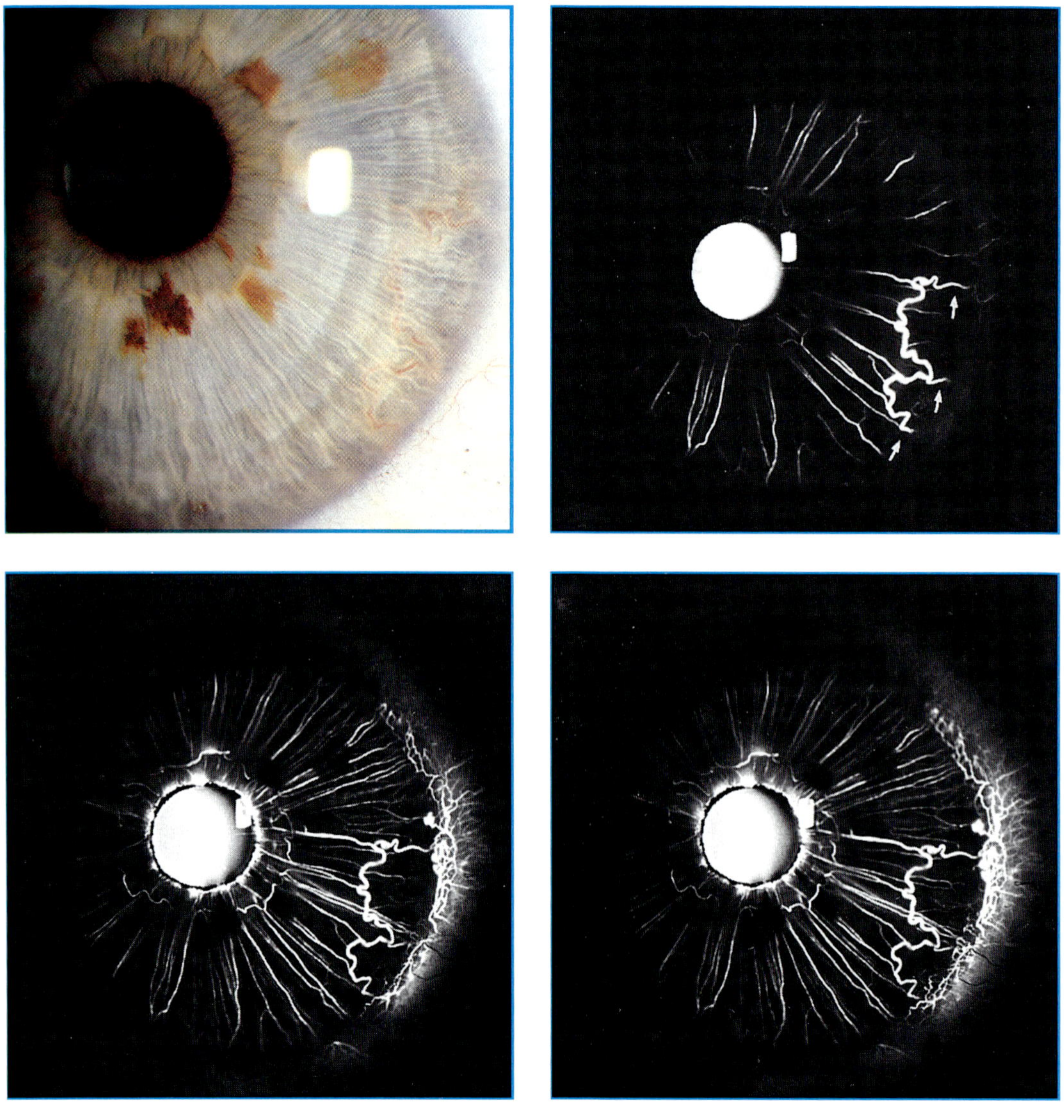

a) *b)*

c) *d)*

*Fig. **4.3**,6 - Three arterial afferents starting from the root of the iris (arrows) combine to form the large transverse vessel seen biomicroscopally (a) in the lower portion of the right hemi-iris. Arteries run out radially from this towards the pupillary border (b,c,d: iris fluorescein angiographic phases).*

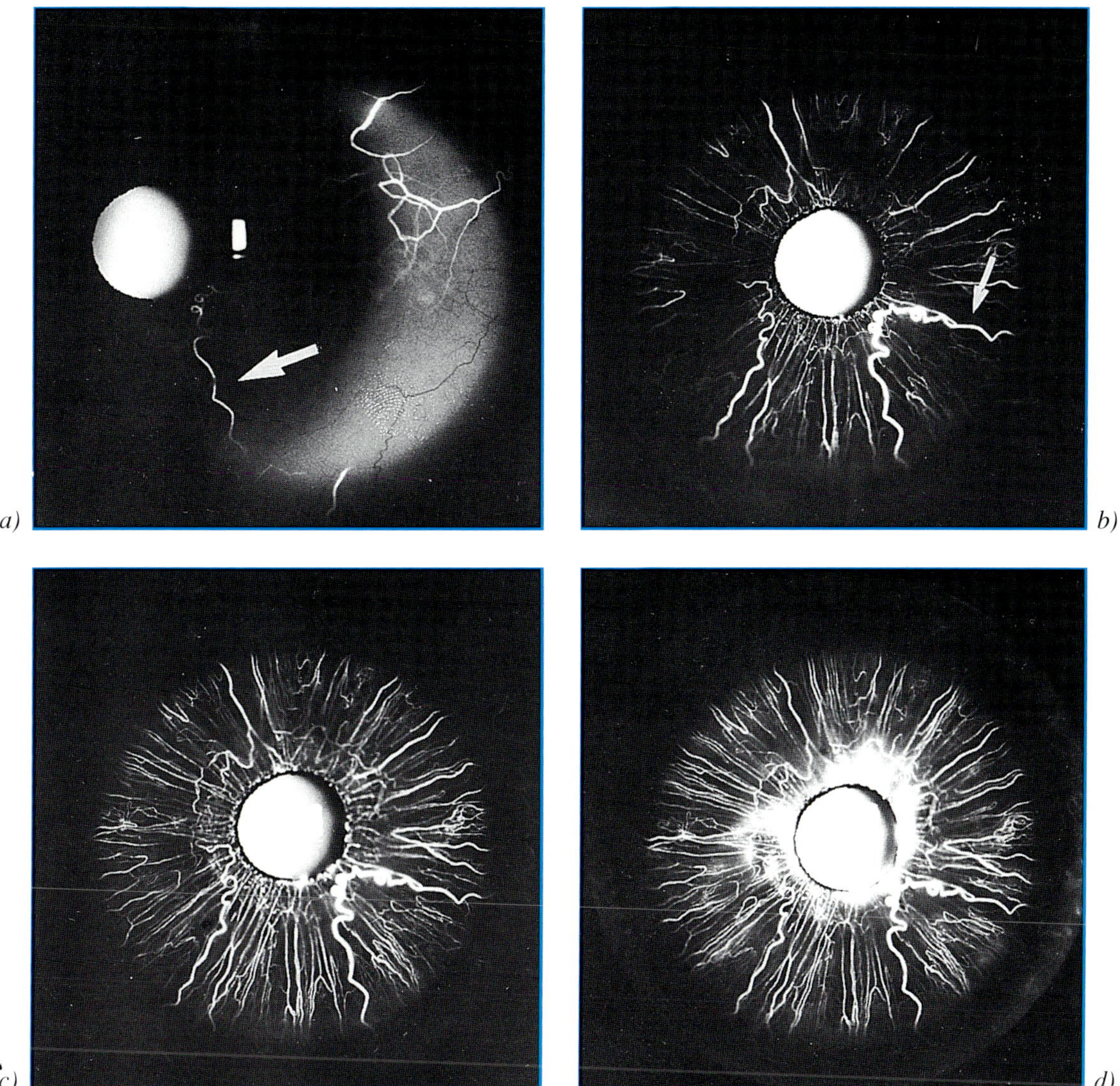

*Fig. **4.3**,7 - Iris fluorescein angiographic phases (a,b,c,d) in a case of artero-venous shunt. The afferent vessel (large arrow) takes up dye early in the arterial phase (a) before the radial arteries. The efferent segment (small arrow) fluoresces in the artero-venous phase (b). In the venous phase (c) iris vessels fill completely. Even at later times (d) no dye leaks from the vessels connecting the arteries and veins. There is, however, some pupillary margin leakage.*

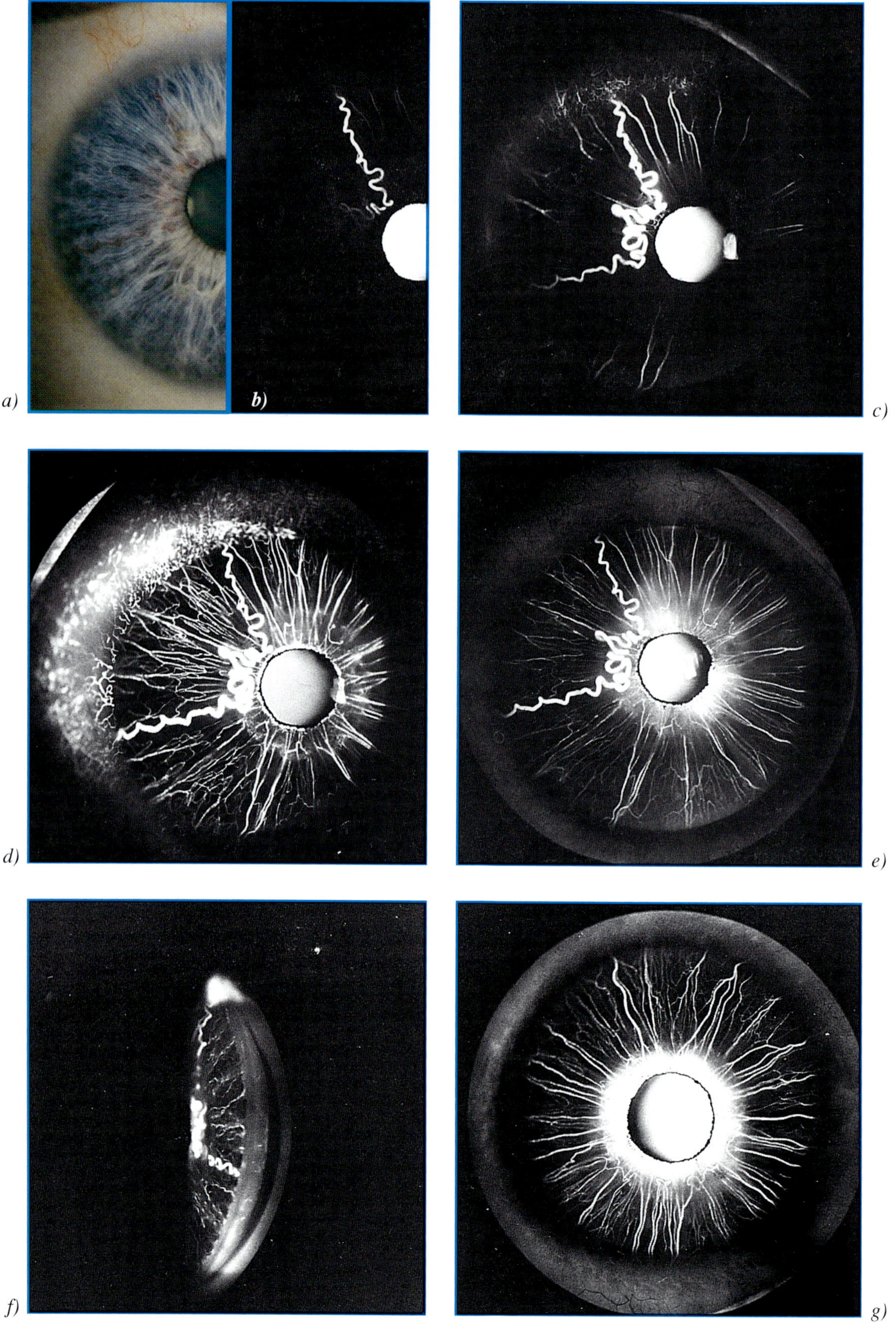

Fig. ***4.3****,8 - A case similar to the one above. The nature of the dilated, tortuous vessels can be seen biomicroscopically (a) but iris fluorescein angiography in its different phases (b,c,d,e) shows that this is an artero-venous shunt. The Goldmann lens (f) can be used to observe that the anomalous vessels stand out in relief against the surface of the stroma. The pupillary margin leakage seen in the late phase (e) - and in both eyes (g) - is age-related.*

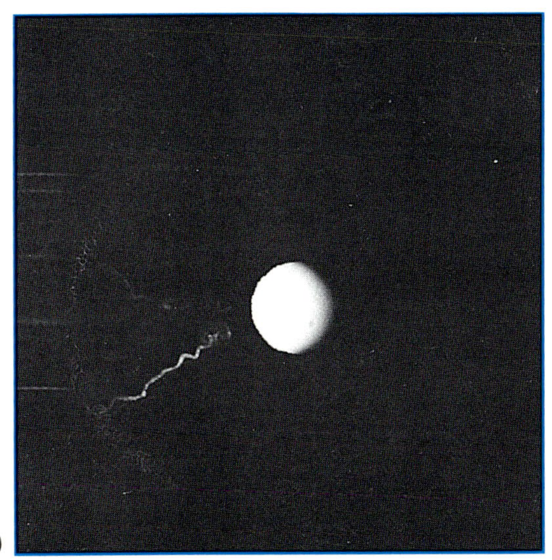

a)

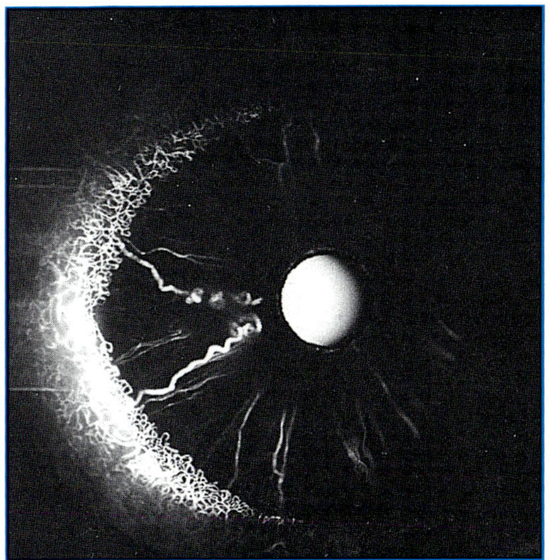

b)

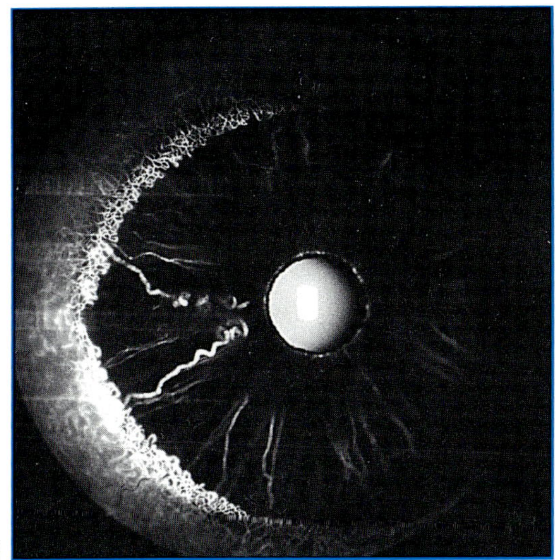

c)

*Fig. **4.3**,9 - Three filling phases (a,b,c) in iris vessels of abnormal caliber and path. In the pupillary portion, it is probably either the excess of pigment or the fact that the vessels run on a deeper plane that makes it impossible to see the point of communication between what looks like the afferent and efferent vessels of an artero-venous shunt.*

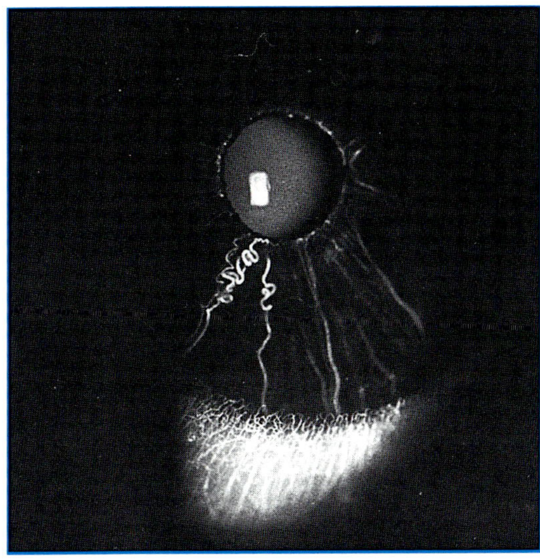

*Fig. **4.3**,10 - Iris fluorescein angiography in a case similar to the one above.*

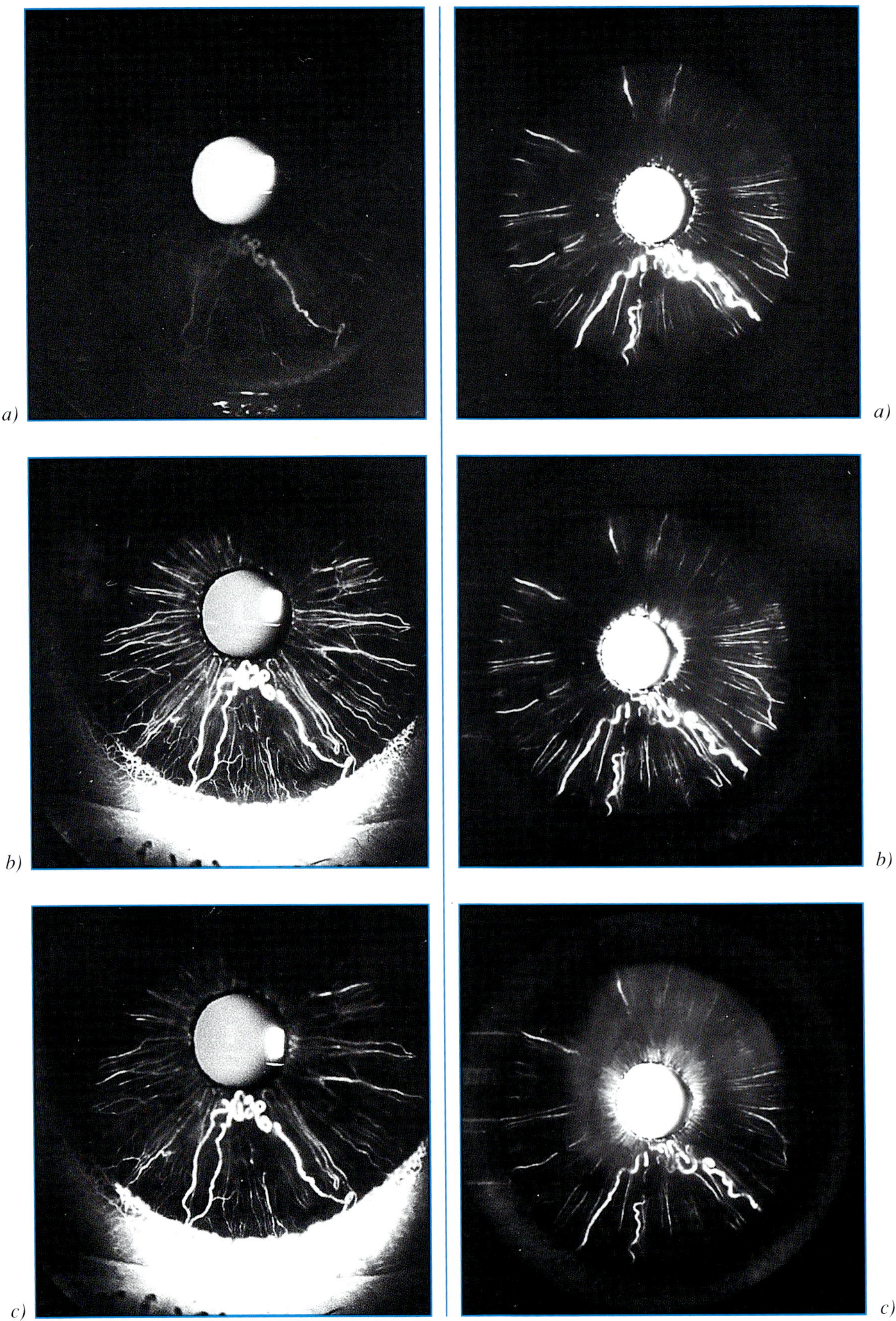

*Fig. **4.3**,11-12 - Two cases of artero-venous shunt involving several iris vessels (a,b,c: fluorangiographic phases). The faint dye leakage from the tortuous congested vessels may partly be an artefact deriving from the fact that since these vessels stand out from the stromal surface they are not sharply focused. Pupillary margin leakage is conspicuous in the case shown in Fig. **4.3**,12.*

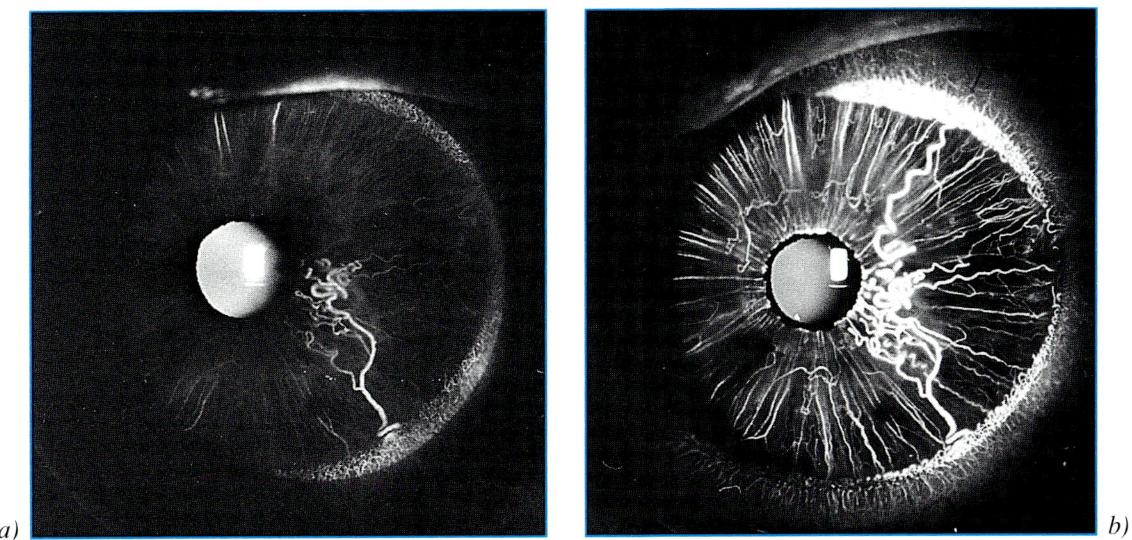

*Fig. **4.3**,13 - A tangle of congested, tortuous iris vessels, anastomosing in loops, and looking like retinal cirsoid aneurysms (early (a) and late (b) iris fluorescein angiographic phases).*

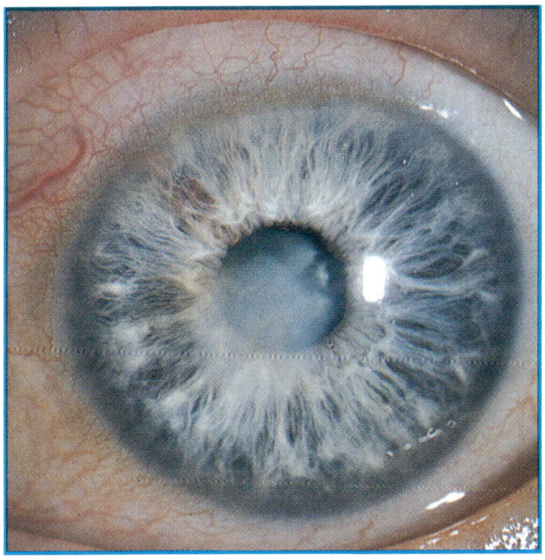

*Fig. **4.3**,14 - A case similar to the one above: biomicroscopy (a) and iris fluorescein angiographic phases (b,c). The blood-iris barrier is damaged throughout.*

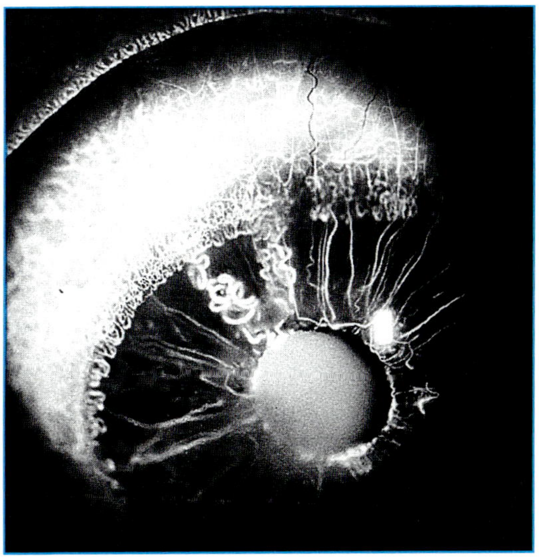

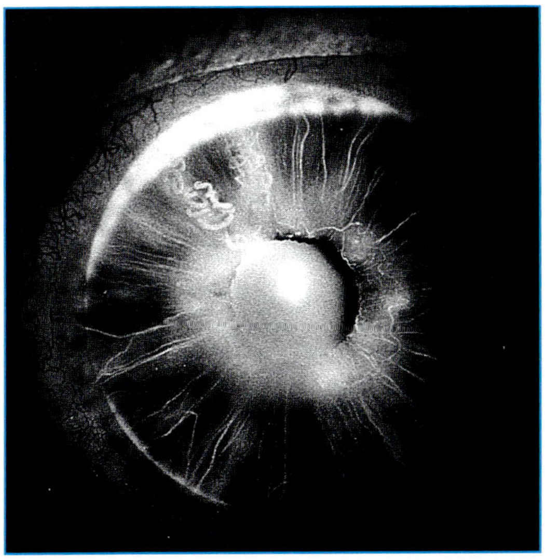

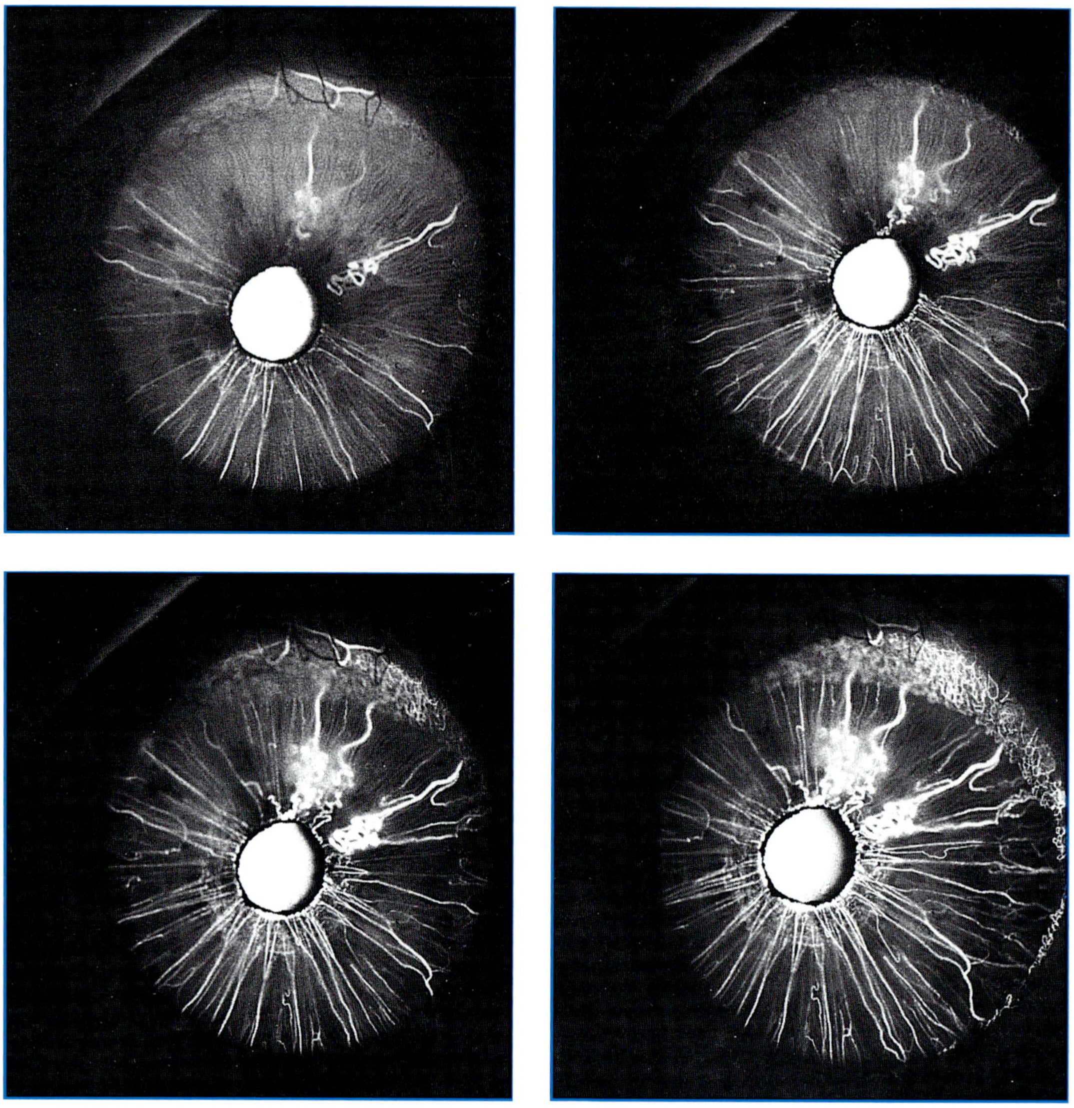

a) *b)*

c) *d)*

*Fig. **4.3**,15 - Iris fluorescein angiographic phases in a case of double artero-venous shunt (a,b,c,d). Perfusion delays and defects are seen in the iris sector where the vascular anomalies are, suggesting that some rheological disorder might explain the shunts.*

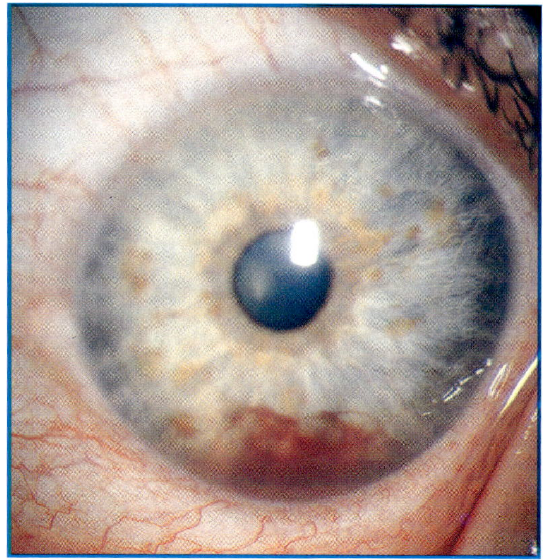

*Fig. **4.3**,16 - Biomicroscopy in a case of spontaneous hyphema.*

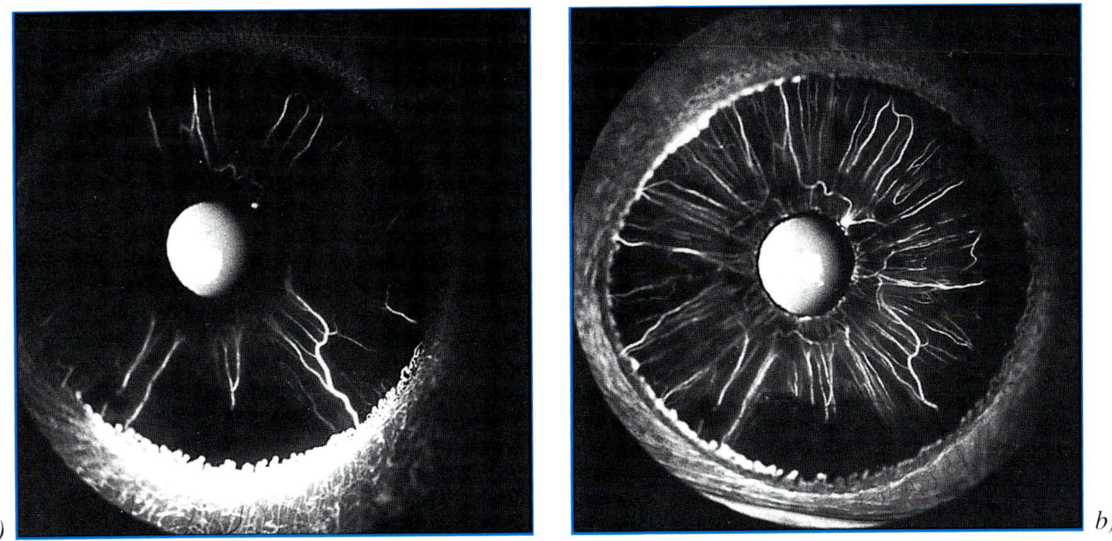

a) b)

*Fig. **4.3**,17 - Same case as in the previous figure. Iris fluorescein angiography, done a few days later, shows an early spot of hyperfluorescence (a) at pupillary margin, growing brighter and larger in the later phase (b). This was interpreted as a microhemangioma. Hypofluorescence in the lower sectors of the iris is due to the masking effect of blood still present.*

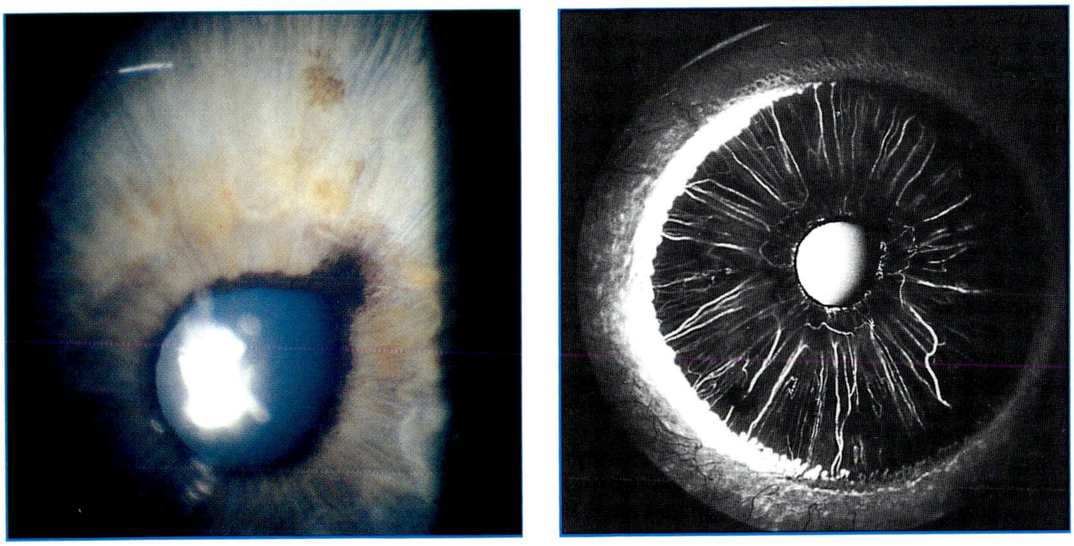

a) b)

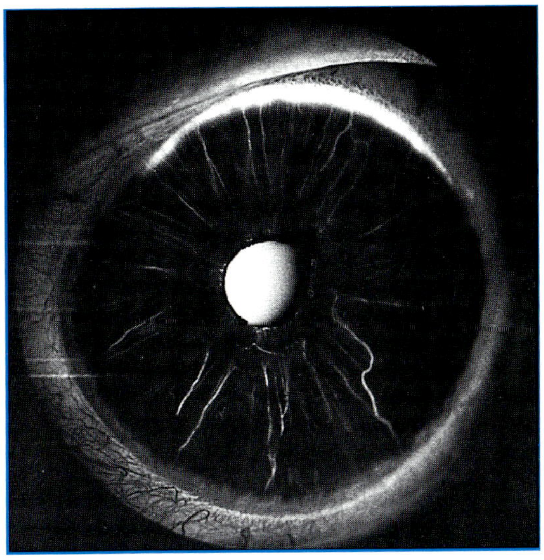

c)

*Fig. **4.3**,18 - Same case as in Figs. **4.3**,16 and **4.3**,17 after direct laser photocoagulation of the vascular tuft at the pupillary margin (a: biomicroscopy; b,c: iris fluorescein angiographic phases).*

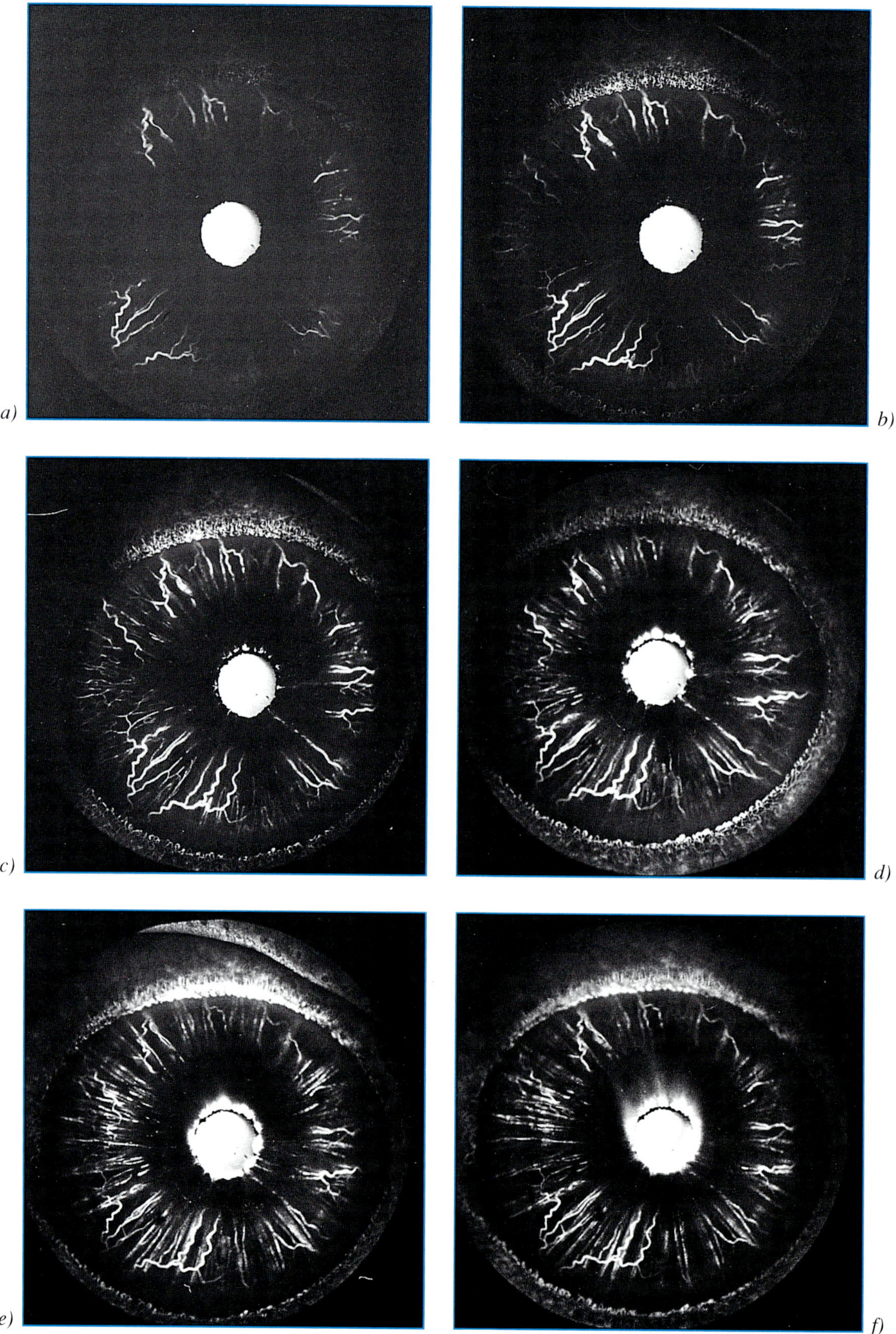

*Fig. **4.3**,19 - Iris fluorescein angiographic phases (a,b,c,d,e,f) in a diabetic patient with marked congestion throughout the vascular network of the iris. The radial vessels appear dilated and run tortuously. Initial neovascularization can be seen at the pupillary margin, causing hyperfluorescent spots which become bigger and brighter in later phases, until they join up in a fluorescent ring which leaks dye in the last phases (f).*

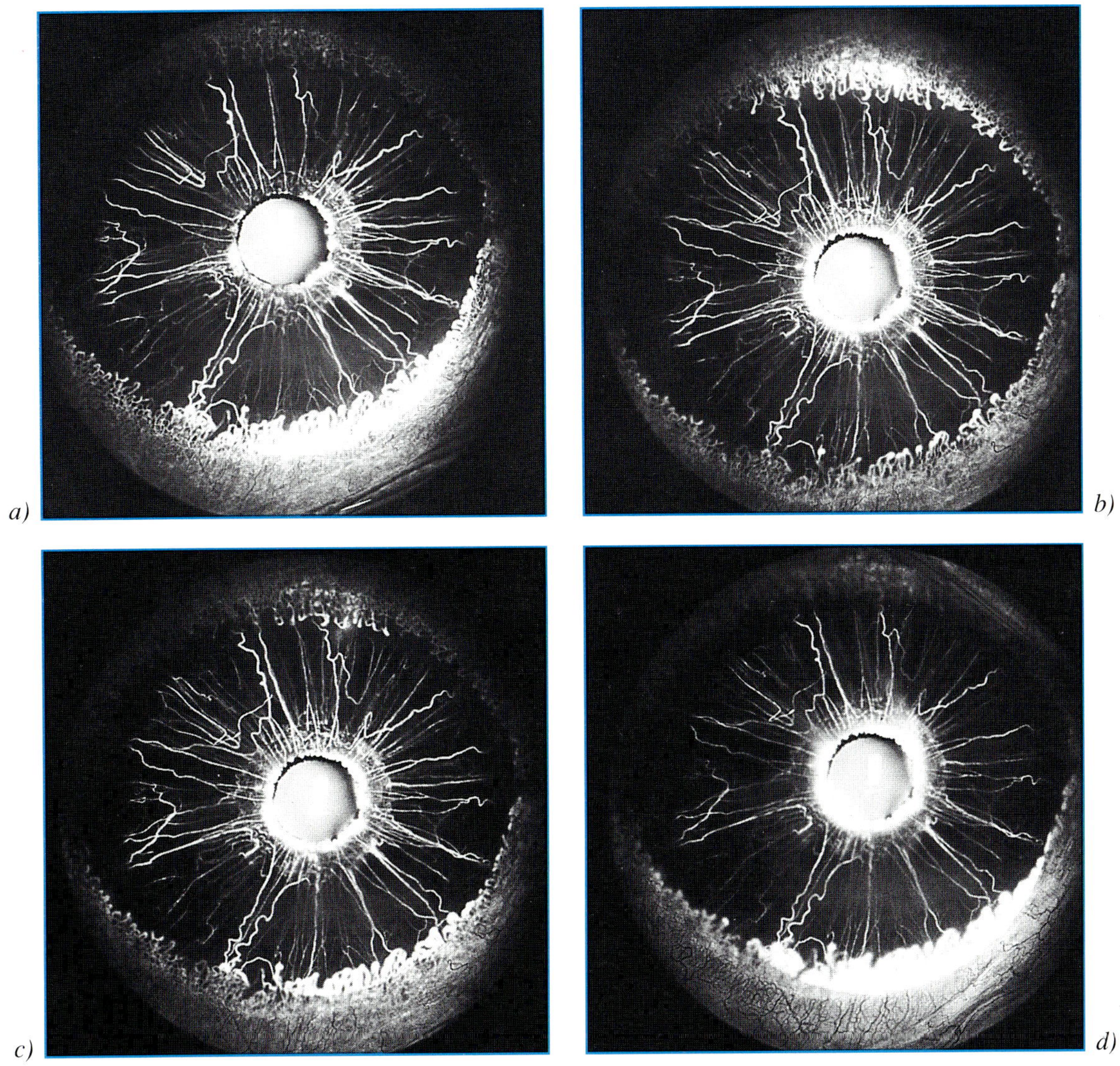

a) b)

c) d)

Fig. ***4.3****,20 - Another iris fluorescein angiographic picture of new vessels at the pupillary border (phases a,b,c,d). The radial network seems to be thinned and the radial vessels present are tortuous but there is no paravascular leakage.*

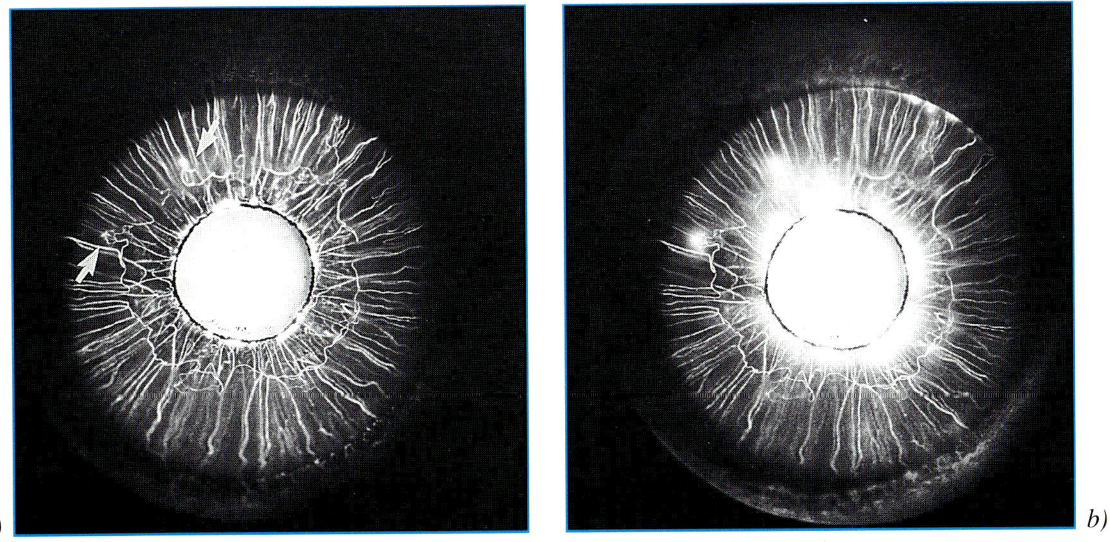

a) b)

Fig. ***4.3****,21 - Early rubeosis of the pupillary border with initial stromal neovascular tufts (arrows). On account of their abnormal permeability, the dye leaks from the walls of the new vessels (early (a) and late (b) iris fluorescein angiographic phases).*

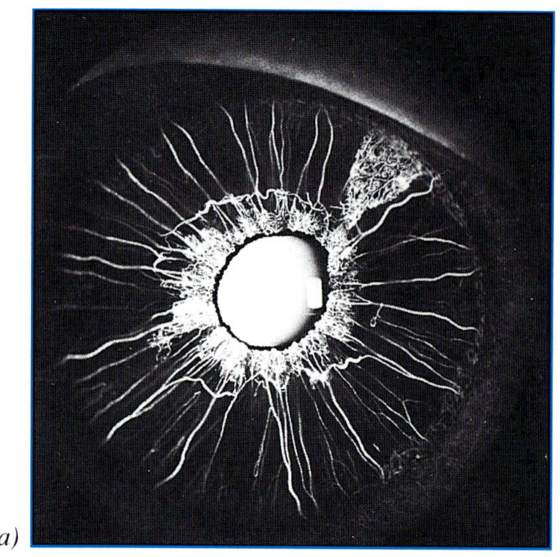

a)

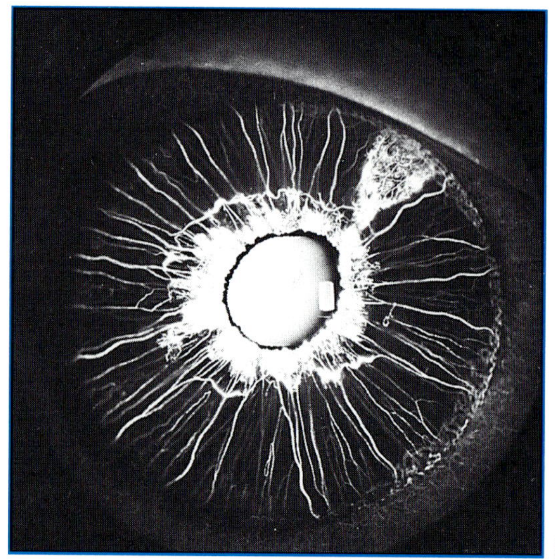

b)

*Fig. **4.3**,22 - Iris fluorescein angiographic phases (a,b,c,d) in a case of diabetic proliferative iridopathy with new* →

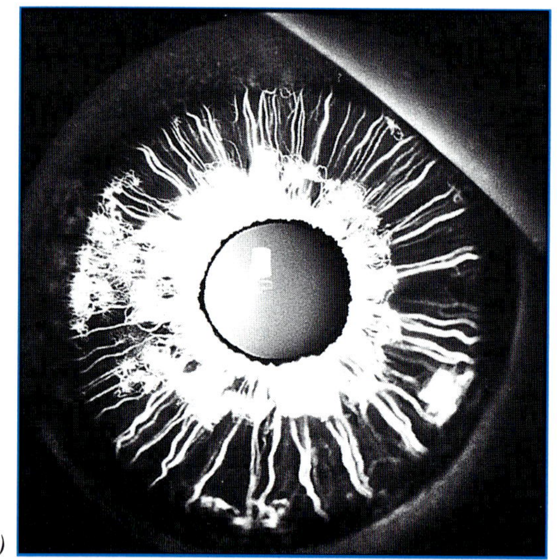

a)

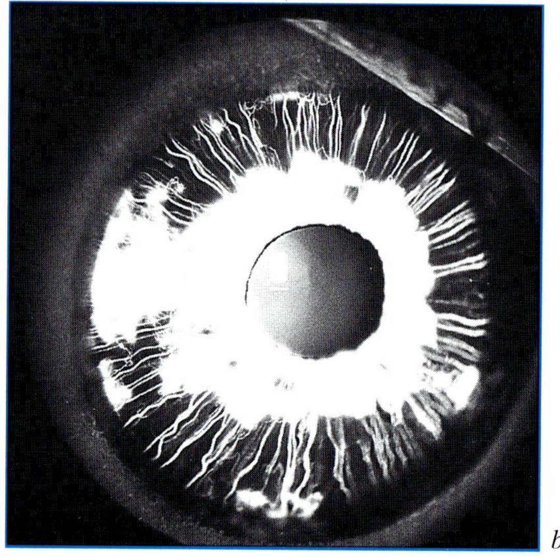

b)

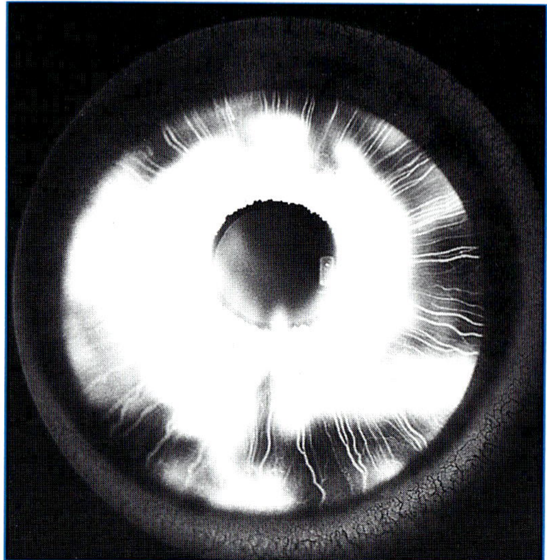

c)

*Fig. **4.3**,23 - Another iris fluorescein angiographic picture of proliferative iridopathy in a patient with retinal angiomatosis. The early phases (a) are essential markers of the precise site and extent of neovascular growth. In this case the conspicuous new vessels at the margin partly merge with those starting from the iris root. Dye leakage from the anomalous vessels subsequently covers (b) all the neovascular network and in the later phase (c) involves the whole of the anterior chamber.*

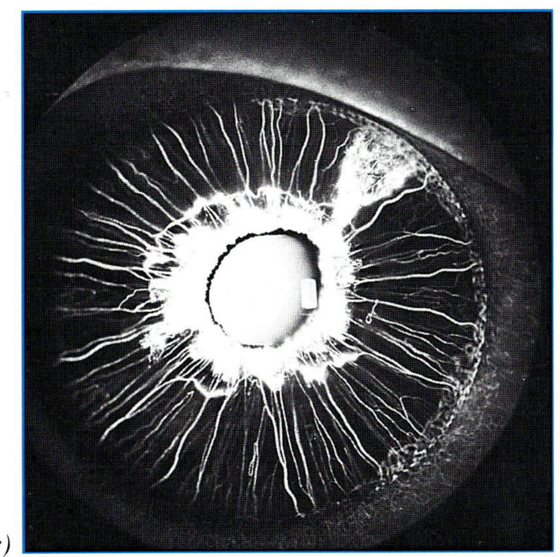
c)

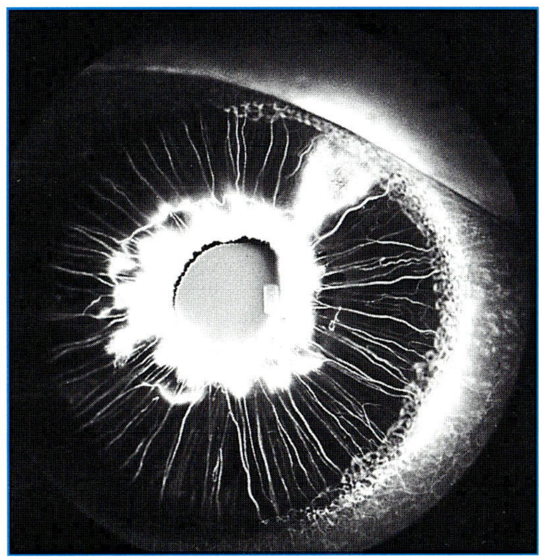
d)

vessels throughout the pars pupillaris and in a segment of the superior ciliary portion.
←

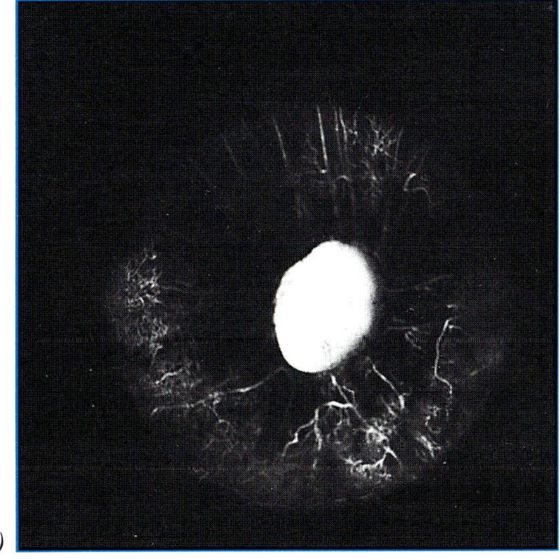
a)

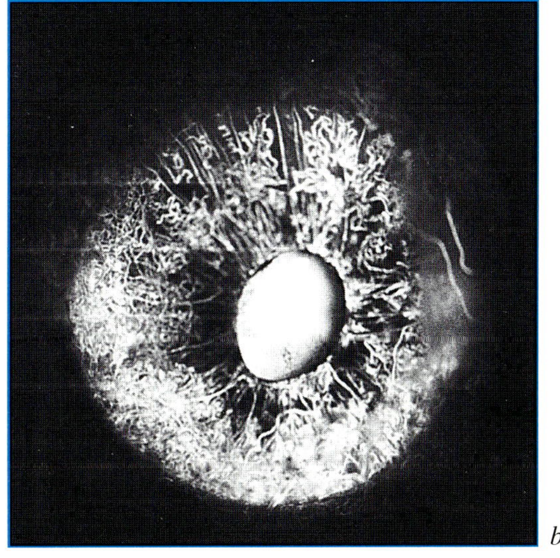
b)

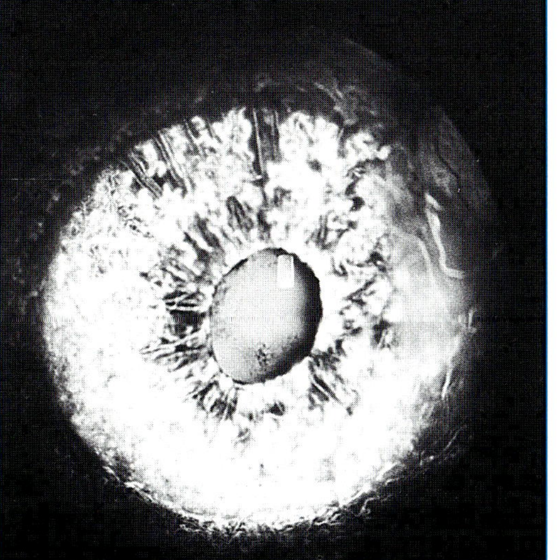
c)

Fig. ***4.3****,24 - New vessels over the whole surface of the iris in a diabetic patient; iris fluorescein angiographic filling phases (a,b,c).*

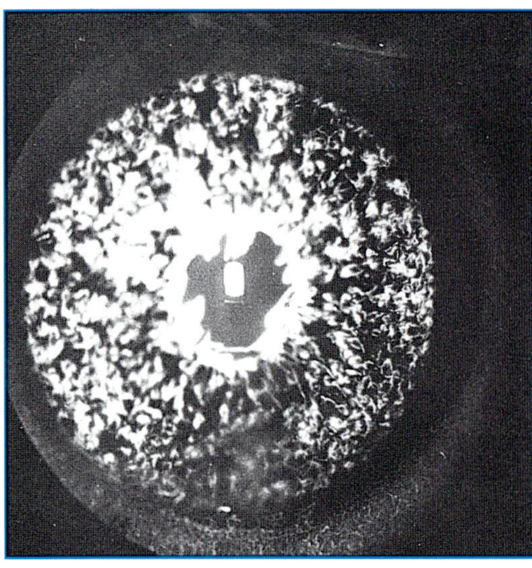

*Fig. **4.3**,25 - Iris fluorescein angiography showing marked rubeosis of the pupillary margin and stroma in a patient with anterior uveitis.*

a) 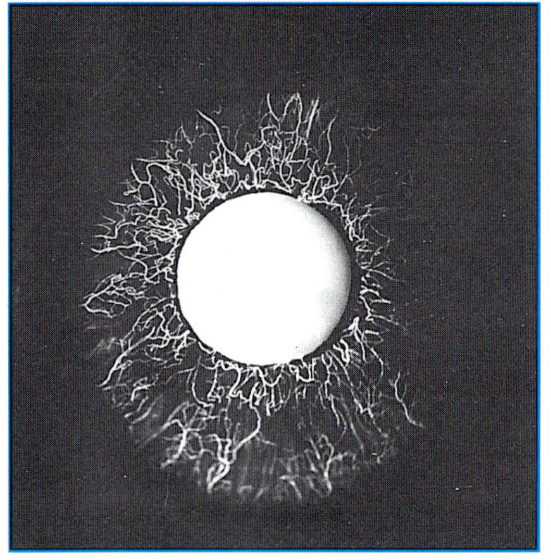

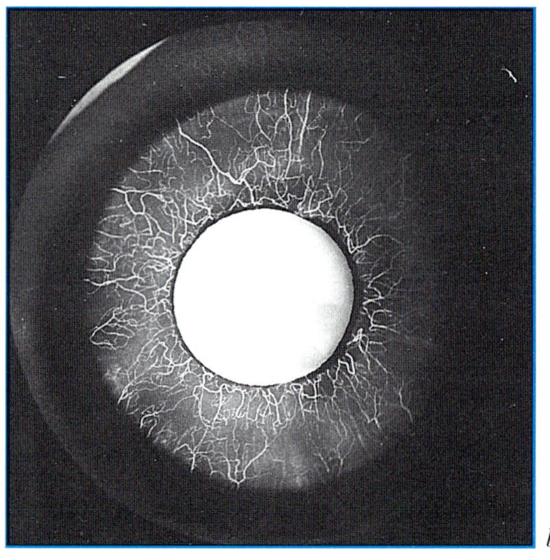 *b)*

*Fig. **4.3**,26 - Early (a) and late (b) iris fluorescein angiographic phases in a patient with central retinal vein occlusion with ischemic capillaropathy. The pattern of iris vessels is upturned and they are replaced by a fine, intricate network of vessels running anomalously, with no dye leakage.*

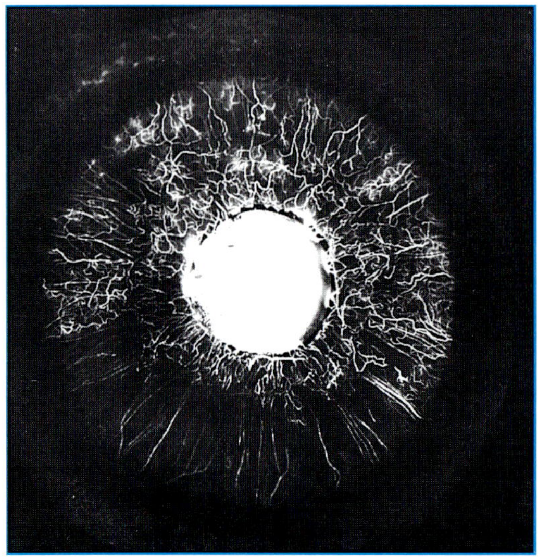

*Fig. **4.3**,27 - Another iris fluorescein angiographic picture from a case of central retinal vein occlusion. Only the vessels in the lower sectors of the ciliary part appear normal. In the remainder of the iris the vessels are anarchic and there are small hyperfluorescent spots due to neovascular tufts.*

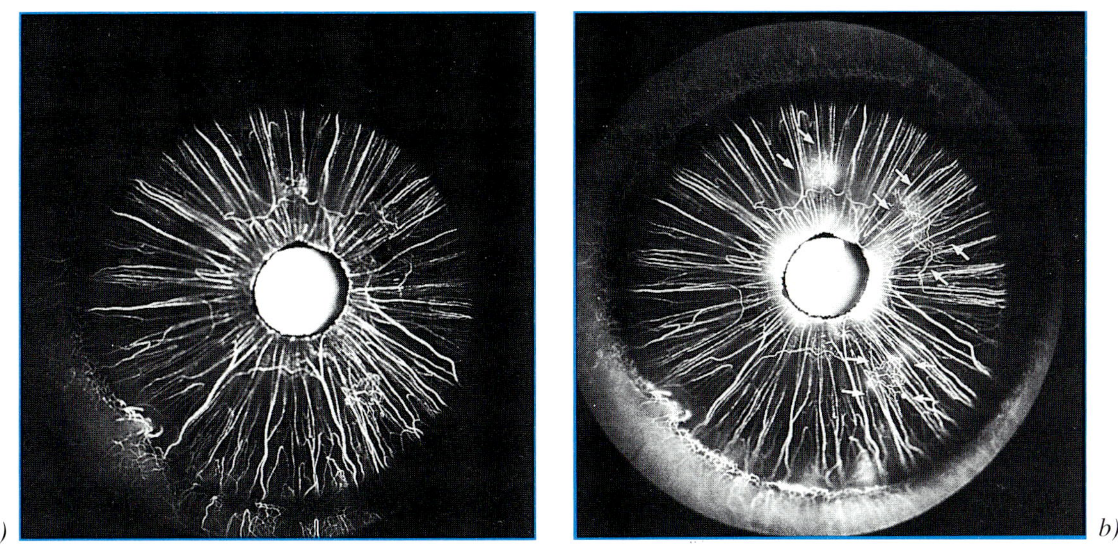

a) b)

*Fig. **4.3**,28 - Iris fluorescein angiographic phases in a patient with diabetes mellitus. Anomalous vascular tufts can be seen (arrows), taking up dye early (a) and leaking it to a limited extent in later phases (b). These could be interpreted as impending neovascular tufts or alterations preceding the onset of overt rubeosis iridis.*

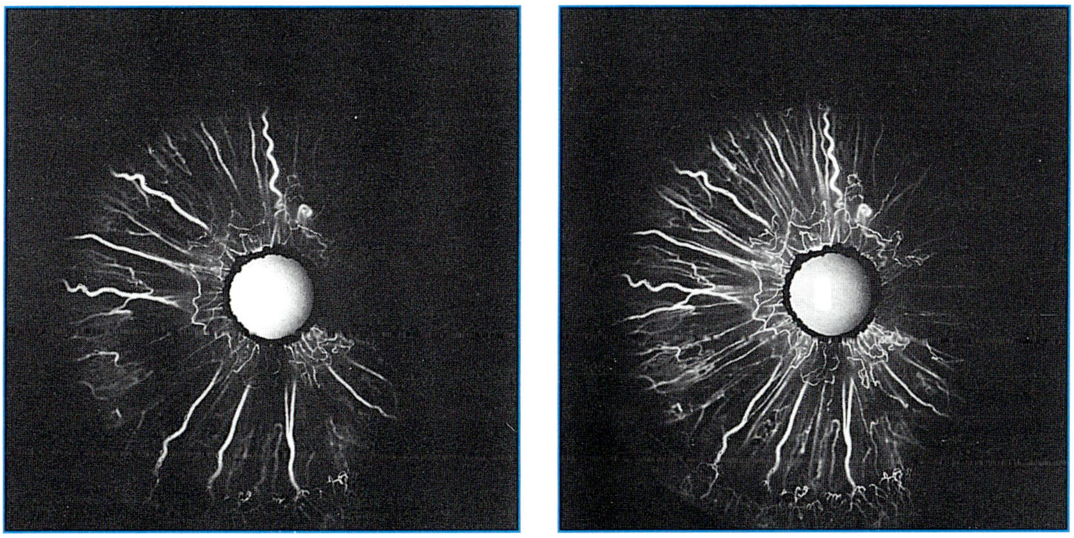

a) b)

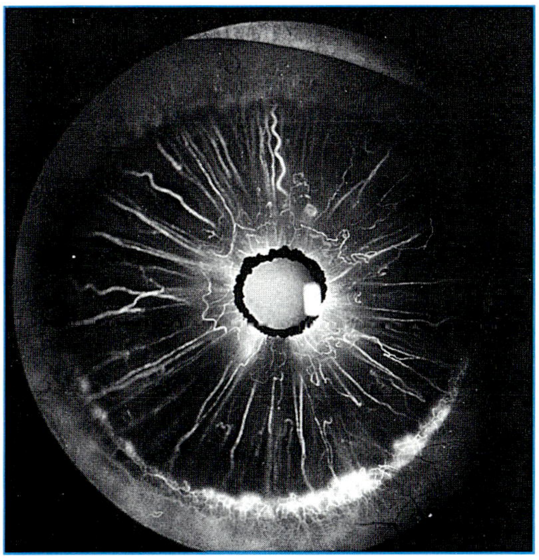

c)

*Fig. **4.3**,29 - Iris fluorescein angiographic examination (phases: a,b,c) in a patient with diabetes mellitus. Filling delays and anomalous radial vessels (dilated or smaller than normal) were seen, and branches of the minor arterial circle of the iris. Pupillary leakage was mainly from the border (c) and was partially masked by ectropion uveae.*

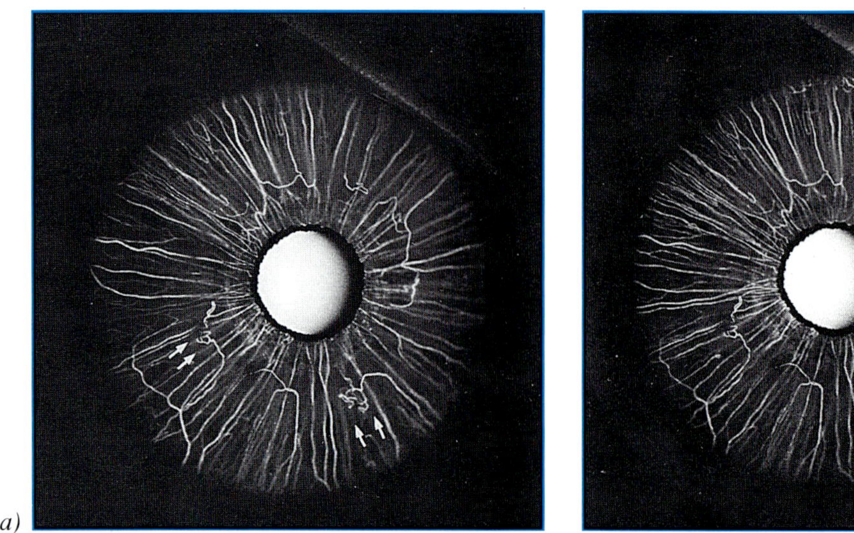

a) b)

*Fig. **4.3**,30 - Iris fluorescein angiographic examination (a, early phase; b, late phase) shows morphological and dynamic anomalies in the iris vessels, not detectable by other techniques. In this case the minor arterial circle of the iris is not complete and has small arborizing branchlets (small arrows), with increased vascular permeability in one circumscribed segment (large arrow).*

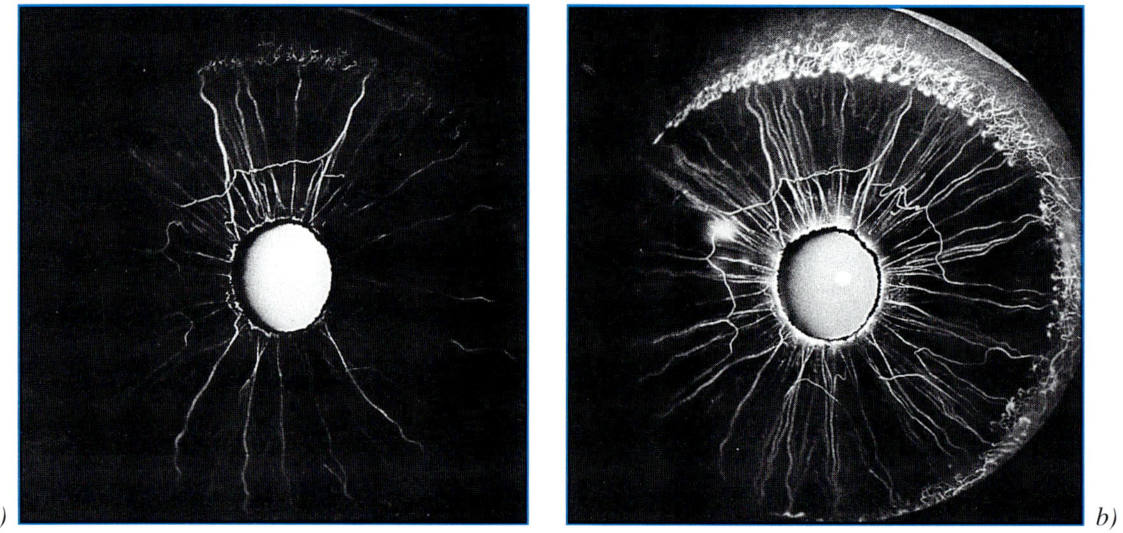

a) b)

*Fig. **4.3**,31 - Hyperfluorescence from iris vessels (b) is not always detectable at the earlier angiographic times (a).*

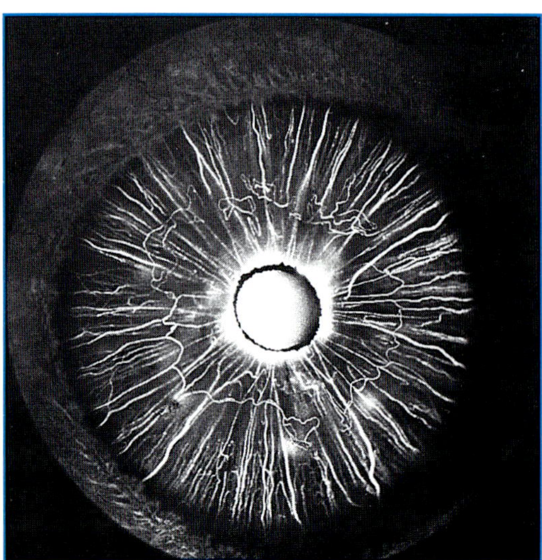

*Fig. **4.3**,32 - Another case of pupillary and extrapupillary dye leakage. Pupillary margin leakage may simply be age-related but rupture of the blood-iris barrier of stromal vessels is always pathological.*

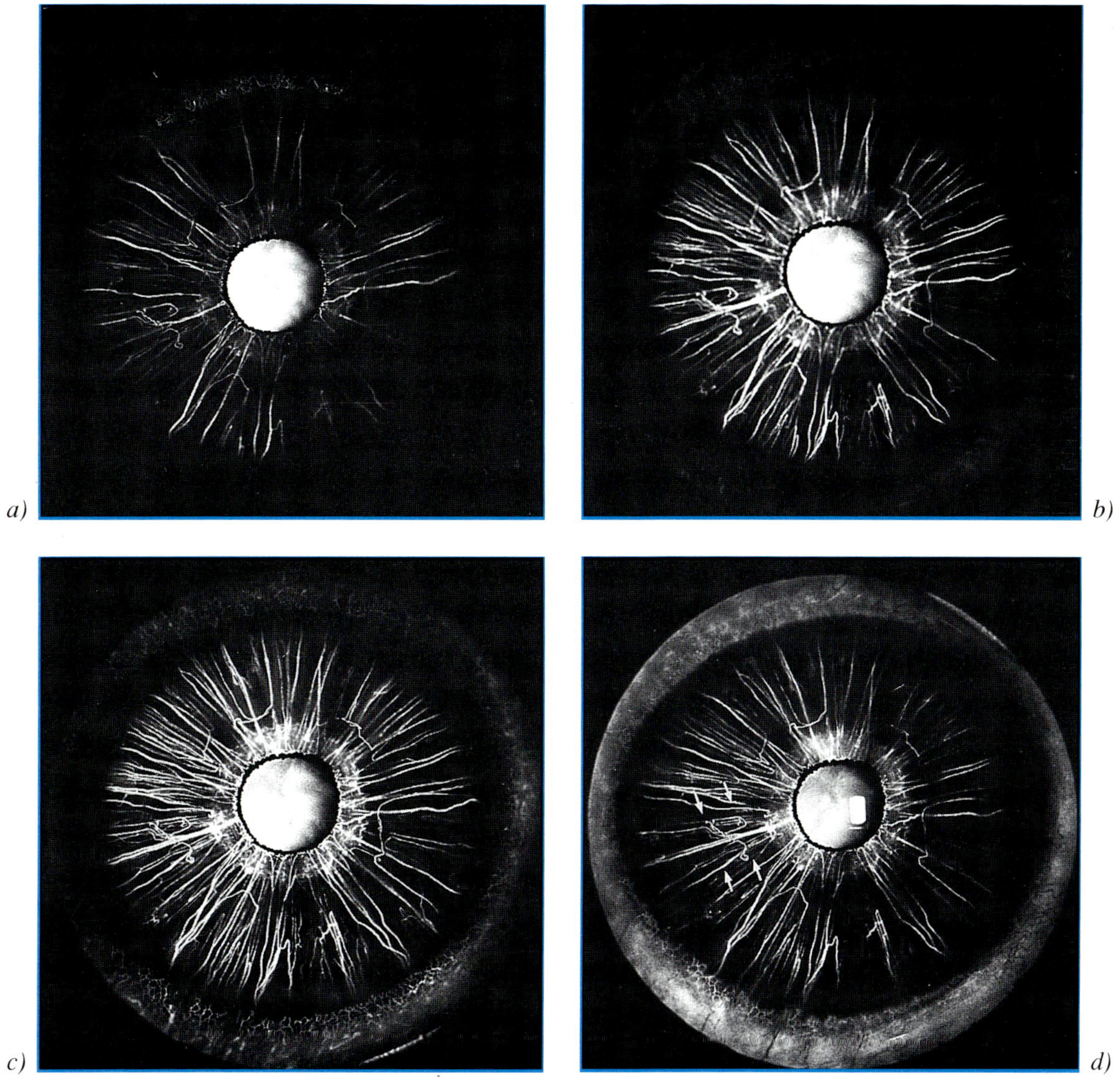

*Fig. **4.3**,33 - Anomalous vascular tangle (arrows) with scant dye leakage. Some increase in vascular permeability is seen in the pupillary portion (filling phases: a,b,c,d).*

R. Brancato, F. Bandello, R. Lattanzio
Atlas of Iris
Fluorescein Angiography
Kugler & Ghedini Publications 1995

Chapter 4.4

Diabetic microangiopathy

Among the systemic diseases that can cause problems in the eyes, diabetes mellitus is the most important, on account of the frequency and the severity of the lesions it causes. The consequences of vascular complications are the main cause of the high morbidity associated with this disease. Diabetic vascular diseases affect not only the large and medium-caliber vessels, but even the small vessels in all organs, causing the specific lesions of diabetic microangiopathy. In the eyes, microangiopathy gives rise to diabetic retinopathy - well known - but also to diabetic iridopathy.

Vascular changes in the iris, of varying degrees of severity, are frequent in diabetic patients and a study by Demeler and Sautter in 1978 estimated them at around 92% by fluoroiridography.[(47)] This extremely high proportion included a large percentage (67%) of patients who only presented dye leakage to the pupillary margin but, as has already been noted, this can be considered physiological in subjects over 40 years old.

In 1928 Salus[(119)] coined the term *rubeosis iridis* to define iris neovascularization. He was not its discoverer, though, as at the start of this century it was already considered a terminal ocular sign in long-standing diabetics.

How frequently rubeosis iridis is recognised depends on the diagnostic method employed. The mean prevalence observed with the biomicroscope varies in different studies from 1 to 17% among unselected diabetic patients.[(5,111,129)] The percentages are much higher among patients who already have proliferative diabetic retinopathy.[(95,96,97,111)]

In a study in Lombardia (Italy), the prevalence of rubeosis iridis was 1.7% in a sample of 1162 subjects extracted by randomisation from a total population of 17704 diabetics, as representative of all the strata of duration of the disease (Fig.**4.4**,1).[(60)]

Rubeosis iridis is found much more frequently by fluorescence angiography of the iris. This method shows up iris neovessels well before they can be detected with the biomicroscope (Fig.**4.4**,2).[(13,79,80,101,102,103)]

Rubeosis iridis is by no means the only problem afflicting the diabetic iris. Alterations may range from simple rupture of the blood-retinal barrier to neovessels in the pupillary border or stroma, or both, and from there on to the devastating situation of neovascular glaucoma.[(37)] Iris fluorescein angiography gives a precise picture of the morphology and vascular dynamics of iris vessels; it shows up vascular anomalies and alterations to permeability that are hard to assess biomicroscopically (Figs. **4.4**,3-5).

In 1968 Jensen and Lundbaek were the first to use this method to analyse the early stages of diabetic iridopathy, and reported that dye leakage was observed in long-standing diabetic patients long before any new vessels could be seen in the iris with the biomicroscope.[(79,80)] Ehrenberg[(51)] and Bandello[(13)] subsequently confirmed that iris fluorescein angiography shows up diabetic iridopathy in a much higher percentage of cases than the biomicroscope.

Iris angiographic studies to date all report a high prevalence of various alterations to the iris among diabetic patients; only Deodati[48] found completely normal iris angiograms in a large number of diabetic subjects.

Biomicroscopic findings of rubeosis iridis

Biomicroscopic findings in rubeosis iridis can be divided into three stages.[62]

In the *first stage*, close observation shows initial ectasia and neovascular tufts distributed separately in various zones of the pupillary border (Figs. **4.4**,6,7) and, sometimes, at the irido-corneal angle (Fig. **4.4**,8). The new vessels, visible on the anterior surface of the iris, are thin-walled and the blood can be seen flowing inside them. They appear as fine, tortuous, red streaks, running irregularly over the surface of the iris, in contrast with the uniform, deeper paths of the normal vessels (Fig. **4.4**,9).

In the *second stage* the neovessel tufts tend to become more extensive and confluent (Fig. **4.4**,10). Connective tissue proliferates to support them, giving rise to areas of atrophy in the iris; as this extends over the anterior surface of the iris, it gives it a smooth, flat look.

In the *third stage*, peripheral anterior synechiae gradually develop, completely closing off the aqueous humor drainage system, thus giving rise to neovascular glaucoma. The newly formed fibrovascular tissue, with its rich content of myofibroblasts, retracts, deforming the pupillary margin until it assumes a position of fixed mid-midriasis (Fig. **4.4**,11). Atrophy of the dilator and sphincter muscles has been demonstrated. The iris loses its sphincter function, the posterior pigment epithelium is drawn toward the anterior surface of the iris, until it becomes visible as a fine dark band around the border (ectropion uveae) (Fig. **4.4**,12). A vascular membrane may even form in the pupil, eventually occluding it (Fig. **4.4**,13). Once this stage has been reached, in 25% of cases rupture of a newly formed vessel may lead to hyphema (Fig.**4.4**,14).[62] This explains why neovascular glaucoma used in the past to be known as "hemorrhagic glaucoma".[75]

In their anatomical structure, the new vessels vary in diameter, sometimes being larger than normal iris vessels. Unlike arteries and normal veins, these vessels' walls are made up of only a fine endothelial layer, with no or only very little adventitia. Electron microscopy shows there is a thick basement membrane and small spaces between one endothelial cell and the next. This is one reason why the new vessels are so highly permeable to fluorescein (Fig.**4.4**,15).[112,127]

Iris fluorescein angiographic classification of diabetic iridopathy

Cited here are some of the most widely used classifications proposed for iris fluorescein angiographic findings in diabetic iridopathy.

Friedurg's classification:[60]

Grade 1	leakage from the pupillary border
Grade 2	stromal leakage
Grade 3	neovascularization of the iris

Zakov-Lewis's classification:[137]

Grade 0	no fluorescein leakage
Grade 1	leakage from the pupillary border
Grade 2	profuse leakage (at the pupillary sphincter, the dye passing into the anterior chamber in 5 min)
Grade 3	neovascular tufts (rubeosis) at the pupillary sphincter and in 1-2 quadrants of the stroma, with leakage and staining of stromal vessels
Grade 4	neovascularization of the pupillary sphincter and in 3-4 quadrants of the stroma.

Laatikainen's classification:[88]

Grade 1	dilatations of the peripupillary vessels with dye leakage
Grade 2	early neovascularization mainly in the anterior chamber angle
Grade 3	prominent rubeosis with or without neovascular glaucoma (arborizing new vessels are more prominent and grow out of the angle covering more of the iris surface)
Grade 4	florid rubeosis.

Moyenin-Bonnet's classification:[106]

Grade 0	no dye leakage
Grade 1	leakage from the pupillary border into 1-2 quadrants, but not to the stroma
Grade 2	leakage from the pupillary border into 3-4 quadrants, but not to the stroma
Grade 3	leakage from all around the pupillary border and stromal spread in 1-2 quadrants
Grade 4	leakage from all around the pupillary border and stromal spread in 3-4 quadrants.

Ehremberg's classification:[51]

Grade 0	no iris new vessels
Grade 1	neovascular tufts in 1-2 quadrants of the pupillary sphincter
Grade 2	neovascular tufts in 3-4 quadrants of the pupillary sphincter
Grade 3	neovascularization in 1-2 quadrants of the stroma of the iris
Grade 4	neovascularization in 3-4 quadrants of the stroma of the iris
Grade 5	diffuse new vessel formation in the stroma of the iris with neovascular glaucoma.

Brancato's classification:[37]

Non-proliferative diabetic iridopathy (exudative diabetic iridopathy)

Grade 0	no dye leakage
Grade 1	leakage from the pupillary border (mild exudative iridopathy)
Grade 2	leakage from the border and from stromal vessels (marked exudative iridopathy)

Proliferative diabetic iridopathy (Fig. **4.4**,16)

Grade 0	no neovascularization
Grade 1	neovascularization at the pupillary border
Grade 2	neovascularization at the border and on the surface of the iris (stroma and iridocorneal angle)
Grade 3	neovascular glaucoma.

None of the iris angiographic anomalies listed can actually be considered pathognomonic of diabetic iridopathy as they are all seen in many other systemic and ocular pathologies. As mentioned earlier, it is physiological for an elderly subject to present dye leakage at the pupillary border, and this cannot be distinguished from the leakage caused by initial diabetic microangiopathy. The iris angiographic picture of neovascular glaucoma in advanced proliferative diabetic iridopathy is likewise comparable to that encountered in other pathologies that present extensive areas of retinal nonperfusion - as we shall see later. Iris angiographic alterations must thus be assessed carefully, taking account of all the patient's other data (history and clinical findings) so as to establish correctly which kind of iris lesion is related to the diabetes.

It is worth stressing that iris alterations arising during diabetes only lead to neovascular glaucoma in a small percentage of cases. The epidemiological study we conducted in Lombardia, referred to earlier, found a prevalence of 0.5% of neovascular glaucoma.[(60)] The various grades of diabetic iridopathy should thus not be considered as stages of development leading inevitably to neovascular glaucoma. They should be viewed more as alterations correlated with the diabetes and often also with the retinopathy,[(31,38,98)] which may get worse, but which may remain stationary or even regress (Figs. **4.4**,17,18). Regression in particular may be achieved in response to well-planned treatment of retinal lesions.

There are no estimates of the iris fluorescein angiographic prevalence of rubeosis iridis in the diabetic population. The only published data suffer major limitations arising from the selection of patients. Demeler, for example, in an iris angiographic study on 75 diabetic patients, found that 23.6% of the cases presented rubeosis iridis.[(47)] The prevalence of proliferative diabetic retinopathy among these same subjects (usually associated with iris neovascularization) reached 41%, i.e. much higher than the real prevalence of proliferative retinopathy in an unselected diabetic population (7.3%).[(60)]

Baggesen[(11)] estimated the iris fluorescein angiographic prevalence of rubeosis at 32.9% in a population of 82 diabetics with mean age 38.5 years and mean duration of the disease 15.4 years. However, the prevalence of the various forms of concomitant diabetic retinopathy in this population was not specified.

Bilateral rubeosis diagnosed by iris fluorescein angiography has been reported on various occasions, with different frequencies: 5%;[(75)] 8.6%;[(97)] 28.5%[(40)] and 76%.[(110)] The striking differences are probably related to differences in the populations considered. Iris neovascularization in both eyes should always alert the examiner to the possibility of a diabetic pathogenesis[(62)] since few other causes give rise to bilateral lesions.

Iris fluorescein angiographic alterations in non-proliferative diabetic iridopathy

Dye leakage at the pupillary border

The mildest vascular lesion likely to be seen in the iris of patients with diabetes mellitus is dilated peripupillary capillaries which let the dye leak through, giving rise to slight, short-lasting fluorescence around the pupil (Figs. **4.4**,19,20). Once the dye bolus has passed through, the hyperfluorescence at the border tends to diminish and disappear, a diffuse veil remaining in the anterior chamber. This is due to endothelial alteration in the capillaries of the pars pupillaris, which causes peripupillary leakage similar to that seen in the elderly. These are, however, isolated alterations of capillary permeability, due to non-specific lesions to the vessel wall. At the same age, though, this lesion is more frequent among diabetic than normal subjects.[11] Peripupillary dye leakage is not seen in young patients with recent diabetes. There are unfortunately no studies analysing how long it takes for this alteration to appear.

Peripupillary leakage is the initial, most benign and frequent form of diabetic iridopathy, and has sometimes been defined diabetic iridopathy "simplex".[47] This alteration is often associated with irregular or slow filling of the radial arteries (Fig. **4.4**,21), but at this stage there are no areas of the iris that fail to fill.[88,89]

Leakage from the pupillary border is seen in from 67%[47] to 92%[1] of diabetic patients, according to different reports. It is worth noting that in the second caselist the patients' mean age was well below 50 years so clearly the vascular anomaly was not due to old age.

Leakage from the pupillary border is seen in 77% of diabetic patients without retinopathy, and it is mostly a non-proliferative form among those with retinopathy. All cases with proliferative diabetic retinopathy present pupillary border leakage but only in 6% of these cases is it the sole sign of alteration to the iris - there are almost always more serious anomalies.[1] Another study,[11] on the other hand, claims this alteration is to be found in 46% of patients with diabetic retinopathy, regardless of the grade.

Leakage at the pupillary border is thus not a serious alteration, and is generally seen in not too severe cases of diabetic retinopathy (without vast ischemic areas on the retina). It may remain unchanged for years and does not usually represent an immediate risk of neovascular glaucoma.

Dye leakage at the pupillary border and stroma of the iris

More marked dye leakage at the pupillary border and from the stromal vessels too indicates more serious vascular impairment (Fig. **4.4**,22).[11] Extrapupillary leakage is always pathological, and is never seen in an iris angiogram from a normal subject.[83] Ehremberg maintains that stromal leakage of this type is an indicator of the risk of development towards more severe forms of diabetic iridopathy (Fig. **4.4**,23).[51]

Iris fluorescein angiographic alterations in proliferative diabetic iridopathy

Neovascularization at the pupillary border

Small vascular "buds" around the pupillary border, not detectable with the biomicroscope, filling rapidly with dye and leaking equally promptly and diffusely, are early expressions of neovascularization, characteristic of proliferative diabetic iridopathy (Figs. **4.4**,24-27). These new-formed vessels must be analysed in the early angiographic phases, before they are hidden by dye leakage (Fig. **4.4**,28). The early stages in the iris angiogram are important for distinguishing the alterations typical of the first stages of diabetic iridopathy (e.g., pupillary border leakage) from actual processes of neovascularization.

The new vessels start at the pupillary border and form a tangled web running out in all directions towards the periphery of the iris. They look like fluorescent dots and streaks, becoming gradually larger and more intense, until they close up - completely or not - in a glowing ring around the pupillary border (Figs. **4.4**,29,30). Larger neovascular networks around the pupillary border, visible with the biomicroscope, may give rise to highly visible dye fluorescence and leakage in the iris angiogram (Figs. **4.4**,31-34).

Peripupillary neovascular buds are characteristic of, though not specific to diabetes. They have also been described as isolated findings or in other ocular and systemic diseases (Fig. **4.4**,35).

Neovascularization at the pupillary border and stroma of the iris

In the more advanced stages of rubeosis iridis the new vessels, of increasing caliber, form an irregular network that tends to spread gradually over the anterior surface of the iris (Figs. **4.4**,36-42). These new vessels differ from normal radial vessels in that they form a tortuous, irregular path (Figs. **4.4**,43,44), and fluorescein leaks through promptly into the anterior chamber, making it impossible to see the iris vessels in later angiographic stages (Figs. **4.4**,45-48).

New vessels can be seen even in a hyperpigmented iris as they are nearer to the surface than the stroma, which only partially impedes the view of their characteristic hyperfluorescence (Figs. **4.4**,49-52).

As neovascular proliferation progresses, the radial vessels, particularly the arteries, start to become tortuous too and leak dye.[88] Marked, generalized leakage is often seen from the radial vessels, preceding or coinciding with neovascular glaucoma (Figs. **4.4**,53-55).

Neovascularization at the iridocorneal angle

New vessels are considered by some authors[88] to start at the angle, near the iris root. At this level they can be seen sooner with the gonioscope and even better by using the gonioscopic lens during angiographic examination (Fig. **4.4**,55). In the early stages the angle remains mostly open and intraocular pressure is normal; the new vessels, however, increasingly take over the angle which gradually closes (Figs. **4.4**,56-63).

Neovascular glaucoma

With the onset of neovascular glaucoma the already severe picture described for proliferative diabetic iridopathy is aggravated by irreversible intraocular hypertension (Figs. **4.4**,64-68).

Rupture of a newly formed vessel may give rise to hyphema which, depending on its severity, may cause varying degrees of masking in the iris angiogram (Fig **4.4**,69). Iris fluorescein angiography cannot identify the stage immediately preceding the onset of hypertension, but marked, diffuse iris leakage, or the clinical finding of pupillary retractions, ectropion uveae, or hyperplasia of the pigment epithelium, are all poor prognostic signs.[83]

Iris fluorescein angiographic circulation times in diabetic patients

No significant differences have been found between the arm-iris and artero-venous iris angiographic circulation times in diabetic and normal subjects.[11] However, the time between fluorescence appearing in the anulus major and in the pupillary border is significantly shorter in diabetics,[11,60,120] more so in patients with vascular leakage than those without, or without retinopathy. In rubeosis iridis the iris arterial filling time is reduced from 3.8 sec. ± 1.0 to 2.5 sec. ± 1.2.[83]

Thus, whereas angiographic circulation times in the retina are increased in rubeosis, in the iris the rate of perfusion seems to be accelerated.[60,120] It thus appears that the hemodynamics of the iris are related more to local factors than to the systemic diabetic vasculopathy.

Relations between iris angiographic findings, patient's age and type and duration of diabetes mellitus

Analysis of the iris fluorescein angiographic patterns in relation to various parameters in a diabetic patient shows that dye leakage from the iris increases linearly with age.[11] The graphic **4.4**,I illustrates this relationship between the iris neovascularization and age, as found in an iris angiographic study on 100 eyes in 78 diabetic patients.[31]

The patient's age has a significant effect on the incidence and severity of iris neovascularization.[31] The high prevalence of proliferative diabetic iridopathy in the population considered in this study was related to the type of concomitant retinopathy (ischemic with or without papillary and/or retinal proliferation). A higher incidence of rubeosis iridis and its more advanced stages was seen among type II diabetes patients, who generally tend to be older than type I patients.[31]

There are nevertheless some authors[47] who maintain that diabetic iridopathy is not related to the patient's age. Some find a significant correlation between rubeosis iridis and the duration of the disease.[11,12,47]

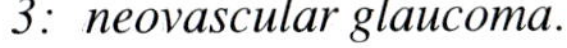

*Graphic **4.4**,I - Relation between iris neovascularization and patient's age.*
0: no neovascularization
1: neovascularization of the pupillary border
2: neovascularization of the pupillary border and surface of the iris
3: neovascular glaucoma.

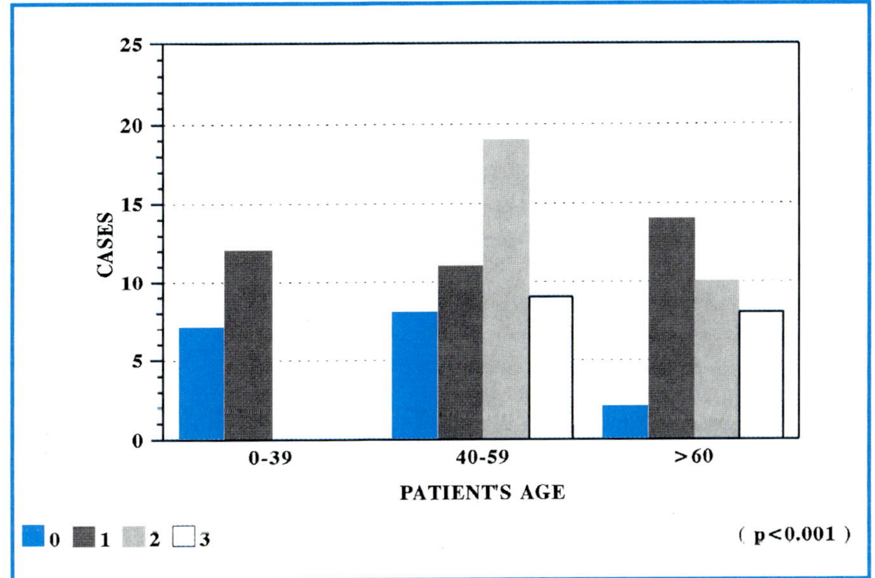

Relation between iridopathy and diabetic retinopathy

The most interesting correlation is between iridopathy and diabetic retinopathy. Patients with retinopathy - according to some reports[47] - generally have some degree of iridopathy. Others, however, have observed patients with iridopathy but no ophthalmoscopically detectable retinopathy.[1] It thus appears that the iris and retinal lesions do not appear in synchrony and that in rare cases the former may precede the latter.[47] Iris fluorescein angiography, by showing up iris alterations unlikely to be detected with the biomicroscope, provides an early indication of vascular lesions due to diabetes mellitus.[47]

Patients without retinopathy may have non-proliferative iridopathy; those with non-proliferative retinopathy mainly presented comparable iris alterations, whereas patients with retinal neovascularization may present either proliferative or non-proliferative iridopathy.[1,47]

Rubeosis iridis and proliferative diabetic retinopathy are often associated. The incidence of iris neovascularization is high in patients with ischemic and proliferative retinal alterations.[29,31,38,40,75,95,96,97,98,109,110,124] The incidence of clinically appreciable rubeosis in patients with proliferative diabetic retinopathy is assessed differently in various studies, ranging from 29%,[137] to 43%[95-97] and even 60%.[108,111]

The prevalence is clearly even higher when the diagnosis is based on iris angiographic findings. A study of 100 eyes with ischemic diabetic retinopathy, with or without papillary and/or retinal proliferation, studied by this technique, found 83% had neovascularization of the iris .[31] In the same study, with the aim of assessing the relation between ischemic diabetic retinopathy and iris neovascularization, the angiographically detectable lesions to the iris were assessed in relation to the extent of retinal ischemia in the corresponding retinal angiography. Retinal ischemia was divided arbitrarily into three stages of severity (Fig. **4.4**,70):[31]

1) grade 1: peripheral ischemia up to the vorticose veins;
2) grade 2: peripheral ischemia up to the temporal vascular arcades;
3) grade 3: ischemia extending from the periphery right into the vascular arcades.

This investigation found a significant correlation between the extent of retinal ischemic damage and the severity of iris neovascularization (see Fig. **4.4**,16). In the eyes classified as group 3 the more advanced stages of diabetic iridopathy were more frequent, up to neovascular glaucoma (Graphic **4.4**,II).

This study also found:

1) a significant relation between neovascularization of the optic disc and rubeosis iridis;
2) a non-significant correlation between retinal neovascularization and rubeosis iridis.[31]

It must be borne in mind that patients frequently present ischemic or proliferative diabetic retinopathy without neovascular glaucoma.[89,95-97] In conclusion, therefore, there is a close relation between the new vessels of the iris and the extent of retinal ischemia which, in turn, appears responsible for the onset of retinal and papillary neovascularization.[116]

*Graphic **4.4**,2 - Relationship between retinal ischemia and rubeosis iridis.*

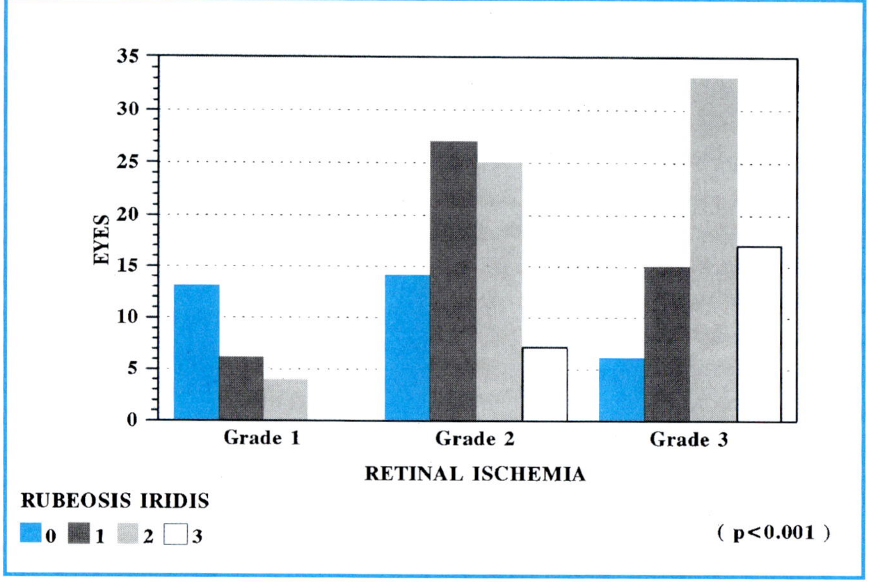

In order to assess the relationship between diabetic iris and retinal microangiopathy, we evaluated 225 eyes of 117 diabetic patients without dioptric media opacities.[14] Each patient underwent an iris and retinal fluorescein angiography. The angiograms were used to classify each eye according to the degree of diabetic iridopathy and diabetic retinopathy present.

The diabetic iridopathy classification employed was as follows:
1) absence of diabetic iridopathy (NoDI);
2) non-proliferative diabetic iridopathy (NPDI);
3) proliferative diabetic iridopathy (PDI);
4) neovascular glaucoma (NVG).

The diabetic retinopathy classification was as follows:
1) absence of diabetic retinopathy (NoDR);
2) background diabetic retinopathy (BDR);
3) pre-proliferative diabetic retinopathy(PPDR);
4) proliferative diabetic retinopathy (PDR).

The results of our study are summarized in the tables **4.4**,I, II. The sensivity of iris flu-

Table 4.4,I: Relationship between DI groups and DR groups in all the patients of the study

	NoDI		NPDI		PDI		NVG		Total	
	n.	%	n.	%	n.	%	n.	%	n.	%
NoDR	44	31	6	43	0	0	0	0	50	22
BDR	48	34	2	15	0	0	0	0	50	22
PPDR	29	21	3	21	25	37	0	0	57	26
PDR	20	14	3	21	43	63	2	100	68	30
Total	141	100	14	100	68	100	2	100	225	100

Table 4.4,II: Relationship between serious forms of DI and serious forms of DR in the study group

	NoDI/NPDI		PDI/NVG		Total	
	n.	%	n.	%	n.	%
NoDR/BDR	100	65	0	0	100	44
PPDR/PDR	55	35	70	100	125	56
Total	155	100	70	100	225	100

orescein angiography in detecting and assessing diabetic retinopathy of any level turned out to be 44.5%, the specificity 88%, the positive predictive value 92.8%, and the negative value 31.2%. Fluoroiridographic detection of iris new vessels turned out to have a sensitivity of 56% and a specificity of 100% in the assessment of pre-proliferative and proliferative diabetic retinopathy. The positive predictive value was 100% and the negative value 65%.

We used also iris fluorescein angiography as gold-standard against which to test the ability of iris biomicroscopy to show up diabetic iridopathy.[13] One hundred and forteen eyes of 63 diabetic patients affected by pre-proliferative or proliferative diabetic retinopathy (the diabetic retinopathy groups with a high risk of developing diabetic iridopathy) were considered.

The diabetic iridopathy fluorangiographic classification used was as follows:
1) absence of diabetic iridopathy (NoDI);
2) non-proliferative diabetic iridopathy (NPDI);
3) proliferative diabetic iridopathy (PDI).

The results of this study are summarized in the table **4.4**,III. The sensitivity of biomi-

Table 4.4,III: Relationship between biomicroscopic and fluorescein angiographic findings

Iris fluorescein angiography	Biomicoscopy				Total	
	No new vessels		New vessels			
	n.	%	n.	%	n.	%
NoDI	33	50	2	4	35	31
NPDI	7	11	1	2	8	7
PDI	26	39	45	94	71	62
Total	66	100	48	100	114	100

croscopy in detecting diabetic iridopathy turned out to be 57%, while the specificity was 94%. The positive predictive value was 93% and the negative predictive value 50%.

Our study proved that biomicroscopy accurately detects when diabetic iridopathy is absent; when this pathology is present, however, there is a high probability that the biomicroscopic test will be less precise in the detection of iris lesions.

Pathogenesis of rubeosis iridis

Further research is still needed to clarify the pathogenesis of rubeosis iridis, but various theories have been proposed. The most plausible one suggests that the causal factor is a vasoactive substance produced by the retina in conditions of hypoxia.[8,9,61,99,115,126,134] Though still not identified, this substance has been suggested as the cause of neovascular proliferation in various pathologies, all involving ischemic damage to the retina. This angiogenic factor, spreading anteriorly through the vitreous, subsequently causes new vessels formation in the iris as well as the retina.

Despite much research[2,3,4,15,16,18,19,63,66,67,76,77,121,123] the nature of this proposed substance remains to be elucidated, and no satisfactory experimental model is yet available.[24,56,57,64] There is ample evidence in its favour, starting with the higher incidence of iris neovascularization among patients operated for vitrectomy or cataract removal (and among the latter iris new vessels seem more frequent after intracapsular than extracapsular extraction).[62,65,113,137] These findings suggested that the vitreous and lens may serve as a barrier to the passage of the vasoproliferative factor from the posterior to the anterior segment of the eye.[20,21,104] A factor has in fact been identified in the vitreous that inhibits neovascularization.[18,19,39,66,68]

This theory thus considers retinal and iris neovascular proliferation as two consequences of the action of the same vasoformative substance.

As already mentioned, dye leakage and iris new vessel formation like the pattern seen in diabetes mellitus have also been reported in patients with ischemic of the Central Retinal Vein Occlusion (CRVO)[43,90,131] and Central Retinal Artery Occlusion (CRAO).[82,83,84] This is another point in favour of a correlation between ischemia of the posterior segment of the eye and iris neovascularization.[89] One more definitely important point in this regard is the time it takes for retinal ischemic damage to occur. When it happens fast, as in CRVO, the probability of neovascularization is less. The risk is in fact higher in ischemic diabetic retinopathy and CRVO with ischemic capillaropathy.[83]

Schulze[121] criticises the theory of a vasoformative factor of retinal origin, pointing out that the neovascular development should in that case extend toward zones where the concentration of the factor is highest, i.e. the posterior segment of the eye. Schulze therefore postulates that it is ischemia not of the retina but of the iris itself that causes the iris neovascularization.

It is in fact sometimes possible by iris fluorescein angiography to identify a process of ischemia of the iris accompanying the neovascularization (Fig. **4.4**,71).[31] This would agree with the observations reported by Morone et al. who used this technique to investigate preparations of uvea from diabetic subjects, and found unperfused areas in the iris. These ischemic areas may thus act as stimuli for new vessels proliferation, as happens in the retina.[105] Other investigations of diabetic iridopathy,[88] however, have failed to find any such unperfused areas in the iris.

Gartner and Henkind[62] stressed the peculiarities of the iris' nutrition system, by which oxygen is supplied through the aqueous humor which carries it from blood in the ciliary body, but in certain cases of iris neovascularization the ciliary body is atrophic. The retinal circulation is another source of oxygen, which diffuses through the vitreous. In cases with vascular problems in the retina (such as proliferative diabetic retinopathy, CRVO or CRAO, etc.) this source dries up too. Iris neovascularization can then be considered a response to the hypoxia affecting various districts - the ciliary body, retina and iris.

Another theory on rubeosis iridis suggests localized iris pathology influenced by unknown factors. Supporting this is the finding of marked exudation, linked to altered permeability of the iris stromal vessels, preceding the onset of neovascularization. In the pre-proliferative phase of diabetic iridopathy, diffuse hyperfluorescence is often seen in fluorescein angiograms - as we have mentioned - starting from the pupillary microcirculation and iris stromal vessels, and leading, in time, to the appearance of new vessels.[31] It is difficult, in the present state of knowledge, to define the relations between exudative and ischemic iridopathy. Probably both - through still unknown and presumably different mechanisms - can lead to rubeosis iridis.[31]

The fact that the incidence of iris neovascularization rises with age and is higher in type II diabetes mellitus (typical of adults) might reflect some sort of existing iris degeneration, creating favourable conditions for the iris to respond to the vasoformative stimulus from the retina. In elderly patients a larger retinal ischemic area corresponds to more severe rubeosis. In young subjects even extensive areas of ischemic retina do not cause iris neovascularization. This might be because in young people the vitreous adheres closely to the retina, and has not normally undergone any of the degenerative processes encountered in elderly patients, so it could inhibit the hypothetical retinal vasoproliferative factor. Therefore in the elderly, especially the aphakic patient, whose protection mechanisms are physiologically inadequate, even small areas of retinal ischemia may give rise to extensive iris neovascularization (Fig. **4.4**,72).[31]

Another pathogenic hypothesis suggests that besides tissue hypoxia, accumulation of metabolites - mainly mucoproteins[112] and acid mucopolysaccharides[74] - plays a causal role in rubeosis. Breakdown products in the vitreous would then induce inflammation in the anterior uvea too. This would lead to alterations to the iris vessels which might contribute to new vessel formation. There are in fact experimental[54,122,123] and clinical studies showing that inflammation can induce rubeosis iridis.

The last theory put forward to provide one single mechanism to explain the various types of neovascularization observed in the different parts of the eye is control by the nervous system.[45] It is too early to confirm this suggestion on the basis of the few studies to date.

The pathogenesis of rubeosis still poses many questions: What role does ischemia of the anterior and posterior segment play? Are they both necessary for new iris vessels to develop in diabetic patients?[88]

Neovascularization of the iris in diabetes mellitus and central retinal vein occlusion

The clinical and angiographic pictures of rubeosis iridis are - as we have already mentioned - substantially comparable, regardless of the underlying pathology.[25,59,86,97,121] However, some differences are detectable between rubeosis due to diabetes and the form caused by CRVO.[83]

In diabetes mellitus neovascularization starts at the pupillary border, whereas in CRVO it starts near the iris root.[59].In diabetes iris fluorescein angiography shows the new vessels filling promptly with dye - already in the arterial phase - whereas in CRVO cases the dye only becomes visible in the venous phase. In diabetic rubeosis the new vessels look like numerous fine capillaries, whereas in CRVO they are fewer but larger in diameter, and thicker-walled.[47] These angiographic findings in the iris have been confirmed experimentally by histological studies with microvascular silicone injections into enucleated eyes.[81]

Therapy of rubeosis iridis

The main therapeutic approach to rubeosis iridis is prevention, by panretinal photocoagulation of the causal elements. There is no known medical or surgical therapy that affects the natural history of rubeosis. The eye tolerates the iris neovascularization until neovascular glaucoma arises. Once the angle is closed no medical therapy has any effect.

The congestive effect of miotics aggravates the situation in an eye with neovascularization of the iris; midriatics have symptomatic activity - on the pain - but no anatomical effect.

Local steroids can be employed[50,71] to relieve pain and reduce the inflammation, and carbonic anhydrase inhibitors,[75] by reducing the production of aqueous humor, lower the intraocular pressure (IOP). Beta-blockers may be used topically for the same purpose. Retrobulbar injections of alcohol can provide pain relief.[100]

There are reports of regression of new vessels after "adrenalectomy",[114] hypophysectomy[108] or section of the pituitary peduncle.[97] However, these are all radical approaches that are hard to recommend on account of their numerous side effects.

Simmons[125] sustained that neovascular glaucoma could be prevented by direct argon laser treatment of the new vessels crossing the scleral spur, if done before the angle was closed by synechiae.

Various surgical therapies have been proposed to deal with iris neovascularization (iridectomy, fistulization, cyclodialysis, destruction of the ciliary bodies by trans-scleral cryocoagulation or trans-scleral laser photocoagulation, and others). However, all these techniques give questionable or downright unsatisfactory results. Cyclocryotherapy may lower IOP and relieve pain but the improvement is often only short-lasting.[26,55] Overdosage - always a possibility with this treatment - may cause phthisis bulbi.

Good results on pain and IOP have been reported recently using the continuous-wave (CW) Nd:YAG laser for trans-scleral coagulation of the ciliary bodies.[10,17,32,33,34,49,52,53,72] This is referred to as contact trans-scleral cyclophotocoagulation and involves placing the end of the optical fiber in contact with the sclera. This method exploits the transparency of the scleral tissue to the Nd:YAG laser's 1064 nm radiation, which is transmitted well along optical fibres.

The use of optical fibres offers several advantages:

- scleral transparency is increased by the optical fibre pressing on it, which has the effect of "squeezing" out the moisture from the tissue;
- the compression also has an ischemic effect on the underlying stroma of the ciliary body. This results in a reduction of heat loss by conduction;
- the optical fibre permits better control of the exact position in relation to the corneal flap. The target tissue is the pigment epithelium which contains large amounts of melanin.

Scattering of the radiation when it meets the stroma of the ciliary bodies is important for the photocoagulative effect.

Histological examination of the lesions caused by this technique was reported first in animals, and recently in human eyes too. There are several possible pathophysiological bases for the hypotonic effect, but the photodestruction of the secretory apparatus appears fundamental. It has been suggested that the stromal stretching that accompanies the process of repair has an effect of cyclodiastasis which causes the aqueous to pass behind the choroid or even to filter through the sclera. Finally, it has recently been suggested that inflammation is the cause not only of the short-term hypotonic effect but also - as it becomes chronic - of the longer-term effect.

The pain relief seems to be achieved through reduction of the IOP but also as a result of destruction of the sensitive nerve endings.

It thus appears that therapy of rubeosis and neovascular glaucoma gives largely disappointing results and is mainly useful in reducing pain.

Prevention of iris neovascularization, by photocoagulation of all the ischemic areas on the retina, must thus be the ophtlamologist's main objective. Panretinal photocoagulation does appear to give a response in cases of neovascular glaucoma, but the duration and validity of this effect remain to be demonstrated.[36,132] Iris fluorescein angiography is important in that it permits very early identification of new vessels, thus making it possible to establish which subjects are at risk of developing this serious complication.

Retinal photocoagulation in rubeosis iridis

In a high percentage of cases panretinal photocoagulation results in regression of the iris neovascularization.[22,28,42,70,78,87,89,107,117,128,132] Photocoagulation of proliferative diabetic retinopathy can be useful as prevention or therapy of rubeosis (Fig. **4.4**,73). If done before neovascular glaucoma arises, photocoagulation can obliterate the new vessels and achieve regression of the iris lesions (Figs. **4.4**,74-76). The iris fluorescein angiogram after laser treatment of retinal ischemic areas shows less vascular congestion and less dye leakage into radial vessels and residual new vessels (Figs. **4.4**,77-79).

Panretinal photocoagulation seems to have more evident beneficial effects in rubeosis secondary to diabetes mellitus than in forms due to ischemic CRVO.[125] The regression of iris new vessels in proliferative diabetic retinopathy treated by panretinal photocoagulation is correlated - according to some reports - with destruction of the retinal ischemic areas where the vasoformative factor is believed to originate.[18,31,82,83]

Other mechanisms too are suggested to explain this finding. Bonnet,[27] in agreement with Shimizu,[124] found neovascularization of the optic disc in 93.8% of patients with proliferative diabetic retinopathy (with confluent ischemic areas) and rubeosis iridis. In view of the fact that the papillary new vessels are anatomically connected with the ciliary circulation, he suggested these vessels were in fact "stealing" blood, not in the retina but in the ciliary bodies. This further reduction of the blood supply to the iris would in itself constitute an ischemic stimulus to the formation of new vessels. Bonnet also noted that panretinal photocoagulation, by destroying part of the choriocapillaris, might end up rerouting a considerable amount of blood to the anterior chamber, reducing hypoxia there.

Glaser and Patz[(69)] pointed out that the laser's destructive effect was more evident on the photoreceptor-pigment epithelium complex which alone consumes two-thirds of total retinal oxygen. By destroying the photoreceptor layer, photocoagulation leaves more oxygen to reach the inner layers of the retina which suffer most from the hypoxia caused by capillary occlusion and which appear to be the producers of the vasoformative factor. The supply of oxygen from the choroid would thus be increased by photocoagulation.

Peyman, Spitznas and Straasma, on the other hand, sustain that photocoagulation of the retinal pigment epithelium results in new metabolic exchange channels being opened between the retina and choroid.[(118)]

Wolbarsht and Landers suggest that vascular tone modulates ocular neovascularization.[(92,135)] Panretinal photocoagulation raises the oxygen pressure in the retina, causing arteriolar vasoconstriction and involution of the new vessels. This theory is borne out by a study by Wilson et al. on how the caliber of retinal vessels is reduced after panretinal photocoagulation.[(133)]

Another theory has it that coagulative necrosis results in release of a substance that inhibits neovascularization.[(107)]

Whatever the mechanism eventually turns out to be, it is certain that photocoagulation of retinal ischemic areas does reduce the tendency of diabetic iridopathy to develop into neovascular glaucoma. Results are disappointing in eyes where the opacity is such that correct, complete photocoagulative treatment is impossible. Indirect treatment by trans-scleral cryocoagulation and contact trans-scleral photocoagulation with the CW Nd:YAG laser destroys the retinal ischemic areas effectively but not always completely.[(35)]

Iris fluorescein angiography is essential as a means of following the regression of the iris neovascularization and assessing the efficacy of retinal photocoagulation (Fig. **4.4**,80).

Natural course of rubeosis iridis

In patients with rubeosis iridis, neovascular glaucoma may develop at a rate related to the type and severity of the underlying disease (Figs. **4.4**,81,82).[(62,83)] In CRVO, as we mentioned earlier, glaucoma develops sooner.[(126)] In diabetics, for reasons that are still not clear, the new vessel formation may stop at any stage, remaining unchanged for years, and even regress.[(71,86,97,109,125)] In such cases it is possible that fibrotic tissue contracts and covers the new vessels, which do in fact seem to disappear.[(62)] The caliber of the neovascular channels may become smaller, but fluorescein angiographic examination confirms they are still there (Fig. **4.4**,83). While some new vessels appear to be obliterated, others may be detected in different parts of the iris (Figs. **4.4**,84,85). It has been proposed[(125)] that the new vessels stop forming and even regress spontaneously in relation to the destruction of retinal tissue as the lesions progress: the retina, in complete disorder or even destroyed, is no longer able to release the hypothetical vasoformative factor responsible for the development of iris new vessels. Thus a stage of involution-atrophy of the lesions is produced in the iris too, similar to the frequently terminal stage in the retina (Figs. **4.4**,86,87).

References

1 Algvere P, Kornacki B: Fluorescein angiography of the iris: a correlation of microangiopathy in the iris and retina. Acta Ophthalmol 56: 803, 1978.

2 Anderson DR, Davis EB: Sensitivity of ocular tissue to acute pressure induced ischaemia. Arch Ophthalmol 93: 267, 1975.

3 Anderson DM, Morin JD: Experimental anterior segment necrosis and rubeosis iridis. Can J Ophthalmol 6: 196, 1971.

4 Anderson DM, Morin JD, Hunter WS: Rubeosis iridis. Can J Ophthalmol 6: 183, 1971.

5 Armarly MF, Baloglou PJ: Diabets and the eye. I: Changes in the anterior segment. Arch Ophthalmol 77: 485, 1977.

6 Ashton N: Retinal vascularization in health and disease. Am J Ophthalmol 44: 7, 1957.

7 Ashton N: Diabetic microangiopathy. Adv Ophthalmol 8: 1, 1958.

8 Ashton N: Neovascularization in ocular disease. Trans Ophthalmol Soc UK 81: 145, 1961.

9 Ashton N: Oxygen and the growth and development of retinal vessels. Am J Ophthalmol 62: 412, 1966.

10 Badeeb O, Trope GE, Mortimer CH: Short-term effects of Nd:YAG trans-scleral cyclocoagulation in patients with uncontrolled glaucoma. Br J Ophthalmol 72: 615, 1988.

11 Baggesen LH: Fluorescence angiography of the iris in diabetics and non-diabetics. Acta Ophthalmol 47: 449, 1969.

12 Baggesen LH: Fluorescein angiography of the iris in rubeosis iridis diabetica. Eye Ear Nose Throat Mon 51: 48, 1972.

13 Bandello F, Brancato R, Lattanzio R et al: Biomicroscopy versus fluorescein angiography of the iris in the detection of diabetic iridopathy. Graefe's Arch Clin Exp Ophthalmol 231: 444, 1993.

14 Bandello F, Brancato R, Lattanzio R et al: Relationship between iridopathy and retinopathy in diabetes. Br J Ophthalmol 78: 542, 1994.

15 Barritault D, Arruti C, Courtois Y: Is there a ubiquitous growth factor in the eye? (Proliferation induced in different cell types by eye-derived growth factors). Differentiation 18: 29, 1981.

16 Baum JL, Wise GN: Experimental subretinal neovascularization. Am J Ophthalmol 61: 528, 1966.

17 Beckman H, Sugar SA: Neodymium-YAG laser cyclocoagulation. Arch Ophthalmol 90: 27, 1973.

18 Ben Ezra D: Neovasculogenic ability of prostaglandins, growth factors and synthetic chemoattractans. Am J Ophthalmol 86: 455, 1978.

19 Ben Ezra D: Neovasculogenesis. Triggering factors and possible mechanisms. Surv Ophthalmol 24: 167, 1979.

20 Blankenship G: Preoperative iris rubeosis and diabetic vitrectomy results. Ophthalmology 87: 176, 1980.

21 Blankenship G, Cortez R, Machemer R: The lens and pars plana vitrectomy for diabetic retinopathy complications. Arch Ophthalmol 97: 1263, 1979.

22 Blankenship G, Goodart R: Panretinal photocoagulation influence on vitrectomy results for complications of diabetic retinopathy. Ophthalmology 87: 183, 1980.

23 Blankenship G, Machemer R: Pars plana vitrectomy for the management of severe diabetic retinopathy: an analysis of results five years following surgery. Ophthalmology 85: 553, 1978.

24 Blumenkranz M, Hernandez E: Experimental rubeosis in the rabbit. Inv Ophthalmol Vis Sci 22 (Suppl): 234, 1982.

25 Böhringer HR. Sekundärglaukom mit gefässneubildung auf der iris. Ophthalmologica 123: 211, 1952.

26 Boniuk M: Cryotherapy in neovascular glaucoma. Trans Am Acad Ophthalmol Otolaryngol 78: 337, 1974.

27 Bonnet M: Néo-vaisseaux papillaires dans la rétinopathie diabétique. In Coscas G: La Rétinopathie Diabétique. Proc Symposium International sur la Rétinopathie Diabétique. Paris, 1984. Rev Chibret Ophtalmol 105: 281, 1985.

28 Bonnet M, El Khatib W: The value of fluorescein angiography of the iris in the monitoring of rubeosis iridis treated with panretinal photocoagulation. Bull Mem Soc Fr Ophtalmol 94: 312, 1982.

29 Bonnet M, Jourdain M, Francoz-Taillanter N: Correlation neovaisseaux papillaires-rubeosis iridis. J Fr Ophtalmol 4: 405, 1981.

30 Bonnet P: Rubeosis iridis. Ophthalmologica 118: 575, 1949.

31 Brancato R, Carnevalini A, Pece A et al: Correlazione tra iridopatia e retinopatia diabetica. Atti Congresso Società Italiana Laser in Oftalmologia. Verduci Ed, Milano, 1985.

32 Brancato R, Leoni G, Trabucchi G et al: Probe placement and energy levels in continuous-wave Neodymium-YAG contact trans-scleral cyclophotocoagulation. Arch Ophthalmol 105: 679, 1990.

33 Brancato R, Leoni G, Trabucchi G et al: Contact trans-scleral cyclophotocoagulation with CW Nd:YAG laser in uncontrolled glaucoma. Ophthalmic Surg 20: 547, 1989.

34 Brancato R, Leoni G, Trabucchi G et al: Contact trans-scleral cyclophotocoagulation with CW Nd:YAG laser in uncontrolled glaucoma. Inv Ophthalmol Vis Sci 30 (Suppl): 353, 1989.

35 Brancato R, Leoni G, Trabucchi G et al: Contact trans-scleral irradiation of human chorioretina with continuous-wave Nd:YAG laser. Ophthalmic Res 21: 1, 1989.

36 Brancato R, Menchini U: Microchirurgia laser in Oftalmologia. Ghedini Ed, Milano, 1989.

37 Brancato R, Menchini U, Carnevalini A: Atlante di iridografia a fluorescenza. C.I.C. Ed Int Gruppo Ed Medico, Roma, 1981.

38 Brancato R, Menchini U, Carnevalini A et al: Rubeosis iridis et rétinopathie diabétique. In Coscas G: La rétinopathie Diabétique. Proc Symposium International sur la Rétinopathie Diabétique. Paris, 1984. Rev Chibret Ophtalmol 105: 287, 1985.

39 Brem S, Preis I, Langer R et al: Inhibition of neovascularization by an extract derived from vitreous. Am J Ophthalmol 84: 327, 1977.

40 Bresnick GH, De Venecia G, Myers FL: Retinal ischaemia in diabetic retinopathy. Arch Ophthalmol 93: 1300, 1975.

41 Brown GC, Magargal LE, Federman JL: Ischaemia and neovascularization. Trans Ophthalmol Soc UK 100: 377, 1980.

42 Callahan MA, Hilton GF: Photocoagulation and rubeosis iridis. Am J Ophthalmol 78: 873, 1974.

43 Cappin JM, Whitelocke R: The iris in central retinal vein thrombosis. Proc R Soc Med 67: 1048, 1974.

44 Carnevalini A, Menchini U, Camesasca F et al: Valutazione obiettiva dei fluorangiogrammi di alterazioni vascolari iridee proliferative. Clin Ocul Patol Oc 3: 223, 1988.

45 Cassel GH, Groden LR: New thoughts on ocular neovascularization: a neurally controlled regenerative process? Ann Ophthalmol 16: 138, 1984.

46 Coscas G, Gaudric A: Rubéose de l'iris et glaucome neovasculaire. J Fr Ophtalmol 2: 653, 1979.

47 Demeler U, Sautter H: Irisangiographische untersuchungen bei Patienten mit Diabetes mellitus. Adv Ophthalmol 36: 233, 1978.

48 Deodati F, Bec P, Labro JB: Angiographie fluorescéinique du segment antérieur de l'oeil. Arch Ophtalmol (Paris) 12: 859, 1971.

49 Devenyi RG, Trope GE, Hunter WH et al: Nd:YAG trans-scleral cyclophotocoagulation in human eyes. Ophthalmology 94: 1519, 1987.

50 Drews RC: Corticosteroid management of haemorrhagic glaucoma. Trans Am Acad Ophthalmol Otolaryngol 78: 334, 1974.

51 Ehremberg M, Mc Cuen BW: Rubeosis iridis: preoperative iris fluorescein angiography and periocular steroids. Ophthalmology 91: 321, 1984.

52 England C, Van der Zypen E, Fankhauser F: A comparison of optical methods for trans-scleral cyclophotocoagulation in rabbit eyes produced with the Nd:YAG laser; a morphological, physical and clinical analysis. Lasers & Light Ophthalmol 2: 87, 1988.

53 Fankhauser F, Van der Zypen E, Kwasniewska S: Trans-scleral cyclophotocoagulation using a Nd:YAG laser. Ophthalmic Surg 17: 94, 1986.

54 Federman L, Brown GC, Felberg NT et al: Experimental ocular angiogenesis. Am J Ophthalmol 89: 231, 1980.

55 Feibel RM, Bigger JF: Rubeosis iridis and neovascular glaucoma: evaluation of cyclocryotherapy. Am J Ophthalmol 74: 862, 1972.

56 Folkman J: Tumor angiogenesis: therapeutic implications. N Engl J Med 285: 1182, 1971.

57 Folkman J, Merler E, Abernathy C et al: Isolation of a tumor factor responsible for angiogenesis. J Exp Med 133: 275, 1971.

58 Fralick FB: Rubeosis iridis diabetics. Am J Ophthalmol 28: 123, 1945.

59 Friedburg D: Fluoreszenzangiographie der iris bei diabetiken. Klin Monatsbl Augenheilkd 162: 218, 1973.

60 Garancini P, Micossi P, Valsania P et al: Prevalence of retinopathy in diabetic subjects from out-patient clinics in Lombardy (Italy) and associated risk factors. A multicentre epidemiologic study. Diab Res Clin Pract 6: 129, 1989.

61 Garner A, Kissun RD: Ocular angiogenis in disease states. Trans Ophthalmol Soc UK 100: 381, 1980.

62 Gartner S, Henkind P: Neovascularization of the iris (Rubeosis iridis). Surv Ophthalmol 22: 291, 1978.

63 Gerke E, Spitznas M, Brodde OE: The role of lactic acid in retinal neovascularization. Albrecht von Graefes Arch Klin Ophthalmol 200: 79, 1976.

64 Gimbrone MA, Leapman SB, Cotran RS et al: Tumor angiogenesis; iris neovascularization at a distance from experimental intraocular tumors. J Nat Cancer Inst 50: 219, 1973.

65 Gitter KA, Cohen G: Complication of vitrectomy. In Gitter KA: Current concepts of the vitreous including vitrectomy. CV Mosby, St Louis, 1976.

66 Glaser BM, D'Amore PA, Lutty GA et al: Chemical mediators of intraocular neovascularization. Trans Ophthalmol Soc UK, 100: 369, 1980.

67 Glaser BM, D'Amore PA, Michels RG et al: The demonstration of angiogenic activity from ocular tissue. Ophthalmology 87: 440, 1980.

68 Glaser BM, D'Amore PA, Michels RG et al: Demonstration of vasoproliferative activity from mammalian retina. J Cell Biol 84: 298, 1980.

69 Glaser BM, Patz A: Neovascularization: current concepts. In Little HL, Jack RL, Patz A et al: Diabetic retinopathy. Thieme-Stratton Inc Ed, N.Y. - Stuttgard, 1983.

70 Grange JD, Bonnet M: Retinal pan-photocoagulation and rubeosis iridis. Bull Soc Fr Ophtalmol 78: 607, 1978.

71 Grant WM: Management of neovascular glaucoma. In Leopold IH: Symposium on Ocular Therapy. CV Mosby, St Louis, 1974.

72 Hampton C, Shields B: Trans-scleral Nd:YAG cyclophotocoagulation. A histologic study of human autopsy eyes. Arch Ophthalmol 106: 1121, 1988.

73 Henkind P: Ocular neovascularization. Am J Ophthalmol 85: 287, 1978.

74 Heydenreich A: Zur Klinik und Pathologie der Rubeosis Iridis. Klin Monatsbl Augenheilkd 134: 350, 1959.

75 Hohl RD, Barnett DM: Diabetic hemorrhagic glaucoma. Diabetes 19: 944, 1970.

76 Imre G: Studies of the mechanism of retinal neovascularization: role of lactic acid. Br J Ophthalmol 48: 75, 1964.

77 Imre G: Rubeosis iridis. Acta Medica Acad Scient Hung 27: 205, 1970.

78 Jacobson DR, Murphy RP, Rosenthal AR: The treatment of the angle neovascularization with panretinal photocoagulation. Am J Ophthalmol 86: 1270, 1979.

79 Jensen VA, Lundbaek K: Fluorescence angiography of the iris in recent and long term diabetes: Preliminary communication. Acta Ophthalmol (Kbh) 46: 584, 1968.

80 Jensen VA, Lundbaek K: Fluorescence angiography of the iris in recent and long term diabetes. Diabetologia 4: 161, 1968.

81 Jocson UL: Microvascular injection studies in rubeosis iridis and neovascular glaucoma. Am J Ophthalmol 83: 508, 1977.

82 Kottow M: Iris Angiography in vascular disease of the fundus. Doc Ophthalmol (Proceedings Series) 9: 465, 1976.

83 Kottow M: Anterior segment fluorescein angiography. Williams & Wilkins, Baltimore, 1978.

84 Kottow M, Hendrickson P: Iris angiographic findings in retinal arterial occlusion. Can J Ophthalmol 9: 435, 1974.

85 Kottow M, Metzler U: Stagnation thrombosis: an iris fluorescein angiographic study. Ophthalmologica 171: 192, 1975.

86 Kottow M, Metzler U, Hendrickson P: Iris angiographic findings in retinal vein occlusion. In Cant JS: Vision and circulation. Proc 3rd William Mackenzie Memorial Symposium, Glasgow, 1974. Henry Kimpton Publishers, London, 1976.

87 Krill AE, Archer D, Newell FW: Photocoagulation in complications secondary to branch vein occlusion. Arch Ophthalmol 85: 48, 1971.

88 Laatikainen L: Development and classification of rubeosis iridis in diabetic eye disease. Br J Ophthalmol 63: 150, 1979.

89 Laatikainen L: Preliminary report on effect of retinal panphotocoagulation on rubeosis iridis and neovascular glaucoma. Br J Ophthalmol 61: 278, 1977.

90 Laatikainen L, Black RK: Behaviour of the iris vasculature in central retinal vein occlusion. A fluorescein angiographic study of the vascular response of the retina and the iris. Br J Ophthalmol 61: 272, 1977.

91 Laatikainen L, Kohner EM: Fluorescein angiography and its prognostic significance in central retinal vein occlusion. Br J Ophthalmol 60: 411, 1976.

92 Landers MB, Stefansson E, Wolbarsht ML: Panretinal photocoagulation and retinal oxygenation. Retina 2: 167, 1982.

93 Lewis ML: Iris fluorescein angiography. Dev Ophthalmol (Karger, Basel) 2: 282, 1981.

94 Little HL, Rosenthal AR, Della Porta A et al: The effect of panretinal photocoagulation on rubeosis iridis. Am J Ophthalmol 81: 804, 1976.

95 Madsen PH: Ocular findings in 123 patients with proliferative diabetic retinopathy. I: Changes in the anterior segment of the eye. Doc Ophthalmol 29: 331, 1971.

96 Madsen PH: Rubeosis of the iris and haemorrhagic glaucoma in patients with proliferative diabetic retinopathy. Br J Ophthalmol 55: 368, 1971.

97 Madsen PH: Haemorrhagic glaucoma. Comparative study in diabetic and non-diabetic patients. Br J Ophthalmol 55: 444, 1971.

98 Menchini U, Carnevalini A, Pece A et al: Correlazione fluorangiografica tra lesioni del fondo oculare ed iridopatia diabetica. Atti LXIII Congresso Società Oftalmologica Italiana. Cappelli Ed, Bologna, 1982.

99 Michaelson IC, Campbell ACP: The anatomy of the finer retinal vessels and some observations on their significance in certain retinal disease. Trans Ophthalmol Soc UK 60: 71, 1940.

100 Michels RG, Maumenee AE: Retrobulbar alcohol injection in seeing eyes. Trans Am Acad Ophthalmol Otolaryngol 77: 164, 1973.

101 Mitsui Y, Matsubara M, Kanagawa M: Fluorescence iridocorneal photography. Br J Ophthalmol 53: 505, 1969.

102 Mitsui M, Parel JM, Weder HY et al: Some improved methods of anterior segment fluorescein angiography. I: Basic system. Am J Ophthalmol 74: 1075, 1972.

103 Mitsui M, Weder HJ, Parel JM: Some improved methods of anterior segment fluorescein angiography. II: Simultaneous stereoscopic photographic system. Am J Ophthalmol 76: 54, 1973.

104 Moffat K, Blumenkranz MS, Hernandez E: The lens capsule and rubeosis iridis: an angiographic study. Can J Ophthalmol 19: 130, 1984.

105 Morone G, Tazzi A, Carella G et al: L'uveopathie diabétique. Bull Mem Soc Fr Ophtalmol 95: 343, 1984.

106 Moyenin P, Bonnet M: Angio-fluo irienne dans les rethinopathies diabetiques proliferantes traitees par vitrectomie. Bull Soc Ophtalmol Fr 5: 621, 1987.

107 Murphy RP, Egbert PR: Regression of iris neovascularization following panretinal photocoagulation. Arch Ophthalmol 97: 700, 1979.

108 Ohrt V: Rubeosis iridis diabetica. Acta Ophthalmol 38: 556, 1958.

109 Ohrt V: Glaucoma due to rubeosis iridis diabetica. Ophthalmologica (Basel) 142: 356, 1961.

110 Ohrt V: Rubeosis iridis diabetica. Dan Med Bull 2: 17, 1964.

111 Ohrt V: The frequency of rubeosis iridis in diabetic patients. Acta Ophthalmol 49: 301, 1971.

112 Okamura P, Rohen JW: Elektronmikroskopischer untersuchugen über die rubeosis iridis. Albrecht von Graefes Arch Klin Ophthalmol 182: 53, 1975.

113 Okun E: Pars plana vitrectomy in advanced diabetic retinopathy: a review of 80 consecutive cases managed with the Douvas Roto-Extractor. In Mc Pherson A: New and controversial aspects of vitreoretinal surgery. CV Mosby, St Louis, 1977.

114 Oosterhuis JA, Loewere-Sieger D, Van Goal J: Treatment of diabetic retinopathy by adrenalectomy. Acta Ophthalmol 41: 365, 1963.

115 Patz A: The effect of oxygen on immature retinal vessels. Inv Ophthalmol 4: 988, 1965.

116 Patz A: Clinical and experimantal studies on retinal neovascularization. Am J Ophthalmol 94: 715, 1982.

117 Pavan PR, Folk JC, Weingeist TA et al: Diabetic rubeosis and panretinal photocoagulation: a prospective, controlled, masked trial using iris fluorescein angiography. Arch Ophthalmol 101: 882, 1983.

118 Peyman GA, Spitznas M, Straasma BR: Chorioretinal diffusion of peroxidase before and after photocoagulation. Inv Ophthalmol 10: 489, 1971.

119 Salus R: Rubeosis iridis diabetica, eine bisher unbekannte diabetische irisveränderung. Medsche Klin 7: 256, 1928.

120 Schnicke T: Fluoreszenzangiographie der iris bei patienten mit diabetes mellitus und patienten mit retinaler venenthrombose. Dissertation. Bonn, Rheinische Friedrich-Wilhelms Universität, 1975.

121 Schulze RR: Rubeosis iridis. Am J Ophthalmol 63: 487, 1967.

122 Shabo AL, Maxwell DS: Experimental immunogenic proliferative retinopathy in monkeys. Am J Ophthalmol 83: 471, 1977.

123 Shabo AL, Maxwell DS, Shintaku IP: Experimental immunogenic rubeosis iridis. Inv Ophthalmol 16: 342, 1977.

124 Shimizu K, Kobayashi Y, Muraoka K: Midperipheral fundus involvement in diabetic retinopathy. Ophthalmology 88: 601, 1981.

125 Simmons RJ, Dueker DK, Kimbrough RL et al: Goniophotocoagulation for neovascular glaucoma. Trans Am Acad Ophthalmol Otolaryngol 83: 80, 1977.

126 Smith R: Neovascularization in ocular disease. Trans Ophthalmol Soc UK 81: 125, 1961.

127 Tamura T: Electron microscopic study on the small blood vessels in rubeosis iridis diabetica. Jap J Ophthalmol 13: 65, 1969.

128 Tasman W, Magargal LE, Augsburger JJ: Effects of Argon Laser photocoagulation on rubeosis iridis and angle neovascularization. Ophthalmology 87: 400, 1980.

129 Turianskaya AM: Gonioscopy in patients with diabetes mellitus. Aftol Z 2: 135, 1966.

130 Vannas A: Fluorescein angiography of the vessels of the iris in pseudoexfoliation of the lens capsule, capsular glaucoma and some other forms of glaucoma. Acta Ophthalmol (Kbh) 105: 9, 1969.

131 Vannas S, Raitta C: Microcirculatory disturbances of the occlusive disease of the eye. Doc Ophthalmol 33: 345, 1972.

132 Wand M, Dueker DK, Aiello LM et al: Effects of panretinal photocoagulation on rubeosis iridis, angle neovascularization and neovascular glaucoma. Am J Ophthalmol 86: 332, 1978.

133 Wilson CA, Stefansson E, Klombers L et al: Optic disk neovascularization and retinal vessel diameter in diabetic retinopathy. Am J Ophthalmol 106: 131, 1988.

134 Wise GN: Retinal neovascularization. Trans Am Ophthalmol Soc 54: 729, 1956.

135 Wolbarsht ML, Landers MB: The rational of photocoagulation therapy for proliferative retinopathy: a review and model. Ophthalmol Surg 11: 235, 1980.

136 Wolter JR, Phillips RL: Secondary glaucoma following occlusion of the central retinal artery. Am J Ophthalmol 47: 335, 1959.

137 Zakov ZN, Lewis ML: Iris fluorescein angiography in diabetic vitrectomy patients. Albrecht Von Grafes Arch Klin Exp Ophthalmol 206: 17, 1978.

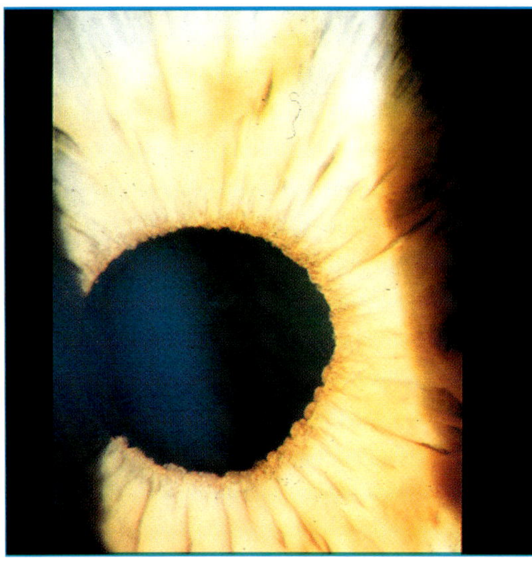

Fig. ***4.4****,1 - New vessels in the pupillary border (biomicroscopic view).*

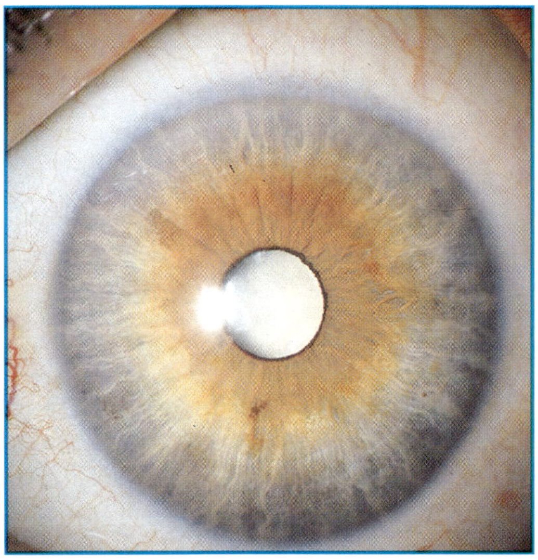

a)

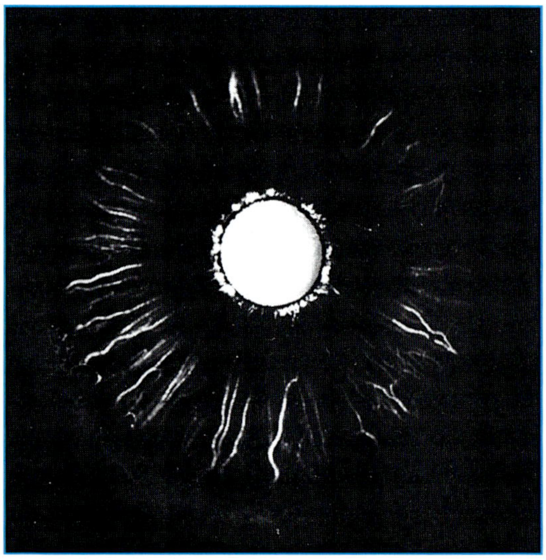

b)

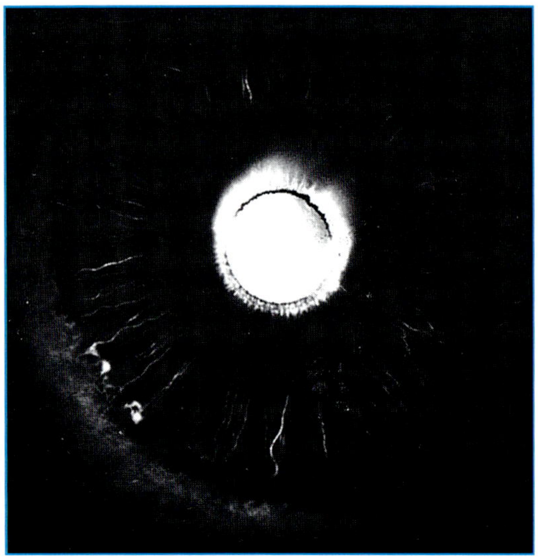

c)

Fig. ***4.4****,2 - Initial neovascularization of the iris not visible by biomicroscopy (a) is shown up well by iris fluorescein angiography: b) early phase; c) late phase.*

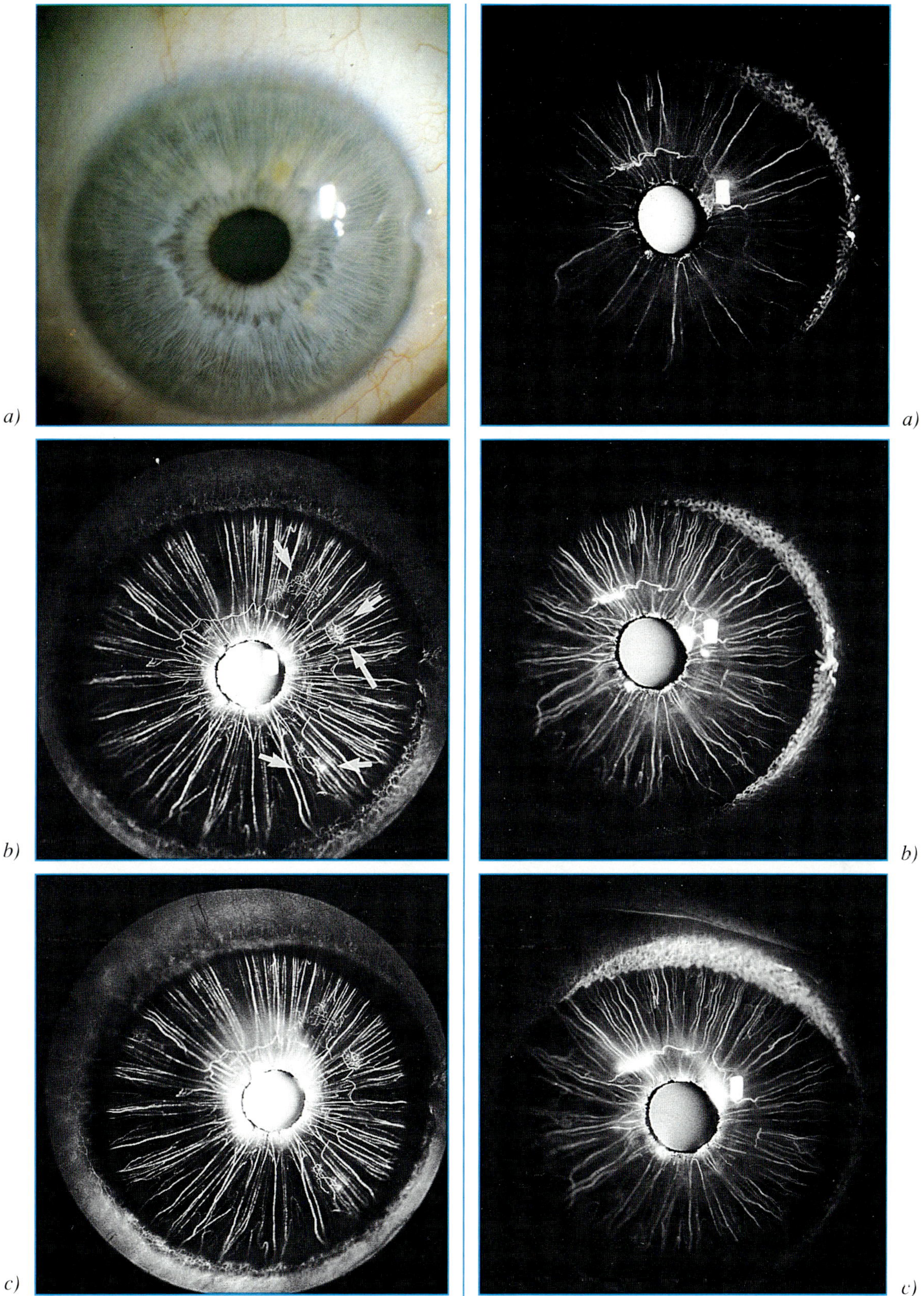

*Fig. **4.4**,3 - Anomalous vessels in the iris (arrows) are not biomicroscopically visible (a) but iris fluorescein angiography shows up them in the early (b) and late (c) phases. These vessels do not leak dye even in the late phases (c).*

*Fig. **4.4**,4 - Successive phases of iris fluorescein angiography (a,b,c) with initial neovascular proliferation of the iris.*

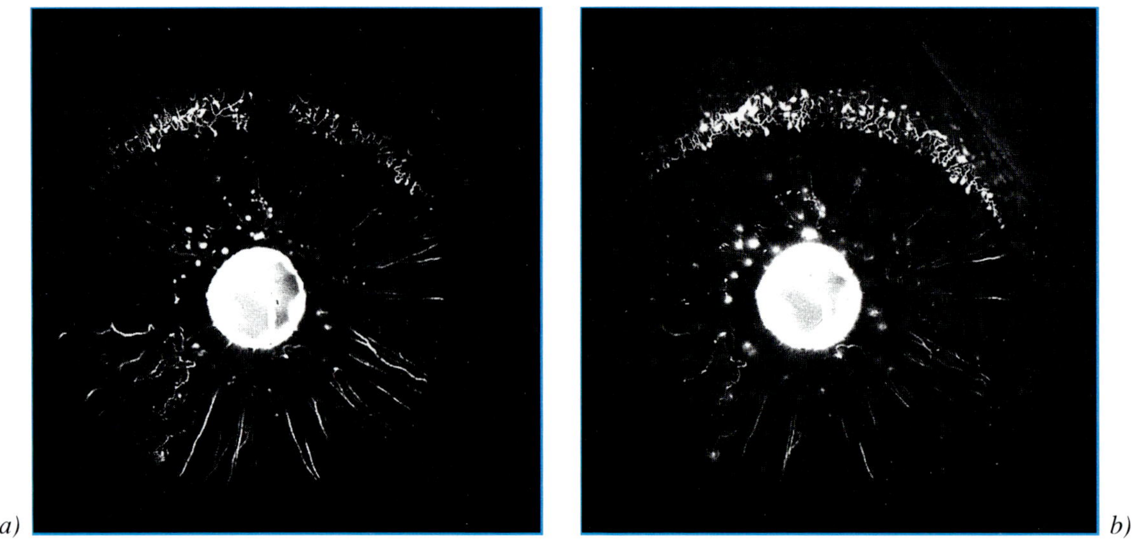

*Fig. **4.4,5** - Iris fluorescein angiographic findings (a, early; b, late) show unusual ectasia and aneurysmatic formations in the pupillary border and stroma of the iris.*

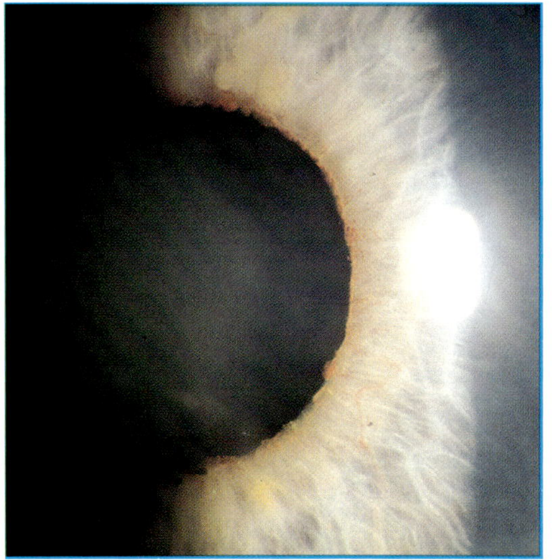

*Fig. **4.4,6** - Iris new vessels (biomicroscopy).*

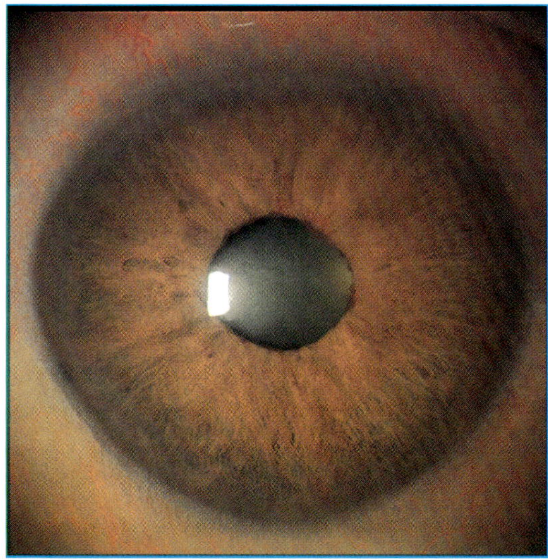

*Fig. **4.4,7** - Another case of iris new vessels (biomicroscopy).*

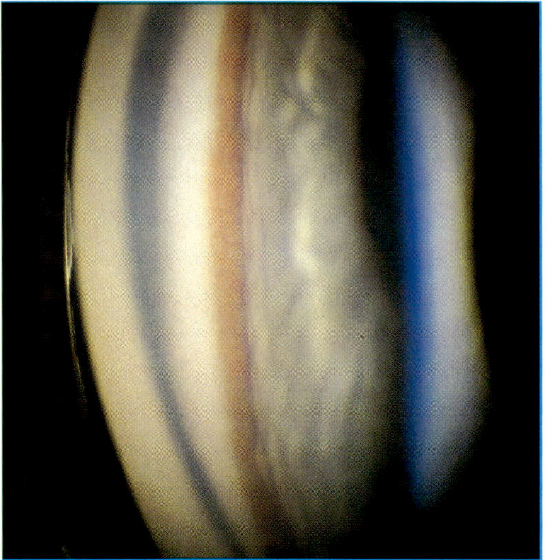

*Fig. **4.4,8** - Neovascular tufts in the iridocorneal angle (gonioscopy).*

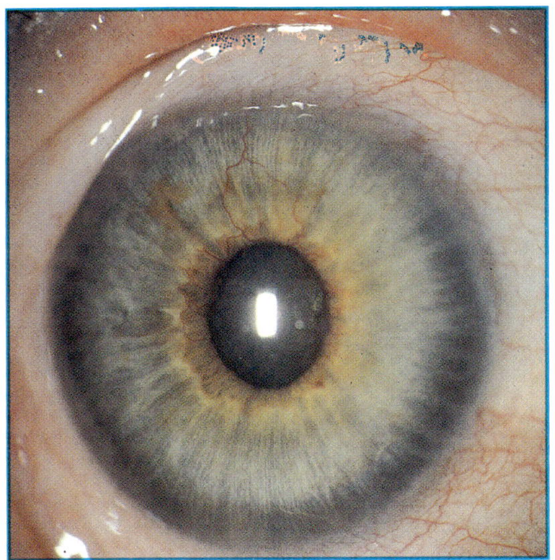

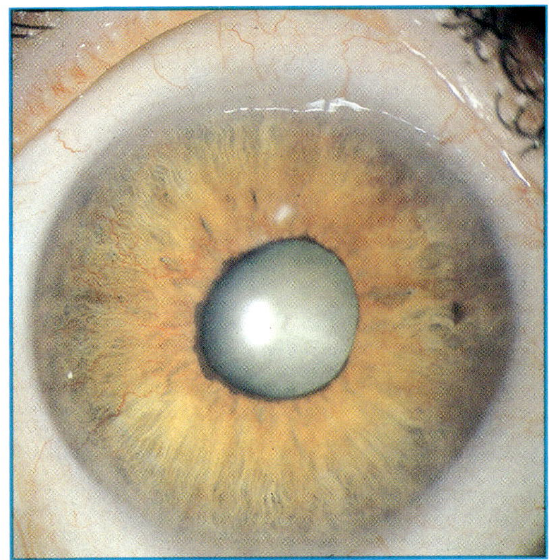

*Figs. **4.4**,9,10 - Seen with the biomicroscope iris new vessels present an anarchic pattern of fine red streaks*

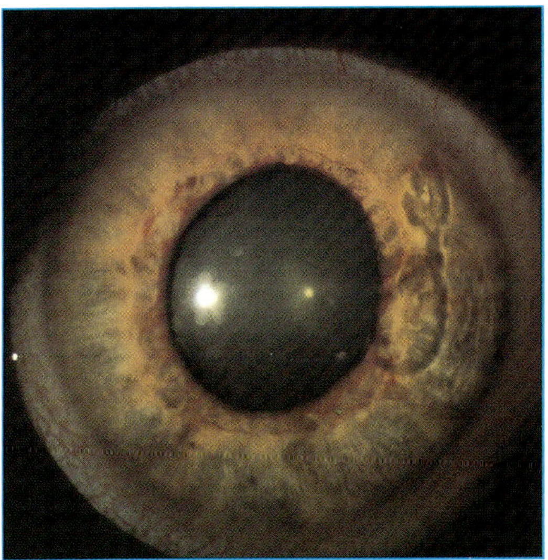

*Fig. **4.4**,11 - Imposing neovascular proliferation over the whole of the surface of the iris in neovascular glaucoma (biomicroscopy). Note the mid-midriatic position of the pupil.*

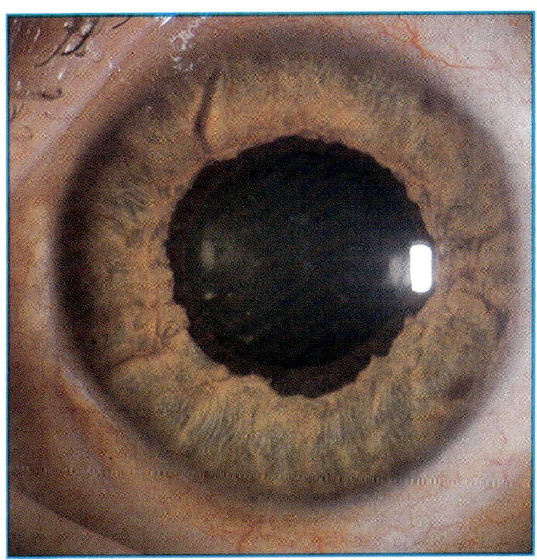

*Fig. **4.4**,12 - Biomicroscopic picture of neovascular glaucoma with ectropion uveae.*

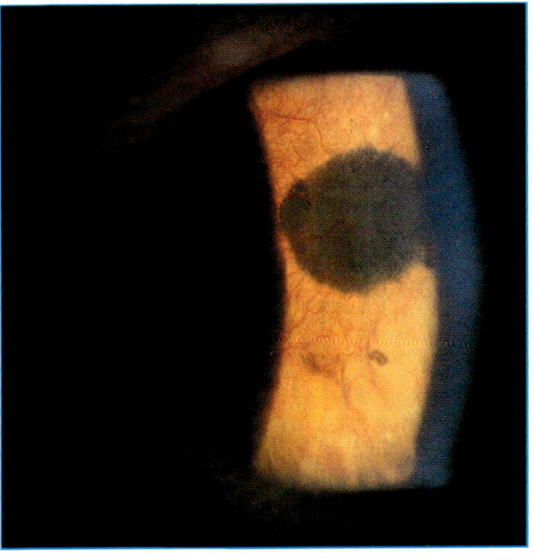

*Fig. **4.4**,13 - Pupillary occlusion in neovascular glaucoma (biomicroscopy).*

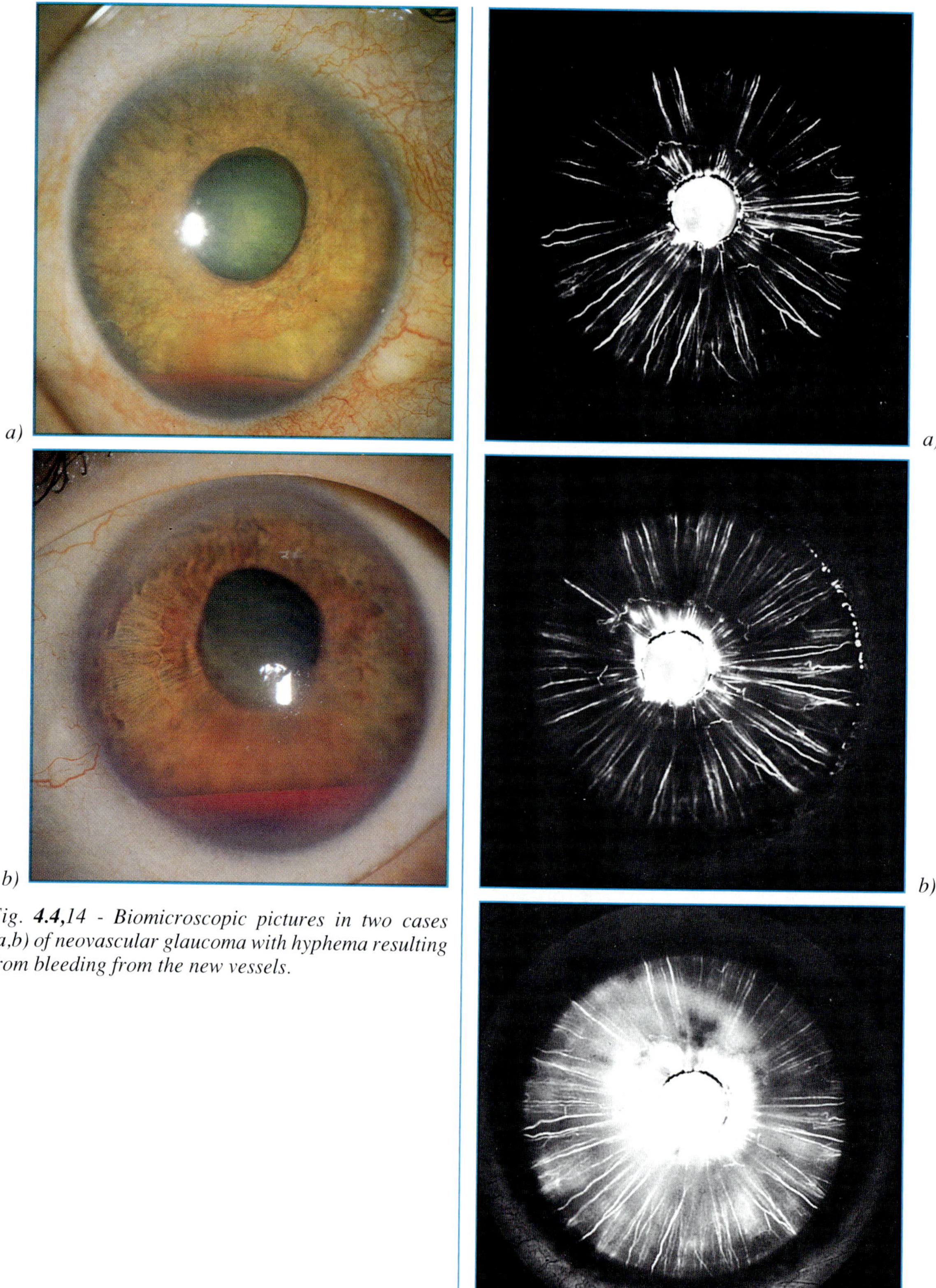

*Fig. **4.4,14** - Biomicroscopic pictures in two cases (a,b) of neovascular glaucoma with hyphema resulting from bleeding from the new vessels.*

*Fig. **4.4,15** - New vessels at the border are easily seen in the early iris fluorescein angiographic stages as hyperfluorescent spots (a). They are responsible in later phases (b) for dye leakage, increasing in subsequent phases (c) to involve the whole surface of the iris.*

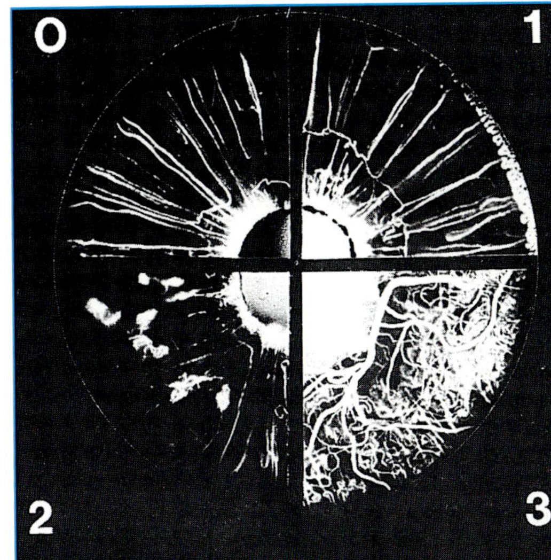

*Fig. **4.4,16** - Fluorescein angiographic classification of proliferative diabetic iridopathy;* [37] *grade 0 - no neovascularization; grade 1 - neovascularization of the pupillary border; grade 2 - neovascularization of the border and stroma; grade 3 - neovascular glaucoma.*

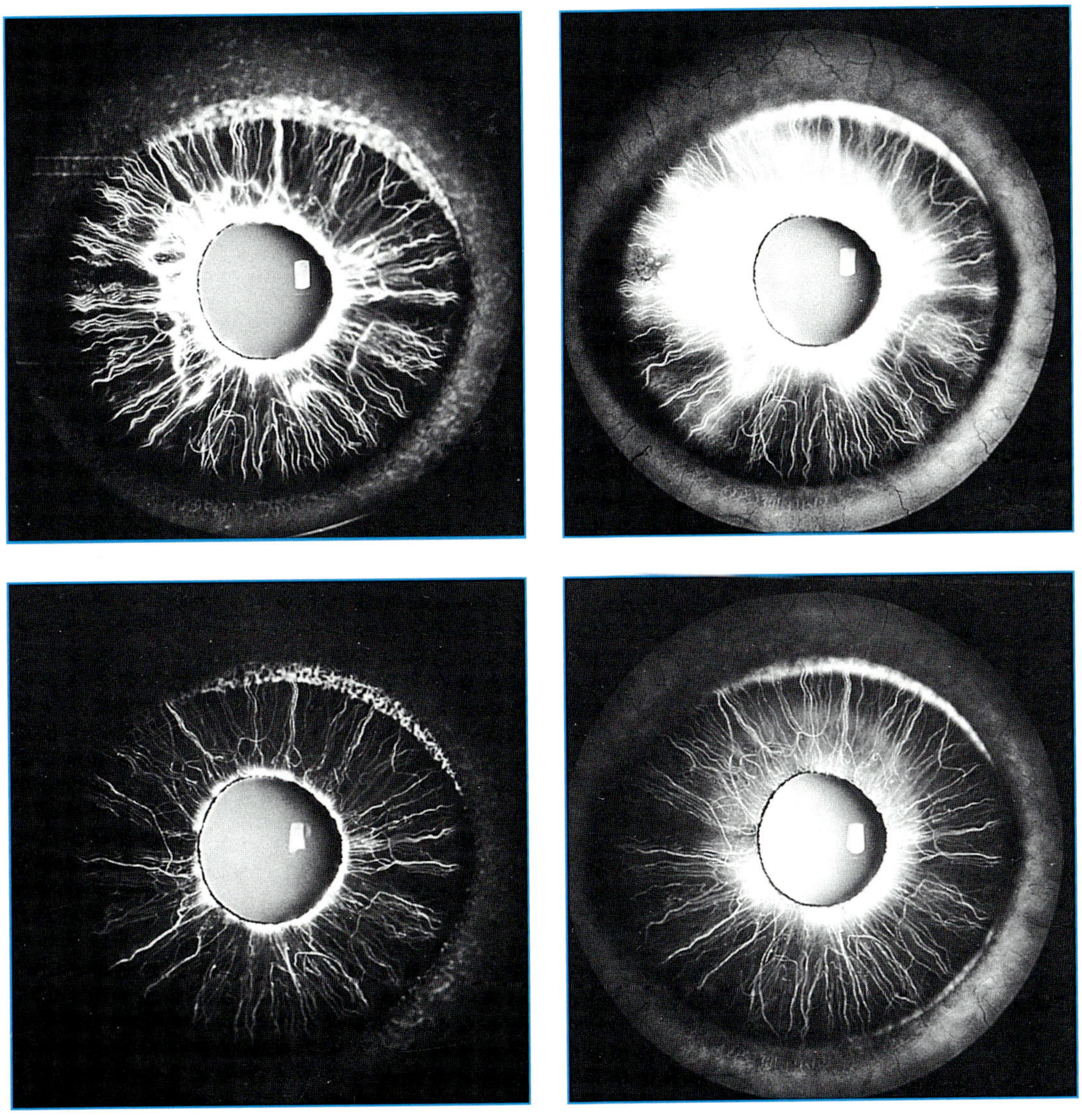

a)

b)

c)

d)

*Fig. **4.4,17** - A case of spontaneous regression (c,d) of iris new vessels (a,b) in a diabetic patient; early (a,c) and late (b,d) iris angiographic phases.*

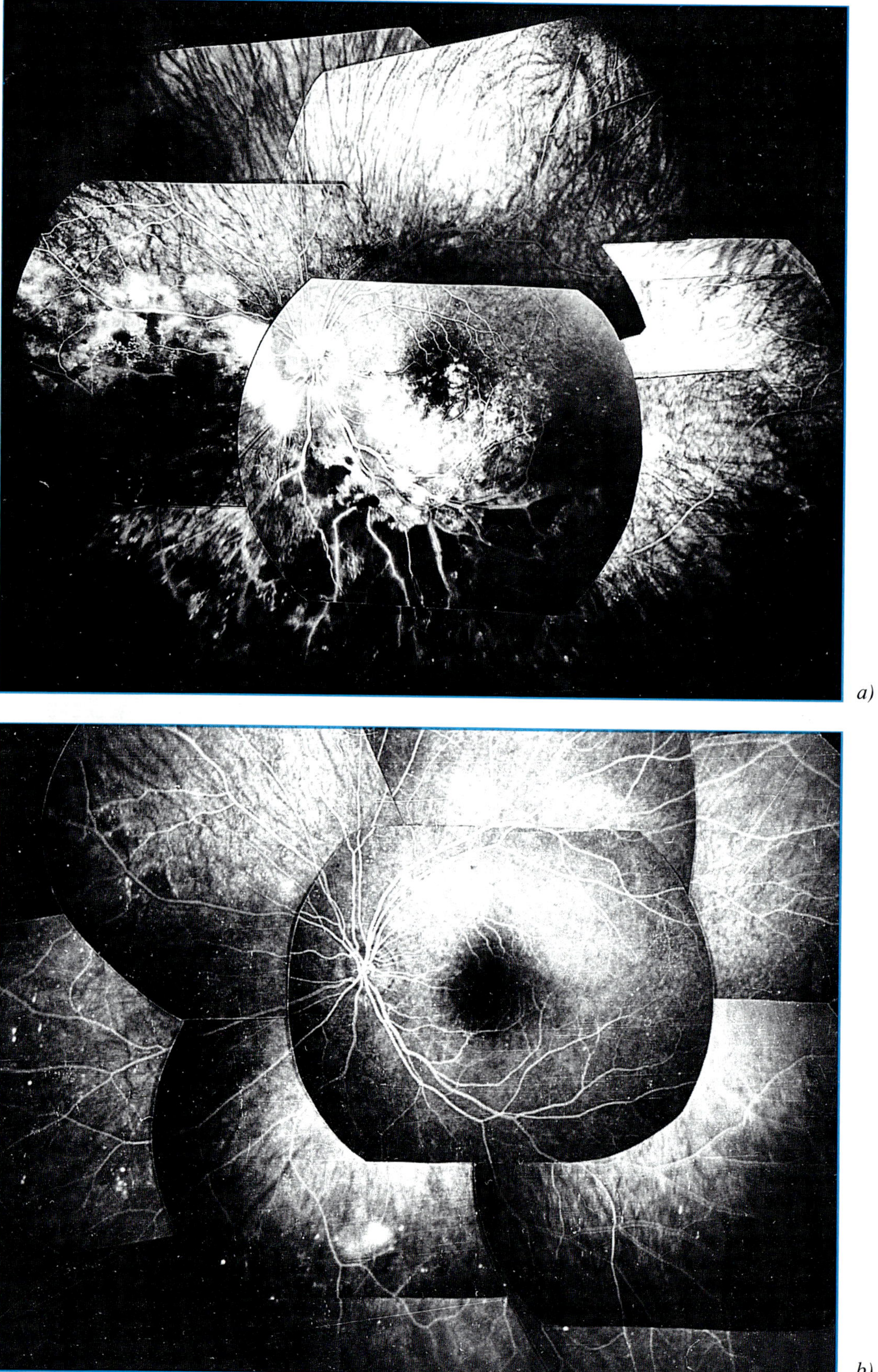

a)

b)

Fig. ***4.4,****18 - Same eye as in Fig.* ***4.4****,17: the epiretinal new vessels (a) have regressed spontaneously (b) (fluorescein angiography).*

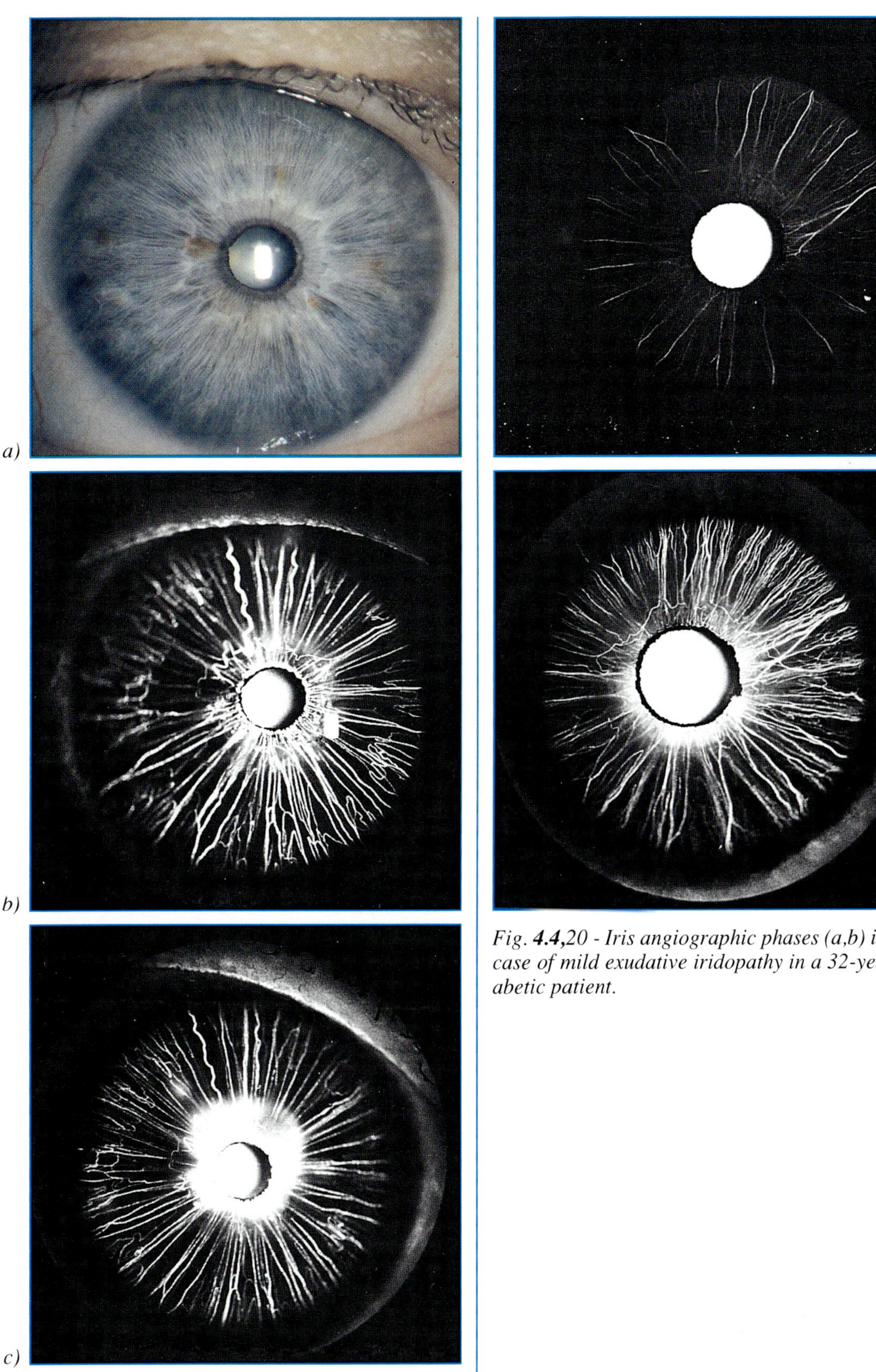

Fig. **4.4**,19 - *Biomicroscopy shows no noteworthy anomalies (a) in this case of mild exudative diabetic iridopathy. However, iris fluorescein angiography shows dye leakage at the pupillary border (b), increasing conspicuously in later phases (c).*

Fig. **4.4**,20 - *Iris angiographic phases (a,b) in another case of mild exudative iridopathy in a 32-year-old diabetic patient.*

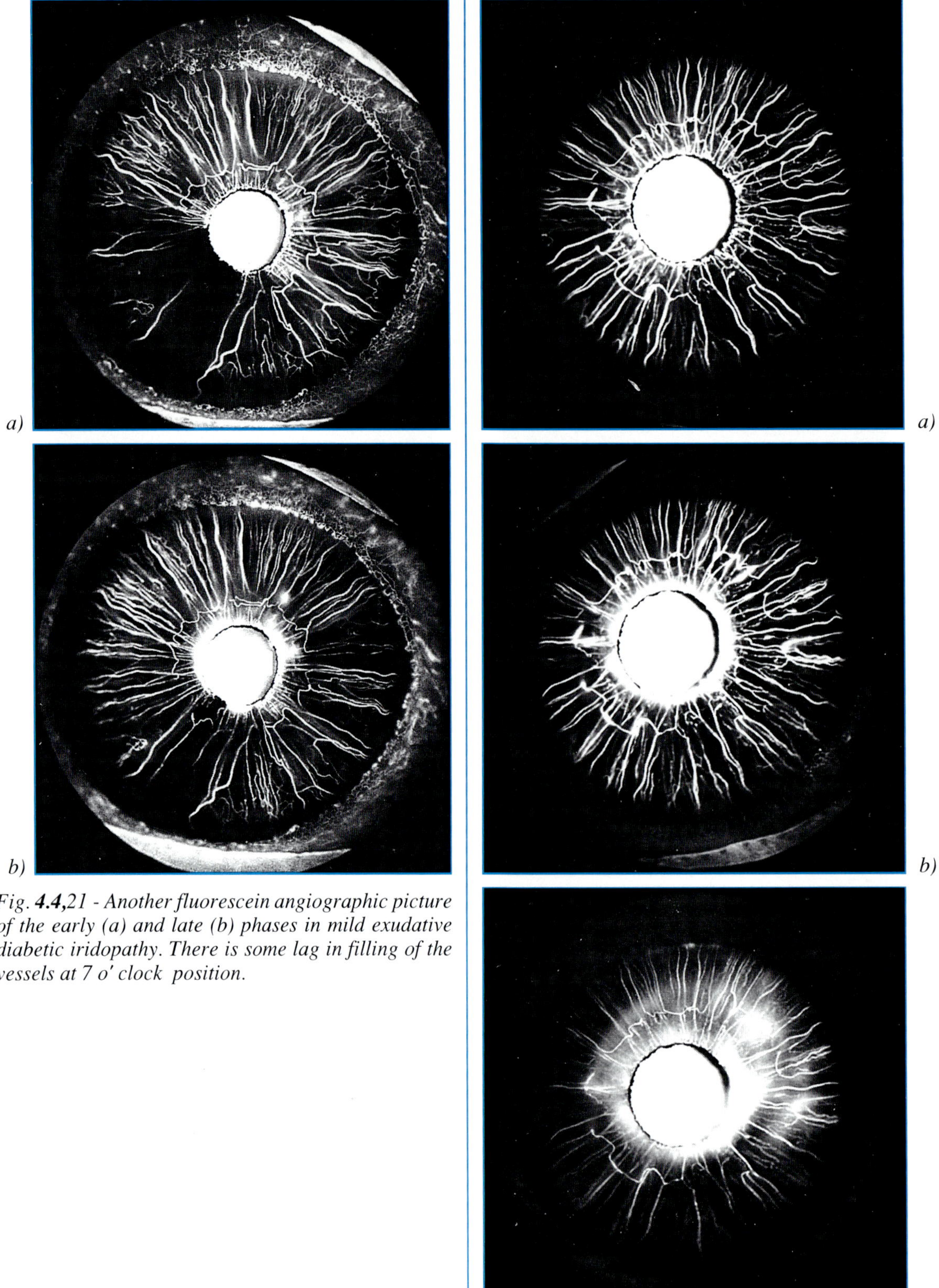

*Fig. **4.4,**21 - Another fluorescein angiographic picture of the early (a) and late (b) phases in mild exudative diabetic iridopathy. There is some lag in filling of the vessels at 7 o' clock position.*

*Fig. **4.4,**22 - Iris fluorescein angiographic phases (a,b,c) in a more severe case of exudative diabetic iridopathy. Dye leakage can be seen in the pupillary border but also at the stromal vessels.*

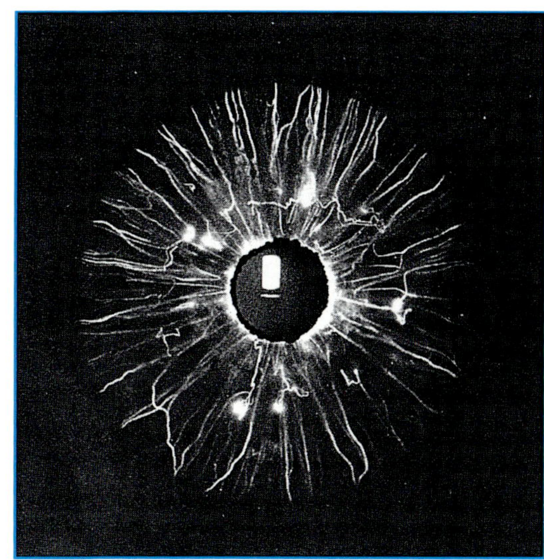

Fig. ***4.4,23*** *- Iris fluorescein angiography shows up alterations in the path of iris vessels. Areas of extrapupillary leakage where there is also microvascular ectasia are indicative of early neovascularization (transition iridopathy known as pre-proliferative).*

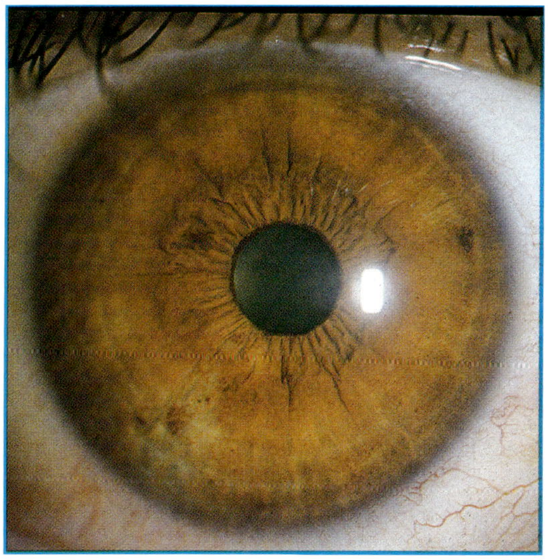

a)

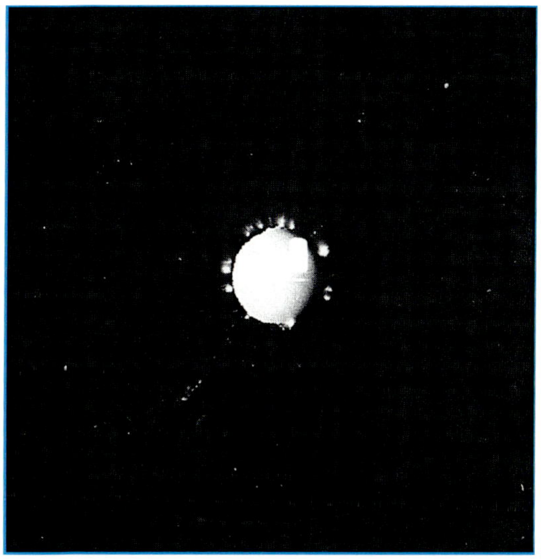

b)

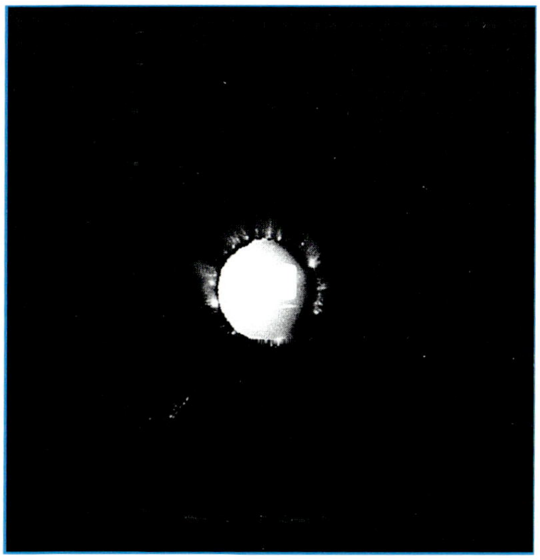

c)

Fig. ***4.4,24*** *- In a highly pigmented iris neovascular buds at the pupillary border are hard to detect with the biomicroscope (a). Iris fluorescein angiography shows them up as spots that take up dye early (b) and leak it in later phases (c).*

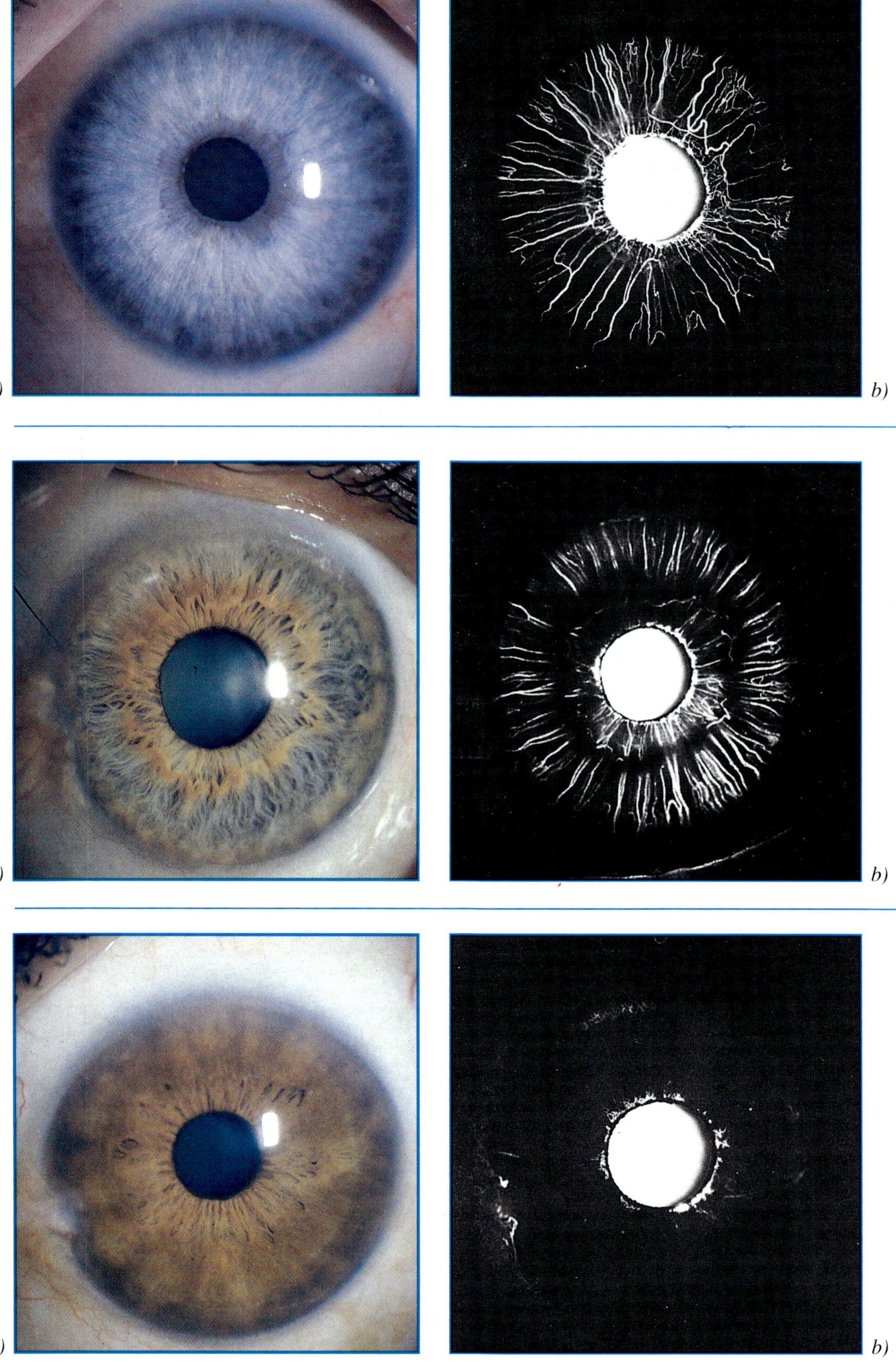

*Figs. **4.4**,25-27 - Three cases of grade 1[37] proliferative diabetic iridopathy in irises with different degrees of pigmentation. The biomicroscope cannot detect neovascular tufts at the pupillary border (a) even in the less* →

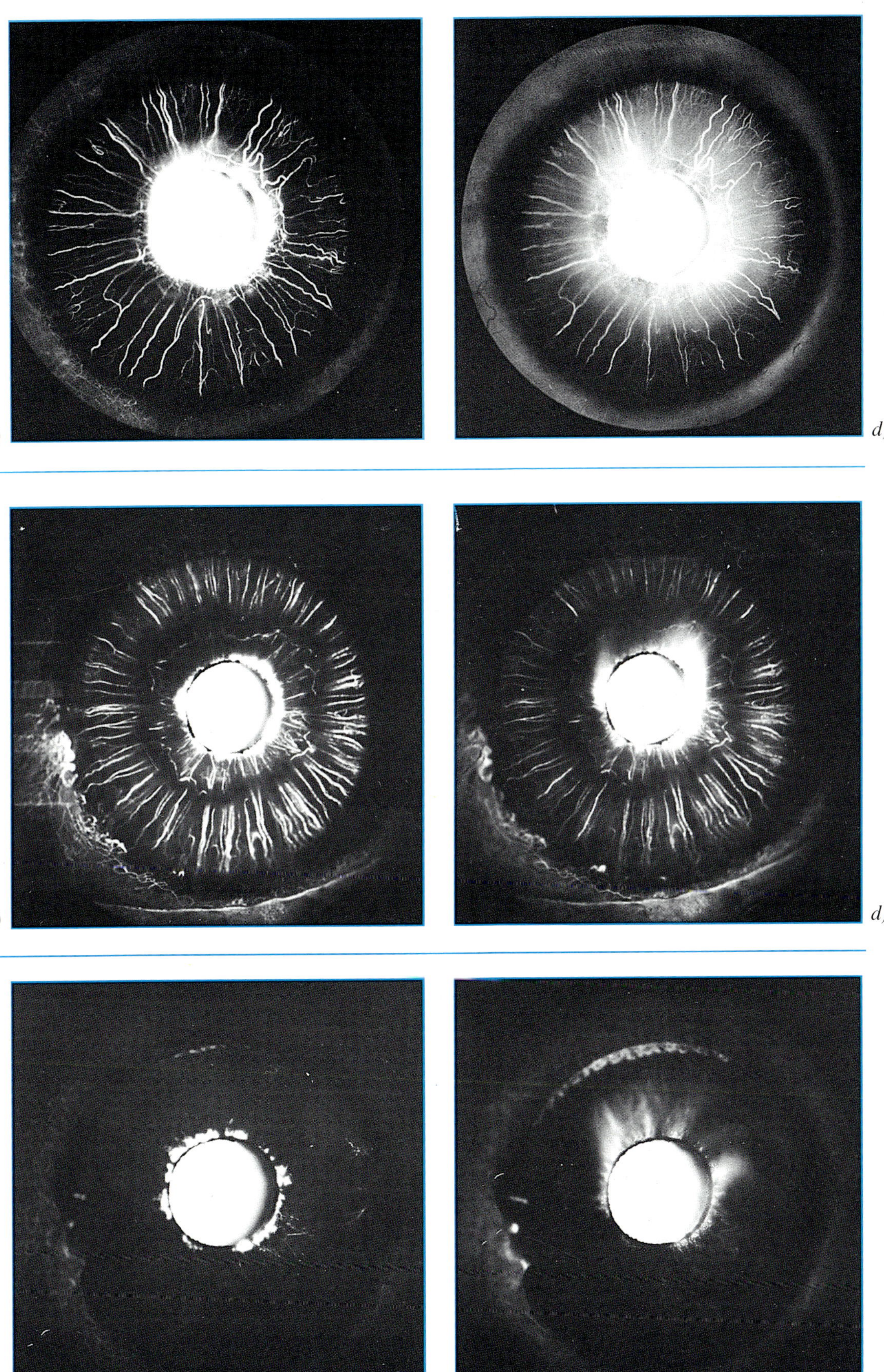

*pigmented irises (Figs.**4.4**,25 and **4.4**,26) whereas fluorescein angiography shows them up clearly in the different phases (b,c,d).*

←

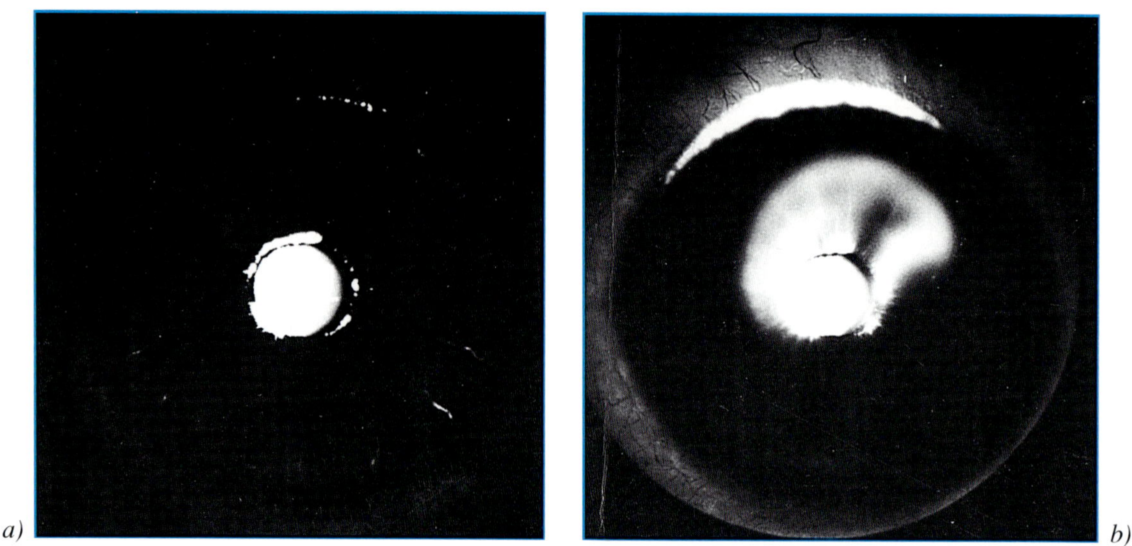

*Fig. **4.4**,28 - Fluorescein angiography in a left eye with new vessels at the pupillary border. These take up fluorescence early (a) and leak it later (b). The dye is then pushed by convection in the aqueous humor to the superotemporal sector of the anterior chamber.*

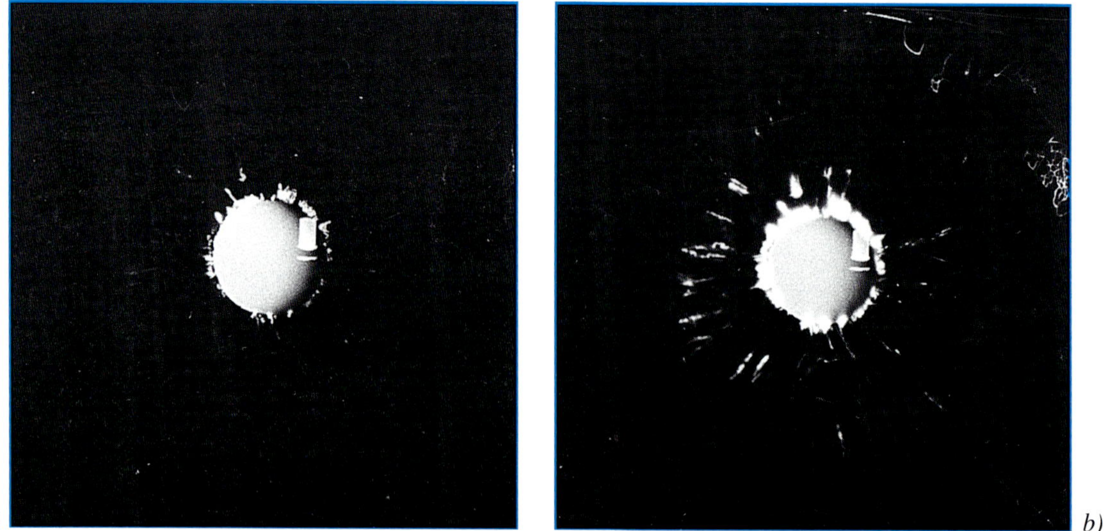

*Fig. **4.4**,29 - Another fluorescein angiography picture of grade 1 proliferative diabetic iridopathy.[37] The new vessels at the pupillary border are seen as spots that fluoresce early (a), becoming gradually more intense and larger in subsequent phases (b) until they are confluent in a glowing peripupillary ring.*

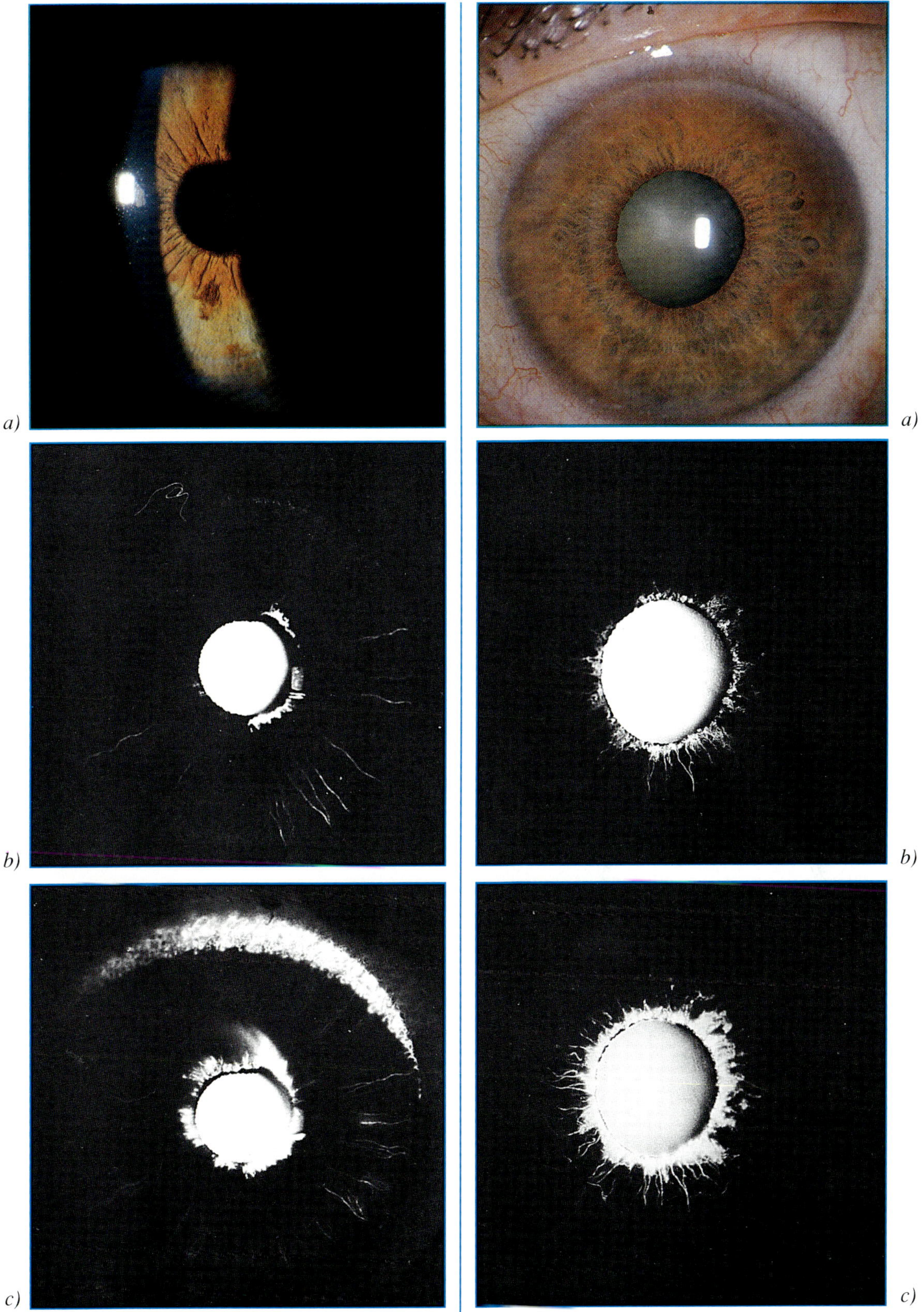

*Fig. **4.4,**30 - Careful biomicroscopic examination (a) shows up these bigger new vessels at the pupillary border; they are easily seen in the fluorescein angiograms (b,c).*

*Fig. **4.4,**31 - Another case of new vessels at the pupillary border: biomicroscopic picture (a) and fluorescein angiograms (b,c).*

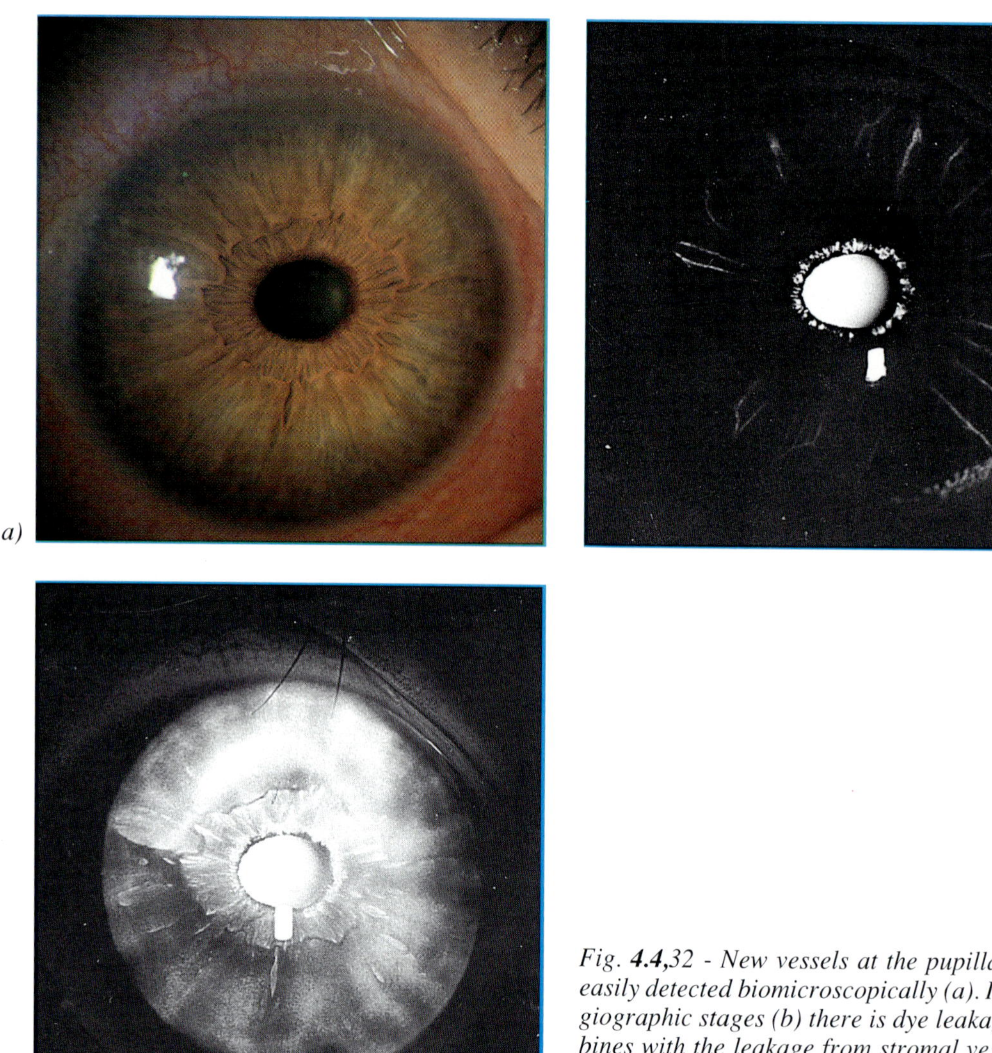

Fig. ***4.4,****32 - New vessels at the pupillary border are easily detected biomicroscopically (a). In the early angiographic stages (b) there is dye leakage which combines with the leakage from stromal vessels to form a diffuse veil of fluorescence in the anterior chamber in later phases (c).*

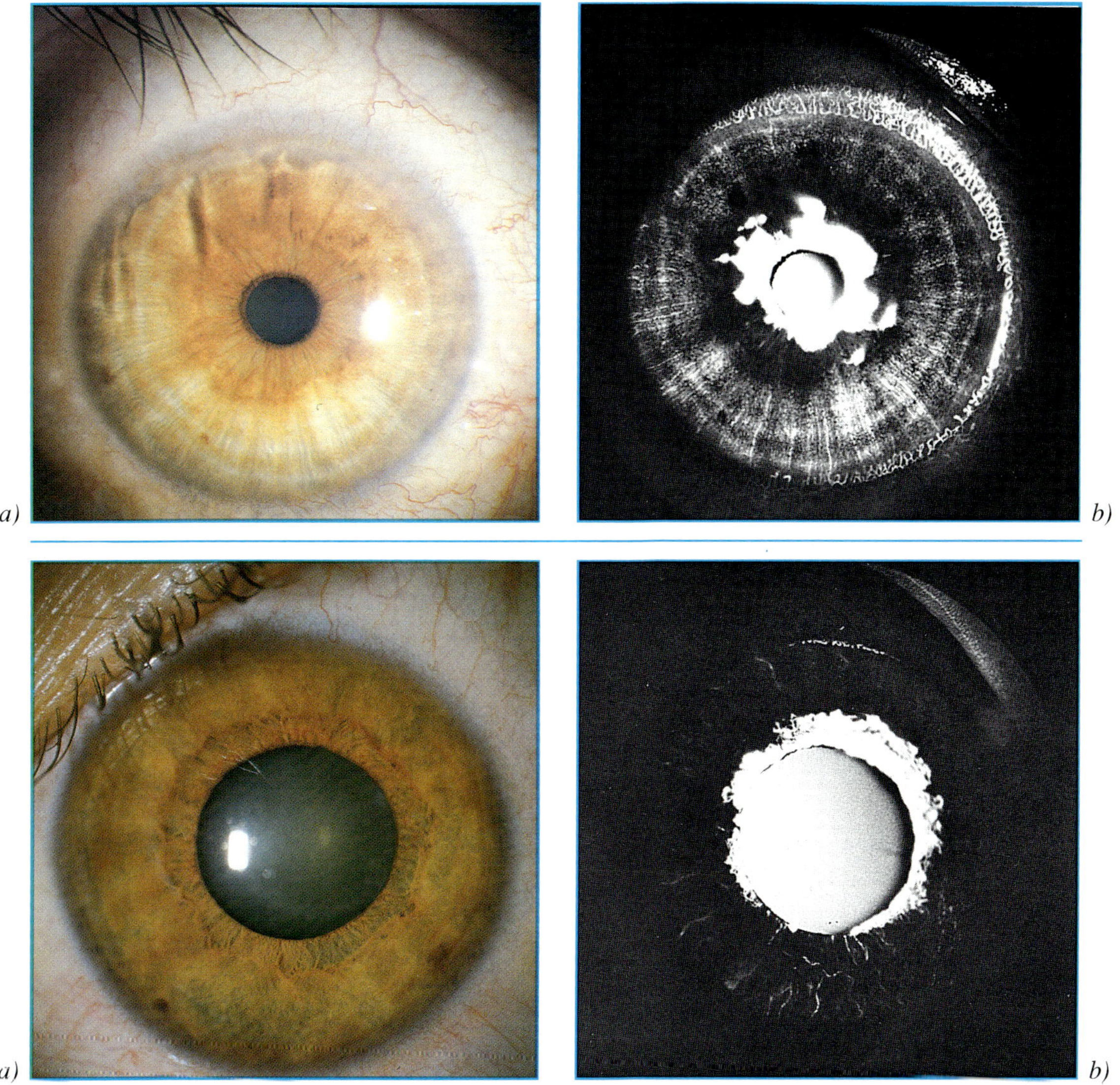

*Figs. **4.4**,33,34 - Two cases of bigger new vessels at the pupillary border seen clearly with the biomicroscope (a) and by fluorescein angiography (b) even in a heavily pigmented iris (Fig.**4.4,** 34).*

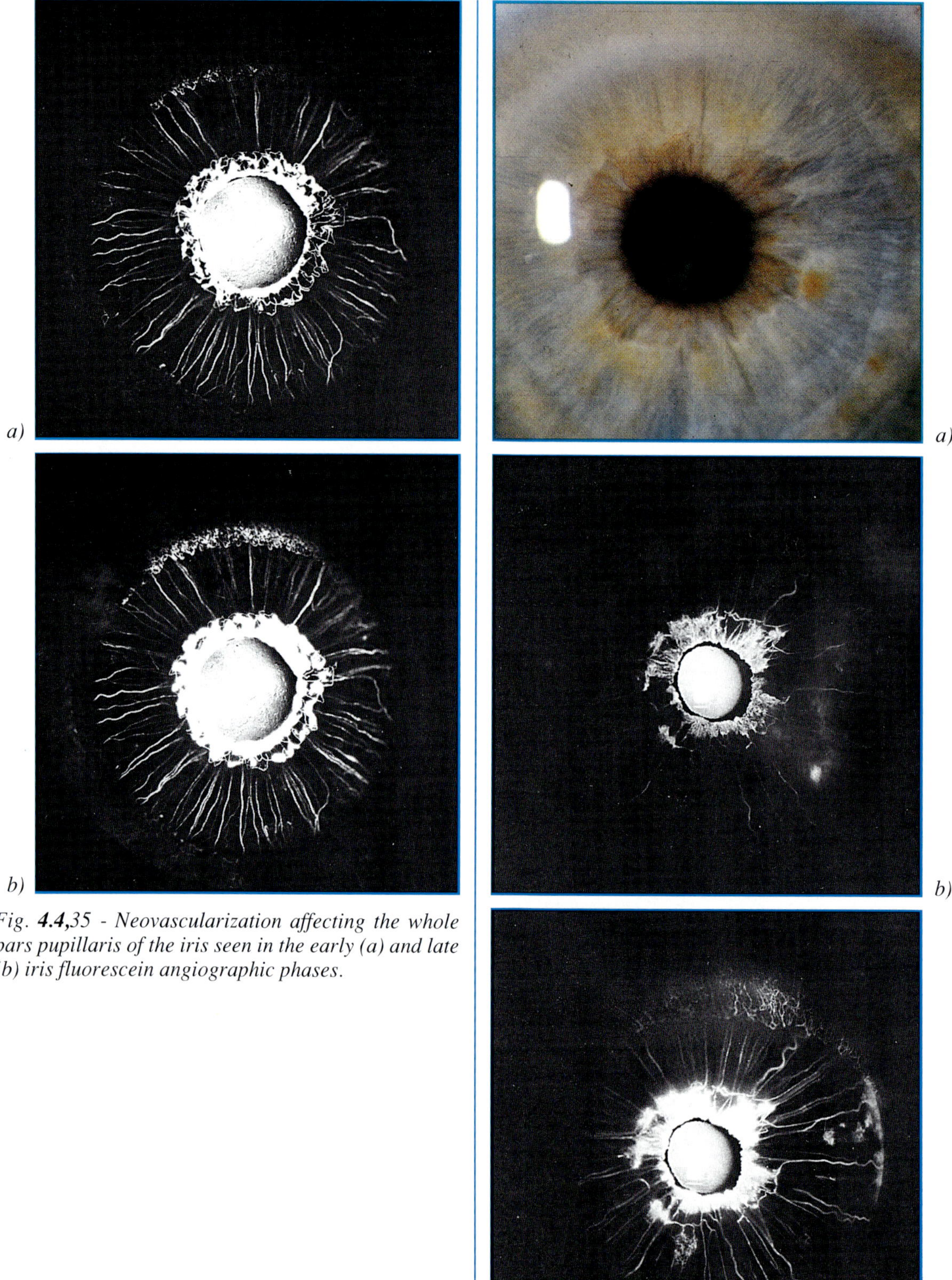

*Fig. **4.4,**35 - Neovascularization affecting the whole pars pupillaris of the iris seen in the early (a) and late (b) iris fluorescein angiographic phases.*

*Fig. **4.4,**36 - Biomicroscopy (a) and fluorescein angiographic phases (b,c) of imposing new vessels at the pupillary border with initial involvement of the stroma and irido-corneal angle.*

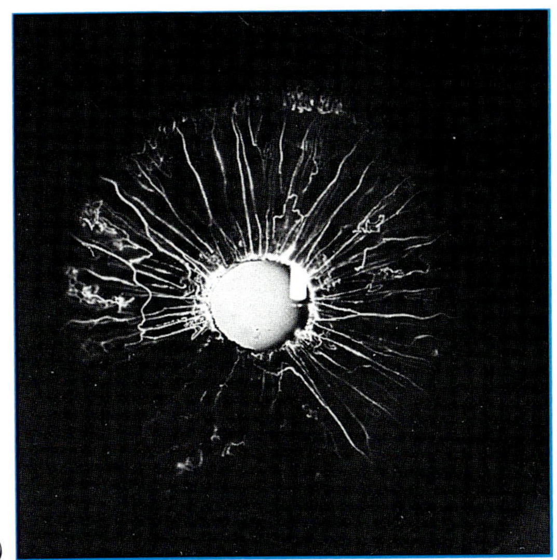
a)

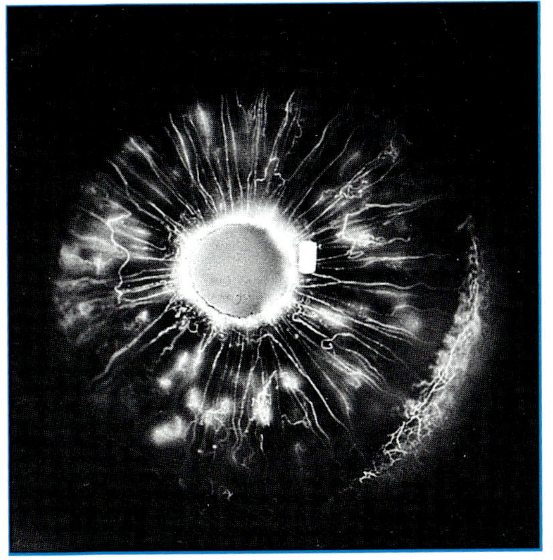
b)

Fig. **4.4**,*37 - New vessels at the border and stroma (early (a) and late (b) fluorescein angiographic findings). In the early phase filling of the vessels in the lower sector is delayed.*

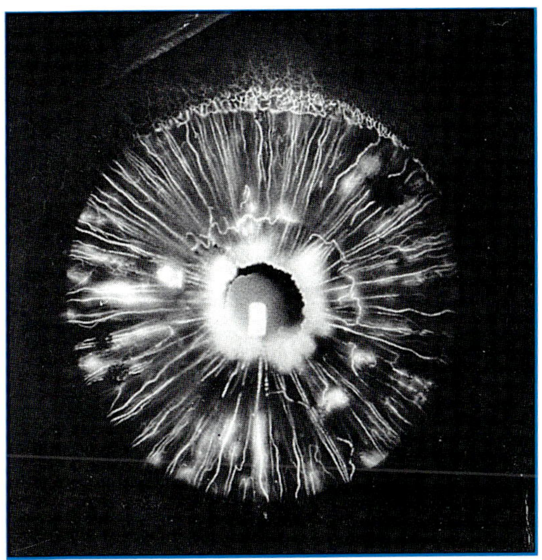

Fig. **4.4**,*38 - Fluorescein angiographic findings of neovascular proliferation at the border and stroma of the iris. Dye leakage can also be seen in radial vessels on account of altered permeability.*

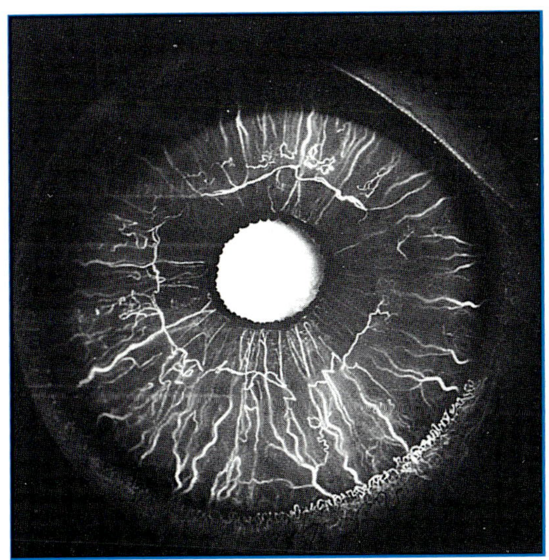
a)

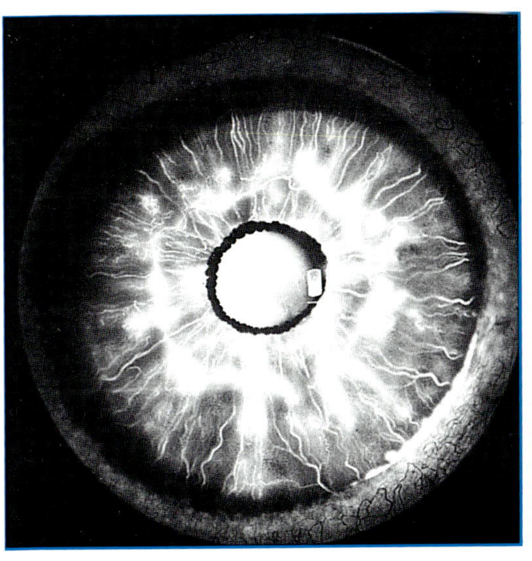
b)

Fig. **4.4**,*39 - Initial new vessels in the stroma of the iris in the early (a) and late (b) angiographic phases. New vessels cannot be seen at the pupillary border probably because they are masked by hyperplasia of the border itself.*

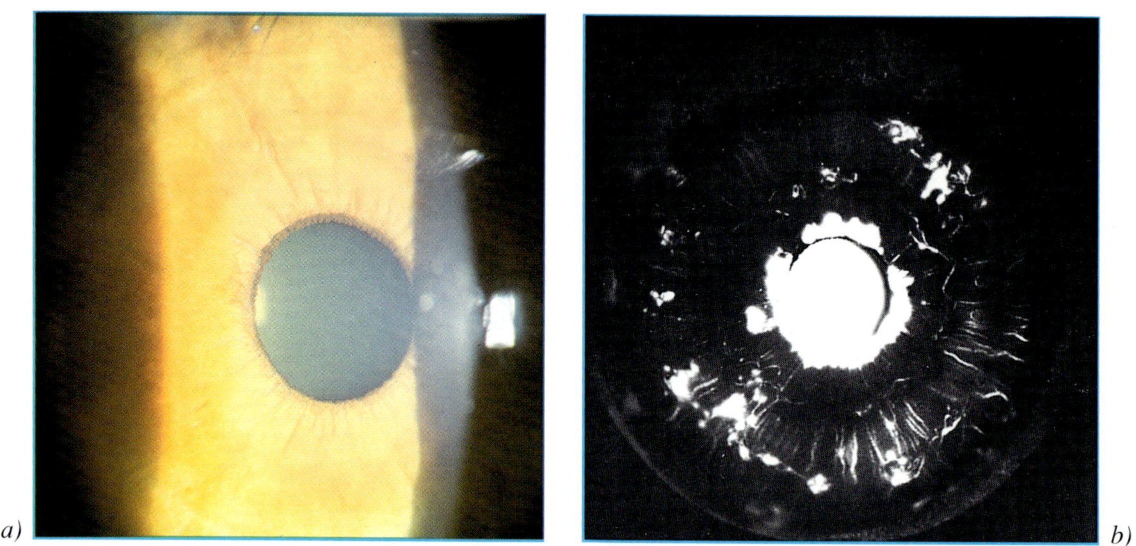

a) b)

Fig. ***4.4,**40 - New vessels at the border and stroma: biomicroscopic (a) and iris fluorescein angiography (b) pictures.*

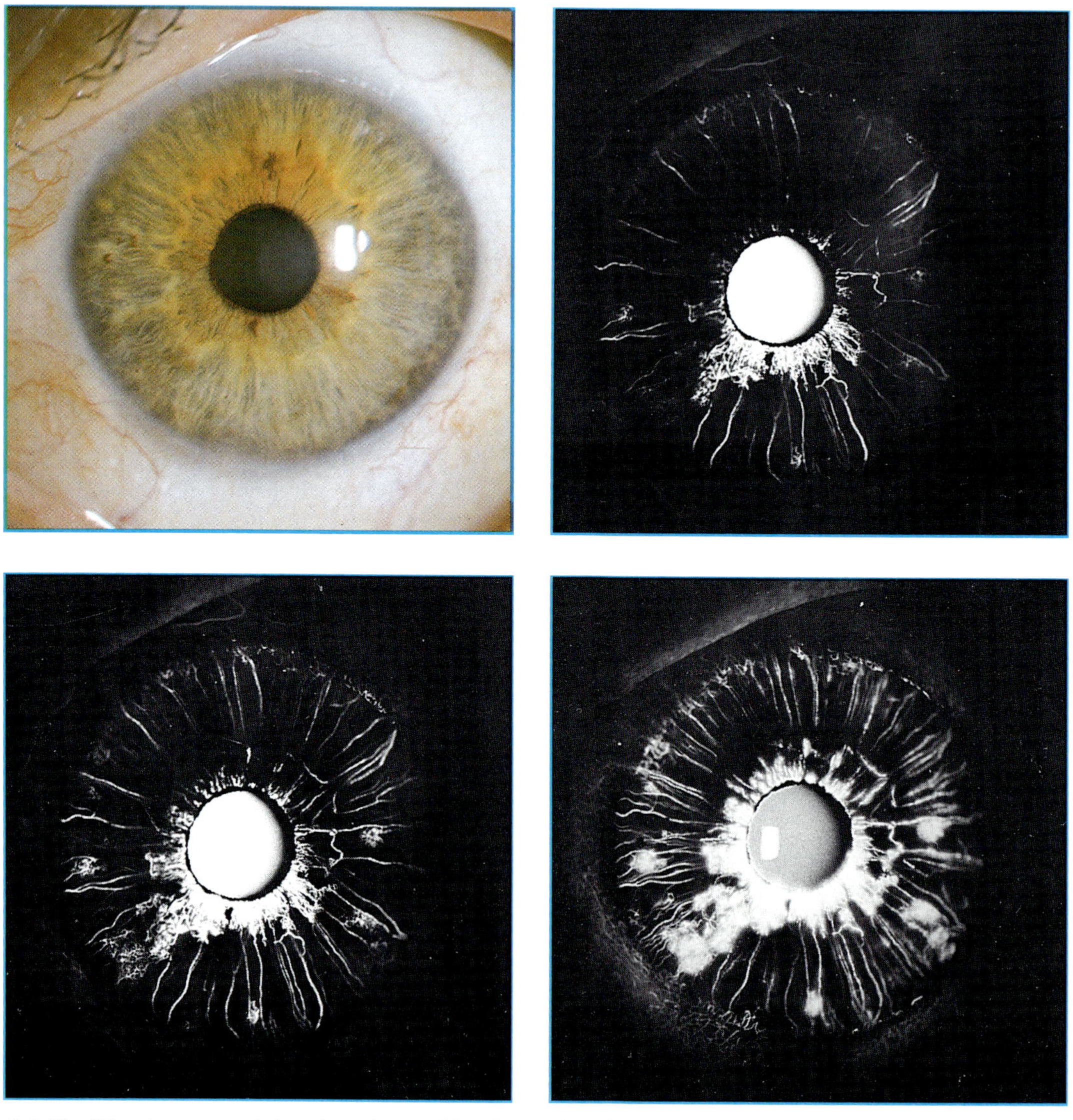

a) b)

c) d)

Fig. ***4.4,**41 - Biomicroscopy (a) and angiographic phases (b,c,d) in another case of grade 2 proliferative diabetic iridopathy*[37] *with new vessels at the border and stroma of the iris.*

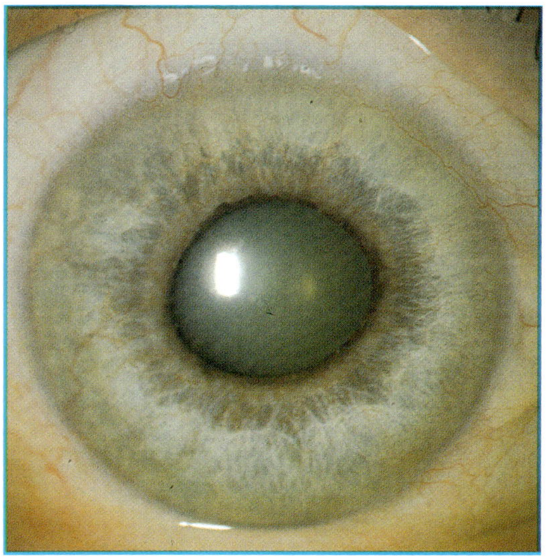

a) 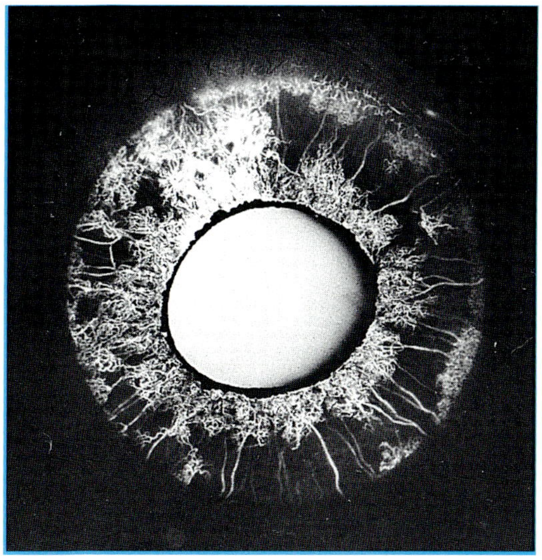 b)

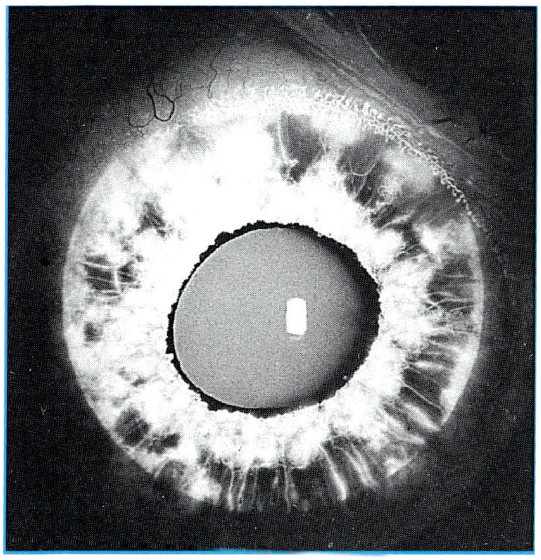

c)

*Fig. **4.4**,42 - Irregular network of new vessels extending over the whole anterior surface of the iris (biomicroscopy (a) and angiographic phases (b,c)).*

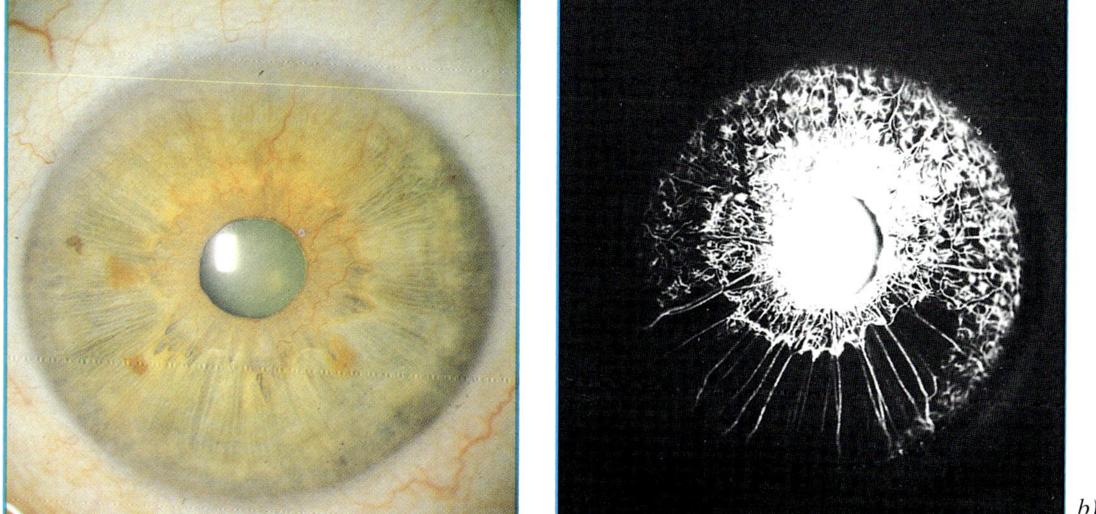

*Fig. **4.4**,43 - Biomicroscopy (a) and fluorescein angiography (b) of new vessels around the whole pupillary border and mainly the superior segments of the stroma.*

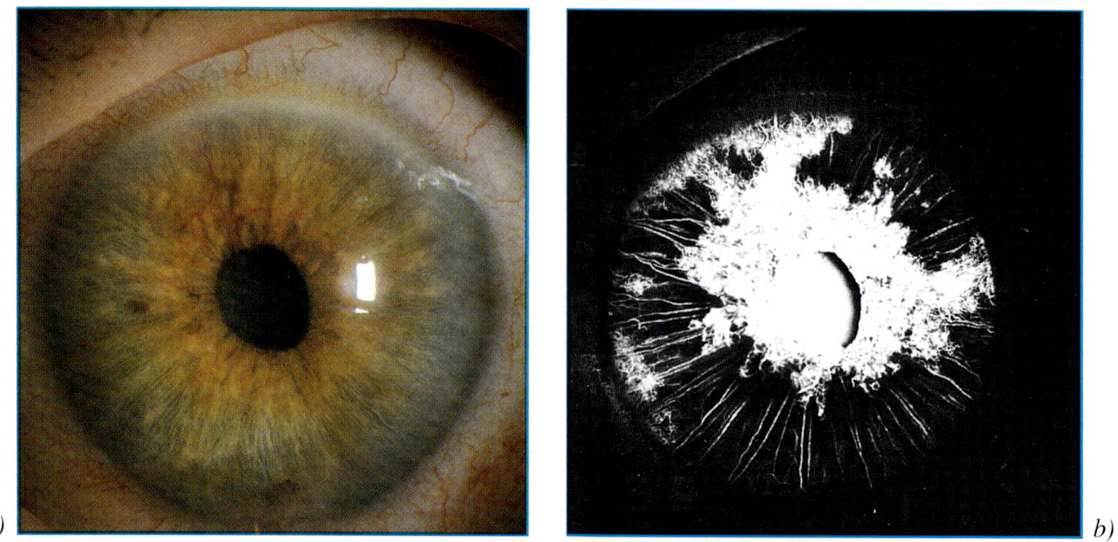

*Fig. **4.4,**44 - Another case of grade 2 proliferative diabetic iridopathy[37] with new vessels at the pupillary border and stroma, visible biomicroscopically (a) and clearly defined by fluorescein angiography (b).*

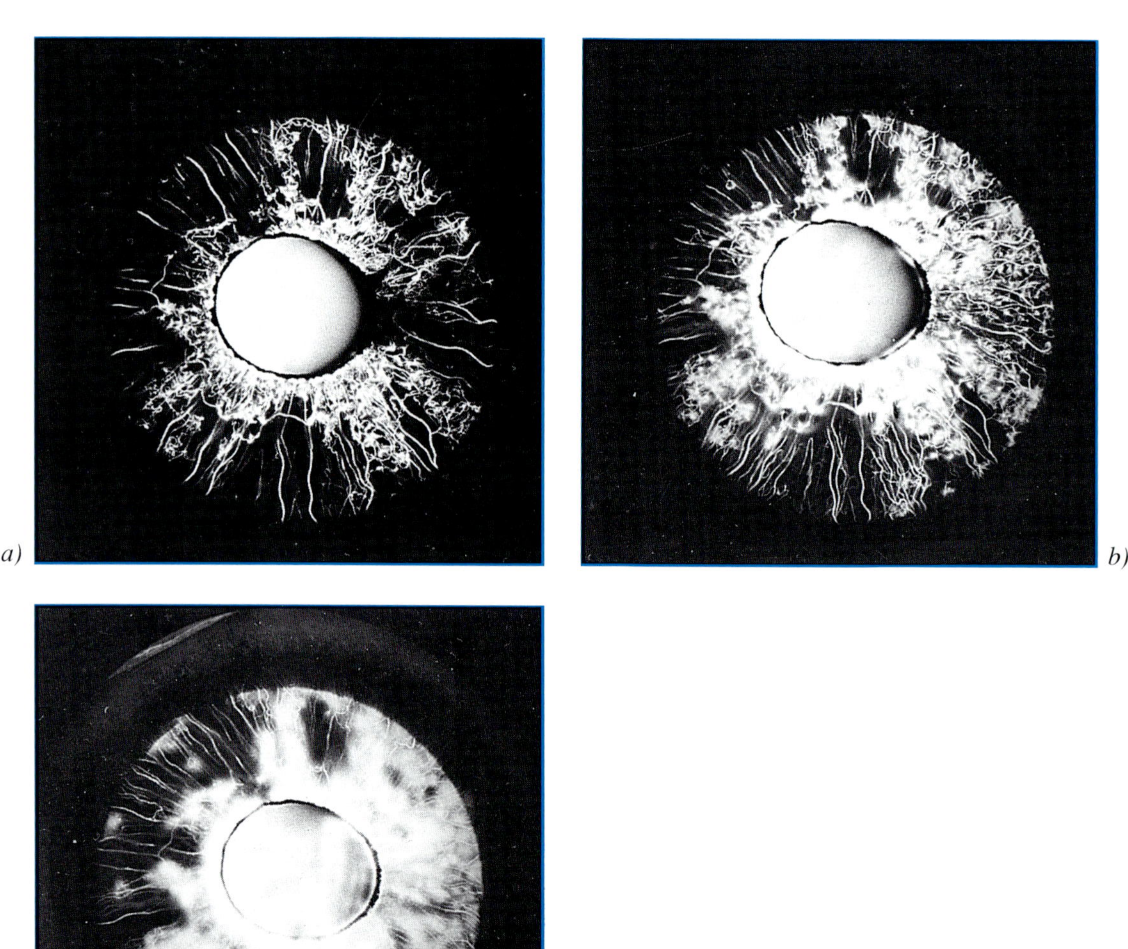

*Fig. **4.4,**45 - Iris fluorescein angiography in a case of proliferative iridopathy. The radial structure is completely upturned and early hyperfluorescence (a) can be seen in the anarchic network of new-formed vessels responsible for the dye leakage (b) that becomes more marked in later phases (c).*

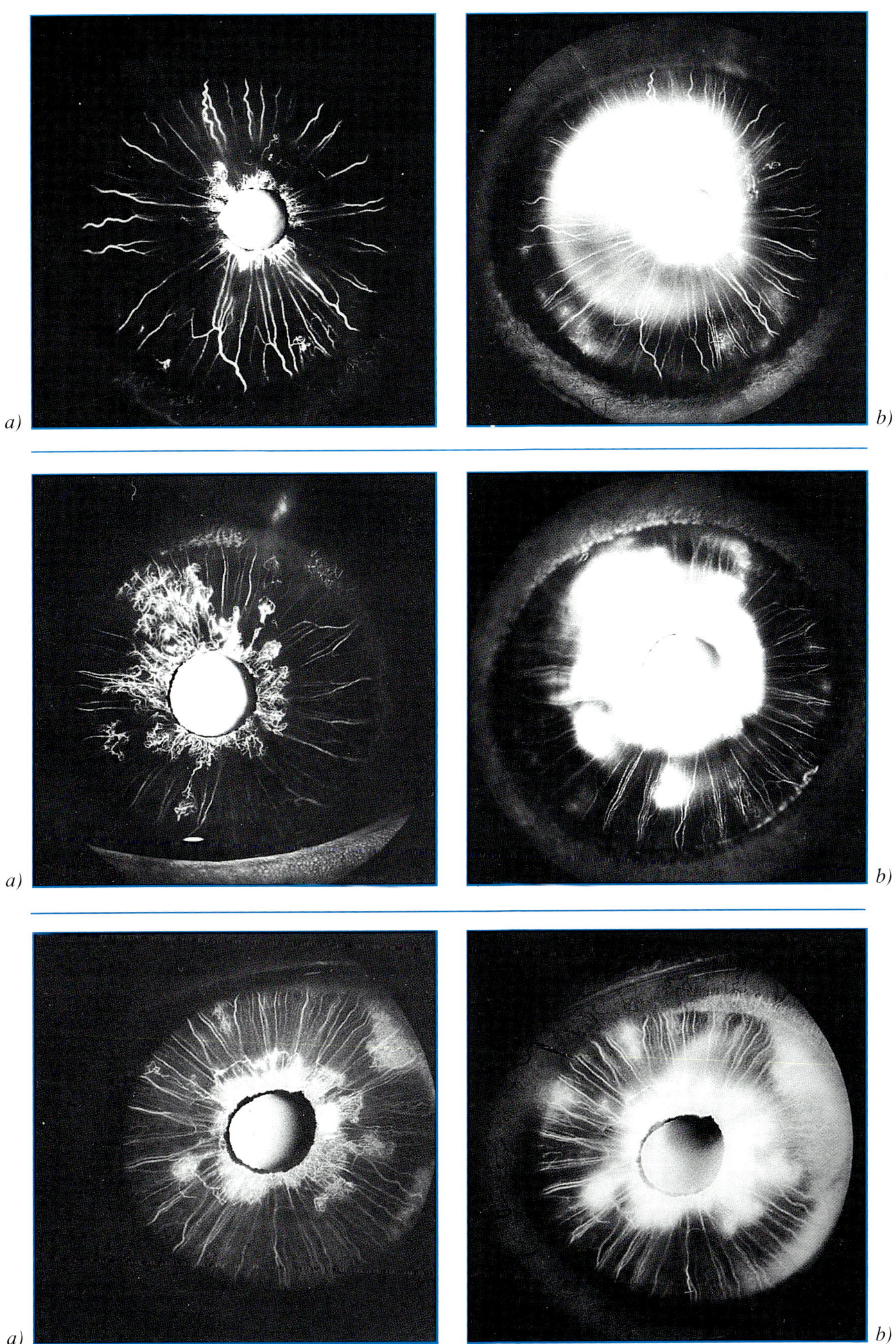

*Figs. **4.4**,46-48 - In these three cases the site and precise extension of new vessels in the iris are clearly visible in the early (a) iris angiographic phases before the dye leakage typical of the later phases (b) makes them harder to see as it covers radial vessels too.*

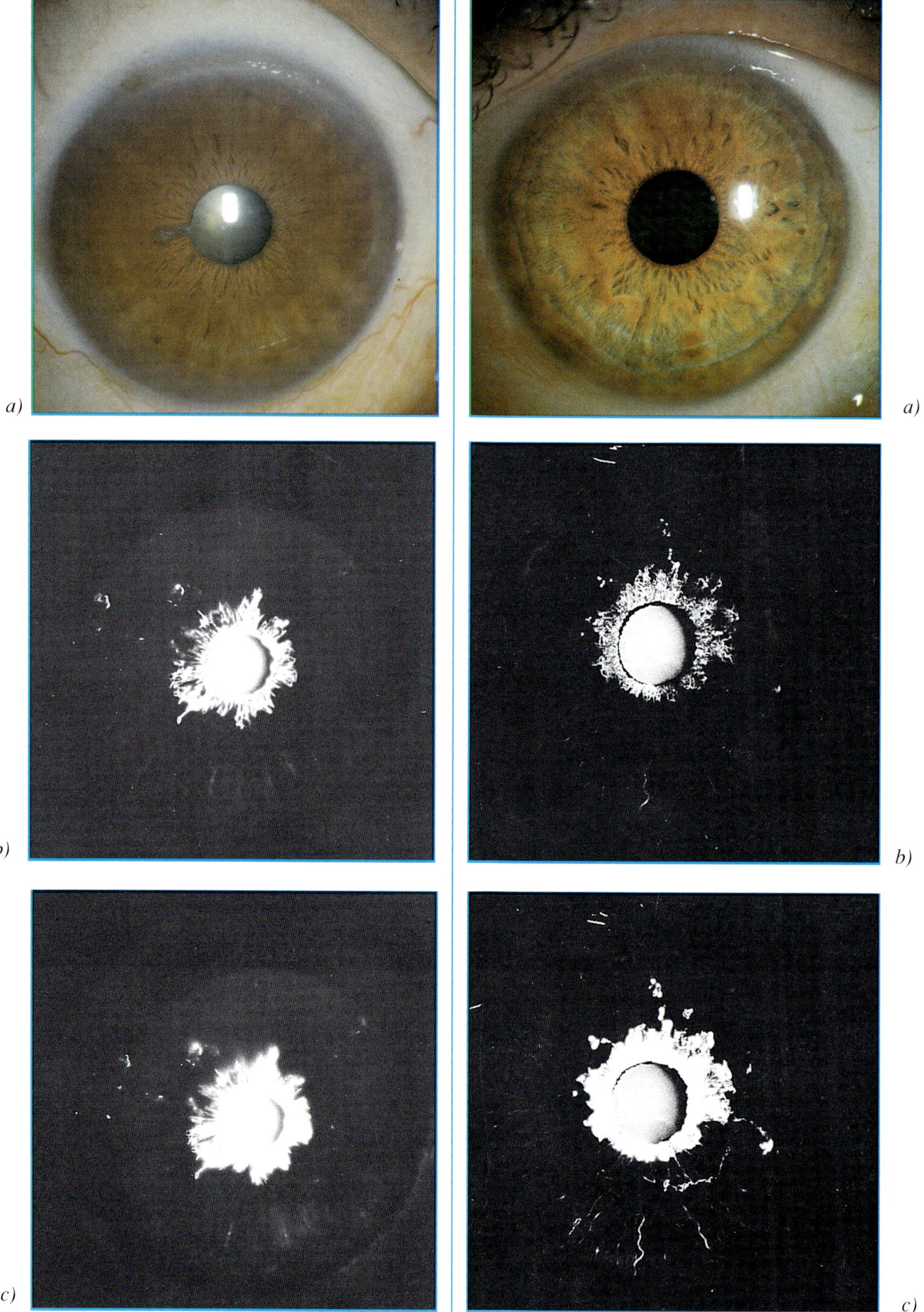

Figs. ***4.4,****49-51 - The pigment in these three dark irises makes it difficult to detect new vessels with the bio-*

→

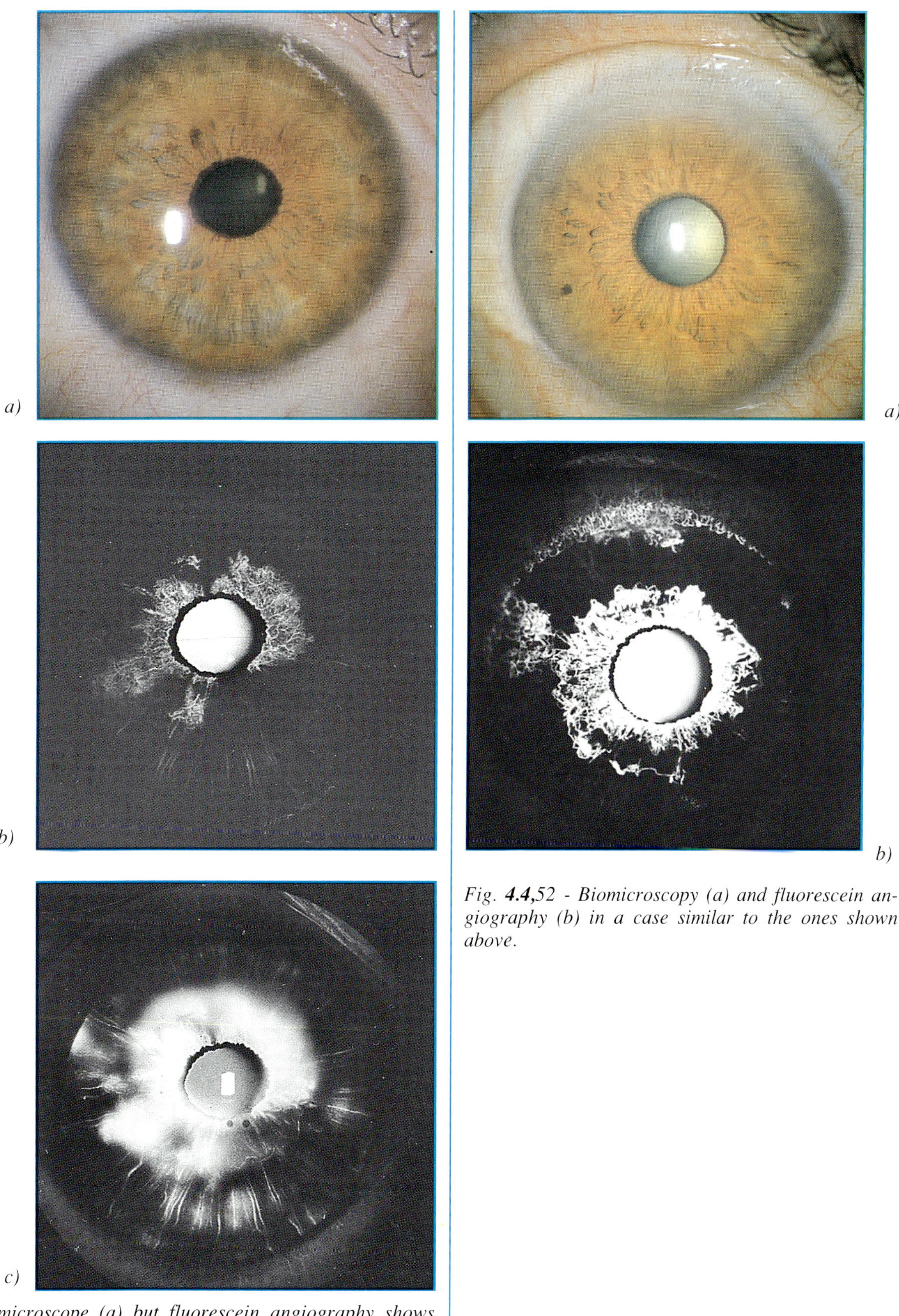

microscope (a) but fluorescein angiography shows them clearly (b,c).

←

*Fig. **4.4**,52 - Biomicroscopy (a) and fluorescein angiography (b) in a case similar to the ones shown above.*

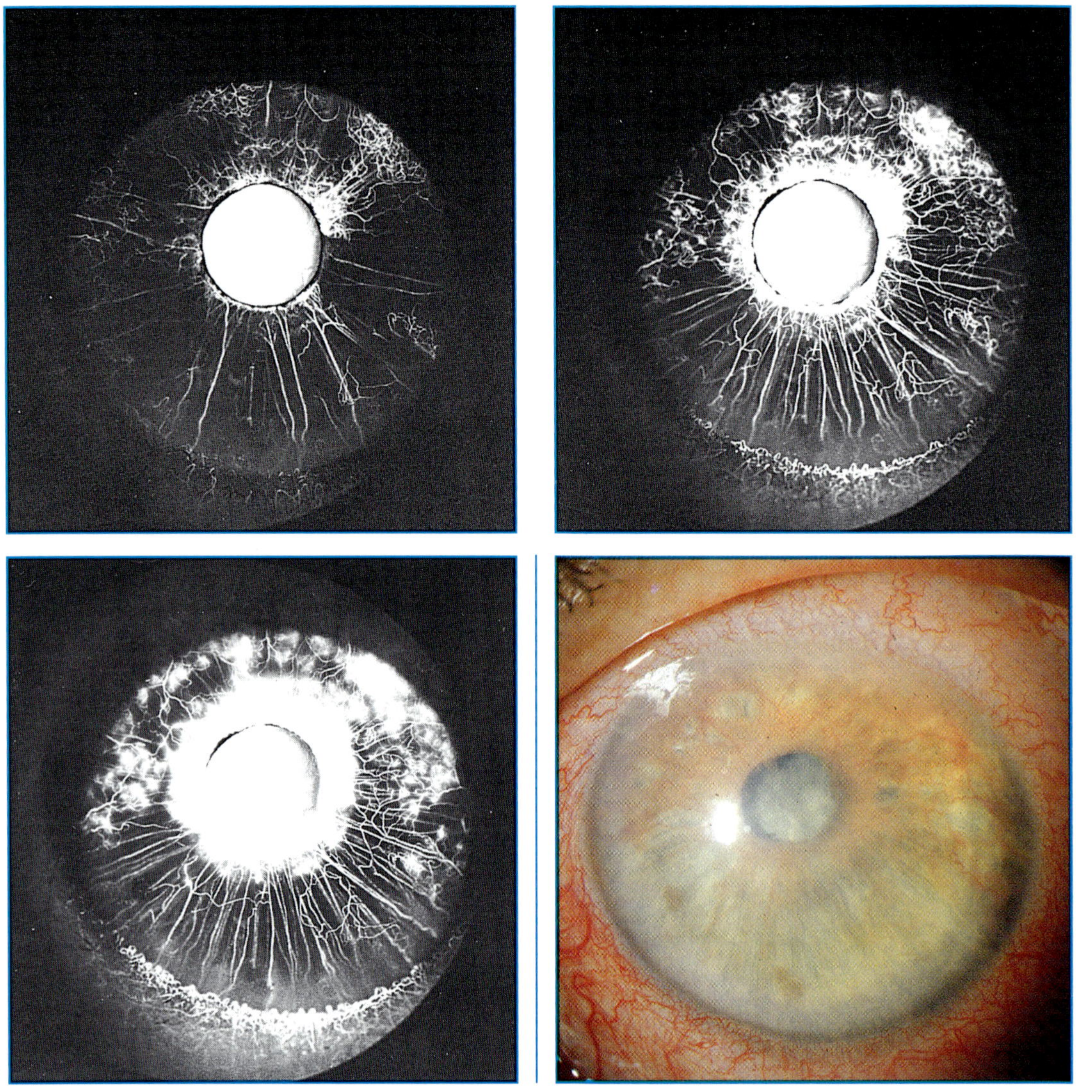

a) b)

c)

*Figs. **4.4**,53,54 - Major neovascularization over most of the surface of the iris (Fig. **4.4**,53a,b,c: serial angiographic phases); five years later neovascularization has become extensive and the typical ocular hypertension of neovascular glaucoma is present (Fig. **4.4**,54, biomicroscopy).*

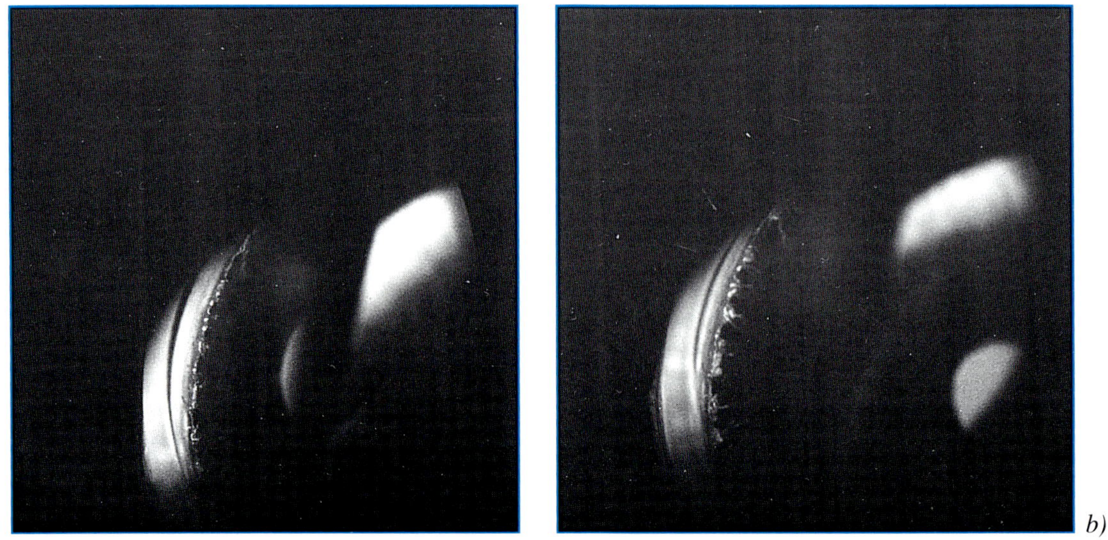

a) b)

*Fig. **4.4**,55 - Angiographic examination using the gonioscopic lens (a,b) shows up new vessels at the iridocorneal angle in their early stages.*

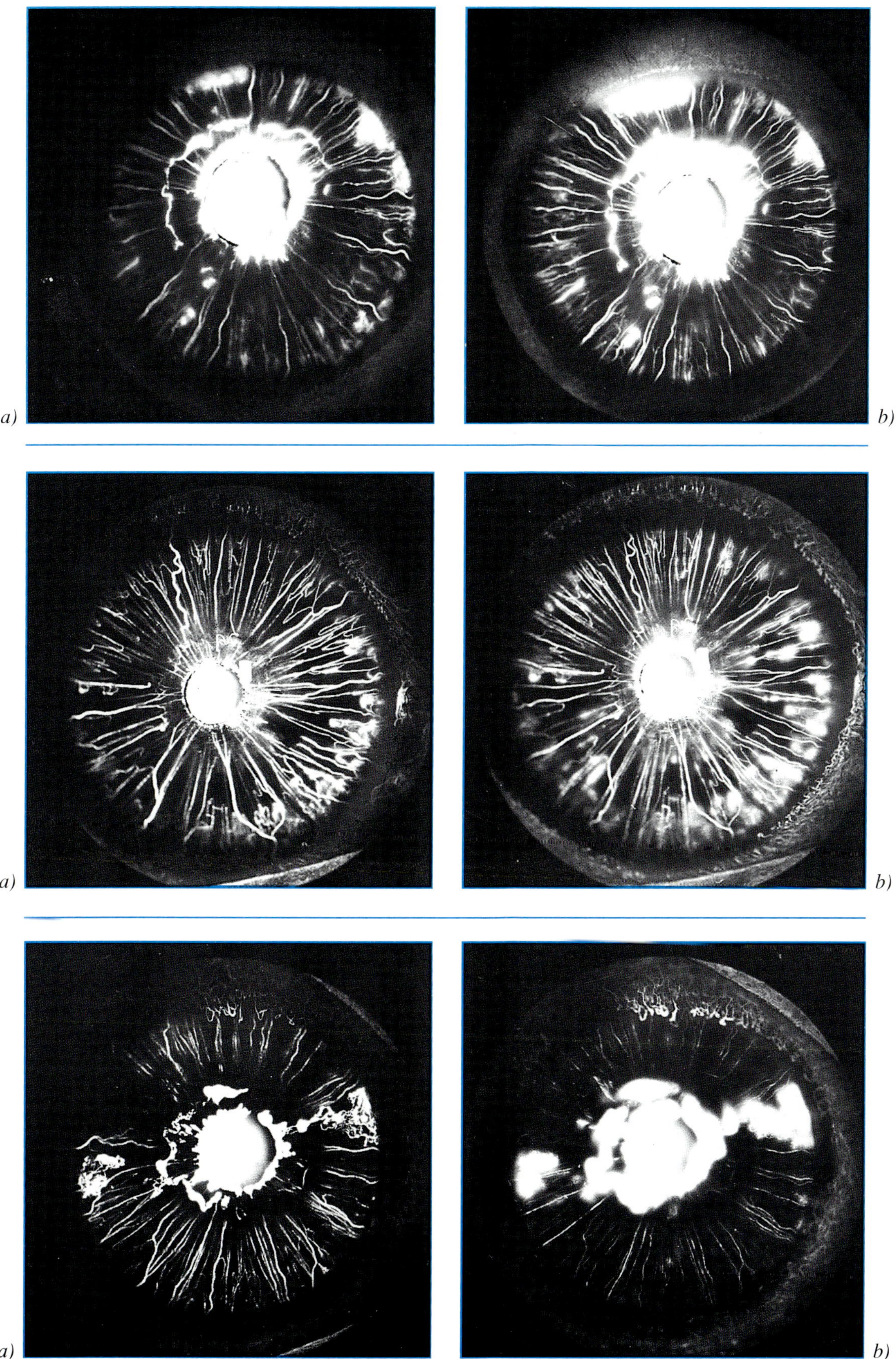

*Figs. **4.4**,56-58 - Early (a) and late (b) fluorescein angiographic phases in three cases of neovascularization at the pupillary border, the stroma and iridocorneal angle.*

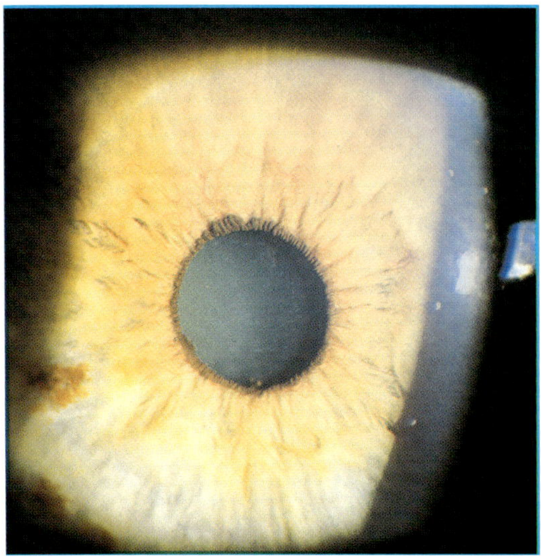

*Fig. **4.4**,59 - Biomicroscopic (a) and angiographic (b,c) pictures in grade 2 proliferative diabetic iridopathy.*[37]

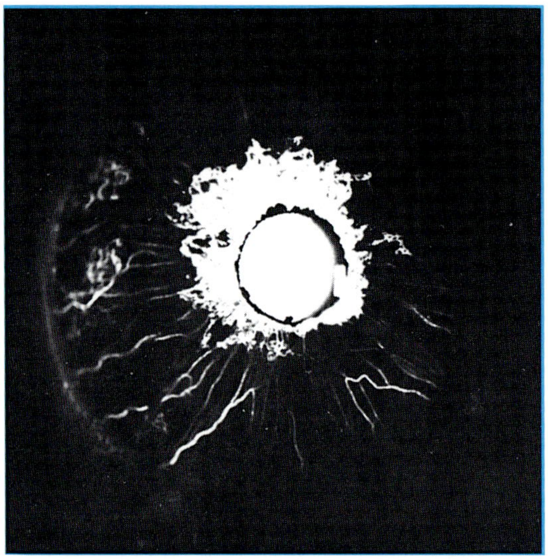

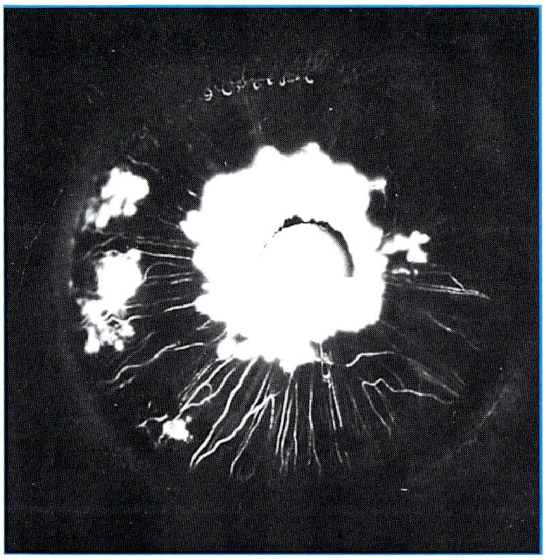

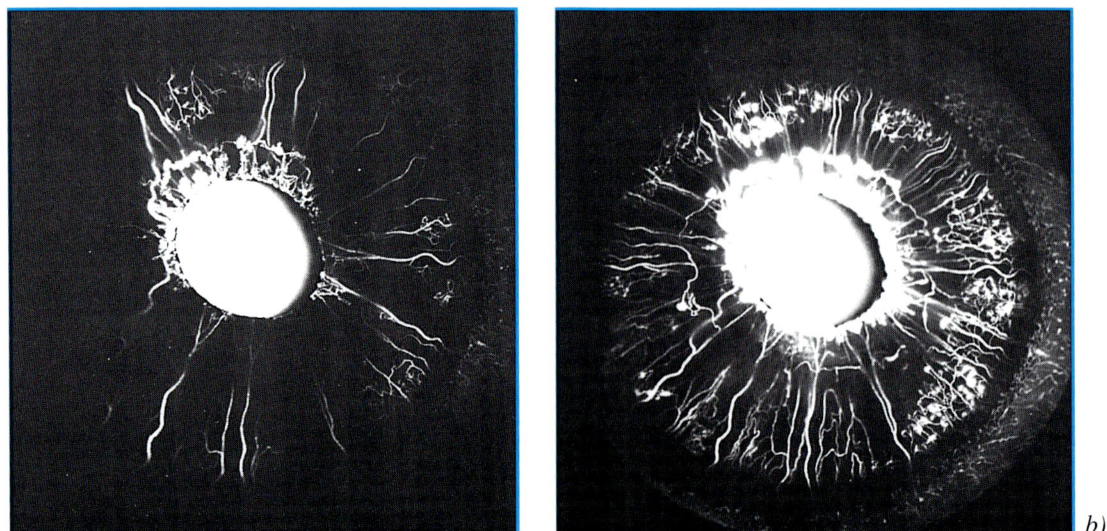

*Fig. **4.4**,60 - Delayed filling and new vessels over the whole surface of the iris in proliferative diabetic iridopathy (early (a) and late (b) fluorescein angiographic phases).*

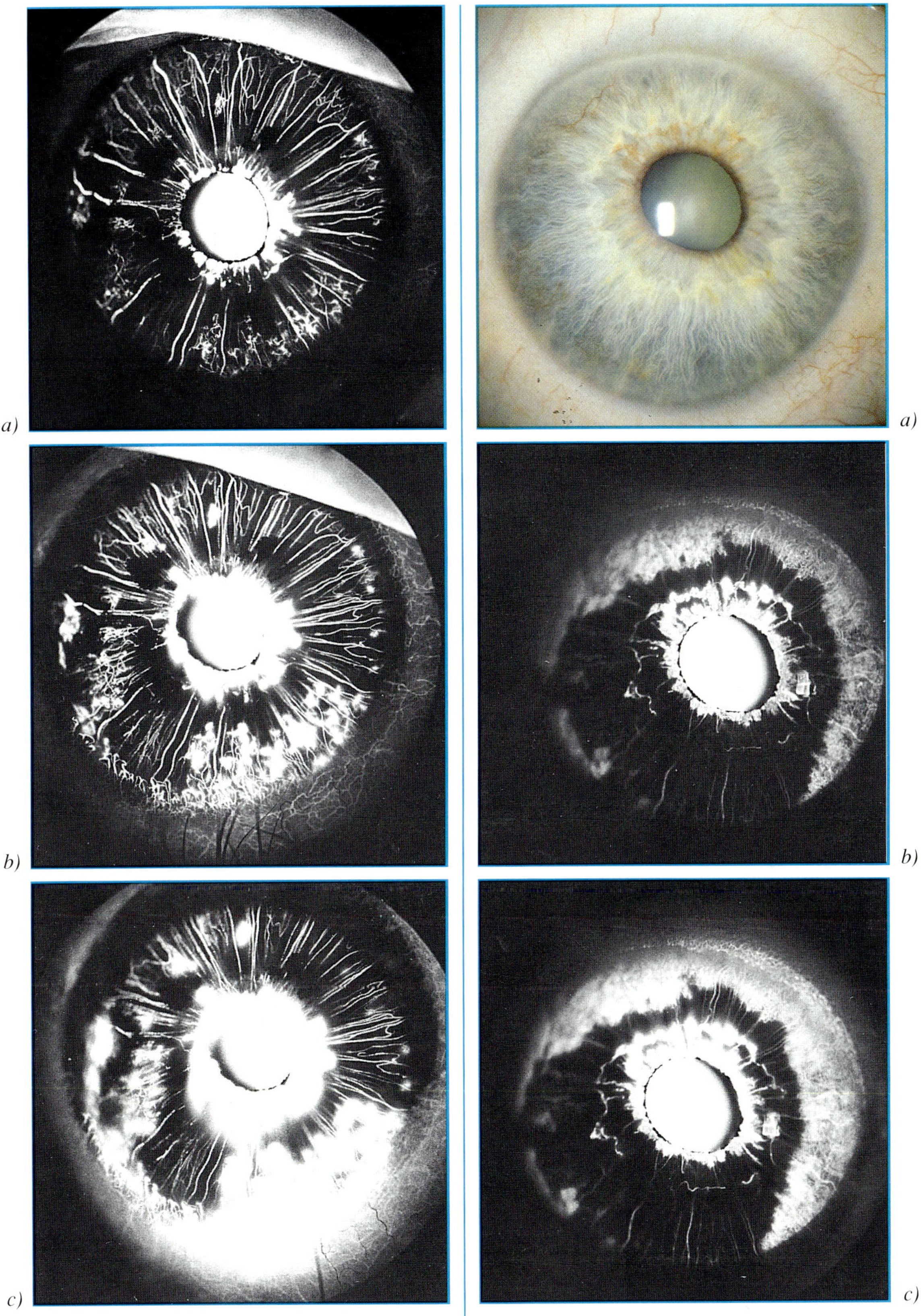

*Fig. **4.4**,61 - New vessels at the border and stroma running into those starting at the root of the iris (fluorescein angiographic phases: a,b,c).*

*Fig. **4.4**,62 - Neovascularization detected with the biomicroscope (a) can be visualized with precision in the fluorescein angiograms (b,c) wherever it is (border, stroma or iris root).*

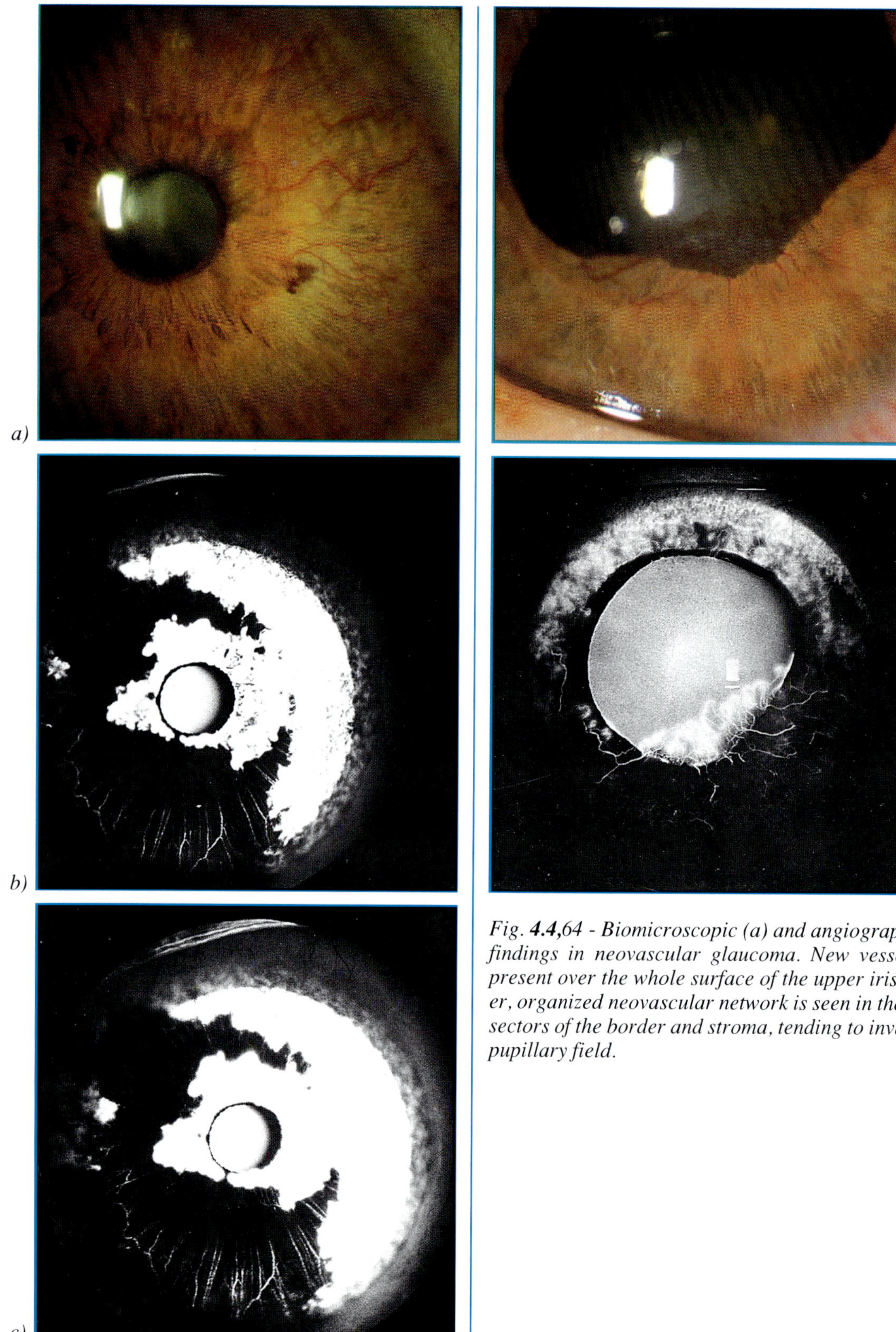

*Fig. **4.4,63** - Imposing neovascularization involving the whole pupillary border, stroma and root of a hemiiris (a: biomicroscopy; b,c: early and late fluorescein angiography).*

*Fig. **4.4,64** - Biomicroscopic (a) and angiographic (b) findings in neovascular glaucoma. New vessels are present over the whole surface of the upper iris. A finer, organized neovascular network is seen in the lower sectors of the border and stroma, tending to invade the pupillary field.*

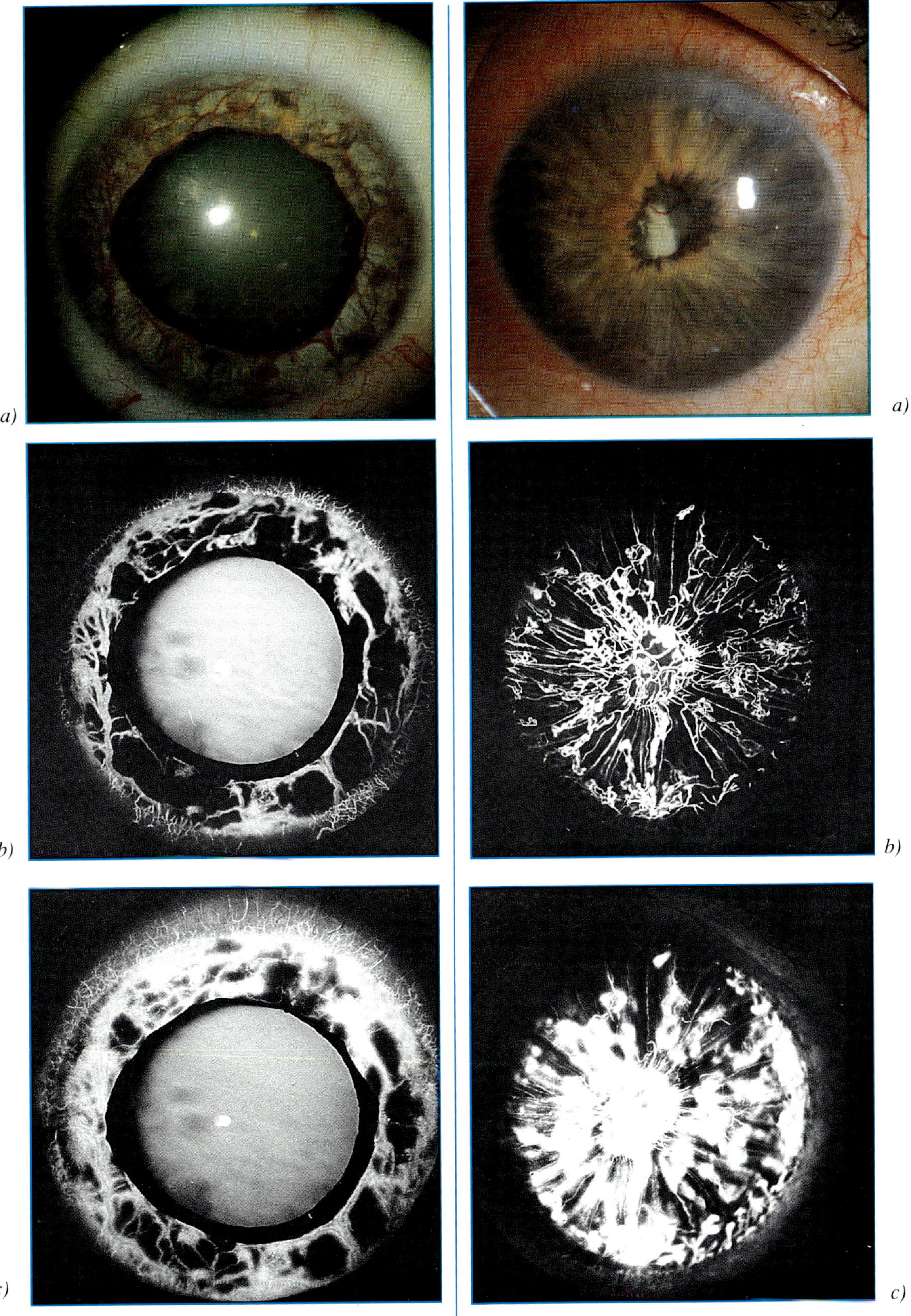

*Fig. **4.4**,65 - Neovascular glaucoma: ectropion uveae detectable with the biomicroscope (a) shows up as hypofluorescence in the angiogram (b,c), with unperfused areas of the iris. Voluminous neovascular trunks take up the dye copiously.*

*Fig. **4.4**,66 - Neovascular glaucoma with pupillary occlusion caused by a dense, intricate neovascular membrane (biomicroscopic (a) and fluorescein angiographic (b,c) pictures).*

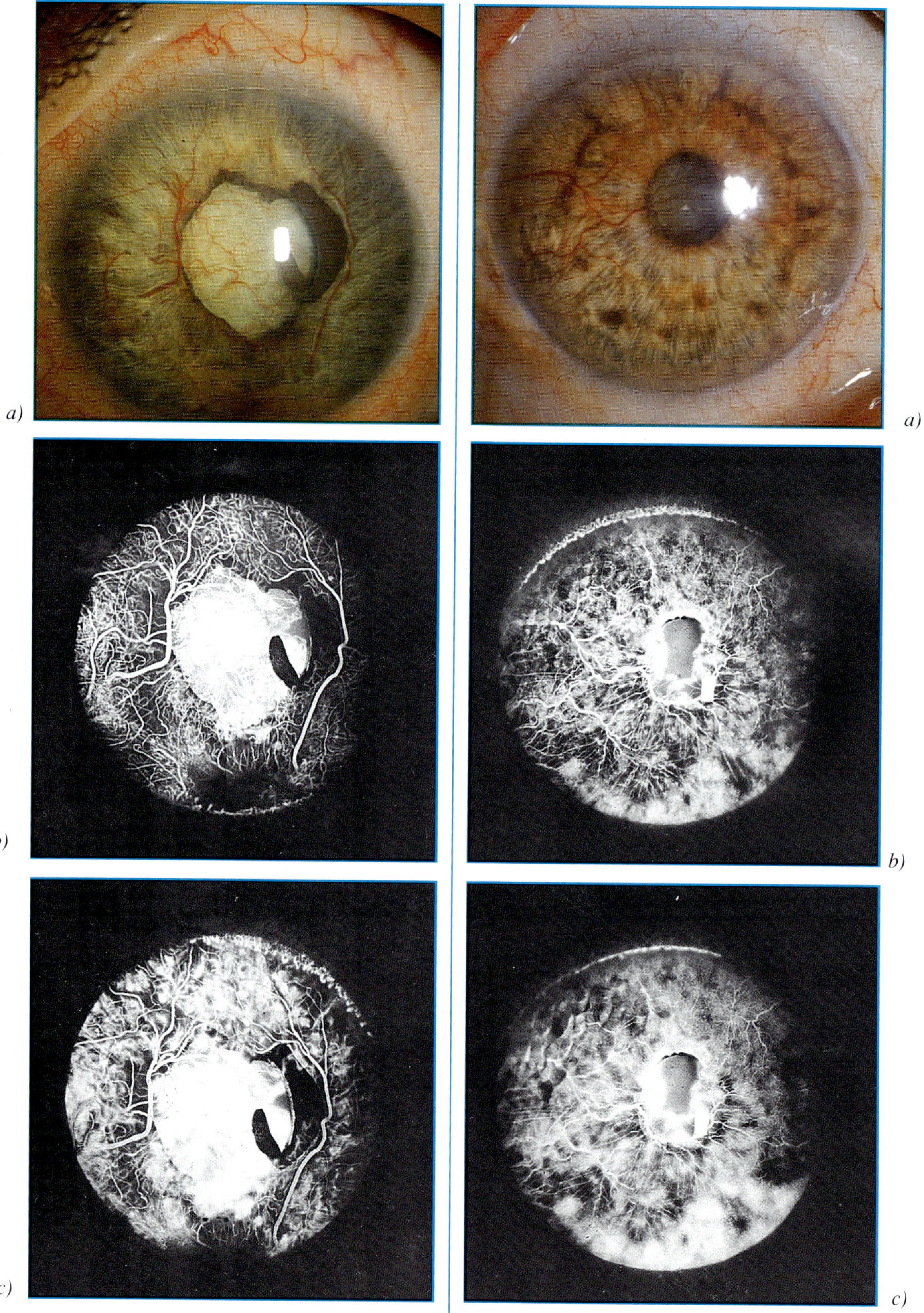

*Fig. **4.4,**67 - Biomicroscopic (a) and fluorescein angiographic (b,c) findings in neovascular glaucoma. The pupil is deformed with partial ectropion uveae, there are voluminous neovascular trunks over the surface of the iris and a dense neoformed network in the pupillary field.*

*Fig. **4.4,**68 - Biomicroscopy (a) and angiographic phases (b,c) in neovascular glaucoma with partial pupillary occlusion.*

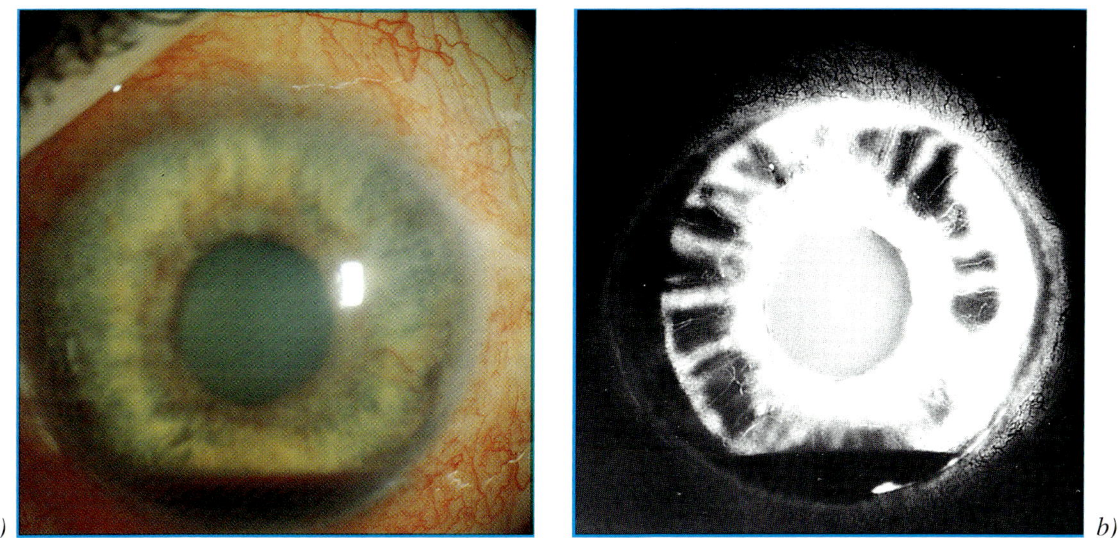

a) b)

*Fig. **4.4**,69 - Biomicroscopic (a) and fluorescein angiographic (b) findings in neovascular glaucoma. Hyphema due to bleeding from new vessels causes the clear-cut hypofluorescence indicating blockage in the lower part of the angiogram.*

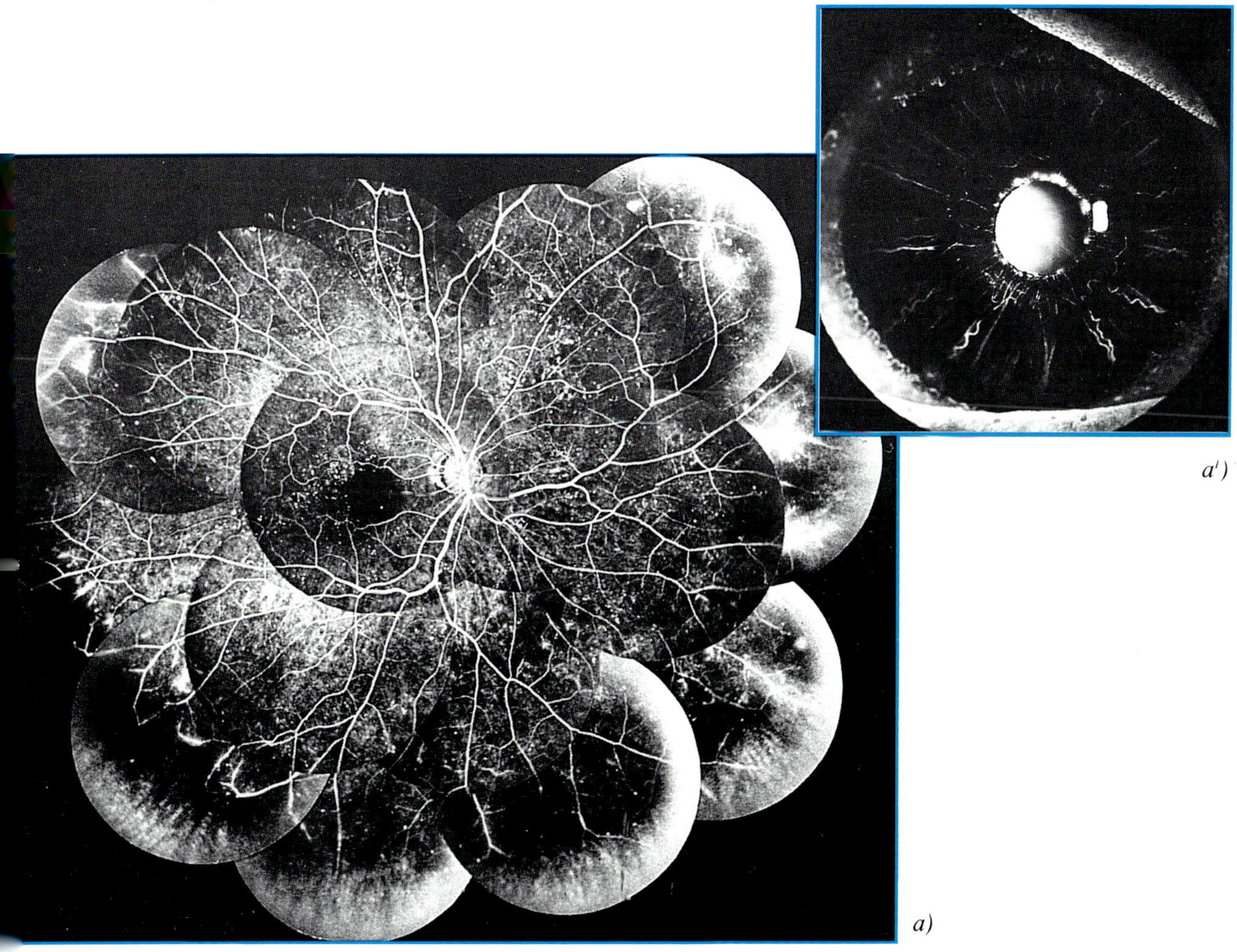

a[1])

a)

*Fig. **4.4**,70 - Panretinal fluorescein angiography in three cases of ischemic diabetic retinopathy of increasing severity: Grade 1: peripheral ischemia up to the vorticose veins (a); Grade 2: peripheral ischemia up to the temporal vascular arcades (b); Grade 3: ischemia reaching from the periphery right into the vascular arcades (c) and correspondent fluoroiridographic pictures (a[1], b[1], c[1] - see next page).*

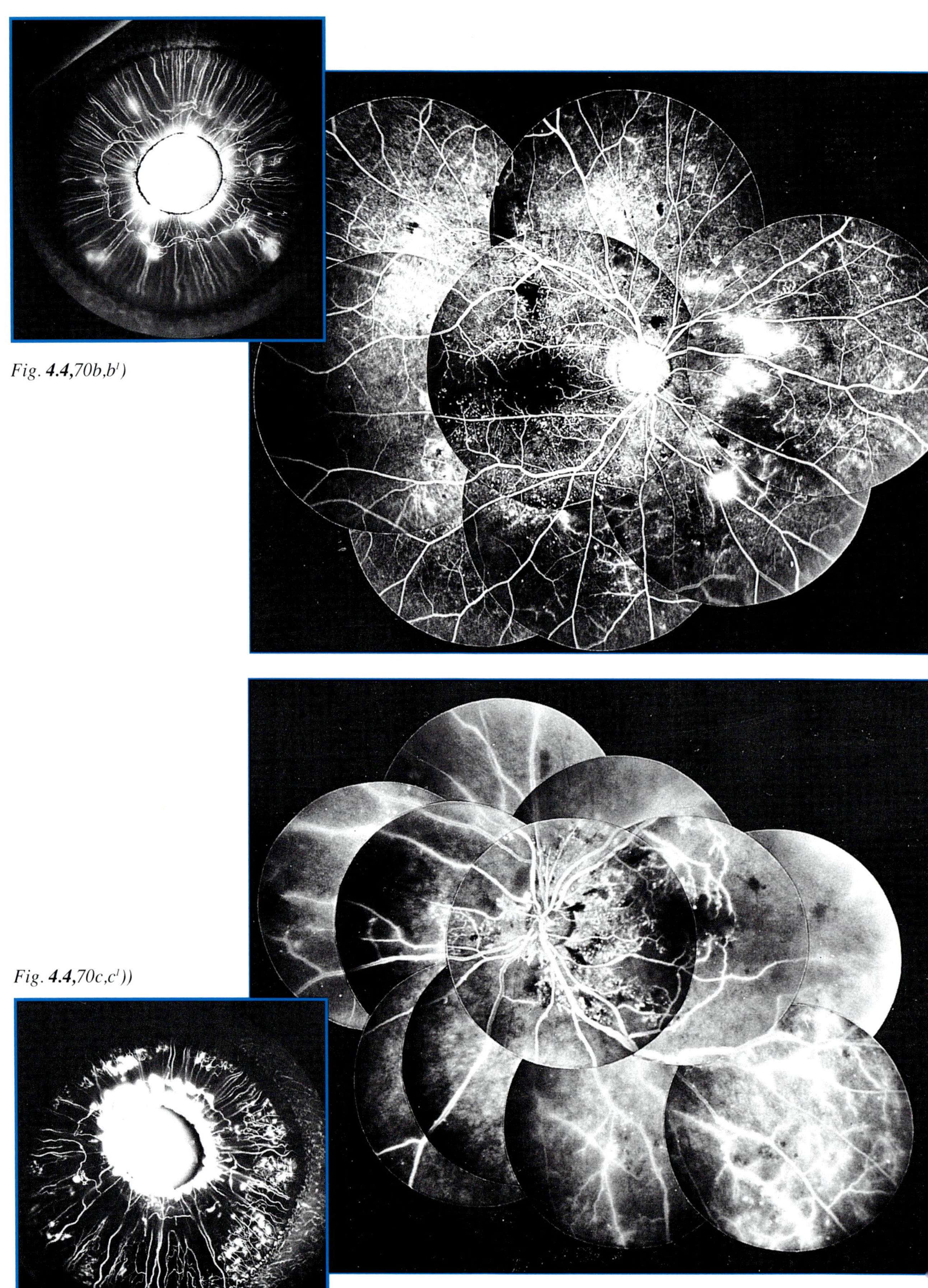

Fig. **4.4**,70b,b[1])

Fig. **4.4**,70c,c[1]))

a) 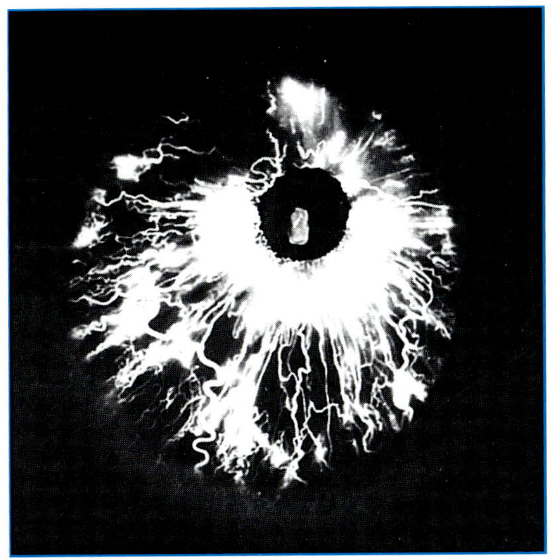
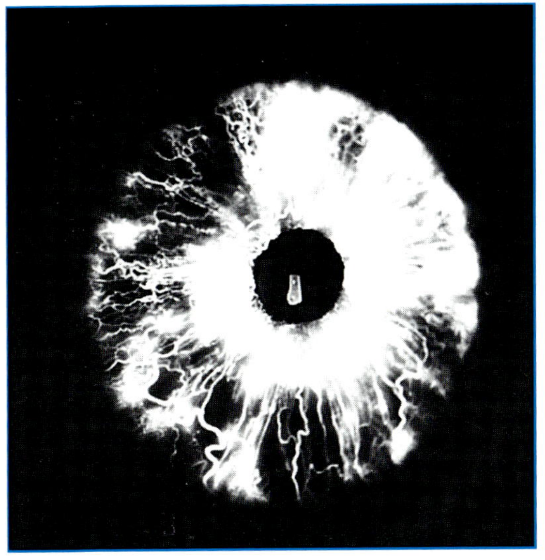 b)

*Fig. **4.4**,71 - Early (a) and late (b) angiographic picture in proliferative diabetic iridopathy. Neovascular proliferation causes hyperfluorescence whereas areas of ischemia on the iris show up as hypofluorescence.*

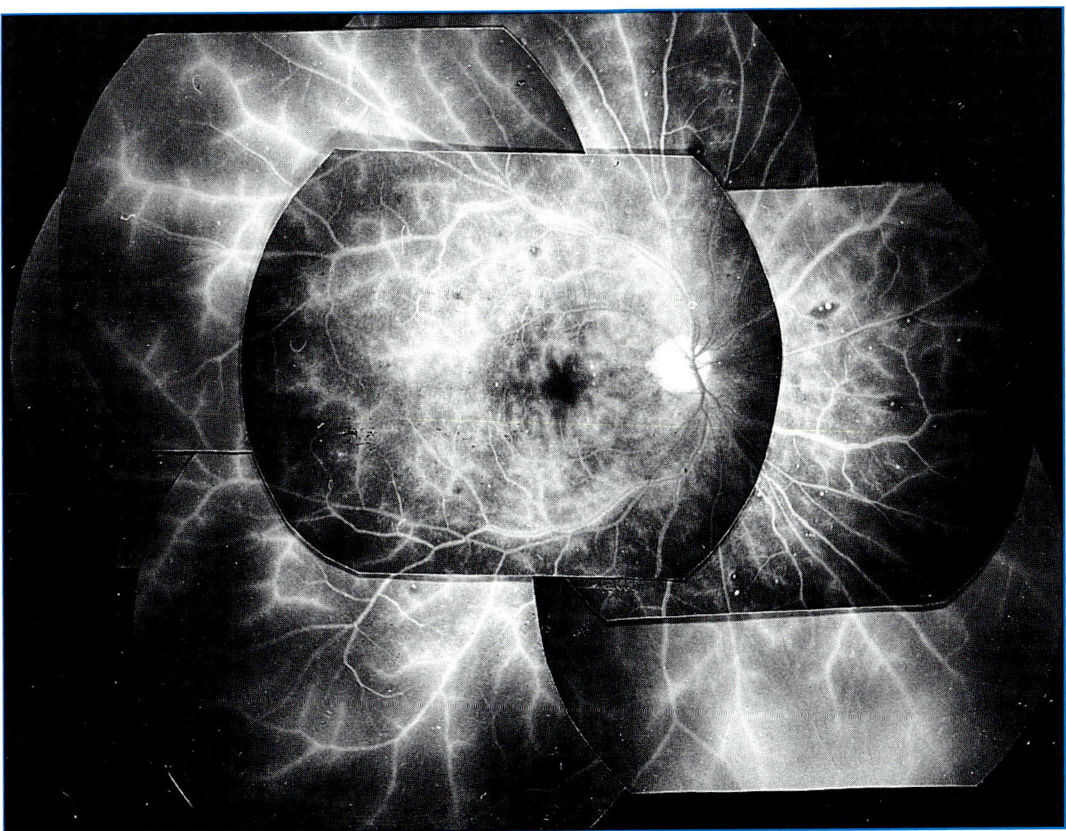

*Fig. **4.4**,72 - Panretinal fluorescein angiography in an elderly diabetic patient. There are confluent areas of capillary nonperfusion which, even when there are no epiretinal new vessels, can become complicated with rubeosis iridis.*

a)

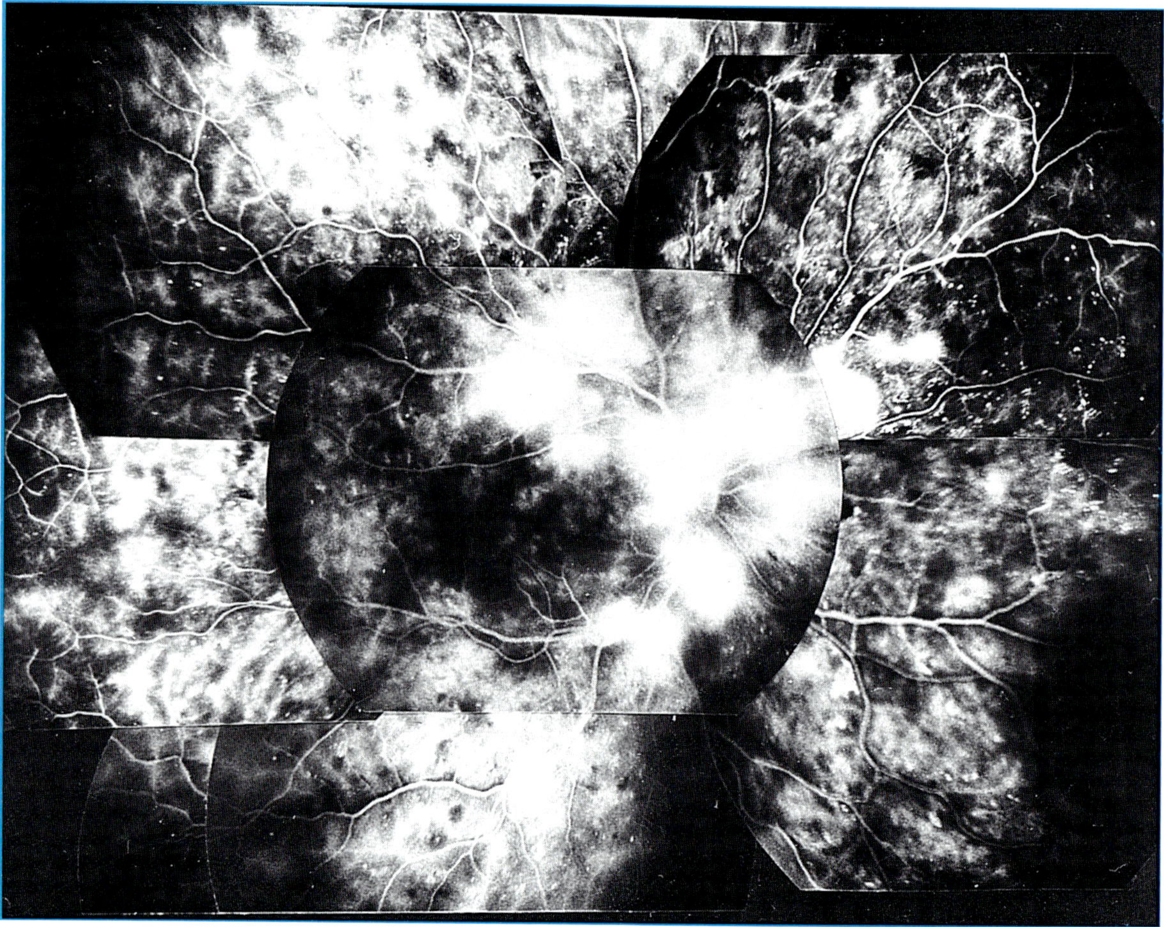

*Fig. **4.4,**73 - Proliferative diabetic retinopathy before (a) and after (b) panretinal-photocoagulation treatment.*

b)

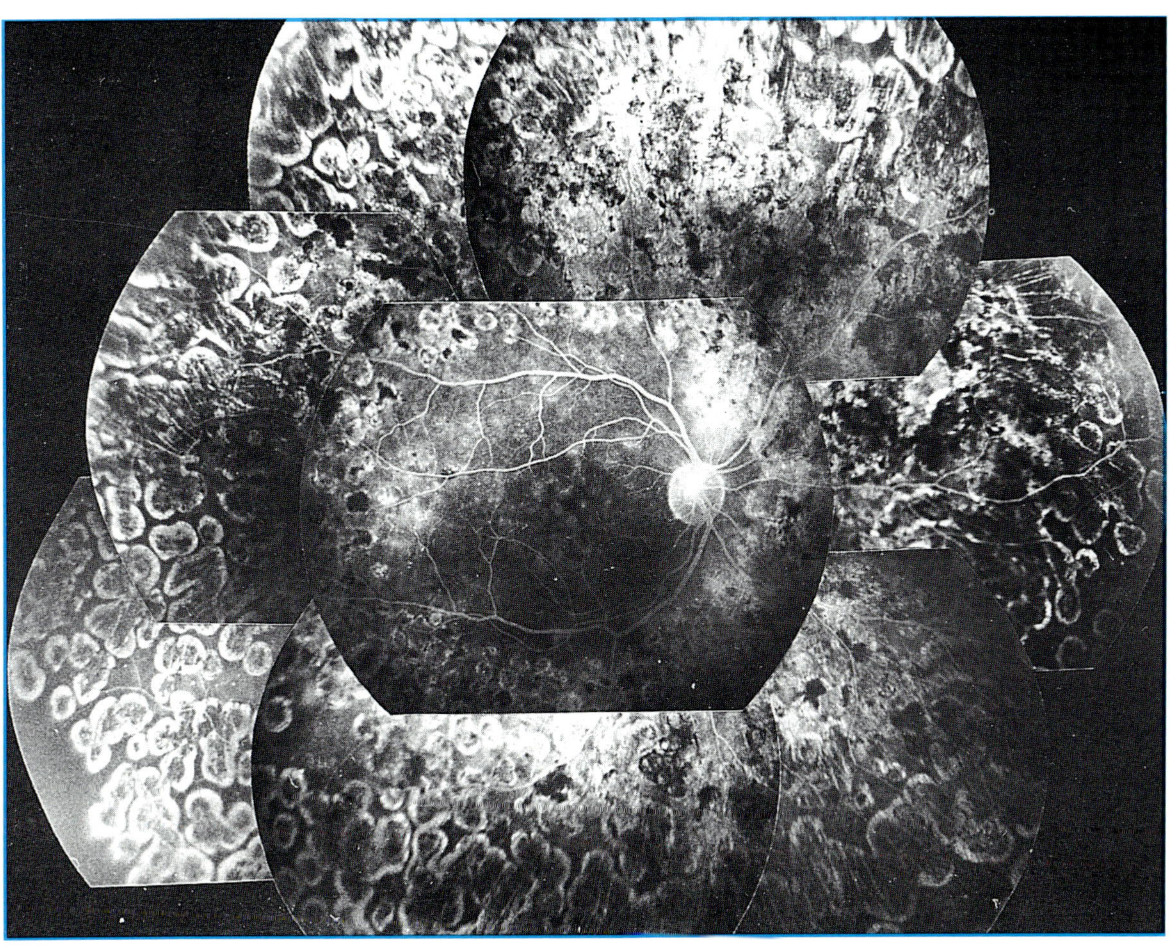

The epiretinal and epipapillary new vessels have regressed completely (fluorescein angiography).

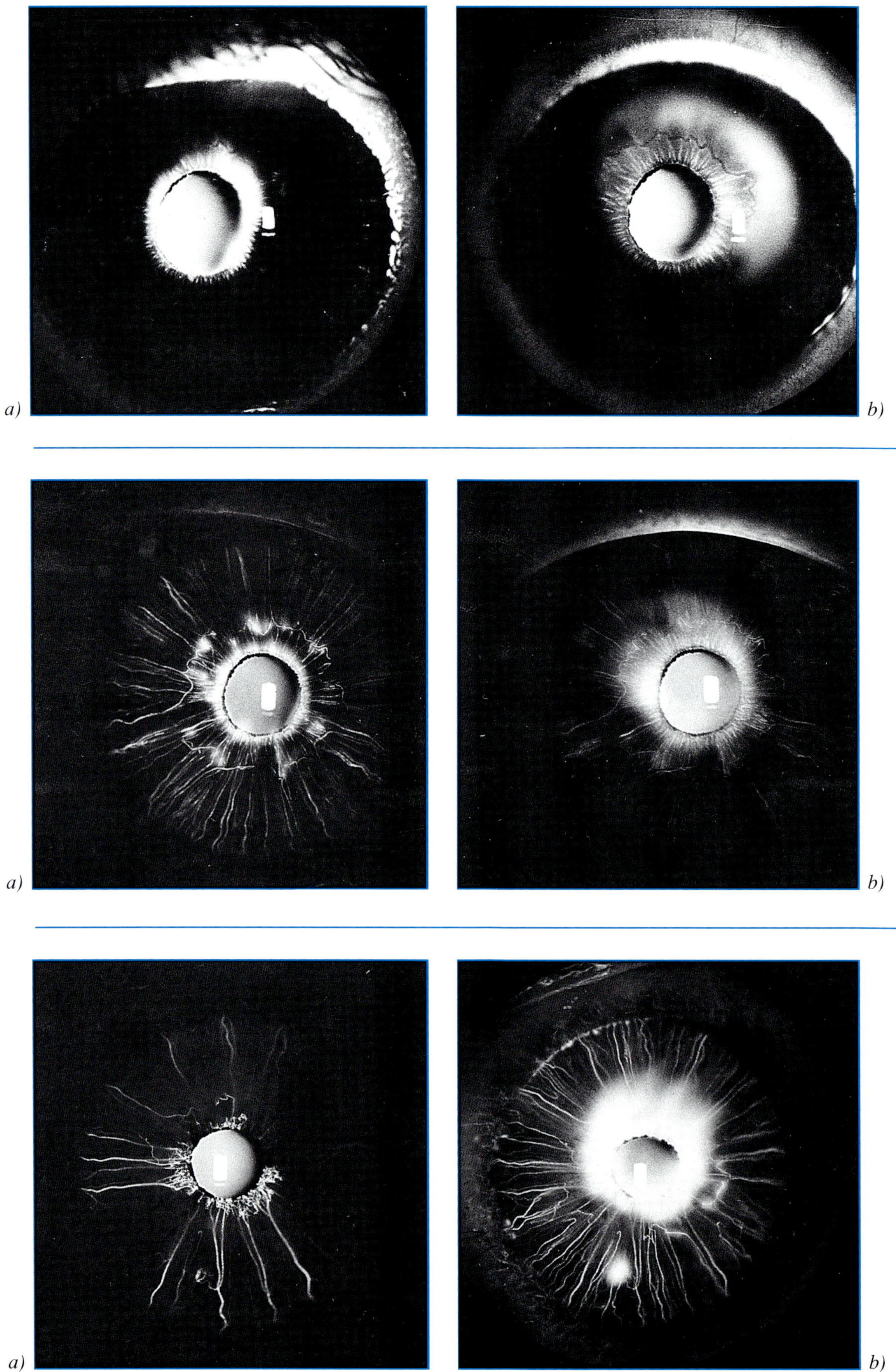

*Figs. **4.4**,74-76 - Different cases of iris new vessels before (a,b) and after (c,d) panretinal photocoagulation,* →

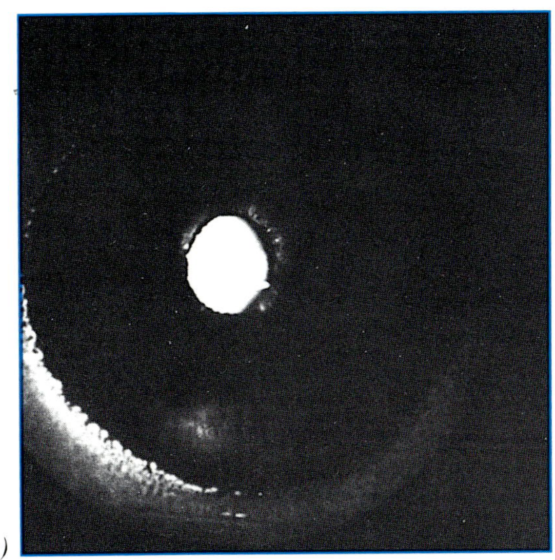
c)

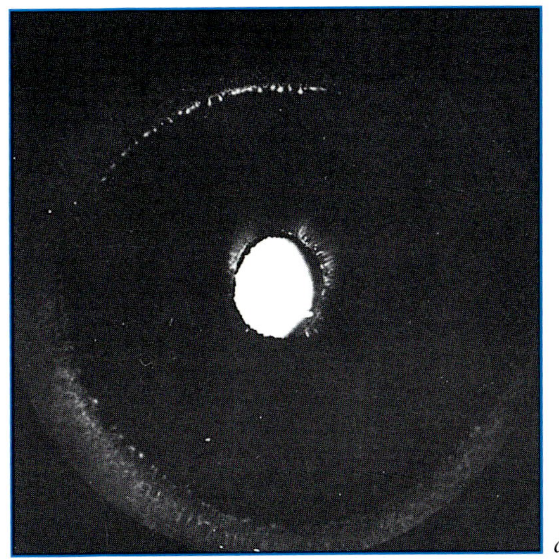
d)

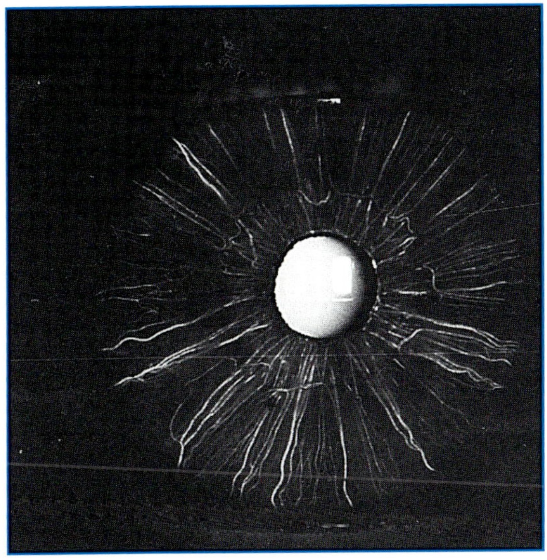
c)

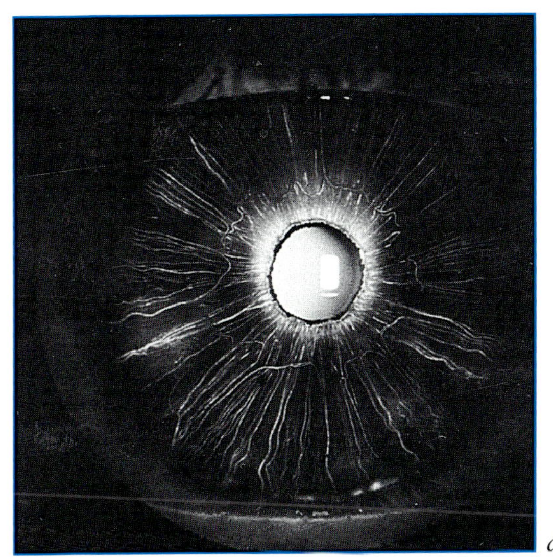
d)

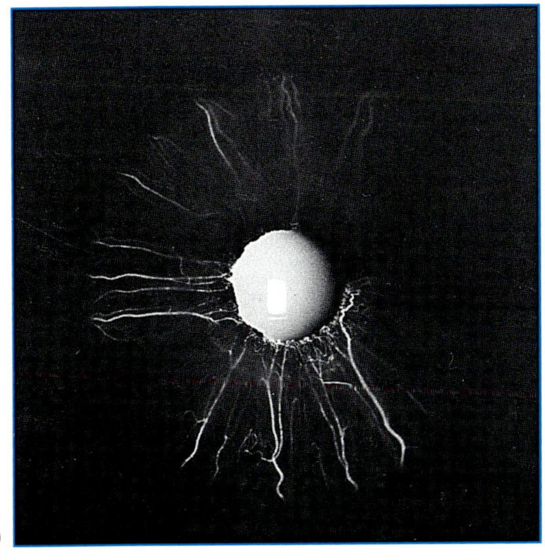
c)

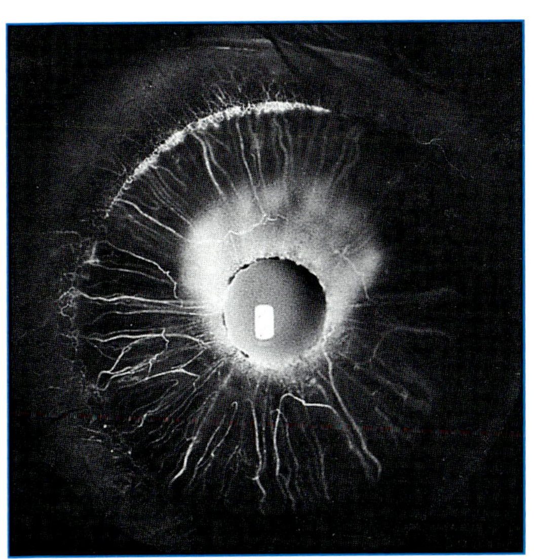
d)

which has resulted in regression (early (a,c) and late (b,d) angiographic pictures).
←

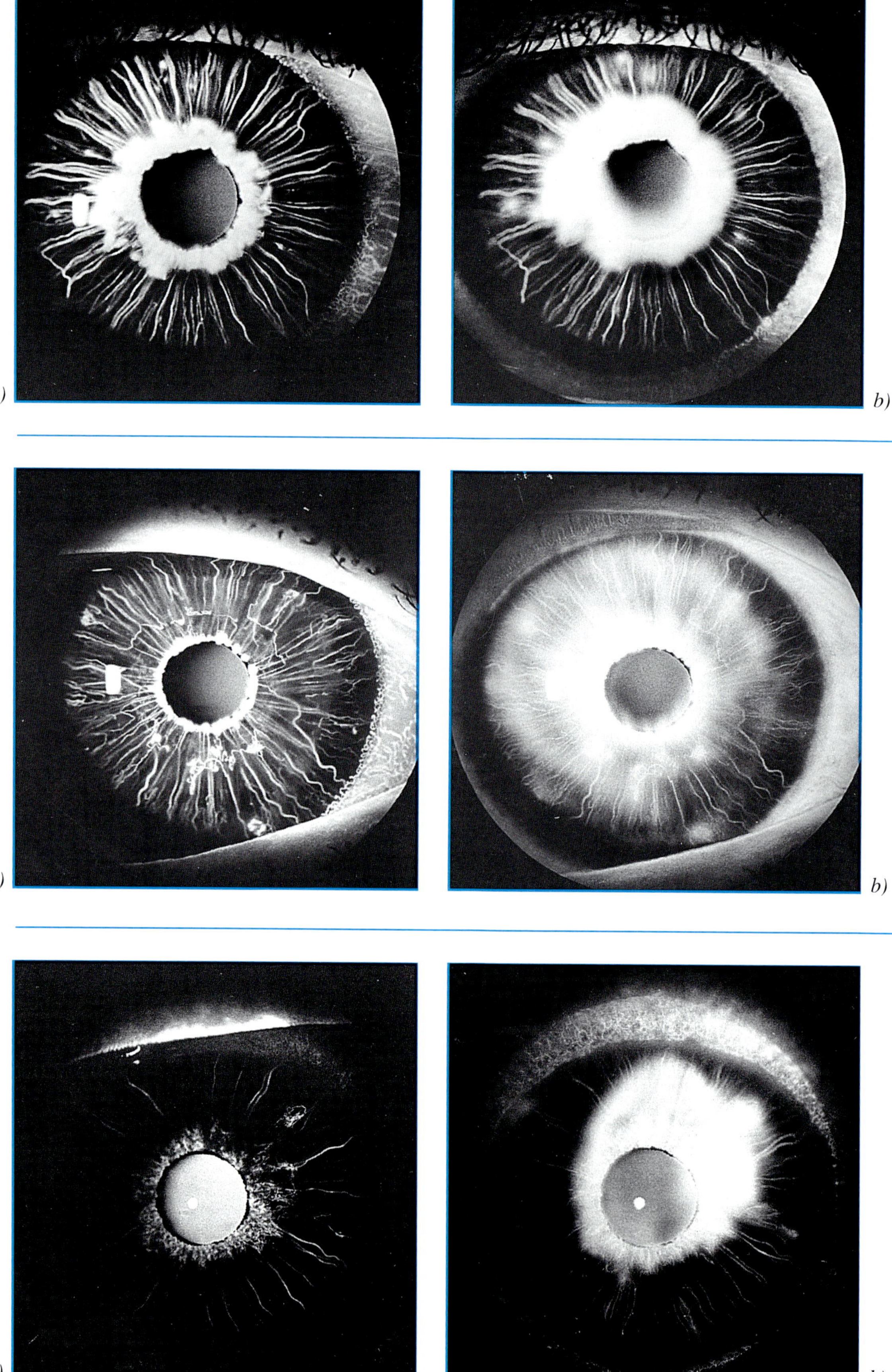

*Figs. **4.4**,77-79 - Three more cases of proliferative diabetic iridopathy before (a,b) and after (c,d) photocoagula-* →

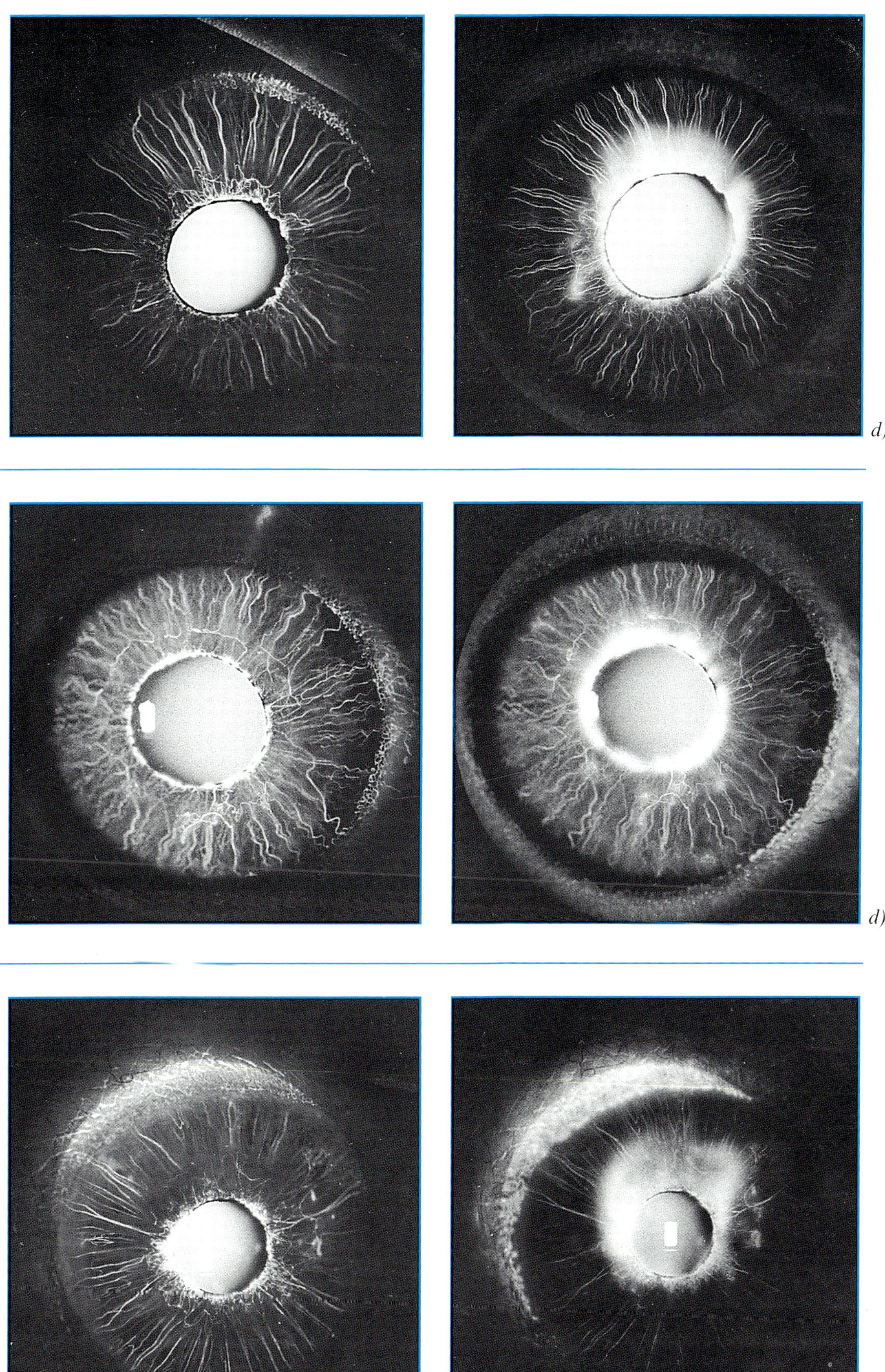

tion of the ischemic retinal areas. Dye leakage from the neovascular buds and radial vessels of the iris is reduced.
←

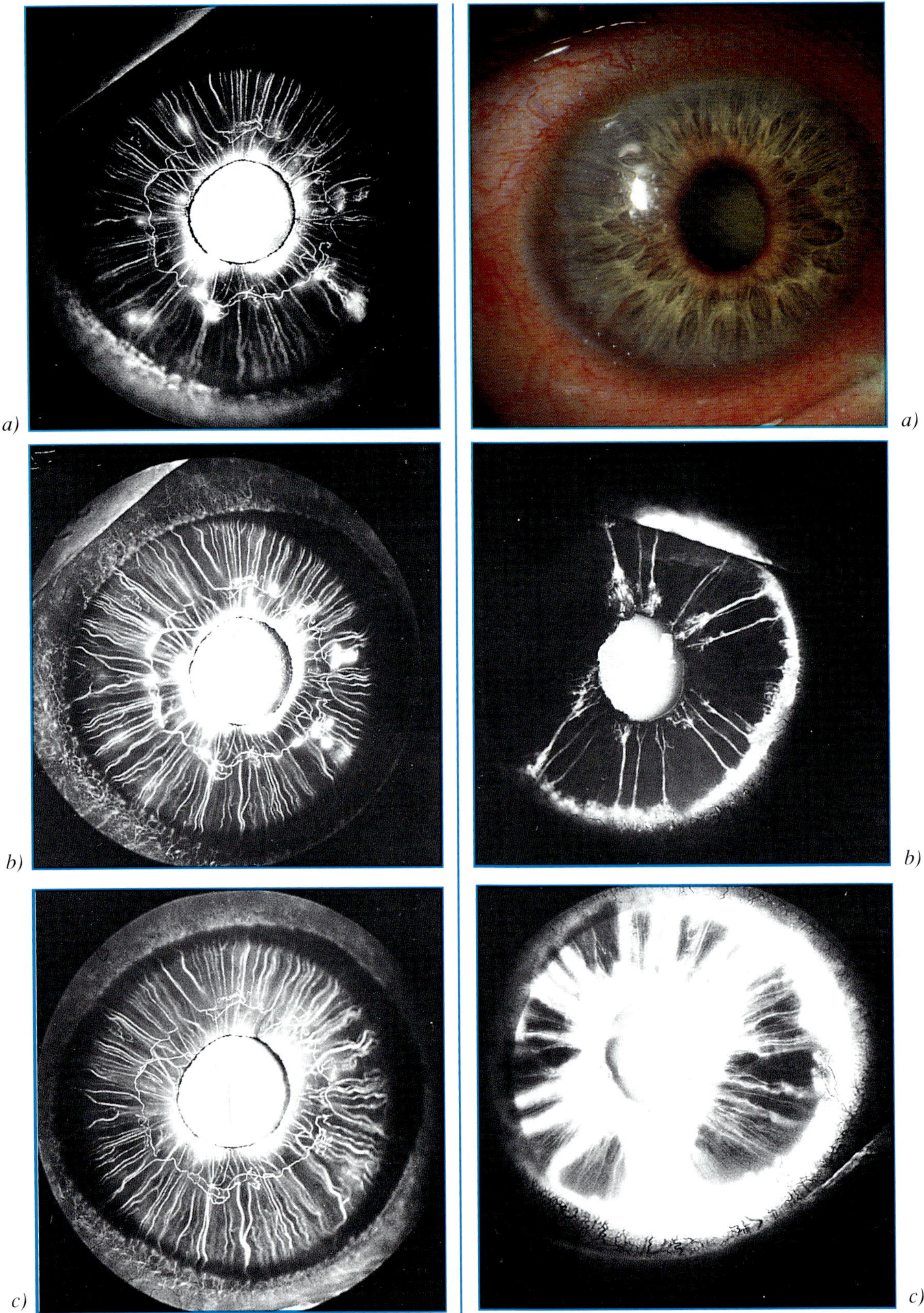

*Fig. **4.4,**80 - Rubeosis iridis before (a) and after (c) photocoagulation of the retina. The lack of regression of the new vessels, seen in the iris fluorescein angiogram (b), indicated the need for further laser treatment which did in fact restore the picture to normal (c).*

*Fig. **4.4,**81 - Hypofluorescence where sectors of the iris are not perfused and hyperfluorescence starting from the congested radial vessels and neovascular buds can be seen in the pupillary part biomicroscopically (a) and in the fluorescein angiograms (b,c).*

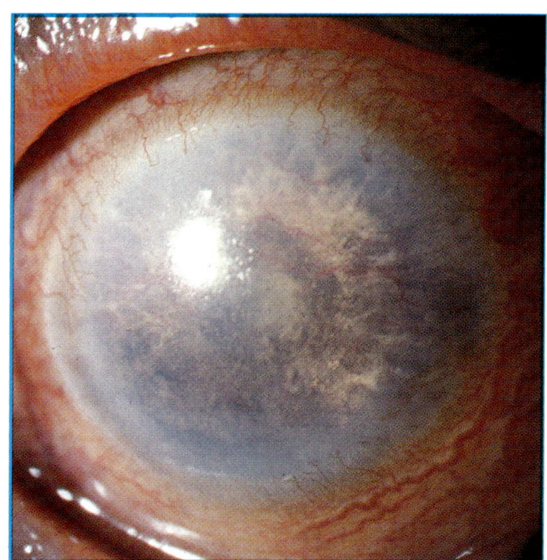

*Fig. **4.4,**82 - Same case as in the previous figure, one year later. Progression of the rubeosis and the onset of intraocular hypertension have combined to give a biomicroscopic picture of neovascular glaucoma.*

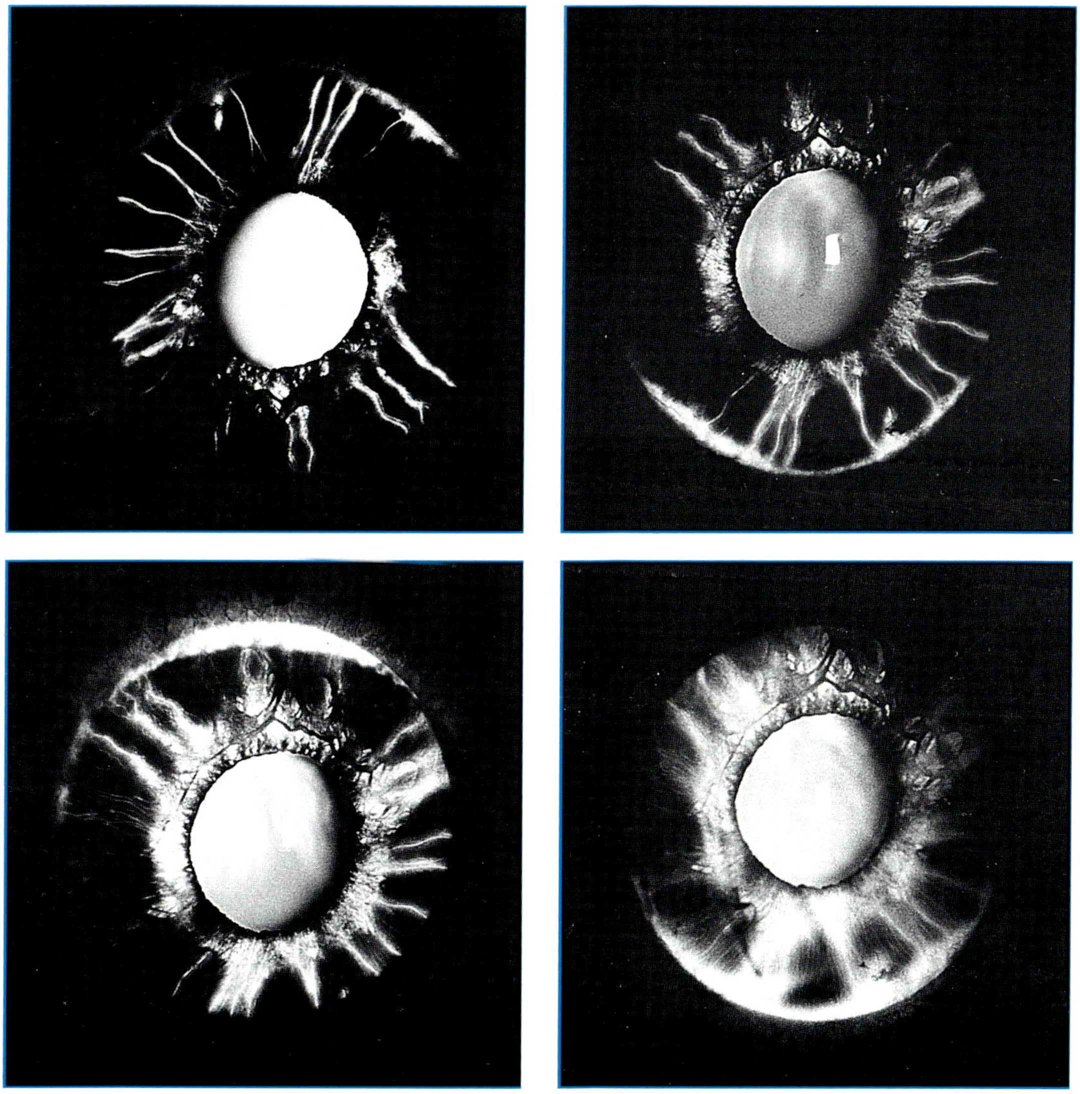

a) b)

c) d)

*Fig. **4.4,**83 - Proliferative iridopathy in the involutive phase illustrated in various fluorescein angiographic stages (a,b,c,d). Confluent areas of ischemia of the iris can be seen, with marked congestion of the residual radial vascular network and dead-end or involuted neovascular tufts.*

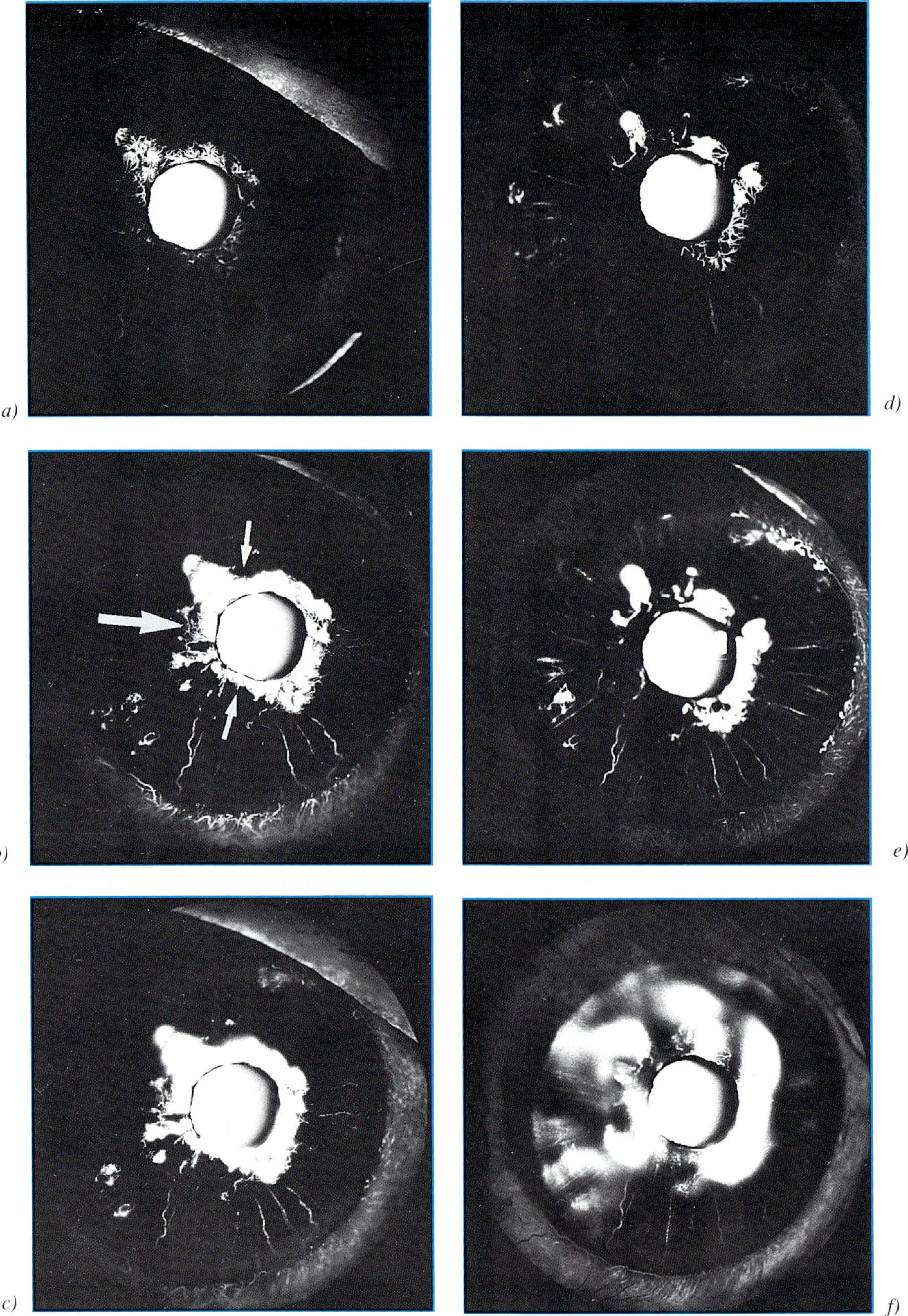

a) d) b) e) c) f)

Fig. ***4.4,****84 - Evolution of rubeosis iridis: fluorescein angiographic examination before (a,b,c) and one year later (d,e,f). Some new vessels are obliterated (arrows) while others proliferate in different parts of the iris.*

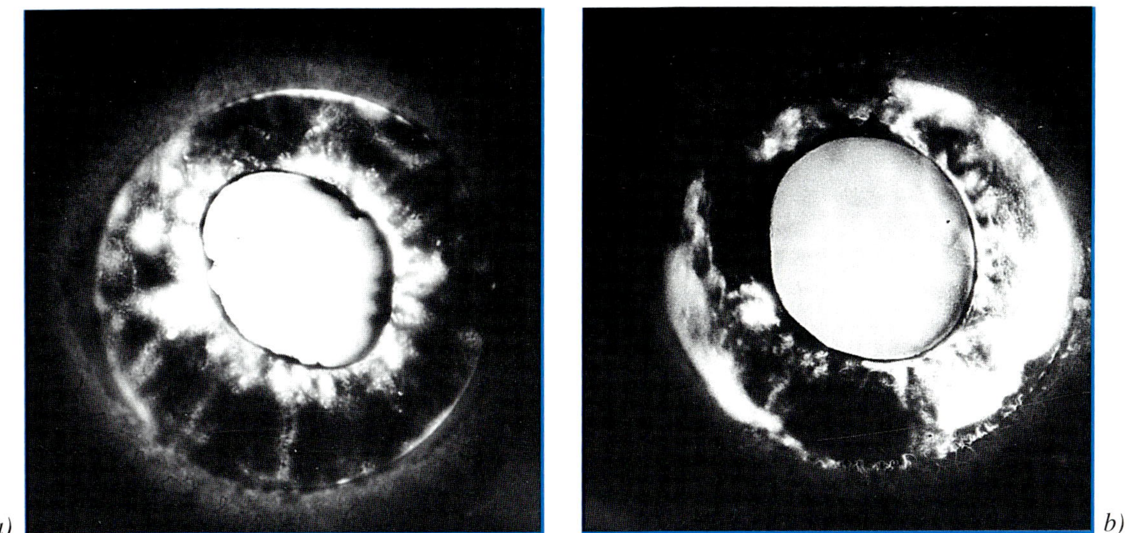

a) b)

*Fig. **4.4,**85 - A case similar to the one above before (a) and eight months later (b).*

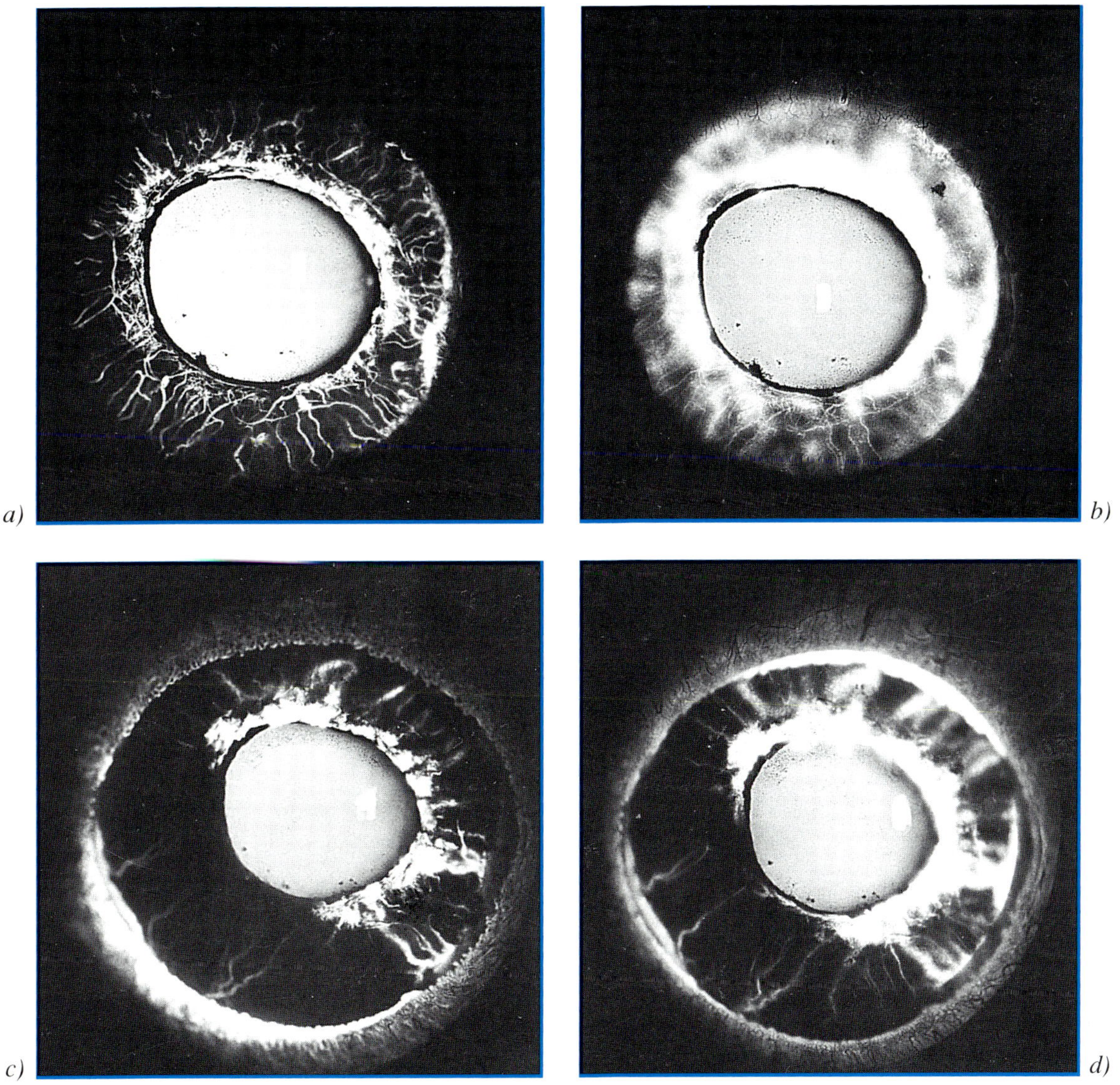

a) b)

c) d)

*Fig. **4.4,**86 - Early (a,c) and late (b,d) angiographic pictures of the same patient before (a,b) and after 15 months (c,d). The radial vascular structure is in disarray and ischemia of the iris has progressed because of inadequate perfusion on account of intraocular hypertension.*

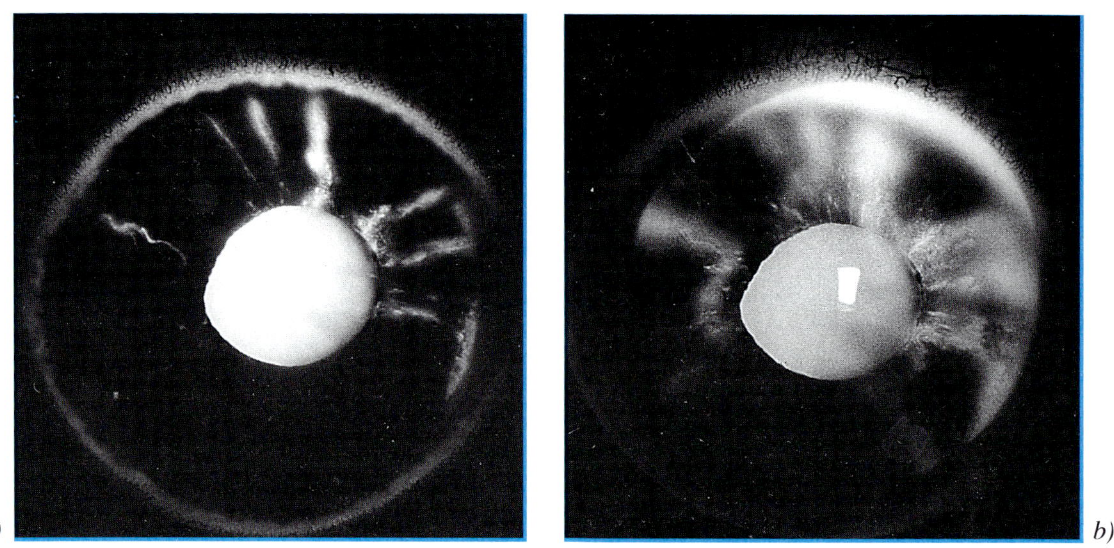

Fig. ***4.4,****87 - Neovascular glaucoma in the involutive-atrophic phase: early (a) and late (b) angiographic pictures. The lack of vascular perfusion is striking.*

R. Brancato, F. Bandello, R. Lattanzio
Atlas of Iris
Fluorescein Angiography
Kugler & Ghedini Publications 1995

Chapter 4.5

Retinal vessel occlusions

Both the arterial and venous systems of the eye may become occluded. Retinal arteries are substantially of the terminal type with few supplementary anastomotic systems, so that occlusion of one of these arteries may result in ischemia in the area it normally supplies. Likewise, venous drainage can be viewed as sectorial, meaning that obstruction of a single vein can cause damage to tissue before collateral drainage has time to develop. Occlusion of a major retinal vessel or any branch thereof can lead to serious complications in the anterior segment of the eye.

Occlusion of retinal veins is more frequent than occlusion of the retinal arteries and often leads to severe complications involving the circulation in the iris. Iris neovascularization is unquestionably the most widely feared consequence of Central Retinal Vein Occlusion (CRVO), and a careful biomicroscopic check must always be made to check for it. Better still, iris fluorescein angiography provides prompter identification of any tendency to rubeosis and neovascular glaucoma. CRVO is in fact the most frequent reason for enucleation in cases of intractable neovascular glaucoma.[90,104]

Retinal Vein Occlusions

Occlusion of the retinal veins is fairly frequent, and small, medium-sized or large veins may be involved. The retinal districts damaged by the lesions, always upstream of the occlusion, may therefore vary in size from small, generally paracentral areas (segmental occlusion) (Fig. **4.5**,1), to a whole quadrant (occlusion of a branch of the central retinal vein: Fig. **4.5**,2), or even half the retina (hemispherical and hemicentral: Fig. **4.5**,3) or all the districts of the retina (central retinal vein occlusion).

Various classification systems have been proposed for CRVO. Hayreh[41] suggested a distinction between retinopathy due to venous stasis (benign form) and hemorrhagic retinopathy (severe form). The main limitation of this approach lies in the fact that in all cases of venous occlusion stasis and hemorrhage tend to coexist. In clinical practice, therefore, it is hard - sometimes impossible - to make a clear distinction between the two forms. Other proposals make a difference between forms with good perfusion and those with poor perfusion.

Konher suggested considering CRVO as a single disorder with various degrees of severity, in a continuum, without distinguishing different clinical forms.[53,55]

Coscas suggested a classification that seems practical from the clinical viewpoint.[22-26] Depending on the ophthalmoscopic and fluorescein angiographic findings, CRVO was divided into three different types of retinal capillaropathy: ischemic, edematous and mixed. There was also a second group of CRVO termed benign without capillary disease, in which retinal involvement was minimal, there was a tendency to spontaneous resolution and no damage to the anterior segment (Fig. **4.5**,4).

Central Retinal Vein Occlusion with ischemic retinal capillaropathy

Ophthalmoscopic examination shows numerous cotton-wool spots, deep stag-horn hemorrhages, papillary and retinal edema. Fluorescein angiography shows extensive areas of retinal ischemia (Figs. **4.5**,5-7). Pathogenically, occlusions of the arteries are also considered to play a role in the onset of ischemic capillaropathy. Neovascularization, when present, is on the retina and head of the optic nerve, though in most cases it is not seen, only appearing at the pupillary margin or at the anterior chamber angle.

Central Retinal Vein Occlusion with edematous retinal capillaropathy

The ophthalmic findings in this form are retinal and papillary edema, venous congestion, fine, mainly superficial "flame" hemorrhages and - rarely - cotton-wool spots. Fluorescein angiography of the retina shows dilatation of the capillary bed and extensive dye leakage with intraretinal dye accumulation. In the late phases of the examination, dye accumulation at the macula confirms the typical cystoid appearance in 50% of cases (Fig. **4.5**,8).

Central Retinal Vein Occlusion with mixed retinal capillaropathy

Fluorescein angiography in this type of CRVO may show areas with dilated capillaries leaking dye, and areas of nonperfusion. The mixed form may present full-blown, or as an aggravation of a previous edematous form. If adequate photocoagulation therapy is not applied, in half the cases epiretinal and epipapillary and even iris neovessels appear.

Coscas proposed classification of the three forms of capillaropathy holds good for branch and hemispheric occlusions.

Various factors dictate the features of venous occlusion and its complications: the site of the occlusion (central or branch), the type of venous obstruction and the degree of concomitant arterial impairment. Different iris anomalies may be associated with different types of retinal vein occlusion. These vary depending on whether the central or a branch vein is occluded, and how much time has elapsed since the occlusion.

It was already known at the beginning of this century that neovascularization of the iris could follow CRVO.[20,21] Today iris fluorescein angiography provides a means of documenting the finer alterations and - in particular - of detecting the initial stages of iris damage before they become clinically evident.[8,9,22-26,73] Several main points should be borne in mind:

1) neovessels of the iris and angle and neovascular glaucoma are generally related to ischemic CRVO;
2) neovessels of the iris are very rare when the retinal capillaropathy is edematous or mixed, and in Branch Retinal Vein Occlusion (BRVO);
3) retinal and/or papillary neovascularization is not normally seen in CRVO, but is noted with ischemic BRVO (Figs. **4.5**,9,10).[8,9,43,44]

The severity and extent of retinal ischemia thus appears to be the main factor influencing the development of ocular neovessels in cases of retinal vein occlusion. The time elapsed from the occlusion is another important detail.

The alterations found on fluorescein angiography of the iris and their relation with the corresponding retinal findings can thus be summarized as follows:

– Normal iris fluorescein angiogram	– recent CRVO – edematous CRVO – edematous or ischemic BRVO of very recent onset

– Dilatation and dye leakage from capillaries	– edematous CRVO – ischemic CRVO
– Dilatation and dye leakage from radial vessels	– ischemic CRVO
– Sectorial dilatation and diffusion	– ischemic BRVO in the same area
– Rubeosis iridis	– ischemic CRVO or BRVO 2-3 months after onset
– Neovascular glaucoma	– not recent ischemic CRVO

This summary shows clearly how the severity of iris involvement is related to the characteristics of the retinal occlusion. The most serious forms of iridopathy (rubeosis and neovascular glaucoma) are in fact only seen after ischemic retinal vein occlusions.

In classifying iridopathy related to venous occlusion, we apply the same criteria as for diabetic iridopathy, under the following headings:[8,9]

Non proliferative diabetic iridopathy *(edematous or exudative)*

Grade 0 no dye leakage

Grade 1 leakage from the pupillary border (mild exudative iridopathy)

Grade 2 leakage from the border and from stromal vessels (marked exudative iridopathy).

Proliferative diabetic iridopathy

Grade 0 no neovascularization

Grade 1 neovascularization at the pupillary border

Grade 2 neovascularization at the border, on the iris stroma and at the iridocorneal angle

Grade 3 neovascular glaucoma.

Detailed analysis of the iris lesions subsequent to occlusions of the retinal veins clarifies the following patterns:

1) In CRVO with edematous capillaropathy, iris fluorescein angiography may indicate normal iris vascularization (Fig. **4.5**,11). In other instances, only vascular dilatation with pupillary dye leakage may be seen. The leakage is generally much more intense and extensive than the physiological pupillary dye leakage expected in subjects over 50-60 years. In other cases of edematous CRVO the greater retinal involvement may be indicated by extrapupillary dye leakage, starting from the radial vessels, which appear dilated, tortuous and congested (Fig. **4.5**,12). This second type of leakage may vary in intensity and extension but it must always be considered pathological, as stressed earlier.

Neovascularization is not normally seen in edematous CRVO.[4,23,25,31,62,68,69,83,113] Iris neovessels were reported in only 1% of cases by Tasman[98] and in 8% by Laatikainen.[64] Magargal described the onset of neovascular glaucoma in one case of edematous CRVO which subsequently became ischemic too.[68,69]

2) In ischemic CRVO pupillary and extrapupillary dye leakage is more marked and frequent (Figs. **4.5**,13,14). A study of our caselists showed that in most instances dye leakage in the iris was mainly sectorial. That same study found that in edematous CRVO dye leakage in the iris, when present, was not sectorial.

Filling delays and defects were described in 25% of cases (Fig. **4.5**,15).[59]

Iris neovascularization may occur in ischemic CRVO, generally leading to rubeosis iridis and neovascular glaucoma. The development towards rubeosis starts, as shown in the summary table, about 2-3 months after the actual occlusion (Figs. **4.5**,16-19).

New vessels in the iris and at the anterior chamber angle were detected in respectively 63 and 52% of cases of ischemic CRVO in our caselist compared to 8 and 7% for papillary and retinal neovessels.[8] Other studies give a range of frequencies for the development of rubeosis iridis - from 58-82%.[12,61-64,67-70,95,98]

The literature offers few studies dealing with the appearance of new vessels at the angle. Smith described 11 cases in 14 eyes with CRVO, seven of which subsequently developed neovascular glaucoma.[96] Hayreh reported neovessels at the angle in 47.4% of his cases of ischemic CRVO.[44]

Neovascularization presents a fluorescein angiographic picture of prompt, massive leakage. With the biomicroscope one initially sees small vessels crossing each other in an irregular peripupillary network, tending gradually to extend anarchically towards the iris root, and generally merging in the mid-periphery with a second capillary mesh originating independently at the angle (Figs. **4.5**,20,21).[56] This is the stage preceding neovascular glaucoma, which clinically involves rapid closure of the angle by newly formed fibrovascular membranes and goniosynechiae, marked inflammation, and the formation of anterior synechiae, followed by iris atrophy with fibrotic retraction causing pupillary deformation and ectropion uveae. The eye is functionally lost, and becomes painful, with irreducible intraocular hypertension, responding poorly to medical and surgical therapy. Often enucleation is the only solution.[16,56,84,85] Ocular hypertension in neovascular glaucoma and the resulting atrophy may, later, give rise to involution of the iris neovessels (Figs. **4.5**,22-27).[19]

The frequency of neovascular glaucoma in different studies ranges from 8 to 50% of cases of CRVO not treated by panretinal photocoagulation. The higher incidence reported by some investigators might be a reflection of the different forms of venous occlusion considered in the different caselists.[4,7,16,17,22,34,53,54,56,62,63,67-69,71,78,79,83,91,95,96,102-105,107,113]

When ischemic CRVO is very recent dye leakage may be seen from the iris vessels, and in such cases it is not necessarily a sign of neovascularization. It has been interpreted as an alteration to the walls of the iris vessels, associated with canalization of shunts that normally are not functional.[56] This is proposed as the cause of the abnormal vascular paths often seen in these patients.

3) In CRVO with mixed retinal capillaropathy the alterations to the iris may differ in character and extent depending on whether the capillaropathy is mainly edematous or mainly ischemic. The more extensive are the areas of capillary nonperfusion in the retina the greater is the risk of iris neovessels.

4) In BRVO iris fluorescein angiography may give virtually normal findings if the occlusion is very recent, regardless of whether it was edematous or ischemic. After a longer lapse, however, edematous and ischemic branch retinal vein occlusions both give a picture of sectorial dilatation and dye leakage in the iris, topographically corresponding to the affected areas of the retina (Fig. **4.5**,28). In one case in which the occlusion involved two contiguous quadrants of the retina, hemicyclic leakage was seen in the iris, corresponding topographically to the location of the occlusion on the retina.[73,74]

Other findings in central or branch retinal vein occlusions are filling delays and defects, always following a sectorial pattern, and - rarely - extrapupillary leakage (Fig. **4.5**,29). Iris neovascularization does not occur after BRVO, according to the findings of numerous studies.[1,2,5,22-26,49,55,77,91,93,97,99] Iris neovessels were found, however, in 1.5% of cases in a study of 130 eyes with BRVO[98] and in 1.6% of cases in another investigation of 191 eyes.[41] Neovascular glaucoma was found in from 2-10% of cases only in three studies of 50, 71 and 48 eyes.[31,68,100]

In Sanborn's study, iris neovascularization and neovascular glaucoma were found in respectively 9 and 3% of cases of hemispheric retinal vein occlusion.[87] Hayreh divided hemispheric occlusions in his caselist into non-ischemic and ischemic. In the first group (66 eyes) there were no cases of iris or angle neovessels, whereas in the second group (31 eyes) they were seen in respectively 12.9 and 6.5% of cases. Neovascular glaucoma was reported only in 3.2 % of the ischemic group.[44]

Fluorescein circulation times in Central Retinal Vein Occlusion

The arm-iris time in particular is usually normal in retinal vein occlusion. Intra-iris times may be shortened, especially when neovessels are present, suggesting there is no stasis in the anterior segment. In fact iris vessels are not crushed, unless secondary to neovascular glaucoma, meaning only in eyes with high intraocular pressure.[62]

Fluorescein abnormalities in Central Retinal Vein Occlusion: order of events

It is hard to define precisely the order of events preceding the onset of neovascular glaucoma, for several reasons:

1) because the events often proceed with such speed;
2) because the patient often comes to observation late, when neovascularization is already under way;
3) because iris fluorescein angiography is not always done immediately.[22,62]

However, the first angiographic sign of severe iris damage is always dilatation of radial vessels and dye leakage from them.[62,104] New vessels only appear after this has happened, growing up around the pupillary margin, as mentioned.[41] New vessels also grow at the anterior chamber angle, and the two neovascular systems grow independently until they meet and merge by anastomosis.

Rubeosis iridis always precedes intraocular hypertension[6,27,58,85,102,103] and is virtually the same as in diabetes mellitus, except that its course is faster and more explosive.

It has also been sustained that iris vessels in CRVO originate typically at the periphery of the iris and move in towards the pupillary region in the form of "sparsely branching vessels", which fluoresce in the late venous phase and leak only limited amounts of dye.[27] Most studies do not specify the time elapsed between CRVO and the growth of iris new vessels.

Cappin et al. distinguished forms that "progress slowly" and others they call "accelerated" in which the iris neovessels appear respectively 13-20 and 8-15 weeks after the occlusion.[16]

Iris neovessels tend to continue progressing although in some cases they may stop developing; only rarely do they regress and when this happens it is probably a response to spontaneous recanalization of the retinal vessels. A tendency towards neovascular glaucoma may become evident three months or so after the occlusion (*Glaucoma at the 100th day*[20,21]) but the interval may range from one month to 3-4 years.[7,34,84,85] It is thus very important to ensure regular biomicroscopic and fluorescein angiographic checks of the iris in the 3-4 months after an occlusion.

An analysis of animal eyes enucleated at different intervals after experimentally induced CRVO (5, 27 and 133 days) indicated three stages in the process of neovascularization of the iris.[81] All the eyes had been examined by fluorescein angiography before enucleation. The first stage was marked by generalized dilatation of iris vessels, dye leakage and proliferation of endothelial cells in the iris stroma. The second stage consisted of active neovascular proliferation, ectropion uveae, anterior peripheral synechiae and intraocular hypertension. Ultrastructural examination showed a shift in the proliferative activity from the endothelial to the stromal cells which, on losing their normal intercellular relations, migrated anteriorly to constitute the extravascular component of the neovessels. In the third phase the neovascular membranes appeared reduced.

Pathogenesis of rubeosis iridis in Central Retinal Vein Occlusion

The fluorescein angiographic findings in CRVO suggest that neovascular proliferation in the iris only arises when there are extensive areas not perfused in the retinal periphery. In fact, neovascular glaucoma does not occur without retinal ischemia. Retinal and/or papillary neovascularization is reported more often - as already specified - in ischemic branch retinal vein occlusion. Rubeosis iridis can therefore only occur when there is ischemia of the retina. Most Authors do in fact sustain[23,53,56,62,93,96] that the ischemic retina provides the stimulus for retinal and iris neovascular proliferation, since "vascular" glaucoma, like retinal neovessels, only develops when there are large areas of retinal nonperfusion.

The nonperfused retina apparently releases an angiogenic substance, still not identified, that can induce the formation of neovessels. This pathogenic hypothesis is borne out by the fact that thorough, prompt photocoagulation to destroy the retinal ischemic areas can result in regression of the neovascularization, even during CRVO (Figs. **4.5**,30-32).[3,6,8,22,23,25,37,39,43,53,56,61,62,65,67,71,86,91,93,96,98,109]

Despite this, regression of neovascularizations in cases of retinal vein occlusion is not achieved as frequently as in diabetic retinopathy. Magargal's study found no cases of neovascular glaucoma in eyes with ischemic CRVO treated by panretinal photocoagulation before iris neovessels were detectable.[67]

Besides the presence of extensive retinal ischemia, other factors too probably facilitate the formation of iris neovessels, including - for instance - the inadequate arterial perfusion, the rapid capillary obstruction, the slowing of venous drainage and the accumulation of metabolites. The common denominator in neovascular glaucoma, however, is certainly the degree and extension of capillary ischemia regardless of whether the retinal occlusion is arterial or venous.

The fact that neovascular glaucoma is rare after central retinal artery occlusion is related to the state of severe anoxia created in the retina: compared to the hypoxia resulting from venous occlusion this is much less of a neovascular stimulus (Fig. **4.5**,33).[23]

It is therefore of prognostic interest to use retinal fluorescein angiography to clarify the type of venous occlusion, so as to identify ischemic forms early, before rubeosis can get under way, and to establish the indication for prompt laser treatment to avoid the most serious complications (Fig. **4.5**,34). Once the eye already has neovascular glaucoma transpupillary or transcleral contact photocoagulation does not improve vision but does definitely reduce neovessels and dye leakage, and often makes enucleation unnecessary.

There are reports of low intraocular pressure after venous occlusion[34,46,78] and it has been suggested[16] that the angiographic alterations to the iris are due to this hypotonus following retinal vein occlusion. However, others sustain that the incidence of neovascular glaucoma is not influenced by hypotonus.[85]

References

1 Archer DB: Natural course of branch retinal vein obstruction. Trans Ophthalmol Soc UK 94: 623, 1974.

2 Archer DB, Ernest JT, Newell FW: Classification of branch retinal vein obstruction. Trans Am Acad Ophthalmol Otolaryngol 78: 148, 1974.

3 Baarsma GS: Simultaneous bilateral fluorescein angiography of the retina and the iris in central retinal vein occlusion. Int Ophthalmol 6: 243, 1983.

4 Blach RK, Hitchings RA, Laatikainen L: Thrombotic glaucoma; prophylaxis and management. Trans Ophthalmol Soc UK 97: 275, 1977.

5 Blakenship GW, Okun E: Retinal tributary vein occlusion; history and management by photocoagulation. Arch Ophthalmol 89: 363, 1973.

6 Bonnet M, El Khatib W: The value of fluorescein angiography of the iris in the monitoring of rubeosis iridis treated with panretinal photocoagulation. Bull Mem Soc Fr Ophtalmol 94: 312, 1982.

7 Braendstrup P: Central retinal vein thrombosis and hemorrhagic glaucoma. Acta Ophthalmologica (Kbh) 35 (Suppl):1, 1950.

8 Brancato R, Menchini U: Microchirurgia laser in Oftalmologia. Ghedini Ed, Milano, 1989.

9 Brancato R, Menchini U, Carnevalini A: Atlante di iridografia a fluorescenza. C.I.C. Ed Int Gruppo Ed Medico, Roma, 1981.

10 Branch Vein Occlusion Study Group: Argon laser scatter photocoagulation for prevention of neovascularization and vitreous hemorrhage in branch vein occlusion. A randomized clinical trial. Arch Ophthalmol 104: 34, 1986.

11 Brooks AM, Gillies WE: The development and management of neovascular glaucoma. Aust NZ J Ophthalmol 18: 179, 1990.

12 Brown GC, Magargal LE, Schachat A et al: Neovascular glaucoma: etiologic considerations. Ophthalmology 91: 315, 1984.

13 Brown GC, Shah HG, Magargal LE et al: Central retinal vein obstruction and carotid artery disease. Ophthalmology 91: 1627, 1984.

14 Calugaro M: La thrombose de la veine centrale de la retine et le glaucome par fermeture de l'angle sans rubeose. J Fr Ophtalmol 10: 519, 1987.

15 Calugaro M: Le resultats d'une enquête sur la survenue du glaucome neovasculaire après occlusion de la veine centrale de la retine. J Fr Ophtalmol 10: 479, 1987.

16 Cappin JM, Whitelocke R: The iris in central retinal vein thrombosis. Proc Roy Soc Med 67: 1048, 1974.

17 Cassady JV: Central retinal vein thrombosis. Am J Ophthalmol 36: 331, 1953.

18 Chandler P, Grant MW: Angle-closure glaucoma secondary to occlusion of the central retinal vein. In Chandler P, Grant MW: Glaucoma. Lea & Febiger, Philadelphia, 1979.

19 Chen V, Moisseicv J, Treister G: Severe ischemic process in a young man with central vein retinal occlusion. Metab Pediatr Syst Ophthalmol 11: 67, 1988.

20 Coats G: Thrombosis of the central vein of the retina. Roy Lond Ophthalmic Hosp Rep 16: 62, 1904.

21 Coats G: Discussions on retinal vascular disease: pathological aspect. Trans Ophthalmol Soc UK 33: 30, 1913.

22 Coscas G: Retinal vein occlusion, classification, indications for laser treatment. In Brihaye M: Laser in Ophthalmology. Bull Soc Belge Ophtalmol, Bruxelles, 1987.

23 Coscas G, Dhermy P: Occlusions veineuses rétiniennes. Masson, Paris, 1978.

24 Coscas G, Gaudric A: Les occlusions des branches veineuses rétiniennes; aspects angiographiques. Conf Lyon Ophtalmol 132: 1977.

25 Coscas G, Gaudric A, Soubrane G et al: Occlusion de la vein centrale de la rétine à type de capillarophatie ischémique et prevention du glaucome néovasculaire. Bull Soc Ophtalmol Fr 77: 923, 1977.

26 Coscas G, Glacet-Bernard A: Occlusions veineuses rétiniennes. Ophtalmologie 10: 1, 1988.

27 Deodati F, Bec P, Labro JB: Angiographie fluorescéinique du segment antérieur de l'oeil. Arch Ophtalmol (Paris) 31: 859, 1971.

28 Detry-Morel M: Vascular glaucoma. J Fr Ophtalmol 4: 177, 1981.

29 Detry-Morel M, Waterschoot MP, Kevers L et al: Neovascular glaucoma secondary to carotid thrombosis. Bull Soc Belge Ophtalmol 199-200: 55, 1982.

30 Dueker OK: Neovascular glaucoma. In Chandler P, Grant MW: Glaucoma. Lea & Febiger, Philadelphia, 1979.

31 Duff IF, Falls HF, Linman JW: Anticoagulant therapy in occlusive vascular disease of the retina. Arch Ophthalmol 46: 601, 1951.

32 Duker JS, Brown GC: The efficacy of panretinal photocoagulation for neovascularization of the iris after central retinal artery obstruction. Ophthalmology 96: 92, 1989.

33 Fantin J, Grandon M: A case of neovascular glaucoma caused by carotid artery occlusion. Bull Soc Ophtalmol Fr 82: 1079, 1982.

34 Gartner S, Henkind P: Neovascularization of the iris (Rubeosis iridis). Surv Ophthalmol 22: 291, 1978.

35 Gaudric A, Coscas G: Rubeosis iridis and neovascular glaucoma. J Fr Ophtalmol 2: 653, 1979.

36 Gold D: Retinal arterial occlusion. Trans Am Acad Ophthalmol Otolaryngol 83: 392, 1977.

37 Gomolin JE: Efficacy of panretinal photocoagulation in central retinal vein occlusion. Ophthalmologica 199: 24, 1989.

38 Gradle HS: The x-ray therapy of retinal vein thrombosis. Am J Ophthalmol 20: 1125, 1937.

39 Grange JD, Bonnet M: Retinal panphotocoagulation and rubeosis iridis. Bull Soc Ophtalmol Fr 78: 607, 1978.

40 Hayreh SS: Central retinal vein occlusion: differential diagnosis and management. Trans Am Acad Ophthalmol Otolaryngol 83: 379, 1977.

41 Hayreh SS: Classification of central retinal vein occlusion. Ophthalmology 90: 458, 1983.

42 Hayreh SS, Hayreh MS: Hemi-central retinal vein occlusion: pathogenesis, clinical features and natural history. Arch Ophthalmol 98: 1600, 1980.

43 Hayreh SS, Klugman MR, Podhajsky P et al: Argon laser panretinal photocoagulation in ischemic central retinal vein occlusion. A 10 years prospective study. Graefe's Arch Clin Exp Ophthalmol 228: 281, 1990.

44 Hayreh SS, Rojas P, Podhajsky P et al: Ocular neovascularization with retinal vascular occlusion. III. Incidence of ocular neovascularization with retinal vascular occlusion. Ophthalmology 90: 488, 1983.

45 Higgings RA: Neovascular glaucoma associated with ocular hypoperfusion secondary to carotid artery disease. Aust J Ophthalmol 12: 155, 1984.

46 Imre G, Bögi J: Hämorrhagisches Glaukom: Entstehungsmechanismus und therapeutische Möglichkeiten. Klin Monatsbl Augenheilkd 183: 326, 1983.

47 Jarez CP, Tso MO, Van Heuven WA et al: Experimental retinal vascular occlusion. II. A clinicophatologic correlation study of simultaneous occlusion of central retinal vein and artery. Int Ophthalmol 9: 77, 1986.

48 Jarez CP, Tso MO, Van Heuven WA et al: Experimental retinal vascular occlusion. III. An ultrastructural study of simultaneous occlusion of central retinal vein and artery. Int Ophthalmol 9: 89, 1986.

49 Joffe L, Goldberg RE, Magargal LE et al: Macular branch vein occlusion. Ophthalmology 87: 91, 1980.

50 Karjalainen K: Occlusion of the central retinal artery and retinal branch arterioles: a clinical tonographic and fluorescein angiographic study of 175 patients. Acta Ophthalmol (Kbh) 109 (Suppl): 1, 1971.

51 Kartasheva EA: Clinical features of thrombotic glaucoma. Can J Ophthalmol 15: 134, 1980.

52 Kearns TP, Hollenhorst RW: Venous stasis retinophaty of occlusive disease of the carotid artery. Mayo Clin Proc 38: 304, 1963.

53 Kohner EM, Laatikainen L, Oughton J: The management of central retinal vein occlusion. Ophthalmology 90: 484, 1983.

54 Kohner EM, Pettit JE, Hamilton AM et al: Streptokinase in central retinal vein occlusion: a controlled critical trial. Br Med J 1: 550, 1976.

55 Kohner EM, Shilling JS: Retinal vein occlusion. In Rose FC: Medical Ophthalmology. CV Mosby, St Louis, 1976.

56 Kottow MH: Anterior segment fluorescein angiography. William & Wilkins, Baltimore, 1978.

57 Kottow M, Hendrickson P: Iris angiographic findings in retinal arterial occlusions. Can J Ophthalmol 9: 435, 1974.

58 Kottow M, Metzler U: Stagnation thrombosis: an iris fluorescein angiographic study. Ophthalmologica 171: 192, 1975.

59 Kottow M, Metzler U, Hendrickson P: Iris angiographic findings in retinal vein occlusion. In Cant JS: Vision and circulation. Proc 3rd William Mackenzie Memorial Symposium, Glasgow, 1974. Henry Kimpton Publishers, London, 1976.

60 Krill AE, Archer D, Newell FW: Photocoagulation in complications secondary to branch vein occlusion. Arch Ophthalmol 85: 48, 1971.

61 Laatikainen L: Preliminary report on effect of retinal panphotocoagulation on rubeosis iridis and neovas-

cular glaucoma. Br J Ophthalmol 61: 278, 1977.

62 Laatikainen L, Blach RH: Behaviour of the iris vasculature in central retinal vein occlusion: a fluorescein angiographic study of the vascular response of the retina and the iris. Br J Ophthalmol 61: 272, 1977.

63 Laatikainen L, Kohner EM: Fluorescein angiography and its prognostic significance in central retinal vein occlusion. Br J Ophthalmol 60: 411, 1976.

64 Laatikainen L, Kohner EM, Khovry D et al: Panretinal photocoagulation in central retinal vein occlusion: a randomised controlled clinical study. Br J Ophthalmol 61: 741, 1977.

65 Little HL, Rosenthal AR, Della Porta A et al: The effect of panretinal photocoagulation on rubeosis iridis and neovascular glaucoma. Br J Ophthalmol 61: 278, 1977.

66 Lodato G, Brancato G: Neovascular glaucoma caused by branch vein occlusion and deficiency of carotid-encephalic circulation: pathogenetic correlation. J Fr Ophtalmol 7: 615, 1984.

67 Magargal LE, Brown GC, Augsburger JJ et al: Efficacy of panretinal photocoagulation in preventing neovascular glaucoma following ischemic central retinal vein obstruction. Ophthalmology 89: 780, 1982.

68 Magargal LE, Brown GC, Augsburger JJ et al: Neovascolar glaucoma following branch retinal vein obstruction. Glaucoma 3: 333, 1981.

69 Magargal LE, Brown GC, Augsburger JJ et al: Neovascular glaucoma following central retinal vein obstruction. Ophthalmology 88: 1095, 1981.

70 Magargal LE, Donoso LA, Sanborn GE: Retinal ischemia and risk of neovascularization following central retinal vein obstruction. Ophthalmology 89: 1241, 1982.

71 May DR, Klein ML, Peyman GA et al: Xenon arc panretinal photocoagulation for central retinal vein occlusion. A randomized prospective study. Br J Ophthalmol 63: 725, 1979.

72 Mc Crary JA: Venous stasis retinophaty of stenotic or occlusive carotid origin. J Clin Neuro Ophthalmol 9: 195, 1989.

73 Menchini U, Antonini E: L'iridografia a fluorescenza in pazienti affetti da occlusione di una branca della vena retinica. Ann Ottalmol Clin Ocul 105: 213, 1979.

74 Menchini U, Antonini E: L'iridografia a fluorescenza in pazienti affetti da occlusione di una branca della vena retinica. Boll Ocul 59: 65, 1980.

75 Mendelsohn AO, Jampol LM, Shoch D: Secondary angle-closure glaucoma after central retinal vein occlusion. Am J Ophthalmol 100: 581, 1985.

76 Metzler U, Kottow M, Weigelin E: Fluoreszenzangiographische untersuchugen über die Umgehung retinaler Gefässverschlusse. Proc XXII Concilium Ophtalmologicum. Paris, 1974. Masson & CIE, Paris, 1976.

77 Michels RG, Gass JDM: The natural course of retinal branch vein obstruction. Trans Am Acad Ophthalmol Otolaryngol 78: 166, 1974.

78 Moore RF: Retinal vein thrombosis: a clinical study of sixty-two cases followed over many years. Br J Ophthalmol (Monogr Suppl): 2, 1924.

79 Moro F: Rilievi sul controllo a distanza delle trombosi venose retiniche. Ann Ottalmol 83: 329, 1957.

80 Myers KJ, Lalleu A: Central retinal vein occlusion and iris neovascularization hemorrhage. J Am Optom Assoc 59: 787, 1988.

81 Nork TM, Tso MO, Duvall J et al: Cellular mechanisms of iris neovascularization secondary to retinal vein occlusion. Arch Ophthalmol 107: 581, 1989.

82 Perrault LE, Zimmerman LE: The occurrence of glaucoma following occlusion of the central retinal artery: a clinicopathologic report of six new cases with a review of the literature. Arch Ophthalmol 61: 845, 1959.

83 Priluck IA, Robertson DM, Hollenhorst RW: Long-term follow-up of occlusion of the central retinal vein in young adults. Am J Ophthalmol 90: 190, 1980.

84 Raitta C: Der Zentralvenen und Netzhautvenenverschluss; ein klinischer Bericht über 400 Fälle, unter besonderer Berücksichtigung des intraokularen Druckes und der späten Fundus veränderungen. Acta Ophthalmol 83 (Suppl): 1, 1965.

85 Raitta C, Vannas S: Fluoresceinangiographie der Irisgefässe nach Zentralvenenverschluss. Albrecht von Graefes Arch Klin Ophthalmol 177: 33, 1969.

86 Riaskoff S: Le role preventif de la photocoagulation retinienne dans le development de glaucome neovasculaire apres occlusion de la veine centrale de la retine. Bull Soc Fr Ophtalmol 90: 87, 1978.

87 Sanborn GE: Characteristics of the hemisferic retinal vein occlusion. Ophthalmology 91: 1616, 1984.

88 Sanborn GE, Symes DJ, Magargal LE: Fundus-iris fluorescein angiography: evaluation of its use in the di-

agnosis of rubeosis iridis. Ann Ophthalmol 18: 52, 1986.

89 Schnicke T: Fluoreszenzangiographie der Iris bei Patienten mit Diabetes Mellitus und Patienten mit retinaler Venenthrombose. Dissertation. Bonn, Rheinische Friedrich-Wilhelms Universitat, 1975.

90 Schulze RR: Rubeosis iridis. Am J Ophthalmol 63: 487, 1967.

91 Sedney SC: Photocoagulation in retinal vein occlusion. Doc Ophthalmol 40: 1, 1976.

92 Shields MB, Ritch R: Classifications and mechanisms. In Ritch R, Shields MB: The secondary glaucoma. CV Mosby, St Louis, 1982.

93 Shilling JS, Kohner EM: New vessels formation in retinal branch vein occlusion. Br J Ophthalmol 60: 810, 1976.

94 Simmons RJ, Thomas JV: Malignant glaucoma. In Ritch R, Shields MB: The secondary glaucoma. CV Mosby, St Louis, 1982.

95 Sinclair SH, Gragoudas ES: Prognosis for rubeosis iridis following central retinal vein occlusion. Br J Ophthalmol 63: 753, 1979.

96 Smith R: Thrombotic glaucoma: a clinico-pathological study. Proc 17th Concilium Ophthalmologicum, 1954, Canada. Churchill, Livingstone, 1955.

97 Snelling JB, Nisbet RM: Retinal branch vein occlusion. Ann Ophthalmol 13: 1273, 1981.

98 Tasman W, Magargal LE, Augsburger JJ: Effects of argon laser photocoagulation on rubeosis iridis and angle neovascularization. Ophthalmology 87: 400, 1980.

99 Trempe CL, Takahashi M, Topilow HW: Vitreous changes in retinal branch vein occlusion. Ophthalmology 88: 681, 1981.

100 Uhthoff W: Zu den arteriellen und venösen Zirculationsstörungen der Netzhaut. Ber Zusammenkunft Dtsch Ophthalmol Ges (Heidelberg) 45: 63, 1925.

101 Vander JF, Brown GC, Benson WE: Iris neovascularization after central retinal artery obstruction despite previous panretinal photocoagulation for diabetic retinophaty. Am J Ophthalmol 109: 464, 1990.

102 Vannas S: Glaucoma due to thrombosis of the central vein of the retina. Ophthalmologica 142: 266, 1961.

103 Vannas S, Orma H: Experience of treating retinal venous occlusion with anticoagulant and antisclerosis therapy. Arch Ophthalmol 58: 812, 1957.

104 Vannas S, Raitta C: Anticoagulant treatment of retinal venous occlusion. Am J Ophthalmol 62: 874, 1966.

105 Vannas S, Raitta C: Microcirculatory disturbances of occlusive diseases of the eye. Doc Ophthalmol 33: 345, 1972.

106 Vannas S, Tarkkanen A: Retinal vein occlusion and glaucoma; tonographic study of the incidence of glaucoma and of its prognostic significance. Br J Ophthalmol 44: 583, 1960.

107 Vidic B, Hiti H, Schuhmann G et al: Verlauf retinaler Venenthrombosen nach Laserkoagulation. Klin Monatsbl Augenheilkd 179: 415, 1981.

108 Wand M: Neovascular glaucoma. In Ritch R, Shields MB: The secondary glaucoma. CV Mosby, St Louis, 1982.

109 Wand M, Dueker DK, Aiello LM: Effects of panretinal photocoagulation on rubeosis iridis angle neovascularization and neovascular glaucoma. Am J Ophthalmol 86: 332, 1978.

110 Waubke T: Glaukomdisposition und Sekundärglaukom bei Thrombosen der Retinagefässe. Klin Monatsbl Augenheilkd 136: 224, 1960.

111 Weiss DI, Shaffer RN, Nehrenberg TR: Neovascular glaucoma, complicating carotid cavernous fistula. Arch Ophthalmol 69: 304, 1963.

112 Wolter JR, Phillips RL: Secondary glaucoma following occlusion of the central retinal artery. Am J Ophthalmol 47: 335, 1959.

113 Zegarra H, Gutman FA, Conforto J: The natural course of central retinal vein occlusion. Ophthalmology 86: 1931, 1979.

114 Zollinger R: Über das Vorkommen von Gefässneubildungen auf der iris. Ophthalmologica 121: 168, 1951.

*Fig. **4.5**,1 - Retinal fluorescein angiographic picture of a branch venous occlusion with edematous capillaropathy.*

*Fig. **4.5**,2 - Green light retinography (a) and fluorescein angiography (b) in a lately occurred branch venous occlusion.*

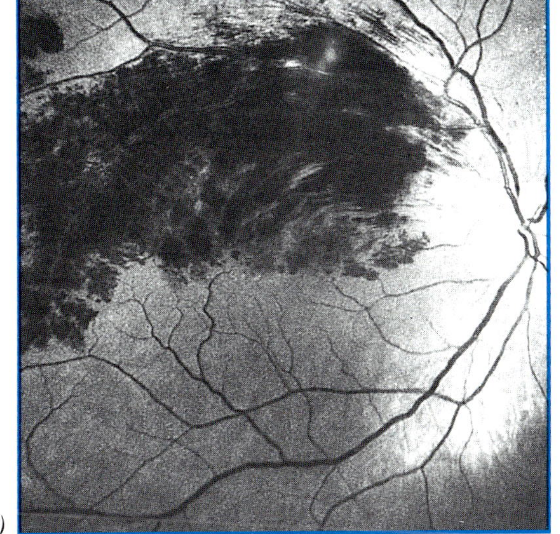

a)

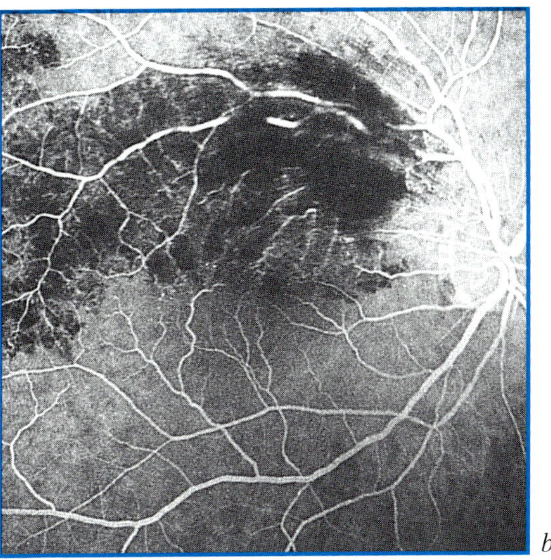

b)

*Fig. **4.5**,3 - Panretinal fluorescein angiography in a patient with hemicentral venous occlusion and ischemic capillaropathy, complicated by hemovitreous masking the lower sectors of the retina.*

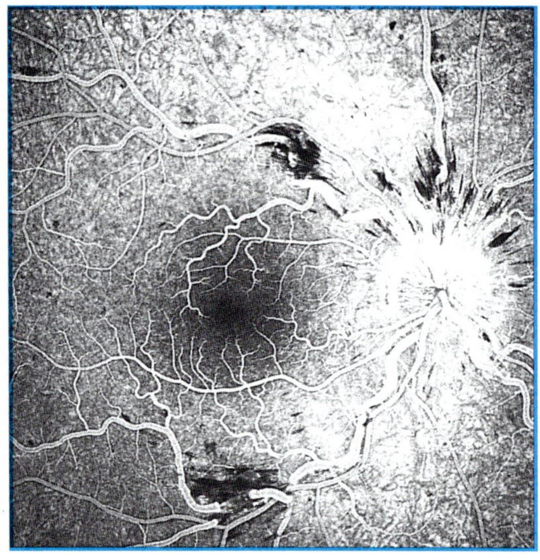

a)

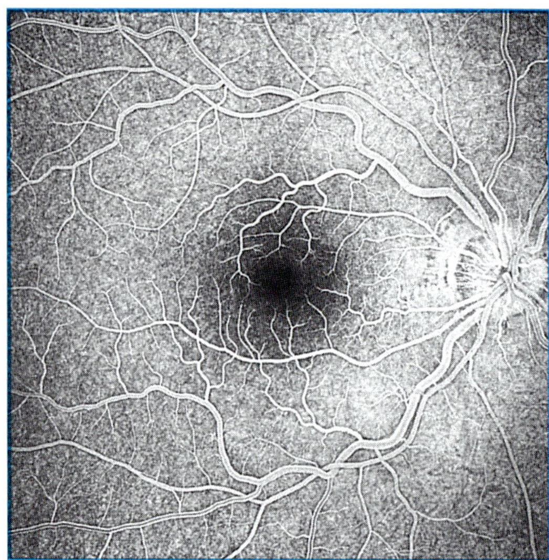

b)

*Fig. **4.5**,4 - Central retinal vein occlusion without capillaropathy (benign form) (a) before and (b) after spontaneous resolution (fluorescein angiographic findings).*

*Fig. **4.5**,5 - The widespread hypofluorescence seen in ischemic central retinal vein occlusion results from the amputations in the microvasculature and from the masking effect of the retinal hemorrhages.*

*Fig. **4.5**,6 - Central retinal vein occlusion with capillary ischemia: panretinal fluorescein angiography.*

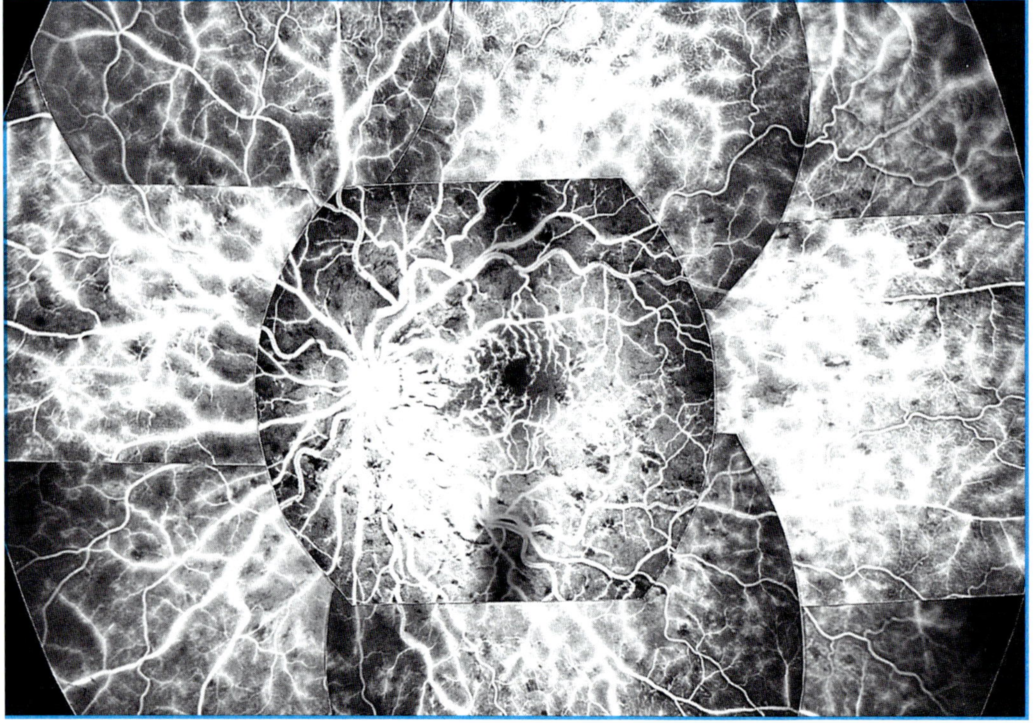

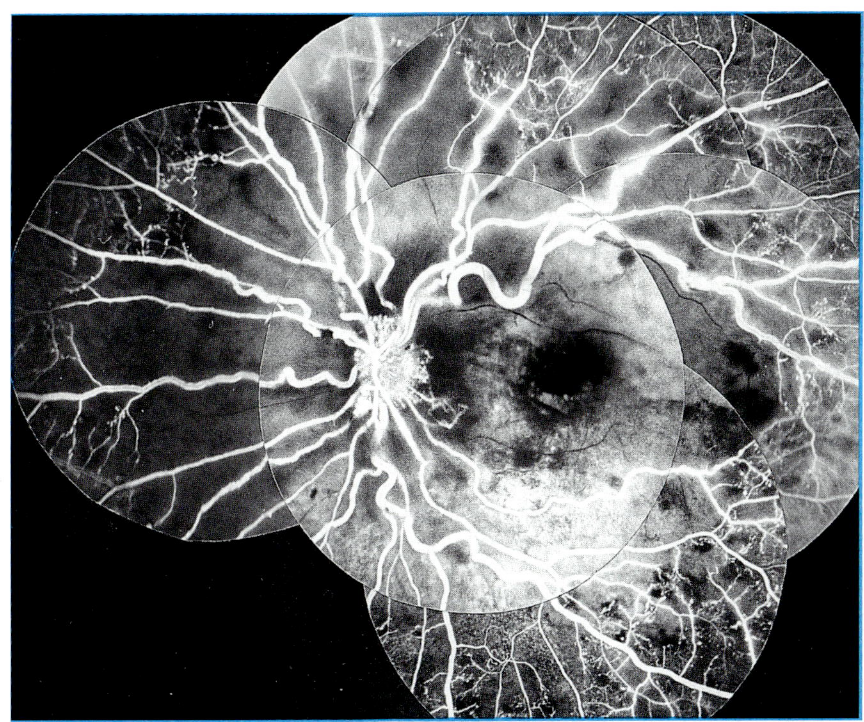

*Fig. **4.5**,7 - Very severe retinal ischemia in a patient with central retinal vein occlusion, involving the macular area too (panretinal fluorescein angiography).*

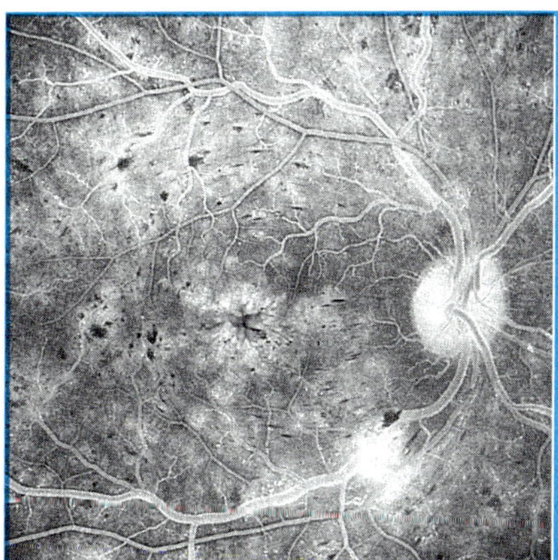

*Fig. **4.5**,8 - Retinal fluorescein angiographic picture in a case of central retinal vein occlusion with edematous capillaropathy.*

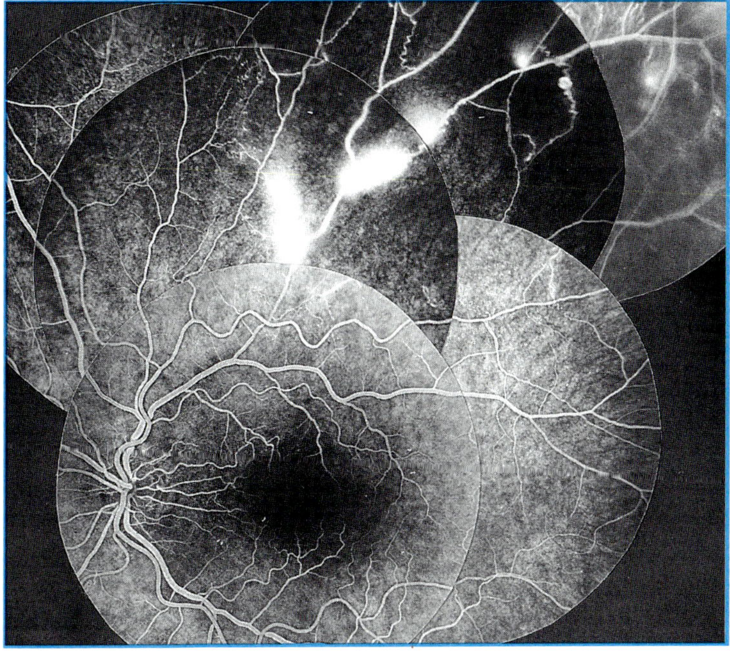

*Fig. **4.5**,9 - Occlusion of the superior temporal branch of the central retinal vein with capillary non perfusion and epiretinal new vessels: fluorescein angiographic picture.*

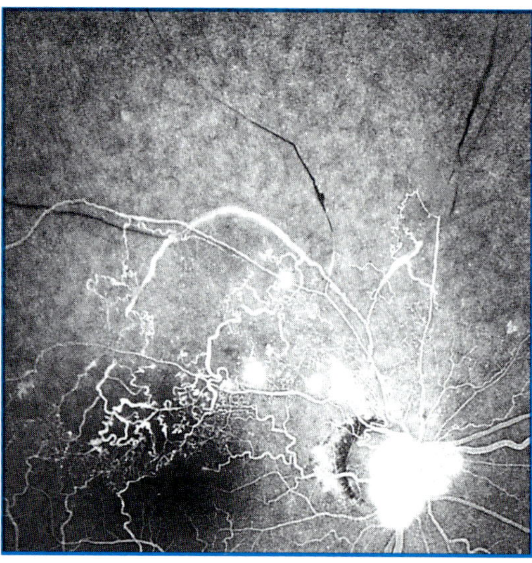

*Fig. **4.5**,10 - Ischemic hemicentral retinal vein occlusion, complicated by papillary neovascularization: fluorescein angiographic picture.*

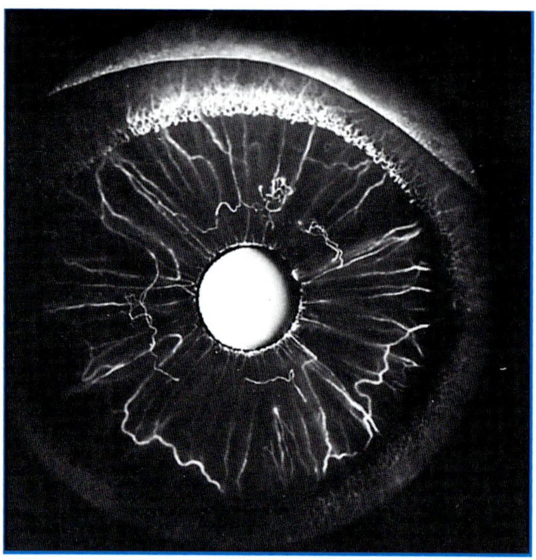

*Fig. **4.5**,11 - In this 62-year-old patient with edematous central retinal vein occlusion, iris fluorescein angiography shows the iris vessels substantially within normal limits.*

a)

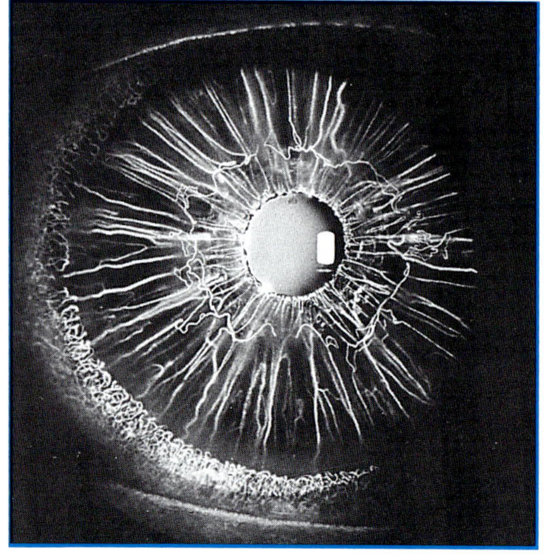

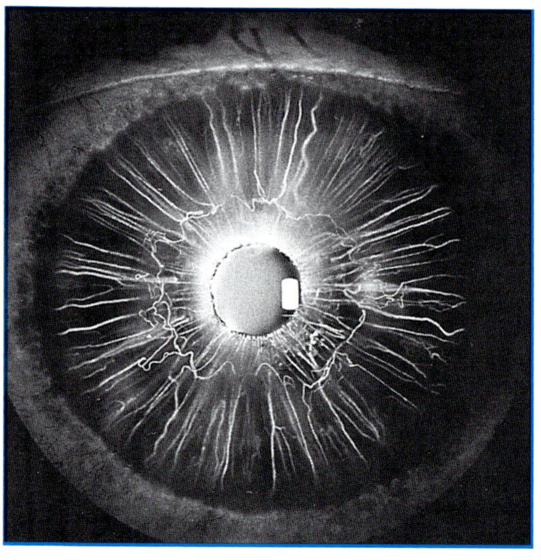

b)

*Fig. **4.5**,12 - Early (a) and late (b) iris fluorescein angiographic findings in a patient with edematous central retinal vein occlusion. There is slight pupillary leakage, with anomalies in the path of the vessels in the pars pupillaris, and congested radial vessels.*

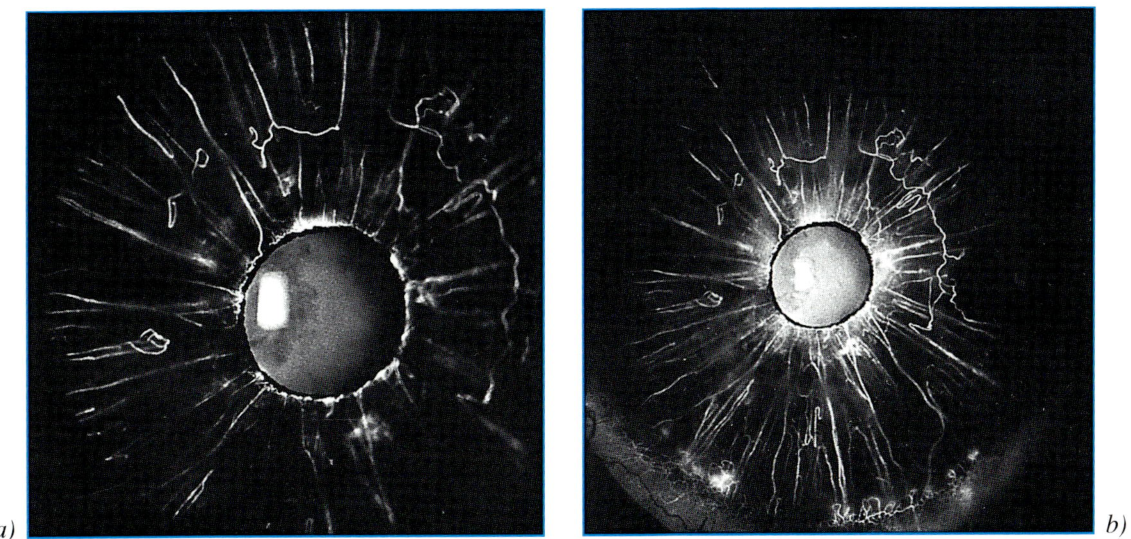

a) b)

*Fig. **4.5**,13 - Early (a) and late (b) iris fluorescein angiographic findings in a patient with ischemic central retinal vein occlusion. There is diffuse pupillary dye leakage and focal areas of extrapupillary spread.*

a) 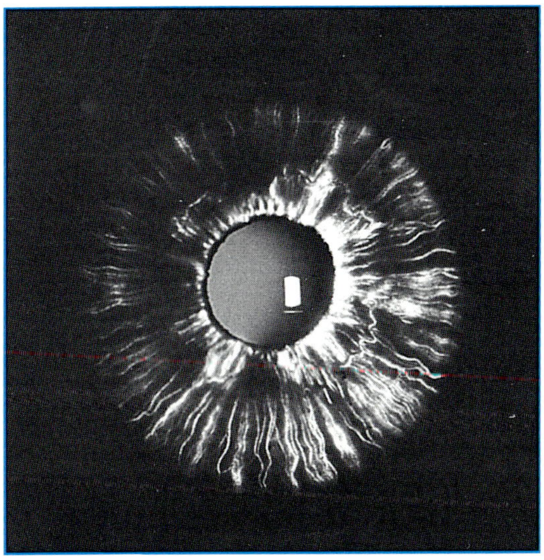 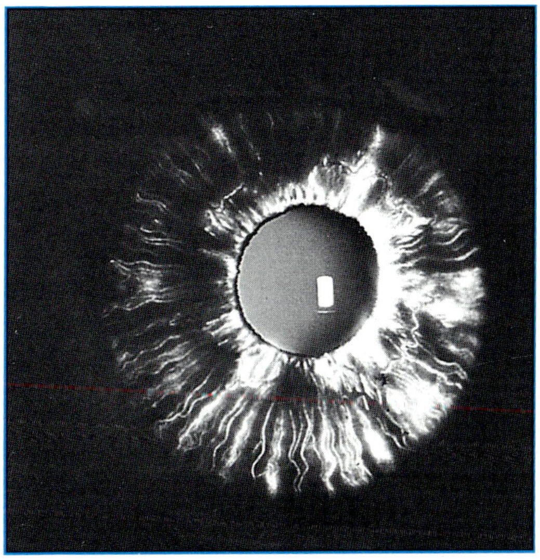 b)

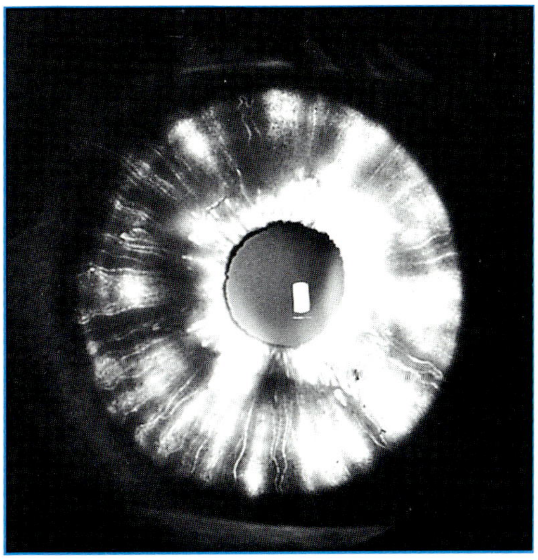

c)

*Fig. **4.5**,14 - A case of ischemic central retinal vein occlusion: iris fluorescein angiography (phases a,b,c) shows pupillary leakage and congested radial vessels, from which dye leaks out copiously.*

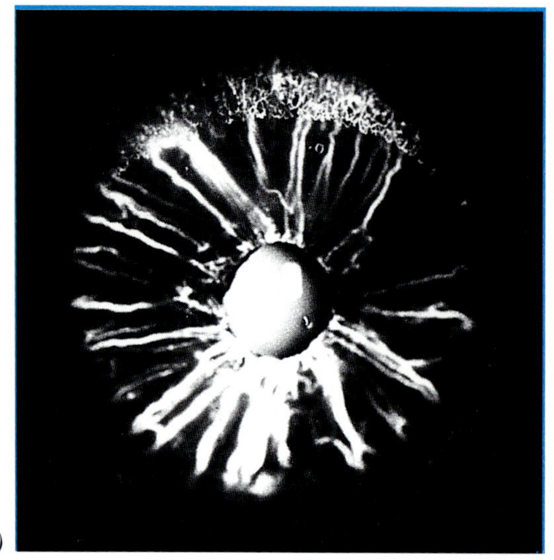
a)

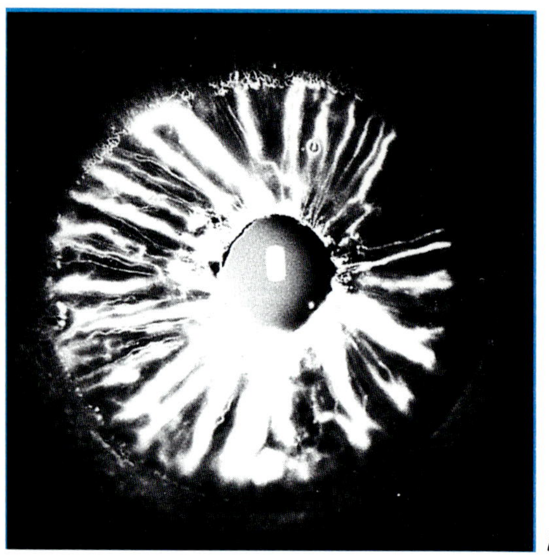
b)

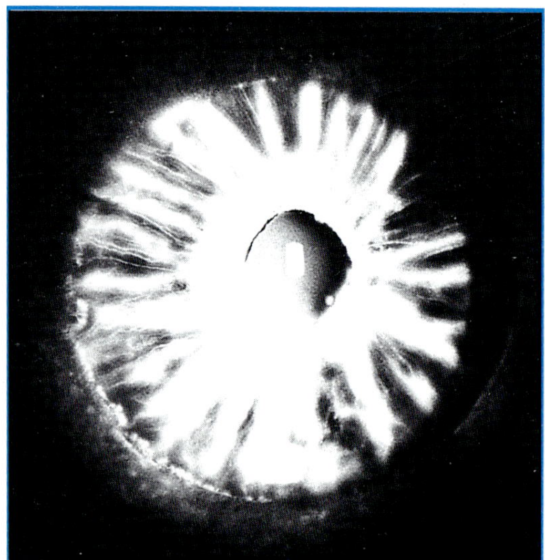
c)

*Fig. **4.5**,15 - Iris fluorescein angiography (phases a,b,c) in a patient with ischemic central retinal vein occlusion. Filling delays and defects are evident, with marked, diffuse leakage particularly from the congested radial vessels, and initial neovascular tufts. This type of iris damage generally precedes neovascular glaucoma.*

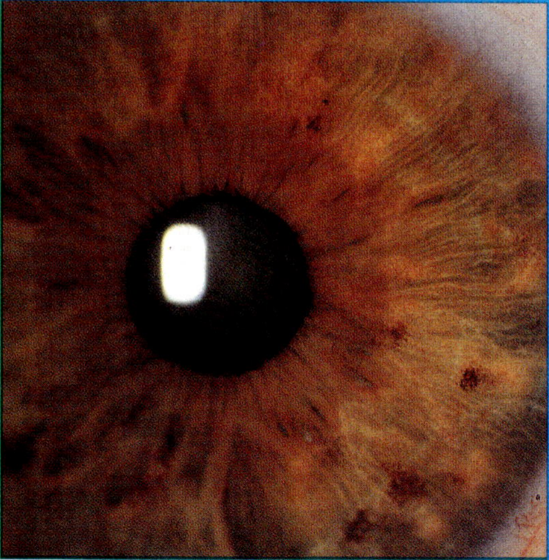

*Fig. **4.5**,16a - Grade 1 proliferative iridopathy [9] in a patient with ischemic central retinal vein occlusion biomicroscopic findings.*

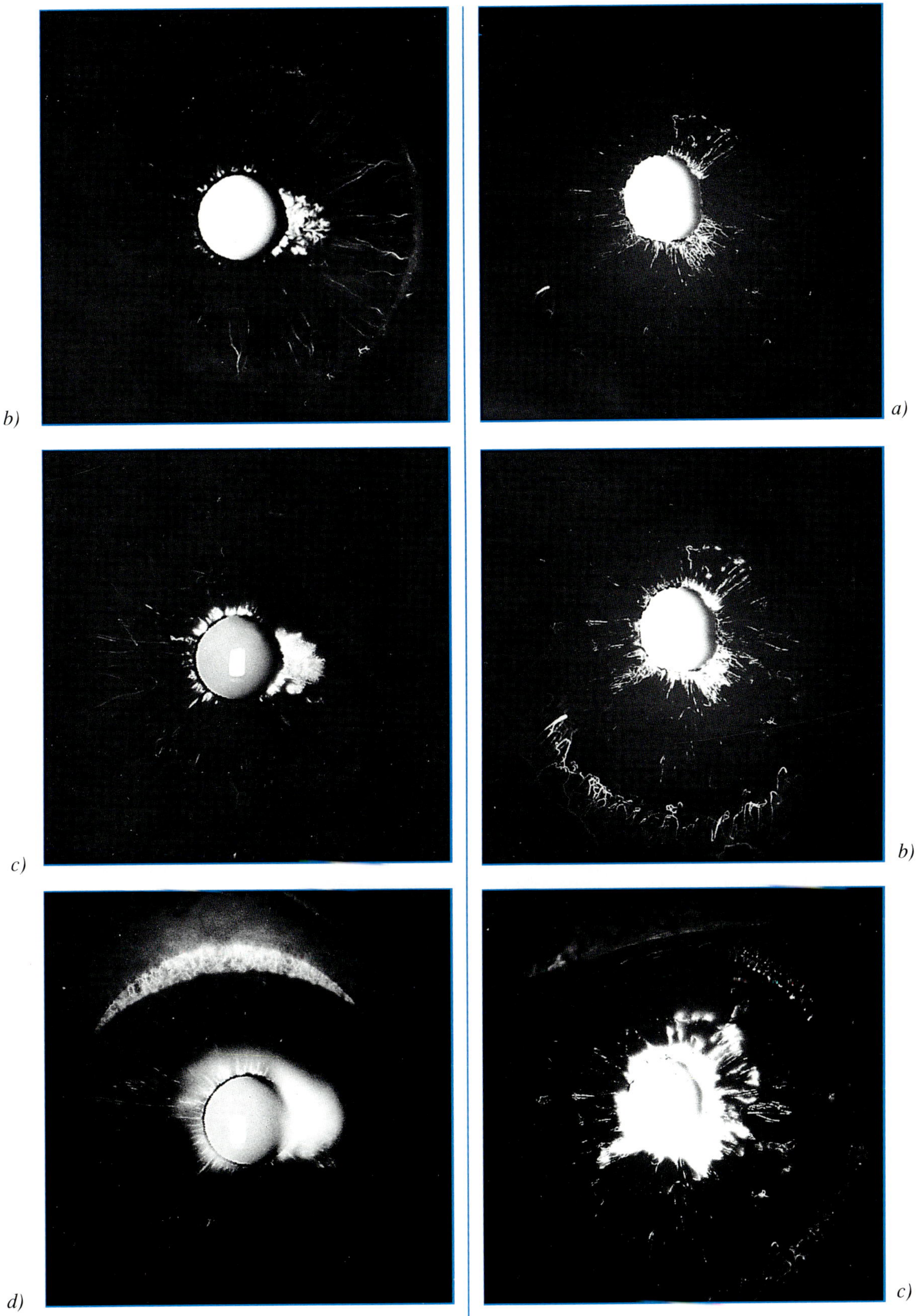

*Fig. **4.5**,16b,c,d - Grade 1 proliferative iridopathy in a patient with ischemic central retinal vein occlusion: iris fluorescein angiographic phases.*

*Fig. **4.5**,17 - New vessels mainly around the pupillary border in a patient with ischemic central retinal vein occlusion (iris fluorescein angiographic phases a,b,c).*

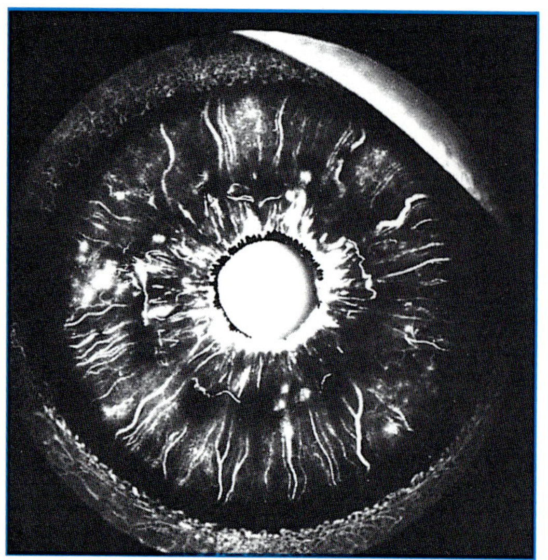
a)

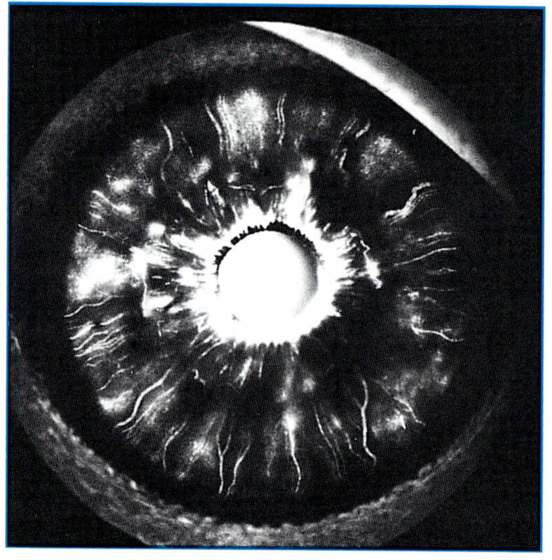
b)

*Fig. **4.5**,18 - Ischemic central retinal vein occlusion. Iris fluorescein angiography (a: early; b: late phase) shows precisely the new vessels around the border and in the stroma.*

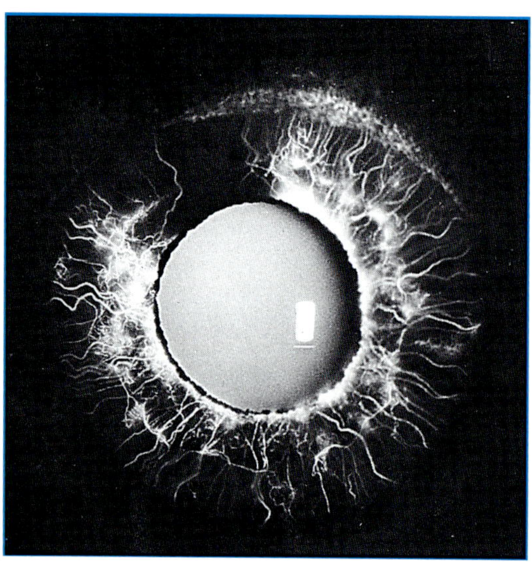

*Fig. **4.5**,19 - Filling defects (10-12 o'clock) and iris new vessels in ischemic central retinal vein occlusion (advanced iris fluorescein angiographic phase).*

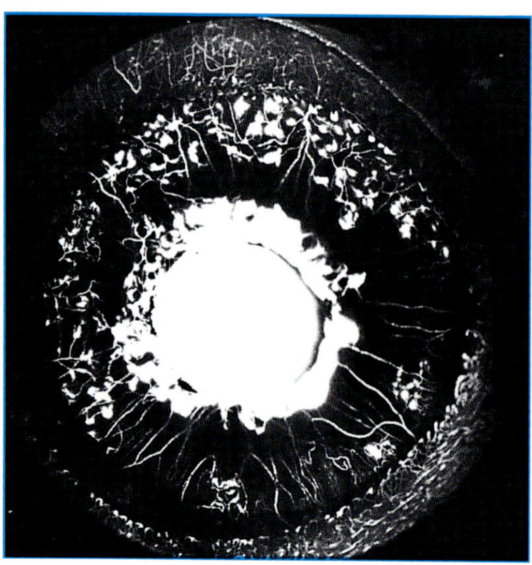

*Fig. **4.5**,20 - Iris fluorescein angiography in this patient with ischemic central retinal vein occlusion shows new vessels around the pupillary border merging in the mid-periphery with a network of new vessels starting from the angle.*

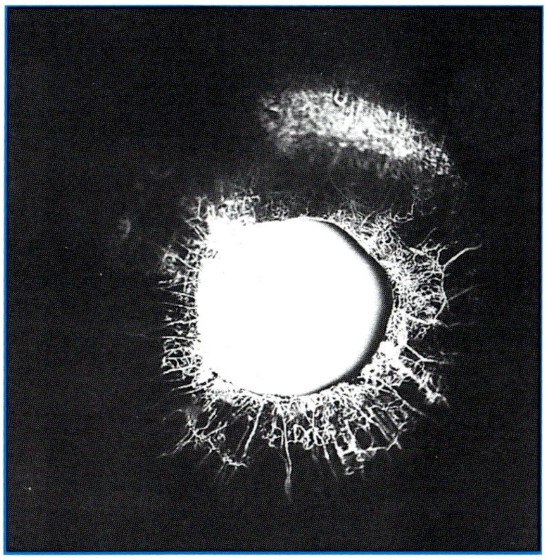

a) 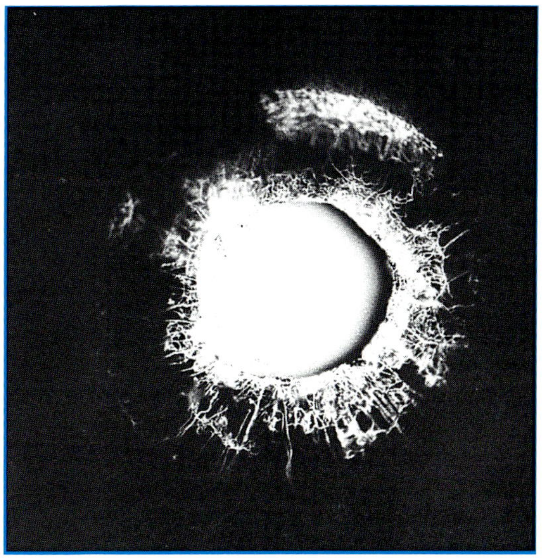 b)

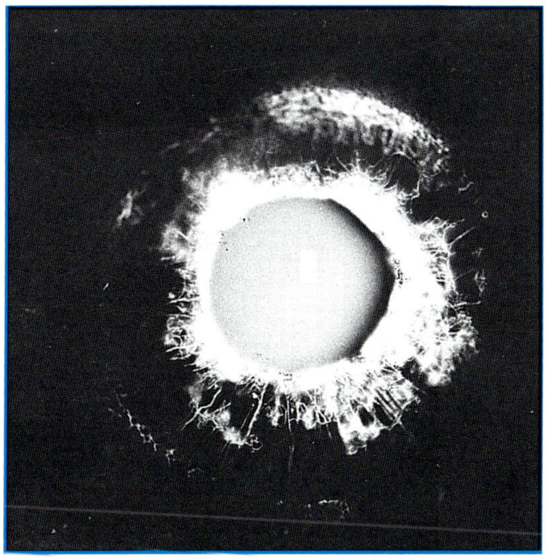

c)

*Fig. **4.5**,21 - Ischemic central retinal vein occlusion: new vessels around the border and in the stroma are clearly seen in the early iris fluorescein angiographic phases (a,b) and leak dye in the later phases (c).*

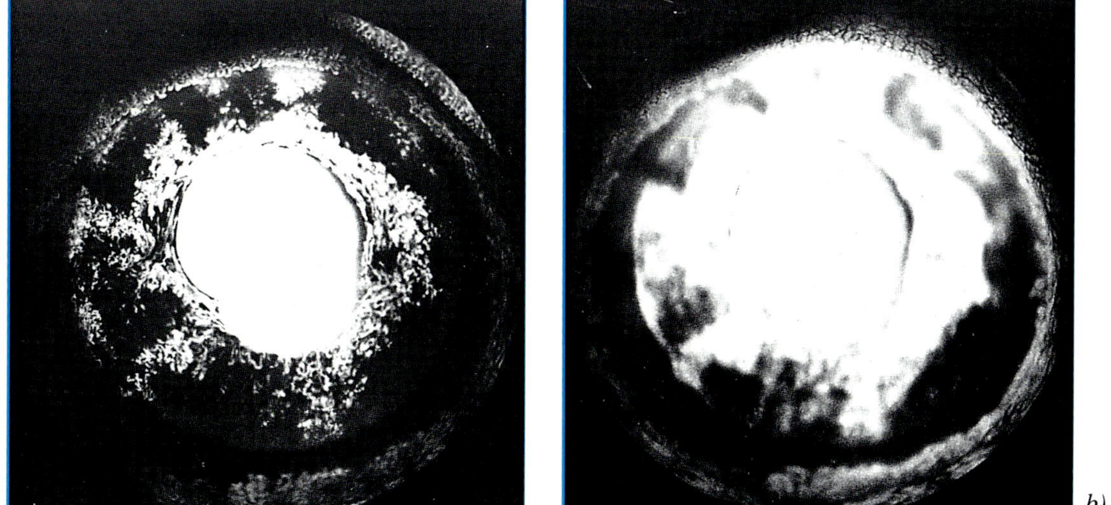

a) b)

*Fig. **4.5**,22 -The early phases (a) of iris fluorescein angiography show up ample areas of the iris without circulation, with dye filling the new vessels around their edges. At later times (b) there is conspicuous dye leakage from these vessels.*

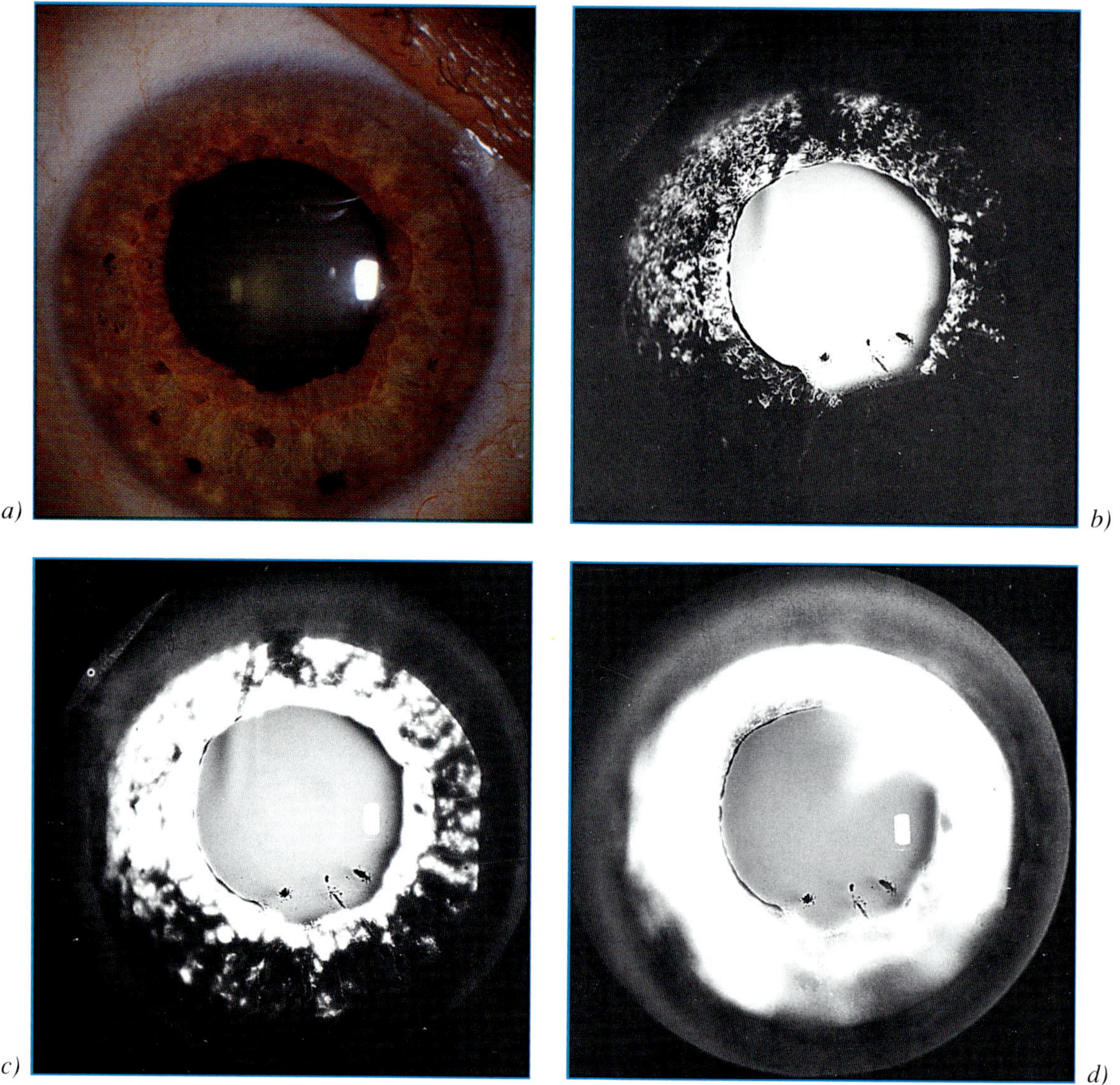

*Fig. **4.5**,23 - Biomicroscopic findings (a) and iris fluorescein angiographic phases (b,c,d) in neovascular glaucoma from ischemic central retinal vein occlusion. An intricate anarchic network of new vessels can be seen over the whole of the surface of the iris, with irido-lenticular synechiae, pupillary deformation and pigment deposits on the anterior lens surface.*

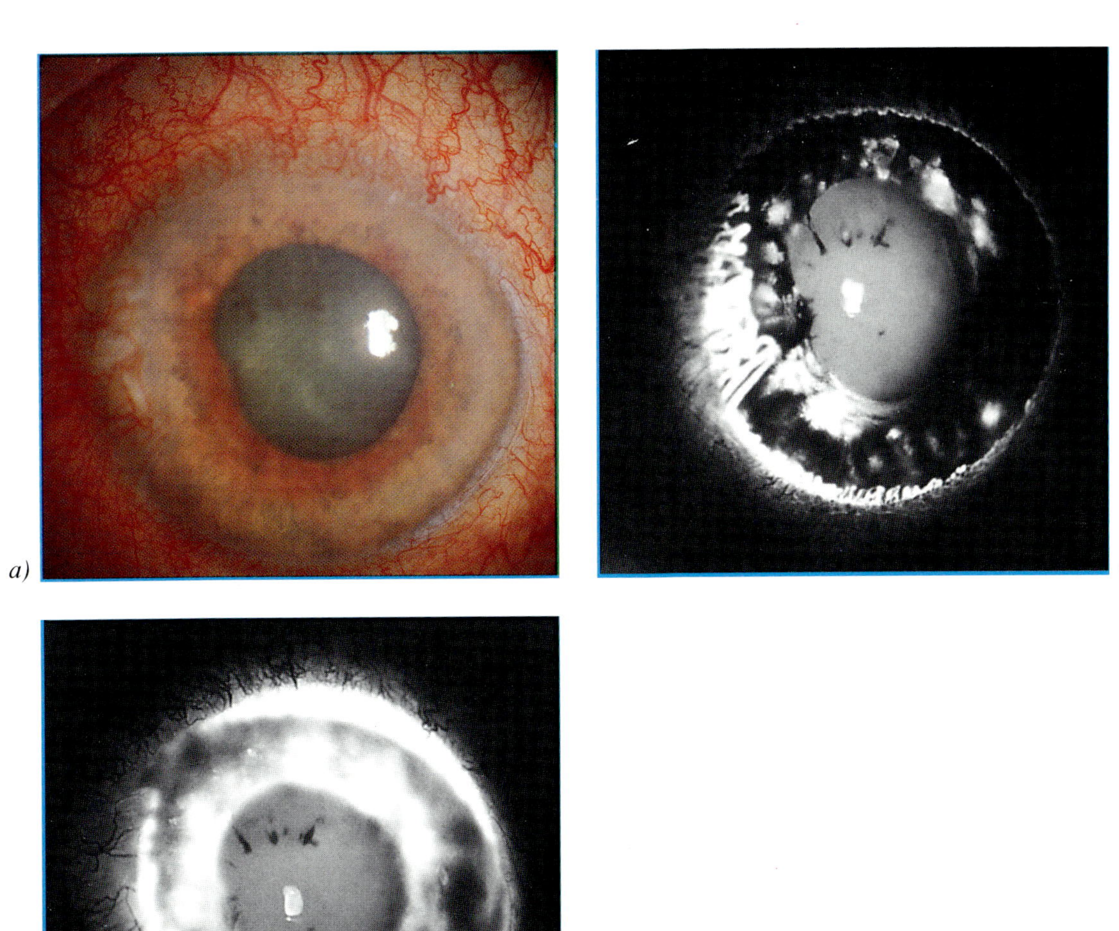

*Fig. **4.5**,24 - Neovascular glaucoma from ischemic central retinal vein occlusion. The pterygium detectable by biomicroscopic examination (a) corresponds on iris fluorescein angiography to early superficial hyperfluorescence (b) and, in the later phases (c), to leakage merging with the dye from the iris new vessels.*

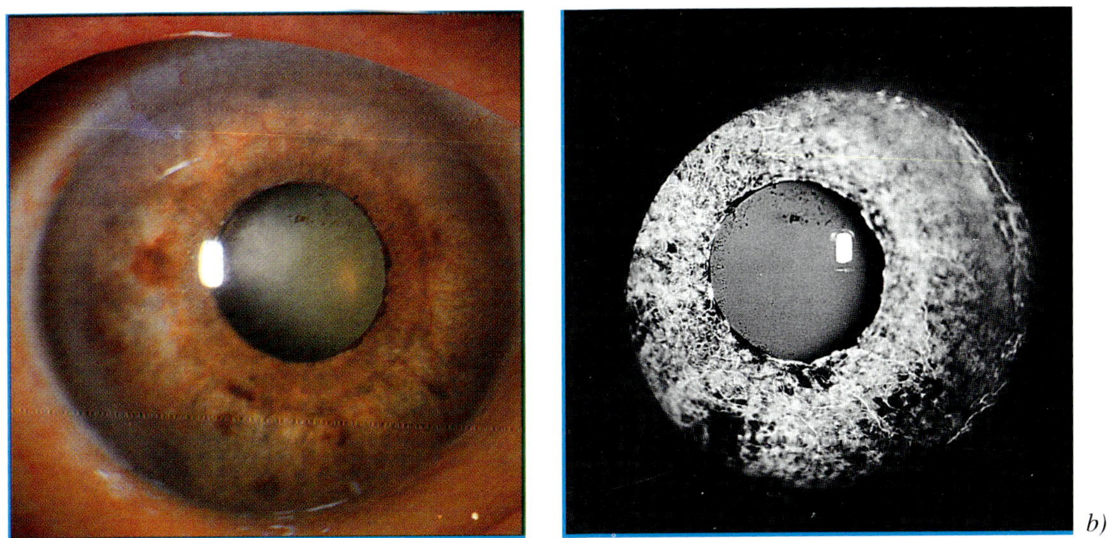

*Fig. **4.5**,25 - Dense neovascular network in neovascular glaucoma from ischemic central retinal vein occlusion. a) Biomicroscopic view, b) iris fluorescein angiography.*

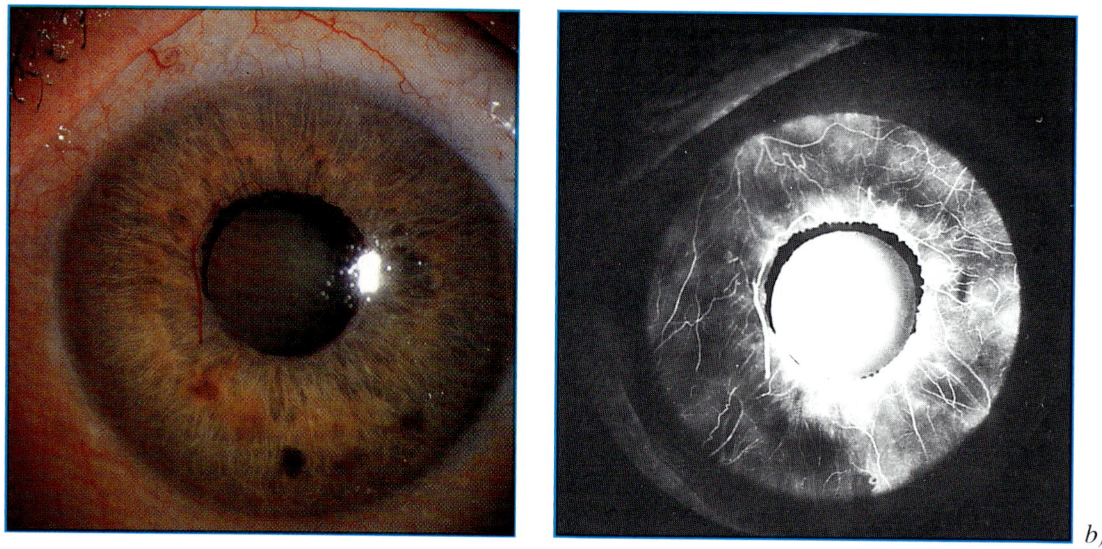

Fig. ***4.5****,26 - Neovascular glaucoma in the involutive-atrophic stage in a case of ischemic central retinal vein occlusion. Corresponding to the biomicroscopically visible ectropion uveae (a), iris fluorescein angiography shows hypofluorescence on account of the masking effect (b). Dye leakage is limited from the large-caliber new vessels.*

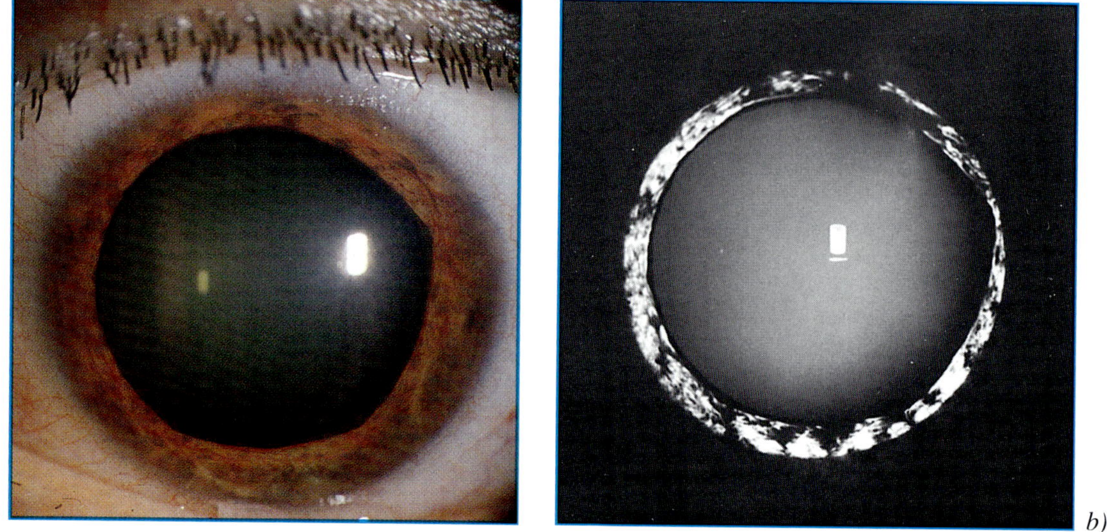

Fig. ***4.5****,27 - Pharmacological midriasis for neovascular glaucoma in ischemic central retinal vein occlusion. a) Biomicroscopic view; b) iris fluorescein angiography, showing clearly the new vessels giving rise to dye leakage.*

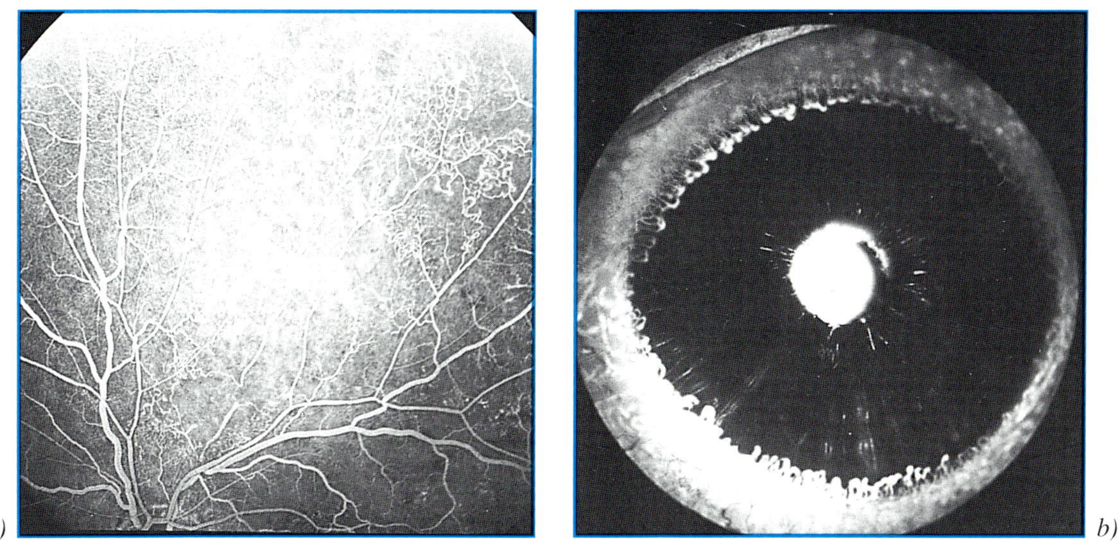

a) b)

*Fig. **4.5**,28 - Dye leakage from the upper sectors of the pupillary border (b), corresponding topographically to the retinal district affected by branch occlusion (a).*

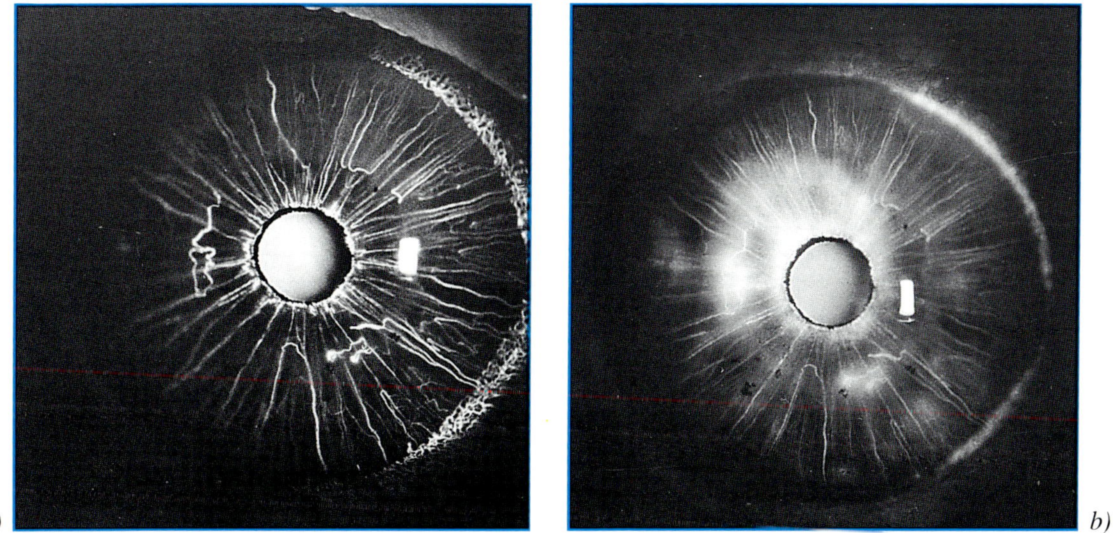

a) b)

*Fig. **4.5**,29 - Early (a) and late (b) iris fluorescein angiographic phases in a case of central retinal vein occlusion with capillary ischemia. There is limited pupillary and extrapupillary leakage, with anomalies in the path and size of the vessels of the iris lesser circle.*

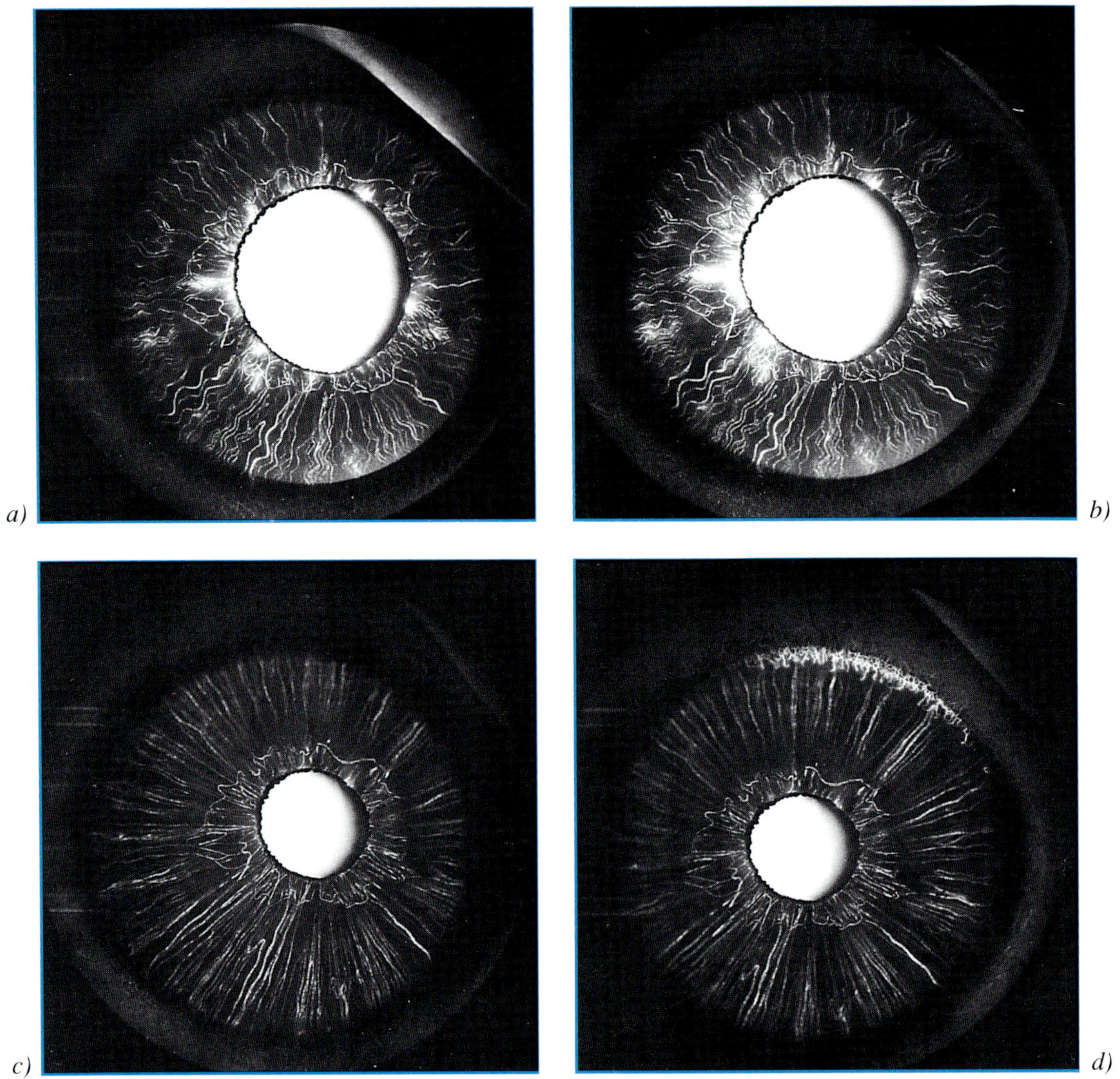

Fig. ***4.5****,30 - Proliferative iridopathy in central retinal vein occlusion before (a,b) and after (c,d) panretinal photocoagulation. Iris new vessels have visibly regressed (iris fluorescein angiography).*

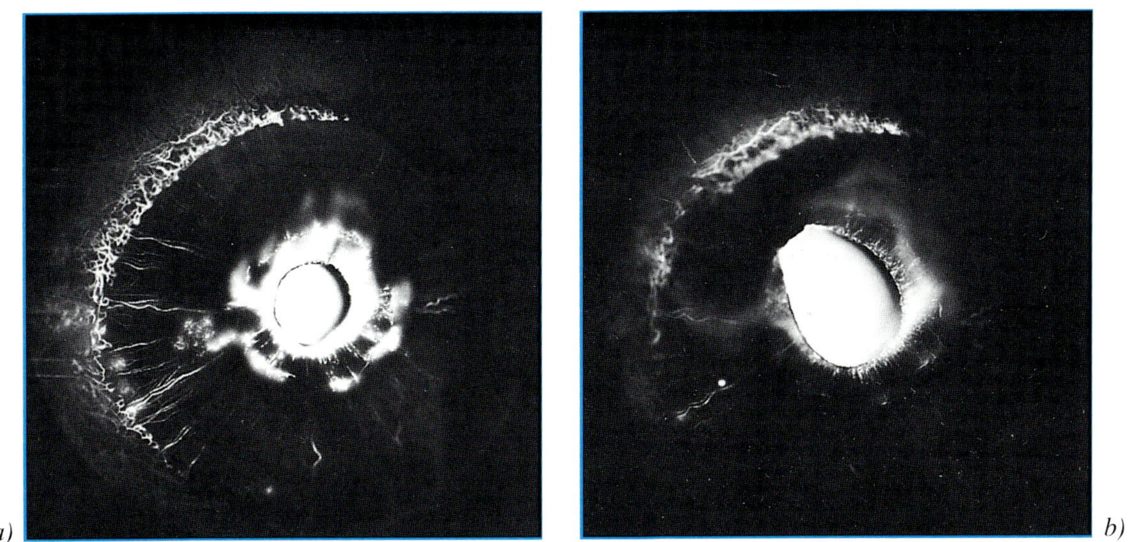

a) b)

*Fig. **4.5**,31 - Iris fluorescein angiography before (a) and after (b) panretinal photocoagulation permits the assessment of iris new vessel regression.*

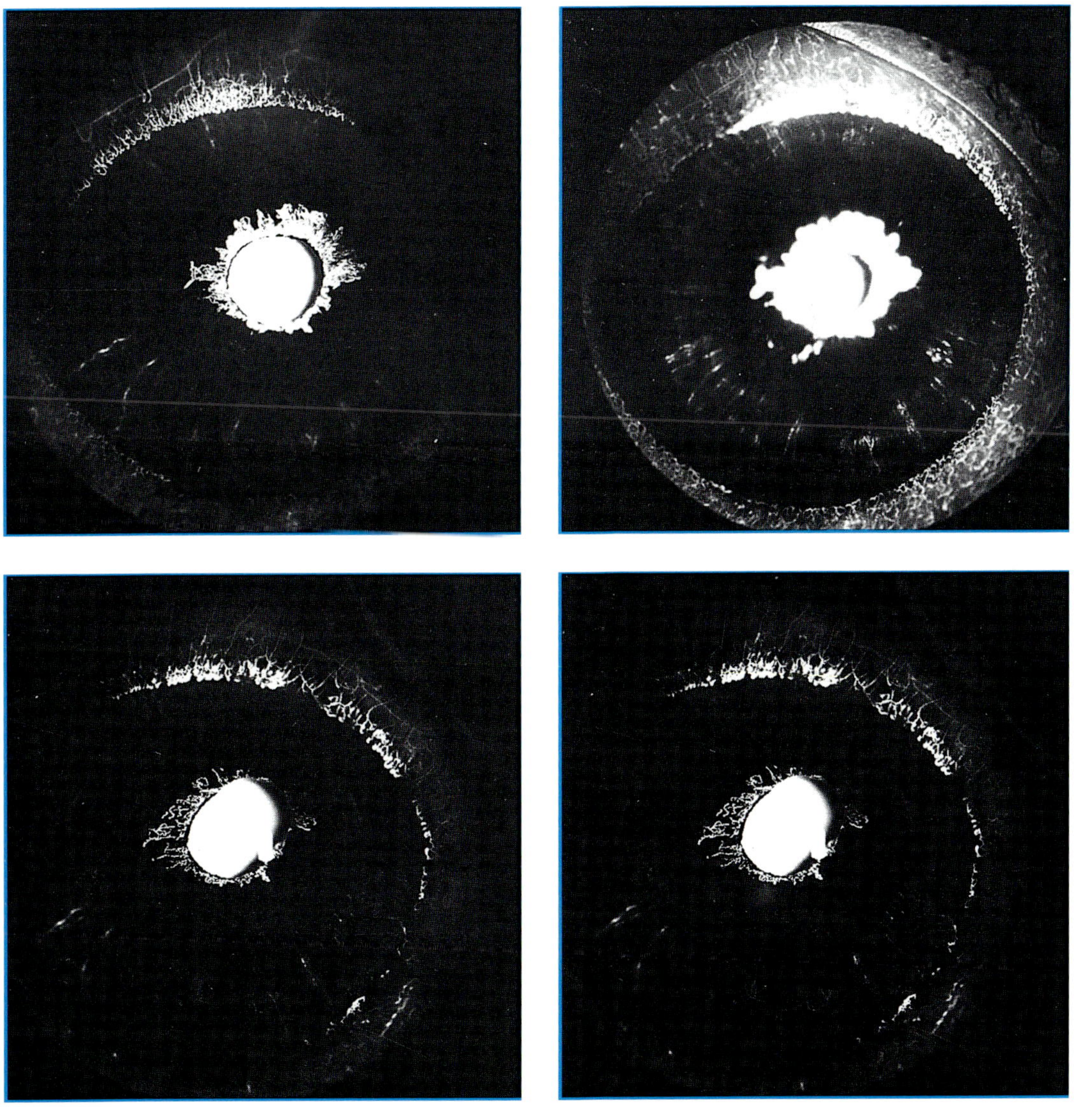

a) b)

c) d)

*Fig. **4.5**,32 - Another case of rubeosis iridis (a,b) from ischemic central retinal vein occlusion which regressed after panretinal photocoagulation (c,d).*

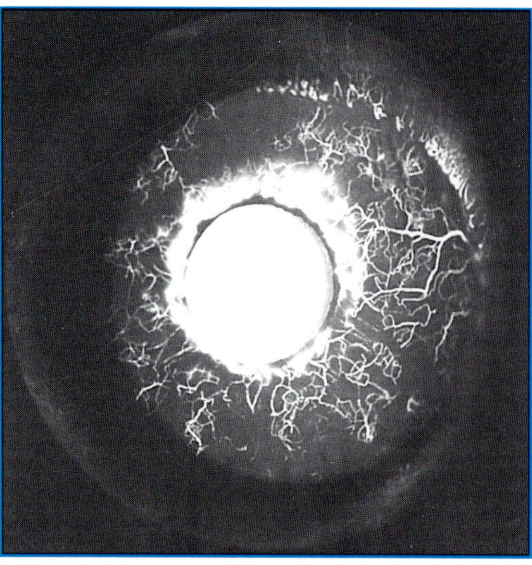

Fig. ***4.5**,33 - Iris fluorescein angiographic findings in a patient with occlusion of the central retinal vein and artery. An intricate neovascular network has taken the place of the iris vascular structure. Iris perfusion defects are evident, indicating the ischemic involvement of the anterior segment.*

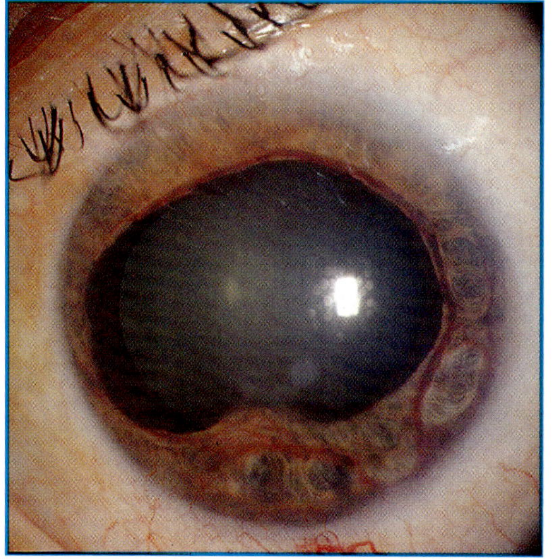

a)

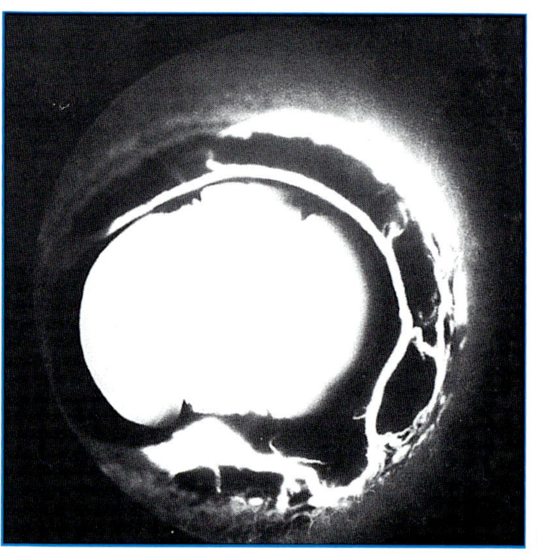

b)

Fig. ***4.5**,34 - Neovascular glaucoma due to ischemic central retinal vein occlusion. The iris fluorescein angiographic picture is dominated by the lack of perfusion and by voluminous new-formed vascular trunks. a) Biomicroscopic findings, b) iris fluorescein angiography. Ectropion uveae and irido-lenticular synechiae are also visible.*

R. Brancato, F. Bandello, R. Lattanzio
Atlas of Iris
Fluorescein Angiography
Kugler & Ghedini Publications 1995

Chapter 4.6

Ocular ischemic syndrome

The Ocular Ischemic Syndrome (OIS), meaning the collection of ocular signs and symptoms arising secondarily to any marked obstruction of the carotid artery, was first described in 1963 by Kearns and Hollenhorst, who called it "venous stasis retinopathy".[37] This term, however, tended to lead to errors as it was also employed to indicate less severe, non-ischemic forms of central retinal vein occlusion.[37] The syndrome has also been known as "ischemic ocular inflammation" and "ischemic oculopathy".

Generally the OIS arises in patients over 50 years old (mean age 65 years),[8,9,41,51,63,68] is more frequent among males[8,51] and is unilateral in 80% of cases.[8] The most frequent symptom, observed in 80-90% of cases, is a reduction of visual acuity;[8,51] this generally happens slowly but progressively, over weeks or months. It may occasionally be sudden and in such cases ophthalmoscopy discloses a foveal cherry-red spot, probably indicating acute embolization of the central retinal artery.

The proportion of patients who report amaurosis fugax varies widely in different caselists - from 5-60%.[8,12,23,28,29,51,55,65,67] Some patients with carotid stenosis report unilateral reduction in vision induced by light and this appears to be secondary to the fact that the choroid circulation cannot keep up with the enhanced retinal metabolic needs in response to exposure to light.[18,21,33]

The extent of reduction of vision reported by patients with OIS varies; in 35% of patients visual acuity is 20/20 or 20/40, 30% fall between 20/50 and 20/400, and the remaining 35% are between finger counting and light perception.[8] The rare cases with no light perception are presumably due to marked ischemia of the posterior segment, often associated with neovascular glaucoma.

From 20-40% report pain[8,51] which may be related to bulbar ischemia or to secondary neovascular glaucoma when present. In fact, the complications resulting from atherosclerotic occlusion of the carotid and the consequent reduced orbital blood flow can affect the anterior segment. The most frequent alterations to this segment are episcleral vascular congestion, corneal edema, band keratopathy, iris atrophy, rubeosis iridis and neovascular glaucoma (Figs. **4.6**,1,2,3).[9,24,30,41,55] Eighteen percent of the eyes analysed in one of these studies had iritis, marked by flare in the anterior chamber.[8]

It is quite frequent to find rubeosis iridis in eyes with OIS and in a study of 51 eyes 66% were found to have it at the first investigation.[8] The % age may in fact be even higher, as many less severe, asymptomatic cases of OIS do not come to the ophthalmologist's attention.

In cases not complicated by iris neovascularization, iris fluorescein angiography may show slight dye leakage at the pupillary margin, filling abnormalities and delays and, though rarely, prominent, dilated arteries.[43] In cases with rubeosis iridis this examination shows aspecific hyperfluorescence corresponding to the neovascular tufts.

In an elderly patient without diabetes, and with no signs of central retinal vein occlusion or other predisposing eye diseases, the finding of rubeosis iridis should suggest OIS. Kearns and Hollenhorst found that two thirds of the patients with OIS that they analysed had rubeosis iridis; half of these had neovascular glaucoma, defined as the association of rubeosis iridis with intraocular pressure more than 22 mmHg.[37] In certain eyes with rubeosis iridis fibrovascular membranes may completely close the angle, even if intraocular pressure is normal or below normal.[32,65] This is presumably related to some perfusion defect in the ciliary bodies and to reduced production of aqueous humor because of the carotid stenosis.[68]

Although it has long been known that carotid stenosis may cause neovascular glaucoma, there are still not many published studies analysing the prevalence of OIS among patients who have neovascular glaucoma. In a study of 208 eyes with this complication, OIS was the sole cause in 12.9%.[10]

Carotid angiography shows that 90% of patients with OIS have marked obstruction (90% or more), generally atherosclerotic, of the ipsilateral internal or common carotid.[8,35,41,55] It is still not clear why only some of the patients with severe carotid stenosis present ischemic retinopathy developing later into rubeosis iridis. The speed of the carotid occlusion, the site of the stenosis, the extent of collateral circulation and the state of the chorioretinal vascularization are all important.[38] It has been reported that a 90% stenosis of the internal carotid artery causes about a 50% pressure drop in the central retinal artery.[35]

In a caselist available to us the most frequent alteration was embolization of the central retinal artery and its branches, and - in two cases - of the cilio-retinal artery.[51]

Some histological reports describe a loss of endothelial cells and especially of pericytes in the retinal vessels of eyes with OIS which would explain the fluorescein leakage from these vessels in angiography.[34,49,50]

The prognosis is not good for eyes with OIS and rubeosis iridis, with severe visual impairment. If the anterior chamber angle is open panretinal photocoagulation may be useful[14,19] in that it may stabilize the retinal situation, but only in a limited number of cases it leads to regression of the iris new vessels. This regression, however, is seen in fewer cases than after panretinal photocoagulation of occluded retinal veins or proliferative diabetic retinopathy.[14,15,19] This may be because the ischemia of the anterior segment is more marked in OIS. Photocoagulation does however slow the course of the rubeosis, or facilitate its reduction in subjects subsequently operated by endarterectomy.

In cases where the new vessels have closed the iridocorneal angle and the eye presents ocular hypertension, cyclocryotherapy, cyclodiathermy and fistulizing techniques may be useful. However, sometimes cyclocryotherapy actually aggravates the ischemia of the anterior segment.[44]

Resolution of the carotid stenosis is the most favourable prognostic factor for visual acuity in patients with OIS.[38,39,59] Vision is stabilized or improved in a good proportion of patients who undergo endarterectomy,[40,59] amounting to 25% according to a study by Sivalingam.[59]

If the angle is closed in an eye with normal intraocular pressure surgical relief of the carotid obstruction may restore correct perfusion to the ciliary bodies, increasing the production of aqueous humor and sometimes considerably raising the intraocular pressure,[12] while still in some cases causing regression of the rubeosis. The rubeosis may also regress when the long posterior ciliary arteries are occluded by an embolus; in the advanced stages of neovascular glaucoma, the new-formed fibrovascular membranes may sometimes strangle the blood supply to the iris, making it avascular.

References

1 Abedin S, Simmons RJ: Neovascular glaucoma in systemic occlusive vascular disease. Ann Ophthalmol 14: 284, 1982.

2 Benson WE, Brown GC, Tasman WS: Diabetes and its ocular complications. WB Saunders, Philadelphia, 1988.

3 Bosley TM: The role of carotid noninvasive tests in stroke prevention. Semin Neurol 6: 194, 1986.

4 Brancato R, Menchini U: Microchirurgia laser in oftalmologia. Ghedini Ed, Milano, 1989.

5 Brown GC: Central retinal vein obstruction: diagnosis and management. In: Reinecke RD: Ophthalmology Annual. Appleton-Century-Crofts, Norwalk, 1985.

6 Brown GC: Anterior ischemic optic neuropathy occurring in association with carotid artery obstruction. J Clin Neuro Ophthalmol 6: 39, 1986.

7 Brown GC: Macular edema in association with severe carotid artery obstruction. Am J Ophthalmol 102: 442, 1986.

8 Brown GC, Magargal LE: The ocular ischemic syndrome: Clinical, fluorescein angiographic and carotid angiographic features. Int Ophthalmol 11: 239, 1988.

9 Brown GC, Magargal LE, Schachat A et al: Neovascular glaucoma. Etiologic considerations. Ophthalmology 91: 315, 1984.

10 Brown GC, Shah HG, Magargal LE et al: Central retinal vein obstruction and carotid artery disease. Ophthalmology 91: 1627, 1984.

11 Brown GC, Magargal LE, Simeone FA et al: Arterial obstruction and ocular neovascularization. Ophthalmology 89: 139, 1982.

12 Bullock JD, Falter RT, Downing JE et al: Ischemic ophthalmia secondary to an ophthalmic artery occlusion. Am J Ophthalmol 74: 486, 1972.

13 Campo RV, Reeser FH: Retinal teleangectasia secondary to bilateral carotid artery occlusion. Arch Ophthalmol 101: 1211, 1983.

14 Carter JE: Panretinal photocoagulation for progressive ocular neovascularization secondary to occlusion of the common carotid artery. Ann Ophthalmol 16: 572, 1984.

15 Coppeto JR, Wand M, Bear L et al: Neovascular glaucoma and carotid artery obstructive disease. Am J Ophthalmol 99: 567, 1985.

16 Cowan CL Jr, Butler G: Ischemic oculopathy. Ann Ophthalmol 12: 1502, 1983.

17 Detry M, Waterschoot MP, Kevers L et al: Neovascular glaucoma secondary to carotid thrombosis. Bull Soc Belge Ophtalmol 199-200: 55, 1982.

18 Donnan GA, Sharbrough FW, Whisnant JP: Carotid occlusive disease. Effect of bright light on visual evoked response. Arch Neurol 39: 687, 1982.

19 Eggleston TF, Bohling CA, Eggleston HC et al: Photocoagulation for ocular ischemia associated with carotid artery occlusion. Ann Ophthalmol 12: 84, 1980.

20 Fantin J, Grandon M: A case of neovascular glaucoma caused by carotid artery occlusion. Bull Soc Ophtalmol Fr 82: 1079, 1982.

21 Furlan AJ, Whisnant JP, Kearns TP: Unilateral visual loss in bright light. An unusual symptom of carotid artery occlusive disease. Arch Neurol 36: 675, 1979.

22 Gartner S, Henkind P: Neovascularization of the iris (Rubeosis iridis). Surv Ophthalmol 22: 291, 1978.

23 Gordon N: Ocular manifestations of internal carotid artery occlusions. Br J Ophthalmol 43: 257, 1959.

24 Green WR, Chan CC, Hutchins GM et al: Central retinal vein occlusion: a prospective histopathologic study of 29 eyes in 28 cases. Retina 1: 27, 1981.

25 Hauch TL, Busuttil RW, Yoshizumi MO: A report of iris neovascularization: an indication for carotid endoarterectomy. Surgery 95: 358, 1984.

26 Hayreh SS: So-called "central retinal vein occlusion". II. Venous stasis retinophaty. Ophthalmologica 172: 14, 1976.

27 Hayreh SS, Podhajsky P: Ocular neovascularization with retinal vascular occlusion. II. Occurrence in cen-

tral and branch retinal artery occlusion. Arch Ophthalmol 100: 1585, 1982.

28 Hedges TR Jr: Ophthalmoscopic findings in internal carotid artery occlusion. Am J Ophthalmol 55: 1007, 1963.

29 Henkind P, Chambers JK: Arterial occlusive disease of the retina. In: Duane TD, Jaeger EA: Clinical Ophthalmology. Harper & Row, Philadelphia, 1985.

30 Higgings RA: Neovascular glaucoma associated with ocular hypoperfusion secondary to carotid artery disease. Aust J Ophthalmol 12: 155, 1984.

31 Hollenhorst RW: Ocular manifestation of insufficiency or thrombosis of the internal carotid artery. Am J Ophthalmol 47: 753, 1979.

32 Huckman MS, Haas J: Reversed flow through the ophthalmic artery as a cause of rubeosis iridis. Am J Ophthalmol 74: 1094, 1972.

33 Jacobs NA, Ridgway AEA: Syndrome of ischaemic ocular inflammation: six cases and a review. Br J Ophthalmol 69: 681, 1985.

34 Kahn M, Green WR, Knox DL et al: Ocular features of carotid occlusive disease. Retina 6: 239, 1986.

35 Kearns TP: Ophthalmology and the carotid artery. Am J Ophthalmol 88: 714, 1979.

36 Kearns TP: Differential diagnosis of central retinal vein obstruction. Ophthalmology 90: 475, 1983.

37 Kearns TP, Hollenhorst RW: Venous-stasis retinopathy of occlusion disease of the carotid artery. Mayo Clin Proc 38: 304, 1963.

38 Kearns TP, Siekert RG, Sundt TM Jr: The ocular aspects of bypass surgery of the carotid artery. Mayo Clin Proc 54: 3, 1979.

39 Kearns TP, Younge BR, Peipgras DG: Resolution of venous stasis retinopathy after carotid artery bypass surgery. Mayo Clin Proc 55: 342, 1980.

40 Kiser WD, Gonder J, Magargal LE et al: Recovery of vision following treatment of the ocular ischemic syndrome. Ann Ophthalmol 15: 305, 1983.

41 Knox DL: Ischemic ocular inflammation. Am J Ophthalmol 60: 995, 1965.

42 Kobayashi S, Hollenhorst RW, Sundt TM Jr: Retinal arterial pressure before and after surgery for carotid artery stenosis. Stroke 2: 569, 1971.

43 Kottow MH: Anterior segment fluorescein angiography. Williams & Wilkins, Baltimore, 1978.

44 Krupin T, Mitchell KB, Becker B: Cyclocryotherapy in neovascular glaucoma. Am J Ophthalmol 86: 24, 1978.

45 Lodato G, Brancato G: Neovascular glaucoma caused by branch vein occlusion and deficiency of carotid-encephalic circulation: pathogenetic correlation. J Fr Ophtalmol 7: 615, 1984.

46 Madsen PH: Venous-stasis retinopathy insufficiency of the ophthalmic artery. Acta Ophthalmol 44: 940, 1966.

47 Magargal LE, Sanborn GE, Zimmerman A: Venous stasis retinopathy associated with embolic obstruction of the central retinal artery. J Clin Neuro Ophthalmol 2: 113, 1982.

48 Mc Crary JA: Venous stasis retinopathy of stenotic or occlusive carotid origin. J Clin Neuro Ophthalmol 9: 195, 1989.

49 Michelson PE, Knox DL, Green WR: Ischemic ocular inflammation: a clinicopathologic case report. Arch Ophthalmol 86: 274, 1971.

50 Michaelson IC: The mode of development of the vascular system of the retina. Trans Ophthalmol Soc UK 68: 137, 1948.

51 Pece A, Menchini U, Chiesa R et al: Neovascular glaucoma and carotid artery obstructive disease: a case report. Ital J Ophthalmol 2: 135, 1988.

52 Pece A, Chiesa R, Minicucci F et al: Aspetti clinici in pazienti affetti da stenosi carotidea sottoposti ad intervento chirurgico. Atti 68 Congresso Società Oftalmologica Italiana, Roma, 1988. Verduci Ed, Roma, 1988.

53 Ridley M, Walker P, Keller A et al: Ocular perfusion in carotid artery disease. Poster presentation, American Academy of Ophthalmology, New Orleans, 1986.

54 Rosenberg PR, Walsh JB, Zimmerman RD: Neovascular glaucoma and carotid bruits. J Clin Neurophthalmol 4: 59, 1984.

55 Sanbor GE, Magargal LE: Carotid artery disease and the eye. In: Duane TD, Jaeger EA: Clinical Ophthalmology. Harper & Row, Philadelphia, 1985.

56 Savino PJ, Glaser JS, Cassady J: Retinal stroke: is the patient at risk? Arch Ophthalmol 95: 1185, 1977.

57 Shaw HE, Holmes MW, Fleisher AS: Regression of ischemic oculopathy after carotid artery by-pass surgery. In: Smith JL: Neuro-ophthalmology focus 1981. Masson, New York, 1981.

58 Sheng FC, Quinones-Baldrich W, Macleder HI et al: Relationship of extracranial carotid occlusive disease and central retinal artery occlusion. Am J Surgery 152: 175, 1986.

59 Sivalingam A, Brown GC, Magargal LE: The ocular ischemic syndrome. III. Visual prognosis and the effect of treatment. Int Ophthalmol 15: 15, 1991.

60 Sivalingam A, Brown GC, Magargal LE et al: The ocular ischemic syndrome. II. Mortality and systemic morbidity. Int Ophthalmol 13: 187, 1989.

61 Smith JL: Unilateral glaucoma in carotid occlusive disease. JAMA 182: 683, 1962.

62 Stefansson E, Coin JT, Lewis WR et al: Central retinal artery occlusion during cardiac catheterization. Am J Ophthalmol 99: 586, 1985.

63 Sturrock GD, Mueller HR: Chronic ocular ischaemia. Br J Ophthalmol 68: 716, 1984.

64 Swan KC, Raaf J: Changes in the eye and orbit following carotid ligation. Trans Am Ophthalmol Soc 49: 435, 1951.

65 Walsh JB: Cardiovascular disorders. In: Duane TD, Jaeger EA: Clinical Ophthalmology. Harper & Row, Philadelphia, 1985.

66 Weiss DI: Vascular insufficiency (neovascular) glaucoma. An integrating pathogenic concept. Trans Ophthalmol Soc UK 97: 280, 1977.

67 Wise GN, Dollery CT, Henkind P: The retinal circulation. Harper & Row, New York, 1971.

68 Young LHY, Appen RE: Ischemic oculopathy: a manifestation of carotid artery disease. Arch Neurol 38: 358, 1981.

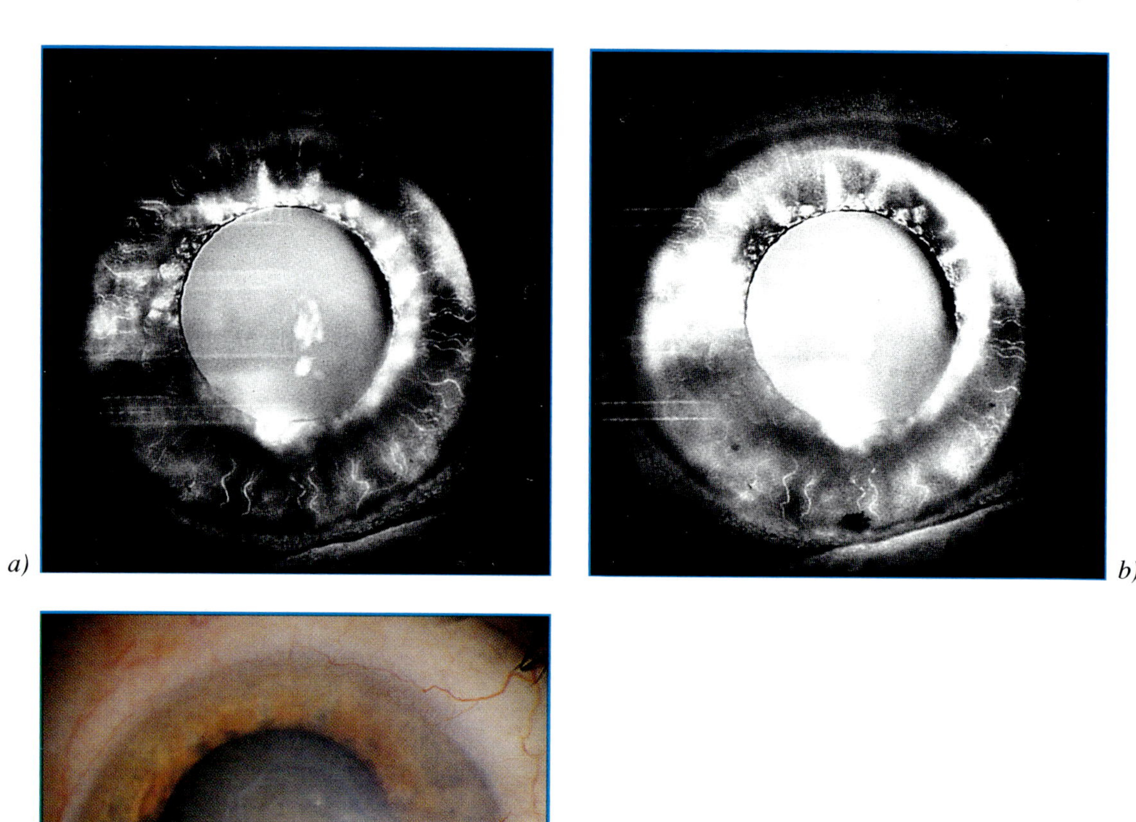

a) b)

c)

*Fig. **4.6**,1 - Rubeosis iridis in a case of ocular ischemic syndrome: a) early and b) late angiographic phases. Two years later the eye developed neovascular glaucoma with corneal edema (c: biomicroscopic picture).*

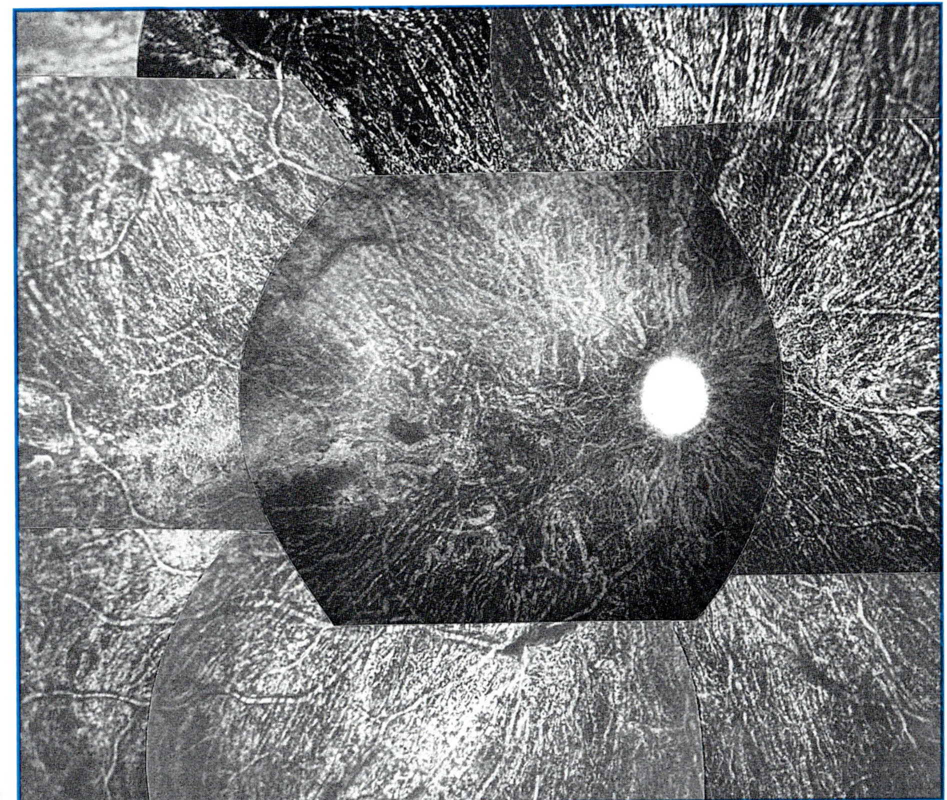

a)

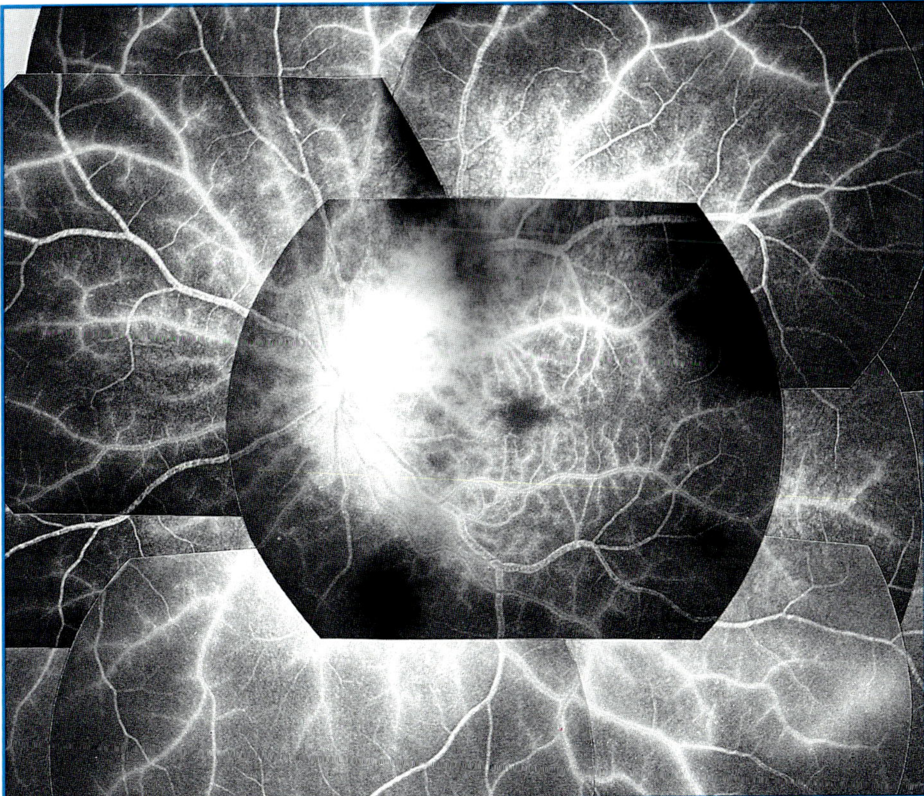

b)

Fig. ***4.6****,2 - Bilateral panretinal fluorescein angiography in a case of Takayasu's disease. In the right eye (a) the vessels are obliterated from narrowing of the common carotid and vertebral arteries, resulting in ischemia of retinal tissues; the absence of retinal pigment epithelium means the choroidal vasculature can be visualized. In the left eye (b) angiography shows widespread retinal capillary non-perfusion and the vessels show marked perivascular leakage (late phase).*

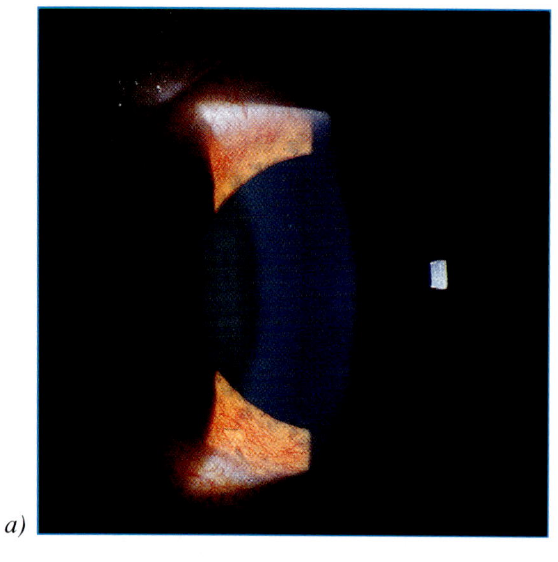
a)

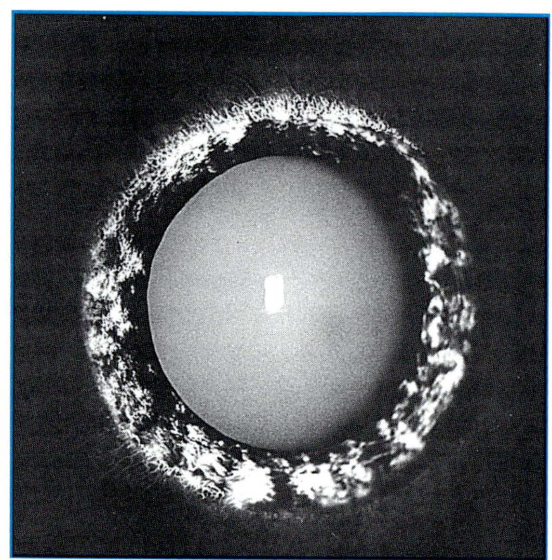
b)

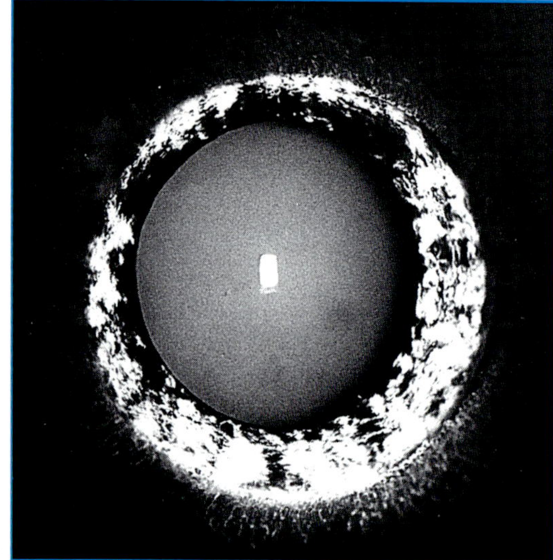
c)

Fig. ***4.6****,3 - Same case as figure* ***4.6****,2: a) biomicroscopy of the right eye with neovascular glaucoma; b,c) fluoroiridographic phases in the left eye, showing new vessels over the whole iris surface. The non-perfused retinal areas of this eye must be laser photocoagulated in order to avoid the onset of neovascular glaucoma.*

R. Brancato, F. Bandello, R. Lattanzio
Atlas of Iris
Fluorescein Angiography
Kugler & Ghedini Publications 1995

Chapter 4.7

Uveitis

Although the iris, ciliary body and choroid may become inflamed separately, on close clinical examination the whole uveal tract is usually found to be involved, reflecting the physiopathological unity of the uveal membrane.

Uveitis can be classified according to various criteria.

Depending on how the condition arises and how long it lasts it may be considered *acute*, *chronic* or *recurrent*.

Again, according to the anatomo-pathological picture, it may be divided into *granulomatous* and *non-granulomatous* forms.

An etiological basis may alternatively be used for classification, although this is often difficult as the causes of the disease may be questionable or - more frequently - simply not known. However, etiological classifications distinguish between *endogenous* and *exogenous* forms. The first group comprises all uveitis related to individual disorders, mostly immunological problems. Exogenous uveitis, on the other hand, may arise from various causes: all sources of infection may lead to uveal inflammation - bacteria (Mycobacterium tuberculosis, Leptospira, Brucella, Mycobacterium leprae, etc.), viruses (Cytomegalovirus, Herpes simplex or zoster, HIV, etc.), fungi (Aspergillus, Candida, etc.), parasites (Toxoplasma, Toxocara canis, Toxocara catis, Histoplasma, Onchocerca volvulus, etc.).

Post-surgical uveitis is a case apart, meaning uveal reactions following surgical manipulation of the globe itself. This category groups bacterial, fungal or anaerobic endophthalmitis, phacogenic or phacoanaphylactic uveitis, Irvine-Gass syndrome, and inflammation induced by intraocular lenses or laser treatments.

The most widely used criteria for classifying uveitis follow the anatomical-topographic system set down by the International Uveitis Study Group (IUSG),[11] which makes the following distinctions:
a) *anterior uveitis* (iritis, anterior cyclitis, irido-cyclitis);
b) *intermediate uveitis* (pars planitis, posterior cyclitis, hyalitis, basal retinochoroiditis);
c) *posterior uveitis* (focal, multifocal and diffuse choroiditis, chorioretinitis, retinochoroiditis, neuro-uveitis, uveopapillitis);
d) *panuveitis* and *endophthalmitis*.

Retinal vasculitis is a separate heading, grouping clinical situations in which the primary lesion is inflammation of the retinal vessels.

Anterior uveitis

Anterior uveitis is the most frequently encountered form and can be divided on the basis of the anatomical features into *iritis, cyclitis* or *irido-cyclitis*.

In the past a distinction was also made between granulomatous or non-granulomatous forms, depending on the anatomo-pathological appearance.

Nowadays, however, they are preferably classified on the basis of genetic typing, as *HLA-B27 positive* or *negative* forms. This histocompatibility antigen is present in a significant proportion of adults with anterior uveitis[50,111] (47% according to Wakenfield[190]). The HLA-B27 antigen has been found in patients with acute and chronic iridocyclitis but not those with chronic cyclitis.[136,137]

Many of the patients with this antigen - though not all - also have a systemic disease known to be closely related to the HLA antigens, etiologically related to ocular inflammation. Mostly these are cases with ankylosing spondylitis; a good percentage, however, has Reiter's syndrome.

Under a separate heading come the *enterogenic* forms such as uveitis occurring with ulcerative colitis or Crohn's disease. There are also various types of uveitis associated with HLA histocompatibility antigens other than the B27 series, such as HLA A29, typical of Birdshot-type chorioretinopathy, and HLA B5 (B51), found in Behçet's disease.

In other cases various types of joint diseases may be associated; these subjects are generally not marked by particular HLA antigens but do have high levels of circulating antinuclear autoantibodies. Often they are young, or males with acute anterior uveitis and juvenile rheumatoid arthritis, or else females with chronic anterior uveitis and juvenile rheumatoid arthritis.[87,127] It thus appears that the population with anterior uveitis is genetically distinct, and predisposed to the disease.[91]

Various causal factors may be involved in *exogenous* anterior uveitis, including toxoplasmosis - generally causing choroiditis; the various forms of syphilitic iritis (roseata, papulosa, nodosa) generally secondary,[7] which may give rise to iris masses[117] or iridoschisis;[147] tubercular iris granulomas; atrophic areas in the iris resulting from certain parasitic infections, leprosy or ophthalmic Herpes zoster.[113]

Retinal vasculitic conditions, such as in Behçet's syndrome, may also be complicated by iridocyclitis, generally not the granulomatous form, and sometimes hypopyon may arise. Chronic nodular iridocyclitis is more common in patients with sarcoidosis.

In some cases of anterior uveitis it is virtually impossible to identify the causal factor. Such *idiopathic* forms may account for 38-52% of all cases of anterior uveitis.[164,190,191] Rothova found that 12.5% of patients with anterior uveitis of unknown etiology had diabetes mellitus, but it was not clear whether these were cases of true inflammation or the expression of ischemic damage to the iris and ciliary body.[164]

Etiological diagnosis of anterior uveitis can thus be problematic and must therefore be based on immuno-histochemical investigations or tests specific for each type of pathology or infection that might be involved.

The pathogenesis of anterior uveitis is also still far from clear. Endogenous inflammatory mediators[165] may take two forms: humoral or tissue factors. Plasma factors include immune complexes that are filtered by the ciliary body and may deposit in the anterior uvea, causing local damage by activating complement. Tissue factors include in particular the prostaglandins, referred to in this context as "irins" on account of their having been isolated experimentally in the iris. These are ubiquitous fatty acids that have been found in larger-than-normal amounts in the aqueous humor of rabbits with anterior uveitis.[3,4] The irins are either released or synthesized ex novo - particularly in the iris - in response to tissue damage.[9]

With an eye to casting light on the nature of these inflammatory mediators, experimental uveitis models have been set up with high prostaglandin levels in the aqueous humor; and the degree of rupture of the blood-iris barrier has been investigated by iris fluorescein angiography.[29,30,84,85,122,148-150,152,153,163,185,195] The results, however, cannot be directly extrapolated to humans on account of the different anatomical features of the human vascular endothelium compared to other species.

Anterior uveitis is generally diagnosed clinically, on the basis of biomicroscopically detectable inflammation in the anterior segment. The main signs are endothelial precipitates and Tyndall's phenomenon. The characteristics of the precipitates - colour, shape, size and site - and of the Tyndall's phenomenon - the flare may be caused by cells or protein - indicate how acute the disease is (Fig. **4.7**,1).

True involvement of the iris may be difficult to establish when inflammation is only mild. There may be vascular engorgement, which used to be referred to as iris hyperemia, and more advanced cases may present petechiae (Fig. **4.7**,2). In the acute phase of the disease vascular dilatation and increased permeability secondary to inflammation cause edema: the iris acts like a wet sponge and its pattern may be blurred. It is not frequent in anterior uveitis, especially in the acute phase, to see iris new vessels with the biomicroscope.

Many patients with anterior uveitis develop cataract on account of the inflammation or the therapy. Other findings reported in anterior uveitis include alterations to the shape, size and dynamics of the pupilla (Figs. **4.7**,3,4). Adhesions may form between the posterior surface of the iris and the anterior capsule of the lens (posterior synechiae). As they become organized these tend to become permanent and may even cut off or occlude the pupil (Fig. **4.7**,5).

Peripheral anterior synechiae between the iris and cornea, at the level of the trabecular meshwork, may close the angle and - especially in chronic iridocyclitis - may give rise to secondary glaucoma, sometimes resulting in serious visual impairment.[16,17] Ocular hypertension may also be caused by pupillary block. In cases of subacute and chronic inflammation, Koëppe nodules may be seen at the pupillary border, with Busacca nodules corresponding to accumulations of epithelioid cells or lymphocytes on the anterior surface of the iris (Fig. **4.7**,6).

Histochemical examination of eyes with anterior uveitis shows not only T-lymphocyte infiltration but also fibronectin, fibrinogen, and immunoglobulins. All these factors help explain the heavy risk of severe inflammatory complications following surgery on eyes with anything other than quiescent uveitis.[131]

Biomicroscopic examination of the signs described forms the basis for diagnosis of anterior uveitis but does not give any information on its etiology. A reliable morphological diagnosis of the type of iridocyclitis can only be made for Fuchs' heterochromic cyclitis. This form presents certain features that make it a clinically distinct condition - only one eye is affected, the heterochromia, absence of synechiae, shape and arrangement of the endothelial precipitates. This condition is therefore dealt with separately.

Iris fluorescein angiographic findings in anterior uveitis

The pathological findings in anterior uveitis described so far are all biomicroscopic. Inflammatory alterations to the anterior uveal tract can in fact be detected perfectly well by this examination. However, initial impairment of the permeability of iris vessels cannot be detected clinically, except indirectly through the finding of Tyndall's phenomenon, which is not always straightforward.

Fluorescein angiography does detect minimal alterations to the permeability of iris vessels, permitting an objective assessment of the degree of rupture of the blood-iris barrier which is always disrupted to some extent in uveitis. The pattern of rupture of the blood-iris barrier provides a map of the uveitis.

Clinical and fluorescein angiographic findings do not always agree. Biomicroscopy in some cases of uveitis shows only mild or extremely localized disease, whereas fluorescein angiography indicates larger-scale problems. The literature offers no comparisons of the sensitivity of fluorescein angiography and clinical investigation in showing up inflammation.

Current knowledge is too limited to enable us to suggest a fluorescein angiographic classification of anterior uveitis that would distinguish the various different forms. It is therefore difficult to summarize the findings reported for anterior uveitis as each published study employed a different basis for classification, or described specific aspects in different forms of uveitis. However, when inflammation is still mild, the main fluorescein angiographic sign is dye leakage from the normal iris vessels, indicative of rupture of the blood-iris barrier. The resulting fluorescence, caused by the abnormal permeability of the endothelium of the iris vessels, may vary in extent. It tends to become more marked in later angiographic phases, until the whole stroma is involved, then spreads to the aqueous and the entire anterior chamber. When it is very marked, it may in later phases of the examination mask the intravascular fluorescence of the iris, making it difficult to see its radial structures. Leakage may be circumscribed, generally first involving the vessels of the pars pupillaris, or diffuse - involving the whole surface of the iris. The spatial distribution of the fluorescence depends on the severity of the inflammation. In severe cases it spreads out to the whole surface of the iris (Figs. **4.7**,7-14). All the inflamed iris vessels however show early, simultaneous fluorescence (Fig. **4.7**,15).[(111)]

Kottow defined anterior uveitis with these iris fluorescein angiographic features as exudative.[(100)] He found that leakage in such cases was more often diffuse, sometimes so marked and prompt that it was not possible to distinguish whether it originated from the posterior chamber and reached the anterior chamber through the pupillary foramen. Generally, however, dye leakage starts from the iris vessels. The ciliary bodies allow only a small amount through, if any.

The dye leakage described here is generally a reversible lesion detected by fluorescein angiography, characteristic of acute forms of anterior uveitis. This leakage tends to diminish as the acute phase regresses although in some cases small fluorescent spots persist around the pupillary border.[(40, 41)] Months after the inflammatory episode, if the condition has not become chronic and there have been no flare-ups, radial and pupillary vessels show normal permeability (Fig. **4.7**,16). Irido-lenticular synechiae may persist, with fibrin clumps, signs of shifting of the iris pigment with dispersion in the anterior chamber, and deposits on the anterior surface of the lens (Figs. **4.7**,17-21).

Iris new vessels are found very rarely during or after acute anterior uveitis since the time and stimulus needed for formation of the neovascular growth factor are lacking.[(40, 41)] More frequent in acute and exudative anterior uveitis are abnormalities of the caliber and path of the iris vessels which appear dilated and sometimes tortuous (Fig. **4.7**,22). Kottow described a denser vascular network, more fluorescent than normal vessels, with dye leakage from small neovascular loops; which with time could gradually develop into rubeosis iridis (Figs. **4.7**,23,24).[(100)]

Hyperfluorescent buds easily mistaken for real neovascular formations are found when anterior uveitis is severe, recurrent or chronic. When inflammation persists for months or years, new vessels do form, their particular features differing with the severity and duration of the disease (Figs. **4.7**,25-28).

The iris fluorescein angiographic findings of new iris vessels in anterior uveitis have been described by Demeler and Laatikainen.[(41,101)] Table **4.7**,I summarizes these findings according to Demeler.[(41)]

Tab. 4.7,I: Angiographic classification of iris new vessels depending on the time and severity of the inflammatory process[41]	
Iris abnormalities	**Inflammatory processes**
1) Small loops, mostly arising near the circolus arteriosus iridis minor, always permeable to fluorescein because of the fenestrate structure of their walls; in the later phases there is diffuse dye leakage into the surrounding iris stroma.	*Chronic uveitis present for months or several years, never in severe acute uveitis; these new vessels develop through a very low-grade growth-stimulating factor by a chronic slowly-burning inflammatory process, not interrupted by severe attacks.*
2) Sprouts arising around the pupillary margin, later being irregularly disseminated over the surface of the iris and finally developing in the chamber-angle leading to closed-angle glaucoma; the typical angiographic pattern of these sprouts is similar to that of brushes or brooms, and they are permeable to fluorescein.	*Severe inflammation and within a very short time (4-6 months); perhaps a very strong growth-stimulating factor leads to this form of neovascularization.*
3) New vessels produced by an actual bifurcation of the original vessels.	*This type of neovascularization would be the consequence of a very low grade stimulating factor present over a long period of time, i.e. 10 years or more.*

Laatikainen[101] described the iris fluorescein angiographic findings of new vessels formed in chronic advanced cases of anterior uveitis as a uniform coarse vascular network covering the whole surface of the iris, giving rise to more profuse leakage in more active disease (Figs. **4.7**,29-32). This network is even present at the angle, though not detectable in the angiogram, in the form of fibrovascular synechiae. The author suggests that this network is different from the arborizing type of neovascularization usually seen in vascular eye diseases such as diabetes mellitus and central retinal vein occlusion, where the new vessels generally originate from the angle and show no tendency to involve the mid-stroma in an early stage. Laatikainen sustains that in vascular diseases the stimulus for the formation of new vessels is more intense, the pathological processes is usually more acute and affects the metabolism of the iris tissue more than in chronic inflammation. Thus in diabetes, for example, or ischemic central retinal vein occlusion, rubeosis iridis may be frequent, varying in degree but always easily detected with the biomicroscope.

In anterior uveitis it is the fibrous component that predominates over neovascular formation and the vascular pattern, according to Laatikainen, resembles the iris fluorescein angiographic anomalies found in chronic capsular glaucoma.[187]

The same investigator described a case of chronic anterior uveitis with clinically detectable rubeosis iridis where, however, some of the leaking vessels were assumed to be probably dilated capillaries rather than newly formed vessels.

Other fluorescein angiographic anomalies described in chronic anterior uveitis complicated by intraocular hypertension include areas of iris hypoperfusion associated with neovascular microalterations,[16,17] or areas of iris atrophy with the iris vascular structure visible (Figs. **4.7**,33,34).[101] Neovascularization of the iris has been described in numerous forms of uveitis including, endophthalmitis,[60] sympathetic ophthalmia,[60] Vogt-Koyanagi syndrome and Eales vasculitis.[12]

Fluorescein angiographic findings in *granulomatous anterior uveitis* merit a separate description. Dye leakage in such cases is marked and diffuse from the radial vessels of the iris and from peripupillary capillaries. Nodules and granulomas may take up fluorescence, their vessels giving a pattern like the "spokes of a wheel", the staining being due to increased extravascular diffusion. In the late phases of the examination leakage is diffuse.[100]

A large iris granuloma may simulate a tumour or cyst but iris fluorescein angiography differentiates it because of the marked effects on the rest of the iris, not affected by the growth.[100] Diagnosis is further aided by the frequent bilateral finding and the multiple lesions in uveitis. The inflammatory nature of the lesion is confirmed by the fact that it becomes smaller in response to steroid therapy.[133]

In granulomatous anterior uveitis the pattern and path of the radial vessels is abnormal in the angiogram: the more tortuous and dilated they are, the more they will leak dye. Filling may be irregular, with perfusion defects. In other areas the capillary network may appear richer than normal, and is generally permeable to the dye. The granuloma may give rise to the formation of secondary cysts.

In other granulomatous forms of uveitis the iris fluorescein angiographic findings are generally similar to those in iridocyclitis with sarcoidosis. Anterior uveitis is one of the ocular manifestations, and is generally bilateral and granulomatous in these cases.[83,134] Monophasic, recurrent and chronic forms are known. The uveitis may occasionally present acutely, but more frequently its onset is insidious, with no or very few subjective symptoms. Iris nodules are characteristic, although they are only found in 11% of subjects with sarcoidosis.[134] They may be found anywhere on the surface of the iris, but most are usually around the pupillary border (Fig. **4.7**,35).

Iris fluorescein angiography shows up nodules even deep in the stroma, so this examination will find more lesions than simple biomicroscopy.

Nodules present a less specific angiographic pattern than in other forms of uveitis, varying in relation to the stage of the disease.[90] In the active stage nodules are "fresh", presenting slight diffuse hyperfluorescence, and surrounded by dilated iris vessels. In late angiographic phases fluorescence is marked over the whole area. Older granulomas are covered or surrounded by a dense network of new vessels, tortuous, irregular and superficial, giving rise to marked dye leakage in the acute phases of the disease. At the end of acute attacks, or between recurrent episodes of uveitis, leakage tends to diminish but the neovascular network persists. Nodules may be visible for years, or may disappear, leaving avascular areas behind them. Exacerbation is marked by intense leakage from old lesions and by new areas of diffusion from fresh nodules.

In highly developed forms small areas of neovascularization or a fibrovascular membrane can be seen covering the whole surface of the iris. Anterior and posterior synechiae may form, and secondary glaucoma may be determined.[16,17]

Generally, the absence of marked leakage from radial vessels agrees with the proliferative nature of iritis due to sarcoidosis, and with the minimal symptomatology observed.[90] Karma,[88,89] however, described cases of panuveitis in sarcoidosis with exudative fibrous features, that led subsequently to bulbar phthisis.

Fuchs' heterochromic iridocyclitis

This disease, first described in 1906 by Fuchs,[57] involves certain clinical aspects that set it apart from the other forms of anterior uveitis. The most characteristic finding is the heterochromia of the iris. Iridocyclitis is unilateral (in the lighter eye), chronic, and involves a tendency to cataract formation (typically beneath the posterior cup), sometimes with intraocular hypertension. The iris tissue appears rarefied, losing density and detail, and is transparent to trans-illumination (*moth-eaten* appearance [158]).

Electron microscope findings include focal areas of depigmentation with degenerative processes in the pigment epithelium; atrophy and fibrosis of the stroma; loss of stromal melanocytes; inflammatory infiltrates; endothelial proliferation and hyalinization causing thickening of the walls and narrowing the caliber of the vessels.[45,67,95,108,118,119,127,128,143,154,189,197]

Iris new vessels have been detected histologically and clinically;[8,154] these may cause hemorrhage in the anterior chamber and in some cases lead to neovascular glaucoma. New vessels have also been seen at the angle and might explain the filiform hemorrhages described after paracentesis in patients with Fuchs' iridocyclitis.[5] However, it has also been suggested that these are not new vessels, but normal iris vessels that become visible on account of the pigment loss.

Peripheral anterior synechiae are a fairly frequent finding.[154] It is not clear whether the occasional intraocular hypertension is secondary to inflammation or caused by the new vessels.[154]

The pathogenesis of this disease is still not understood. Fuchs suggested it was due to vascular insufficiency in the uveal tract.[57] Subsequently the frequent association with chorioretinal scars was noted, comparable to those seen in toxoplasmosis, which led to the theory that iridocyclitis might be a secondary manifestation.[67]

Iridocyclitis is currently believed to be due to an immune dysfunction,[8,42,43,86,166-168] probably involving the humoral component[126,128] which leads to occlusion of the iris vessels. Inflammatory lymphocyte and plasma cell infiltrates have in fact been found in the iris, with reduced suppressor T-cell activity in peripheral blood.[45,67,95,96,108,118,119,127,128,143,154,189,197]

Iris fluorescein angiography showed altered permeability of the blood-iris barrier, resulting in leakage from radial vessels, varying in extent depending on the stage and severity of the disease (Figs. **4.7**,36-40).[8,166-168]

Dye leakage is more frequent in the mid-peripheral parts of the iris.[199-200] There is generally a crown of small fluorescent dots around the pupillary plexus, merging into a ring in the later phases of the examination.[13] Leakage, however, is generally limited, and less marked than in other forms of iridocyclitis.[100]

Typical of Fuchs' iridocyclitis is the slowing of the circulation, leading to perfusion delays and defects (Figs. **4.7**,41,42); these sometimes indicate focal ischemia of the iris in the areas where vascular anomalies show up - described histologically - which are the cause of the iris atrophy in Fuchs' iridocyclitis.[8,166-168] In some cases retrograde filling is seen in the non-perfused areas, starting from adjacent vessels.[8] Iris fluorescein angiography often shows upheaval of the radial vascular structure, with abnormalities of the vessels caliber, path and permeability (Figs. **4.7**,43,44).

In less advanced cases, especially those not complicated by intraocular hypertension, new iris vessels are rare;[13] they are more likely to show up in eyes with angiographically documented iris ischemia.[166-168]

Cases with intraocular hypertension have been reported to present a diffuse veil of transpupillary fluorescence coming from the posterior chamber.[13] This might be due to hyperfunction or altered permeability of the ciliary body, either primary or secondary to the intraocular hypertension. New vessels have never been reported in the contralateral eye; in rare cases some dye leakage may be seen at the pupillary border.[167]

Posner-Schlossman syndrome

In this syndrome, which is a cyclitic-glaucomatous attack, the glaucoma is associated with inflammation confined to the trabecular region.[133] During the acute episodes fine deposits are detectable on the corneal endothelium; sudden ocular hypertension may occur because of reduced out-flow of aqueous humor, and the pupil reacts but midriasis persists. Some time after the attack, permeability of the iris vessels is altered, there are areas where the iris pigment is shifted, and circumscribed zones of atrophy (Figs. **4.7**,45-47).

Intermediate uveitis

These forms of ocular inflammation involve first of all the vitreous and the peripheral retina.[15,73,74,133,171] It is still not clear whether the primary abnormality in intermediate uveitis is the peripheral retinal perivasculitis, or the vitreal inflammation.

Intermediate uveitis amounts to 8% of cases of uveal inflammation;[176] in 70-80% of these cases both eyes are involved, and in one-third of the patients with initially unilateral forms the other eye becomes affected over the years.

Intermediate uveitis does not generally imply a genetic predisposition; no significant associations have been observed with specific HLA haplotypes,[36,194] and familial caselists are rare. This form of uveitis may be seen in patients with intestinal diseases, such as Crohn's disease, ulcerative colitis, Whipple's disease, or demyelinating diseases such as multiple sclerosis. Intermediate uveitis is marked by vitreal and epiretinal peripheral basal exudates (snowballs and snowbanks). These are not real protein exudates and are more probably preretinal fibroglial masses. The other characteristic finding is vitreal infiltration (vitritis), which varies in severity, but may even obscure the retina in very severe cases.

Intermediate uveitis in which there is marked inferior opacity at the pars plana and ora serrata retinae (snowbank), is known as pars planitis;[1] the prognosis for this subgroup is worse, and the vitreal reaction tends to be more marked. Anomalies of the peripheral retinal vessels may give rise even to peripheral neovascularization, leading in some instances to vitreal hemorrhage.[15] Retinal detachment may be induced by contraction of the vitreoretinal membranes.

The anterior segment may present inflammation in some cases; the iris reaction is not usually observed in elderly patients with intermediate uveitis. Younger patients may present Tyndall's phenomenon in the anterior chamber, but never any endothelial deposits. The symptomatology is not usually marked, and the ciliary bodies become involved by contiguity.

Iris fluorescein angiography in intermediate uveitis is thus less useful than in iridocyclitis. Fluorescence secondary to disruption of the blood-iris barrier is rare. A veil of pupillary fluorescence is sometimes noticeable, starting mainly from the posterior chamber, secondary to inflammation of the ciliary bodies; it flows into the anterior chamber through the pupillary foramen.

Posterior uveitis

This heading is taken today to group *choroiditis*, *chorioretinitis*, *retinochoroiditis* and *neurouveitis*. Posterior uveitis may be *focal, multifocal* or *diffuse*.

The most frequent focal form is choroiditis due to Toxoplasma. A differential diagnosis must be made between infections due to Toxocara canis or catis, in which chorioretinal lesions are associated with greater traction, and sometimes with imposing vitreal exudate. Laboratory tests such as ELISA in aqueous humor and serum can clarify the matter. Other situations in which it is easy to make an erroneous diagnosis are syphilitic (rare today) and tubercular granulomatous infections.

There is also a wide range of posterior uveitis forms whose etiology is not known; some of them are now suggested as being due to viruses. Under this heading come the various disorders referred to in clinical practice as multifocal choroiditis,[46] disseminated choroiditis, serpiginous choroiditis, etc. Since it is impossible to classify these forms on any other basis, descriptive criteria are used more for posterior uveitis than for anterior forms. Involvement of the anterior segment may vary in posterior uveitis but when present it is generally marked. As mentioned, toxoplasmosis - and more rarely syphilis and tuberculosis - may all cause iridocyclitis. Multifocal choroiditis is often associated with inflammatory cells in the vitreous, with anterior uveitis or even with panuveitis (Figs. **4.7**,48,49).[46]

Iris fluorescein angiographic findings in posterior uveitis therefore differ, depending on the type of iridocyclitis present (Figs. **4.7**,50-56). Disruption of the blood-iris barrier may differ in extent and severity, and in overt forms dye leakage from iris vessels may be so fast and massive that it is hard to see the radial structure. In some cases the vascular system is so disrupted that a whole anomalous network of neovascular buds may be seen (Figs. **4.7**,57,58).

In posterior uveitis complicated by granulomatous iridocyclitis, iris nodules give different angiographic findings in relation to how long they have been present and how acute the disease is.

Birdshot retinochoroidopathy

Birdshot retinochoroidopathy is an acquired inflammatory disease, normally chronic (with exacerbations and remissions), bilateral, clinically characterized by marked vitreal reaction, anomalies of the retinal vessels, cystoid macular edema and depigmented spots ("multiple, discrete, cream-coloured foci of depigmentation") dotted all over the fundus of the eye (Fig. **4.7**,59).[165] Subretinal neovascularization has been described.[19,133,141,179] The anterior segment is rarely inflamed, or presents only mild inflammation, for example a limited Tyndall phenomenon in the anterior chamber. Iris fluorescein angiography therefore shows up limited dye leakage from iris vessels in some cases, whereas leakage from the pupillary border is more frequent (Figs. **4.7**,60-65).

Sympathetic ophthalmia

This form of granulomatous uveitis appears consequent to a perforating trauma of an eye.[21] Immediately or even some time after a trauma to one eye (the exciting eye) an inflammatory reaction may occur either in that eye of the other one (the sympathizing eye). Eighty percent of cases arise within three months. This is probably an autoimmune reaction.[162]

The condition arises insidiously, is progressive and subject to exacerbations. The reaction may affect the anterior or posterior segment (vitritis, papillitis, macular edema, perivasculitis). Characteristic yellowish-white lesions are seen between the retinal pigment epithelium and Bruch's membrane, tending to become confluent, and corresponding to the Dalen-Fuchs nodules described histologically.[53] Anatomo-pathological findings include diffuse nodular uveal infiltration with lymphocytes and epithelioid cells. A clinical finding of thickening of the iris indicates infiltration.

Although the course of sympathetic ophthalmia may vary, it should always be considered a serious condition. Without adequate treatment it can proceed chronically for 9-12 months, and recurrences are frequent. The introduction of cortisone and immunodepressant therapies has improved the prognosis, but the outcome is always unpredictable.

The iris fluorescein angiographic picture varies with the type and severity (Figs. **4.7**,66,67). This examination is useful for early detection of inflammation in the other eye, and for monitoring the course of the disease and its response to therapy. It is therefore an important auxiliary diagnostic tool, essential when the other eye is known to have suffered traumatic lesions.

Vogt-Koyanagi-Harada syndrome

This form of uveomeningitis is a systemic disorder involving the eyes, ears, skin and meninges. Inflammation of the eyes is generally bilateral from the outset, though in some cases one eye may be affected shortly before the other (Fig. **4.7**,68). The uveitis may involve the posterior or anterior segment, and is generally granulomatous, nodules being found at the pupillary border and iris stroma.

One early finding is a shallow anterior chamber, with a slight increase in intraocular pressure secondary to edematous swelling of the ciliary bodies; on occasion this may have the opposite effect, causing hypotonus. There are some descriptions of new vessels at the angle,[138] though other investigators disagree.[133] The main complication in the anterior segment is the formation of pupillary membranes and cataract.

Iris fluorescein angiographic findings in the Vogt-Koyanagi-Harada syndrome vary in relation to the severity of anterior segment involvement. Dye leakage at the pupillary margin is always seen, sometimes with other, extrapupillary leakage points, indicative of rupture of the blood-iris barrier (Fig. **4.7**,69). Slight hyperfluorescence may be noted in any iris nodules present and in the stroma immediately around them. Histological findings are virtually the same as in sympathetic ophthalmia; once again, the pathogenesis of this syndrome appears to be linked to an immune regulation disorder.[125,135-137,139]

Retinal vasculitis

This heading groups a series of disorders, often idiopathic, in which there is primary inflammation of the retinal vessels. The main objective sign of disease is sheathing of the retinal vessels, with or without other signs of inflammation such as hyalitis, papillitis or, in some instances, anterior uveitis. These retinal vasculitis forms may progress in various ways: they may regress spontaneously or with therapy, with no aftermaths, or they may become recurrent, acute attacks alternating with quiescent periods. Some time after the initial inflammatory episode, hyaline thickening of the vessel wells may be observed, with a narrowing of the lumen, resulting in areas of vascular obliteration and chorioretinal atrophy. The occlusions may affect progressively larger vessels, eventually producing huge ischemic areas in the retina around which new vessels may make their appearance. They may also form around the papilla (Figs. **4.7**,70-72). Alterations to the iris may vary in severity, and neovascular buds may arise here too (Figs. **4.7**,73-77).[14]

Often the retinal manifestations are only one expression of some systemic disorder. Various pathologies may cause vascular retinopathy: Behçet's disease, sarcoidosis, systemic lupus erythematosus, Wegener granulomatosis and polyarteritis nodosa. A certain proportion of cases can only be classified as idiopathic as no cause can be identified and there is no associated systemic pathology. Eales' disease falls into this category.

Behçet's syndrome

This syndrome is diagnosed on the basis of three signs: aphthous oral, genital ulcers and ocular lesions (uveitis). The diagnosis is generally confirmed by the finding of HLA-B51 histocompatibility antigens, detected with statistically significant frequency in this disease.[135]

In Behçet's disease the uveitis may be anterior and posterior; it is bilateral and its onset is explosive, with recurrent acute attacks. The following may be observed simultaneously: episcleritis, keratitis, conjunctivitis, subconjunctival hemorrhage, paralysis of extraocular muscles. Anterior segment involvement is marked, with recurrent iridocyclitis;[203] it is granulomatous and there may be areas of iris atrophy, with hypertonus, neovascularization and - in some cases - neovascular glaucoma. Hypopyon was considered a pathognomonic sign in the past but with the use of antibiotics this has virtually disappeared. Recurrent occlusive retinal vasculitis occurs leading to areas of vascular "amputation", known as capillary drop-out, neovascularization, recurrent vitreal hemorrhage, vitreal contraction and eventually tractional detachment.

Iris fluorescein angiographic findings in Behçet's disease reflect the severity and type of irido-ciliary disorder. Leakage may be found around the pupillary border, and from radial vessels in less serious cases; staining of different degrees and patterns, depending on how acute the disease is, is seen in the iris granulomas visible biomicroscopically; the new vessels at the border and in the stroma show hyperfluorescence. The most severe cases present all the devastating signs of neovascular glaucoma (Figs. **4.7**,78-82).

A fluorescein angiographic study during remission of the disease showed different patterns of leakage; in some cases diffusion started from the posterior chamber, and in other cases from the iris vessels. These different angiographic pictures are related to the different forms this disease may take (with mainly anterior or mainly posterior involvement). Dye leakage, however, is always a sign of persisting vascular damage, regardless of whether the biomicroscopic findings indicate remission.[100]

Eales' disease

This idiopathic condition, probably of autoimmune origin, involves several parts of the retina, and takes the form of occlusive perivasculitis, mainly venous (periphlebitis). The disease usually starts in peripheral vessels, anterior to the equator; vascular obliteration tends then to move gradually into more central zones, affecting larger vessels. Vascular ectasia is followed later by neovascular proliferation forming a characteristic arborizing pattern around the edges of non-perfused areas of the retina (Fig. **4.7**,83). This is the typical picture in the florid stage of the disease, when there may also be endovitreal hemorrhage, secondary retinal detachment, rubeosis iridis and neovascular glaucoma.[14]

Iris fluorescein angiography shows typical findings in Eales' disease complicated by iris neovascularization; hyperfluorescence is seen early at the new vessels, often associated with diffuse leakage from radial vessels, indicative of the disruption of the blood-iris barrier. The angiographic behaviour of the new vessels themselves, however, is not specific, resembling that in other ischemic iridopathies and retinopathies (Fig. **4.7**,84).

Infectious endophthalmitis

These often destructive infectious disorders are caused by pyogenic organisms multiplying inside the eye, giving rise to an inflammatory response that may eventually involve the whole eye - panuveitis.[165]

There are exogenous and endogenous forms of endophthalmitis. Exogenous forms usually follow some form of actual breakage of the globe, such as trauma or surgery. Endophthalmitis of endogenous origin is less frequent and may be the result of microorganisms reaching the eye from other parts of the body. Bacteria, fungi, parasites, virus and other agents may all be causal in endophthalmitis (Figs. **4.7**,85,86).[165-166]

As mentioned, these infections fall into the category of post-surgical uveitis.[109,133] Surgical manipulations of the globe may induce intraocular inflammation, but this alone is not always infectious (Fig **4.7**,87). Patients who already have uveitis may suffer exacerbations after surgery and the reaction may be so severe in some cases as to simulate endophthalmitis. Sometimes it is hard to distinguish an early septic form from a sterile one. Mild inflammation is a common reaction in many patients after cataract extraction, and appears to be mediated by prostaglandins - it is in fact relieved by prostaglandin inhibitors.

Sampling the aqueous and vitreous can be useful as a basis for reliable diagnosis of the type of infection, and for planning specific therapy.[140,157] Iris fluorescein angiography can be useful for assessing the condition of the blood-iris barrier in post-surgical eyes, and for judging the degree of inflammation. Fluorescein angiography should be done before surgery in patients who already have uveitis, so as to verify the indication for surgery (Fig. **4.7**,88). Should the angiogram indicate active uveitis, it is advisable to postpone surgery until angiographic evidence of remission is available, so as to avoid aggravating the condition (see chapter on Surgical Diseases).

Viral diseases

The possibility of a viral etiology of the inflammation is still not clear in many types of uveitis. Viral infection has been demonstrated in certain diseases such as acute retinal necrosis - formerly classified as idiopathic - but not in others, such as the Vogt-Koyanagi-Harada syndrome, whose etiology is still a mystery.

Other diseases currently classified as idiopathic or autoimmune may yet prove to be triggered by a viral infection giving rise to an immune disorder that in turn induces the particular syndrome.[133] There are, however, certain types of eye inflammation known to be caused by a virus. The main forms are described below.

Eye disorders in acquired immune deficiency syndrome (AIDS)

AIDS today is a huge problem, a pandemic extending beyond the limits of any other known in our times. AIDS is the most serious clinical manifestation of infection with human immunodeficiency virus (HIV), of which two types, I and II, have been found so far. AIDS is an enormous challenge for the ophthalmologist who may be the first physician to diagnose the disease since the earliest signs in about 3% of patients involve their eyes. The following main ocular manifestations arise in HIV infection:[35,51,55,56,75-78,82,92,107,112,114,133,151,156,170,172,173,181,188,193]

- retinal microangiopathy with characteristic cotton-wool spots;
- Cytomegalovirus retinitis (the hemorrhagic-edematous and granular forms);
- Toxoplasma, Candida, Treponema, Tuberculosis bacillus, Cryptococcus infections, etc;
- Kaposi's sarcoma of the eyelid or conjunctiva, initially presenting as subconjunctiva-hemorrhage that fails to reabsorb;
- disseminated Herpes zoster of the eyes.

For the time being no iris fluorescein angiographic studies have been published concerning patients with AIDS or other HIV-linked pathologies.

Cytomegalovirus infection

Infection with Cytomegalovirus usually presents as an opportunistic infection in immune-depressed patients.[49,56,133,144,151,173] The infection is often progressive and sometimes destructive. It mainly affects the retina, where there may be two types of clinical sign:[133]

- a perivascular fluffy white lesion with many scattered hemorrhages;
- a more granular-appearing lesion which has few associated hemorrhages and often has a central area of clearing with atrophic retina and stippled retinal pigment epithelium.

Gancyclovir has given satisfactory therapeutic results, but adverse reactions may be heavy (for example serious bone marrow toxicity); these are more marked in immune-deficient subjects, and the drug is incompatible with azidothymidine.[37,78,145]

The iris reaction is visible on iris fluorescein angiography, showing up as a rupture of the blood-iris barrier; this is a constant finding, and is related to the severity of the infection. Tyndall's phenomenon in the anterior chamber may sometimes be conspicuous, making it difficult to distinguish the radial vessels of the iris.

Herpes viral uveitis

Iritis due to Herpes zoster used to be distinguished in two types, exudative and eruptive, but with today's therapeutic options the natural clinical history of the disease has been modified.[42] Iritis may develop early but generally only appears when the skin lesions start to regress. A frequent finding (reported in 74 out of 520 eyes examined by Marsh[113]) is zones of iris atrophy, seen well on trans-illumination. These are circumscribed areas of loss of pigment epithelium; in severe cases, they may become confluent. They are generally triangular, with the base towards the root of the iris. There is not usually stromal damage and sphincter lesion is the cause of the often noted torsion of the iris (Fig. **4.7**,89).

The pathogenic mechanism of the iris atrophy appears to be localized occlusive vasculitis, caused by the virus. This vascular inflammation causes ischemia of the iris, the lesions resembling those of acute glaucoma or necrosis of the anterior segment.

Ischemia has been documented by iris fluorescein angiography, as filling delays or defects in the areas where there is biomicroscopically visible loss of pigment epithelium.[113] In the acute phase of the infection, all iris vessels are markedly dilated with diffuse dye leakage. Some time after the acute stage, small areas of vascular thinning are seen, with filling defects that subsequently develop into whole areas of vascular obliteration. The generalized leakage tends gradually to diminish, and the dilatation only persists in radial vessels at the edges of the areas with loss of pigment epithelium. Sometimes back filling can be seen from neighbouring vessels to the large iris vessels in the atrophic zones. There is almost always leakage around the pupillary border.

Iritis may persist for weeks after the actual infection, not because of viral replication but because of occlusion. Sometimes the ischemia of the iris and ciliary body is so marked that bulbar phthisis may result.[27,69,199]

Herpes simplex infection gives different iris fluorescein angiographic findings: there is no ischemia and no vascular filling defects.[113] Iritis often accompanies herpetic keratitis, a frequent, often recurrent eye infection. In some cases the iritis arises well after the keratitis, but others may suffer repeated episodes of herpetic kerato-uveitis that are highly destructive.

References

1 Aaberg TM: The enigma of pars planitis. Am J Ophthalmol 103: 828, 1987.

2 Abi-Hanna D, Mc Cluskey P, Wakefield D: HLA antigens in the iris and aqueous humor gamma interferon levels in anterior uveitis. Inv Ophthalmol Vis Sci 30: 990, 1989.

3 Ambache N: Irin, a smooth-muscle contracting substance present in rabbit iris. J Phisiol (London) 129: 65, 1955.

4 Ambache N: Properties of irin, a phisiological constituent of the rabbit's iris. J Phisiol (London) 135: 114, 1957.

5 Amsler M, Verrey F: Hétérochromie de Fuchs et fragilité vasculaire. Ophthalmologica 111: 177, 1946.

6 Arffa RC, Schlaegel TF Jr: Chorioretinal scars in Fuchs' heterochromic iridocyclitis. Arch Ophthalmol 102: 1153, 1984.

7 Barthelmess M, Osler S, Volker HE: Iritis and optic nerve meningitis. Initial symptoms of latent syphilis. Klin Monatsbl Augenheilkd 190: 196, 1987.

8 Berger BB, Tessler HH, Kottow MH: Anterior segment ischemia in Fuchs' heterochromic cyclitis. Arch Ophthalmol 98: 499, 1980.

9 Bhattacherjee P: Stimulation of prostaglandin synthetase activity in inflamed ocular tissue of the rabbit. Letter to the editors. Exp Eye Res 24: 215, 1977.

10 Blegvad O: Iridocyclitis and diseases of the joints in children. Acta Ophthalmologica 19: 219, 1941.

11 Bloch-Michel E, Nussenblatt RB: International Uveitis Study Group (I.U.S.G.) reccomendations for the evaluation of intraocular inflammatory diseases. Am J Ophthalmol 103: 234, 1987.

12 Bohringer HR: Sekundarglaukom met Gefässneubildungen auf der iris. Ophthalmologica (Basel) 123: 211, 1952.

13 Brancato R, Frosini R: Aspetti fluoroiridografici della ciclite eterocromica. Ann Ottalmol Clin Ocul 97: 107, 1971.

14 Brancato R, Menchini U, Carnevalini A: Atlante di Iridografia a fluorescenza. C.I.C. Ed Int Gruppo Ed Medico, Roma, 1981.

15 Brockhurst RJ, Schepens CL, Okamura ID: Uveitis II. Peripheral uveitis: clinical description, complications and differential diagnosis. Am J Ophthalmol 49: 1257, 1960.

16 Brooks AM, Gillies WE: Fluorescein angiography of the iris and specular microscopy of the corneal endothelium in some cases of glaucoma secondary to chronic cyclitis. Ophthalmology 95: 1624, 1988.

17 Brooks AM, Grant G, Gillies WE: Changes in the iris vasculature and corneal endothelium in chronic cyclitis. Aust NZ J Ophthalmol 14: 189, 1986.

18 Brown GC, Magargal LE, Schachat A et al: Neovascular glaucoma: etiologic considerations. Ophthalmology 91: 315, 1984.

19 Brucker AJ, Deglin EA, Bene C et al: Subretinal choroidal neovascularization in Birdshot retinochoroidopathy. Am J Ophthalmol 99: 40, 1985.

20 Bryk E: Fluorescein angiography in iritis. Klin Oczna 88: 428, 1986.

21 Chan CC, Benezra D, Hsu SM: Granulomas in sympathetic ophthalmia and sarcoidosis. Immunohistochemical study. Arch Ophthalmol 103: 198, 1985.

22 Chester GH, Black RK, Cleary PE: Inflammation in the region of the vitreous base; pars planitis. Trans Ophthalmol Soc UK 96: 151, 1976.

23 Chignell AH, Easty DL: Iris fluorescein angiography of the globe and anterior segment. Trans Ophthalmol Soc UK 91: 243, 1971.

24 Chylack LT Jr: The ocular manifestations of juvenile rheumatoid arthritis. Arthritis Rheum 20: 217, 1977.

25 Chylack LT Jr, Bienfang DC, Bellows R et al: Ocular manifestations of juvenile rheumatoid arthritis. Am J Ophthalmol 79: 1026, 1975.

26 Cobb B, Smith ME: Fluorescein studies of the iris in pseudoexfoliation of the lens capsula, heterochromic cyclitis and central branch vein occlusion. Acta XXI Concilium Ophthalmologicum, Mexico. Excerpta Medica International Congress Series 222: 953, 1970.

27 Cobo M, Foulks GN, Liesegang T et al: Observations on the natural history of herpes zoster ophthalmicus. Curr Eye Res 6: 195, 1987.

28 Cohen KL, Peiffer RL Jr, Powell DA: Sarcoidosis and ocular disease in a young child. Arch Ophthalmol 99: 422, 1981.

29 Cole DF: The site of breakdown of the blood-aqueous barrier under the influence of vaso-dilatator drugs. Exp Eye Res 19: 591, 1974.

30 Cole DF, Unger WG: Prostaglandins as mediators for the responses of the eye to trauma. Exp Eye Res 17: 357, 1973.

31 Coles RS: Uveitis. In Sorsby A: Modern Ophthalmology. Butter Worths, London, 1964.

32 Crick RP, Hoyle C, Smellie H: The eyes in sarcoidosis. Br J Ophthalmol 45: 461, 1961.

33 Crock J: Clinical syndromes of anterior segment ischaemia. Trans Ophthalmol Soc UK 87: 513, 1967.

34 Cross AG: Uveitis in children. Trans Ophthalmol Soc UK 85: 409, 1965.

35 Croxatto JO, Mestre C, Puente S et al: Nonreactive tuberculosis in a patient with acquired immune deficiency syndrome. Am J Ophthalmol 102: 659, 1986.

36 Culbertson WW, Giles CL, West CW: Familiar pars planitis. Retina 3: 179, 1983.

37 D'Amico DJ, Talamo JH, Felsenstein D et al: Ophthalmoscopic and histologic findings in cytomegalovirus retinitis treated with BW-B759U. Arch Ophthalmol 104: 1788, 1986.

38 Dangel ME, Stark WJ, Michels RG: Surgical management of cataract associated with chronic uveitis. Ophthalmic Surg 14: 145, 1983.

39 De Abreu MT, Belfort R, Hirata PS: Fuchs' heterochromic cyclitis and ocular toxoplasmosis. Am J Ophthalmol 93: 739, 1982.

40 Demeler U: Irisangiographie bei Rubeosis Iridis. Ophthalmologica (Basel) 176: 91, 1978.

41 Demeler U: Value of fluorescein angiography of the iris in uveitis. Trans Ophthalmol Soc UK 101: 380, 1981.

42 Dernouchamps JP, Michiels J: Circulating antigen-antibody complexes in the aqueous humor. In Silverstein AM, O'Connor GR: Immunology and immunopathology of the eye. Masson, New York, 1979.

43 Dernouchamps JP, Vaerman JP, Michiels J et al: Immune complexes in aqueous humor and serum. Am J Ophthalmol 84: 24, 1977.

44 Diamond JG, Kaplan HJ: Uveitis: effects of vitrectomy combined with lensectomy. Trans Am Acad Ophthalmol 86: 1320, 1979.

45 Doughman DJ: Fuchs' heterochromia. Surv Ophthalmol 11: 297, 1966.

46 Dreyer RF, Gass DJ: Multifocal choroiditis and panuveitis. A syndrome that mimics ocular histoplasmosis. Arch Ophthalmol 102: 1176, 1984.

47 Duke-Elder S: System of Ophthalmology. IX. Diseases of the uveal tract. CV Mosby, St Louis, 1966.

48 Edgerton AE: Herpes Zoster ophthalmicus. Report of cases and review of the literature. Arch Ophthalmol 34: 40, 1945.

49 Egbert PR, Pollard RB, Gallaghter JG et al: Cytomegalovirus retinitis in immunosuppressed hosts: II. Ocular manifestations. Ann Intern Med 93: 664, 1980.

50 Ehlers N, Kissmeyer-Nielsen F, Kjerbye KE et al: HLA-27 in acute and chronic uveitis. Lancet 1: 99, 1974.

51 Faber DW, Wiley CA, Lynn GB et al: Role of HIV and CMV in the pathogenesis of retinitis and retinal vasculopathy in AIDS patients. Invest Ophthalmol Vis Sci 33: 2345, 1992.

52 Flynn HW Jr, Davis JL, Culbertson WW: Pars plana lensectomy and vitrectomy for complicated cataracts in juvenile rheumatoid arthritis. Ophthalmology 95: 1114, 1988.

53 Font RL, Fine BS, Messmer E: Light and electron microscopic study of Dalen-Fuchs nodules in sympathetic ophthalmia. Ophthalmology 90: 66, 1983.

54 Franceschetti A: Heterochromic cyclitis. Am J Ophthalmol 29: 50, 1955.

55 Freeman WR, Chen A, Henderly DE et al: Prevalence and significance of acquired immunodeficiency syndrome-related retinal microvasculopathy. Am J Ophthalmol 107: 229, 1989.

56 Freeman WR, Lerner CW, Mines JA et al: A prospective study of the ophthalmologic findings in the acquired immune deficiency syndrome. Am J Ophthalmol 97: 133, 1984.

57 Fuchs E: Veber Komplikationen der Heterochromie. Zeitschrift für Augenheilkunde 15: 191, 1906.

58 Fujikawa LS, Chan CC, Mc Allister C: Retinal vascular endothelium expresses fibronectin and class II histocompatibility complex antigens in experimental autoimmune uveitis. Cell Immunol 98: 139, 1987.

59 Galea P, D'Amato B, Goal KM: Ocular complications in juvenile chronic arthritis. Scott Med J 30: 164, 1985.

60 Gartner S, Henkind P: Neovascularization of the iris (Rubeosis iridis). Surv Ophthalmol 22: 291, 1978.

61 Gass JDM, Olson CL: Sarcoidosis with optic nerve and retinal involvement. Trans Am Acad Ophthalmol Otolaryngol 77: 739, 1973.

62 Gee SS, Tabbara KF: Extracapsular cataract extraction in Fuchs' heterochromic iridocyclitis. Am J Ophthalmol 108: 310, 1989.

63 Georgiades G: Les lesions de l'iris hétérochromique en general. Bull Mem Soc Franc Ophtalmol 77: 465, 1964.

64 Giles CL: Peripheral uveitis and multiple sclerosis. Am J Ophthalmol 70: 17, 1970.

65 Giles CL, Handleman I: Panuveitis presenting symptom of systemic sarcoidosis in a child. J Pediatr Ophthalmol 13: 189, 1976.

66 Godfrey WA, Lindsley CB, Cuppage FE: Localization of IgM in plasma cells in the iris of a patient with iridocyclitis and juvenile rheumatoid arthritis. Arthritis Rheum 24: 1195, 1981.

67 Goldberg MF, Erozan YS, Duke JR et al: Cytopathologic and histopathologic aspects of Fuchs' heterochromic iridocyclitis. Arch Ophthalmol 74: 604, 1965.

68 Hayreh SS, Scott WE: Fluorescein iris angiography. I. Normal pattern. Arch Ophthalmol 96: 1383, 1978.

69 Hedges TR, Albert DM: The progression of the ocular abnormalities of herpes zoster: histopathologic observations of nine cases. Ophthalmology 89: 165, 1982.

70 Helve J, Nieminen H: Simultaneous bilateral fluorescein angiography of the anterior eye. Acta Ophthalmologica 123 (Suppl): 134, 1974.

71 Henkind P, Gottlieb MB: Bilateral internal ophthalmoplegia in a patient with sarcoidosis. Br J Ophthalmol 57: 792, 1973.

72 Henry K, Cantrill H, Fletcher C et al: Use of intravitreal ganciclovir (dihydroxy propoxymethyl guanine) for cytomegalovirus retinitis in a patient with AIDS. Am J Ophthalmol 103: 17, 1987.

73 Hogan MJ, Kimura SJ, Thygeson P: Signs and symptoms of uveitis: I. Anterior uveitis. Am J Ophthalmol 47: 155, 1959.

74 Hogan MJ, Kimura SJ, O'Connor GR: Peripheral retinitis and chronic cyclitis in children. Trans Ophthalmol Soc UK 85: 39, 1965.

75 Holland GN, Pepose JS, Pettit TH et al: Acquired immune deficiency syndrome. Ocular manifestations. Ophthalmology 90: 859, 1983.

76 Holland GN, Engstrom RE Jr, Glasgow BJ et al: Ocular toxoplasmosis in patient with the acquired immunodeficiency syndrome. Am J Ophthalmol 106: 653, 1988.

77 Holland GN: Acquired immundeficiency syndrome and ophthalmology: the first decade. Am J Ophthalmol 114: 86, 1992.

78 Holland GN, Sakamoto MJ, Hardy D et al: Treatment of cytomegalovirus retinopathy in patients with acquired immunodeficiency syndrome. Arch Ophthalmol 104: 1794, 1986.

79 Hoover DL, Khan JA, Giangiacomo JJ: Pediatric ocular sarcoidosis. Surv Ophthalmol 30: 215, 1986.

80 Hoskins HD: Neovascular glaucoma: Current Concepts. Trans Am Acad Opthalmol Otolaryngol 78: 330, 1971.

81 Israel HL, Patrick H, Gottlieb JE et al: Marked elevation of serum angiotensin converting enzyme activity. Clinical correlates. In Grassi C, Rizzato G, Pozzi E: Sarcoidosis and other granulomatous disorders. Elsevier Science Publishers BV, Amsterdam, 1988.

82 Jabs DA, Green WR, Fox R et al: Ocular manifestations of acquired immune deficiency syndrome. Ophthalmology 96: 1092, 1989.

83 Jabs DA, Johns CJ: Ocular involvement in chronic sarcoidosis. Am J Ophthalmol 102: 297, 1986.

84 Jampol LM, Neufeld AH, Sears ML: Pathways for the response of the eye to injury. Invest Ophthalmol 14: 184, 1975.

85 Jampol LM, Rosser MJ, Sears ML: Unusual aspects of progressive essential iris atrophy. Am J Ophthalmol 77: 353, 1974.

86 Johnson O, Leisegang TJ, Brubaker RF: Aqueous humor dynamics in Fuchs' uveitis syndrome. Am J Ophthalmol 95: 783, 1983.

87 Kanski JJ: Juvenile arthritis and uveitis. Surv Ophthalmol 34: 253, 1990.

88 Karma A: Ophthalmic changes in sarcoidosis. Acta Ophthalmol (Kbh) 141: 1, 1979.

89 Karma A, Huhti E, Poukkula A: Course and outcome of ocular sarcoidosis. Am J Ophthalmol 106: 467, 1988.

90 Karma A, Laatikainen L: Fluorescein iris angiography in nodular sarcoid iritis. Int Ophthalmol 3: 97, 1981.

91 Kaufman HE: Genetic inflammatory disease. Editorial. Inv Ophthalmol 13: 555, 1974.

92 Kestelyn P: Ocular problems in AIDS. Int Ophthaloml 14: 165, 1990.

93 Key SN. III, Kimura SJ: Iridocyclitis associated with juvenile rheumatoid arthritis. Am J Ophthalmol 80: 425, 1975.

94 Kimura R: Hyperfluorescent dots in the ciliary body band in patients with granulomatous uveitis. Br J Ophthalmol 66: 322, 1982.

95 Kimura SJ, Hogan MJ, Thygeson P: Fuchs' syndrome of heterochromic cyclitis. Arch Ophthalmol 54: 174, 1955.

96 Kimura SJ, Thygeson P, Hogan MJ: Signs and symptoms of uveitis. I. Classification of the posterior manifestations of uveitis. Am J Ophthalmol 47: 171, 1959.

97 Kishkina VIa, Semenov AD, Kostochkina AV: Results of fluorescein angiography of the iris in surgical treatment of recurrent anterior uveitis. Vestn Oftalmol 106: 33, 1990.

98 Klien BA, Farkas TG: Pseudomelanoma of the iris after Herpes Zoster ophthalmicus. Am J Ophthalmol 57: 392, 1964.

99 Knox DL: Ischemic ocular inflammation. Am J Ophthalmol 60: 995, 1965.

100 Kottow MH: Anterior segment fluorescein angiography. William & Wilkins, Baltimore, 1978.

101 Laatikainen L: Vascular changes in the iris in chronic anterior uveitis. Br J Ophthalmol 63: 145, 1979.

102 Lerman S, Levy C: Heterochromic iritis and secondary neovascular glaucoma. Am J Ophthalmol 57: 479, 1964.

103 Liesegang TJ: Clinical features and prognosis in Fuchs' uveitis syndrome. Arch Ophthalmol 100: 1622, 1982.

104 Lipton NL, Crawford JS, Greenberg ML: Chlorambucil in the treatment of iridocyclitis in juvenile rheumatoid arthritis. J Rheum 8: 141, 1981.

105 Loewenfeld IE, Thompson HS: Fuchs' heterochromic cyclitis: a clinical review of the literature. I. Clinical characteristics of the syndrome. Surv Ophthalmol 17: 394, 1973.

106 Loewenfeld IE, Thompson HS: Fuchs' heterochromic cyclitis: a clinical review of the literature. II. Etiology and mechanisms. Surv Ophthalmol 18: 2, 1973.

107 Macher A, Rodrigues MM, Kaplan W et al: Disseminated bilateral chorioretinitis due to Histoplasma capsulatum in a patient with the acquired immunodeficiency syndrome. Ophthalmology 92: 1159, 1985.

108 Makley TA: Heterochromic cyclitis in identical twins. Am J Ophthalmol 41: 768, 1956.

109 Mandelbaum S, Forster RK: Post-operative endophthalmitis. Int Ophthalmol Clin 2: 95, 1987.

110 Mapstone R: Fluorescein iridography. Br J Ophthalmol 55: 400, 1971.

111 Mapstone R, Woodrow JC: Acute anterior uveitis and HLA-27. Lancet 1: 681, 1974.

112 Marsh RJ: Ocular manifestations of AIDS. Br J Hosp Med 42: 224, 1989.

113 Marsh RJ, Easty DL, Jones BR: Iritis and iris atrophy in Herpes Zoster ophthalmicus. Am J Ophthalmol 78: 255, 1974.

114 Martenet AC: Ocular complications of AIDS. Diagnostic problems. Klin Monatsbl Augenheilkd 200: 555, 1992.

115 Masi R, O'Connor GR, Kimura SJ: Anterior uveitis in geographic or serpiginous choroiditis. Am J Ophthalmol 86: 228, 1978.

116 Matsuo T, Nakayama T, Koyama T et al: Immunological studies of uveitis. III. Cell-mediated immunity to interphotoreceptor retinoid binding protein. Jpn J Ophthalmol 30: 487, 1986.

117 Mc Carron MJ, Albert DM: Iridocyclitis and an iris mass associated with secondary syphilis. Ophthalmology 91: 1264, 1984.

118 McCartney ACE, Bull TB, Spalton DJ: Fuchs' heterochromic cyclitis. An electron microscopy study. Trans Ophthalmol Soc UK 105: 324, 1986.

119 Melamed S, Lahav M, Sandbank U et al: Fuchs' heterochromic iridocyclitis. An electron microscopy study of the iris. Inv Ophthalmol Vis Sci 17: 1193, 1978.

120 Menchini U, Pece A, Carnevalini A et al: Aspetti fluorangiografici delle uveiti. Clin Ocul 4: 282, 1986.

121 Meredith TA: Clinical microbiology of infectious endophthalmitis. In Ryan SJ: Retina. CV Mosby, St Louis, 1989.

122 Miller JD, Eakins KE, Atwal M: The release of PGE2-like activity into aqueous humor after paracentesis and its prevention by aspirin. Inv Ophthalmol 12: 939, 1973.

123 Mills KB, Rosen ES: Intraocular lens implantation following cataract extraction in Fuchs' heterochromic uveitis. Ophthalmic Surg 13: 467, 1982.

124 Mitsui Y, Matsubara M, Kanagawa M: Fluorescence irido-corneal photography. Br J Ophthalmol 53: 505, 1969.

125 Momoeda S: Lymphocite transformation test in Vogt-Koyanagi-Harada syndrome. Acta Soc Ophthalmol Jpn 80: 491, 1976.

126 Murray PI: Immunology of Fuchs' heterochromic cyclitis. In Ferraz de Oliveira LN: Ophthalmology Today. Excerpta Medica, Amsterdam, 1988.

127 Murray PI, Dinning WJ, Rahi AH: Contrasting relations between suppressor cell number and function in acute anterior uveitis and heterochromic cyclitis. Acta Ophthalmol 163 (Suppl): 52, 1984.

128 Murray PI, Mooy CM, Visser De Jong E et al: Immunohistochemical analysis of iris biopsy specimens from patients with Fuchs' heterochromic cyclitis. Am J Ophthalmol 109: 394, 1990.

129 Neufeld AH, Sears ML: Prostaglandin and eye. Prostaglandins 4: 157, 1973.

130 Newsome DA, Green WR, Miller ED et al: Microvascular aspects of acquired immune deficiency syndrome retinopathy. Am J Ophthalmol 98: 590, 1984.

131 Ni M, Chan CC, Nussenblatt RB et al: Iris inflammatory cells, fibronectin, fibrinogen and immunoglobulin in various ocular diseases. Arch Ophthalmol 106: 392, 1988.

132 Nobe JR, Kokoris N, Diddie KR: Lensectomy-vitrectomy in chronic uveitis. Retina 3: 71, 1983.

133 Nussenblatt RB, Palestine AG: Uveitis: fundamentals and clinical practice. Year Book Medical Publishers Inc, Chicago, 1989.

134 Obenauf CD, Shaw HE, Sydnor CF: Sarcoidosis and its ophthalmic manifestations. Am J Ophthalmol 86: 648, 1978.

135 Ohno S: Immunological aspects of Behçet's and Vogt-Koyanagi-Harada diseases. Trans Ophthalmol Soc UK 101: 335, 1981.

136 Ohno S, Char DH, Kimura SJ et al: HLA antigens and antinuclear antibody titers in juvenile chronic iridocyclitis. Br J Ophthalmol 61: 59, 1977.

137 Ohno S, Kimura SJ, O'Connor GR et al: HLA antigens and uveitis. Br J Ophthalmol 61: 62, 1977.

138 Okinami S, Ogino N, Matsumara M et al: Neovascularization at the angle of anterior chamber in cases of uveitis. High incidence in Vogt-Koyanagi-Harada disease. Nippon Ganka Gakkai Zasshi 86: 2186, 1982.

139 Okubo K, Kurimoto S, Okubo K et al: Surface markers of peripherals blood lymphocites in Vogt-Koyanagi-Harada disease. J Clin Lab Immunol 17: 49, 1985.

140 Okumoto M: Laboratory diagnosis of endophthalmitis. Int Ophthalmol Clin 2: 89, 1984.

141 Oosterhuis JA, Renger-van Dijk DH: Birdshot chorioretinopathy. In Ryan SJ, Dawson AK, Little HL: Retinal diseases. Grune & Stratton Inc, Orlando, 1985.

142 Ostler HB, Dawson CR, Schachter J et al: Reiter's syndrome. Am J Ophthalmol 71: 986, 1971.

143 O'Connor GR: Current classification of uveitis. In Saari KM: Uveitis update. Elsevier Science Publishers BV, Amsterdam, 1984.

144 Palestine AG, Rodrigues MM, Macher AM et al: Ophthalmic involvement in the acquired immune deficiency syndrome. Ophthalmology 91: 1092, 1984.

145 Palestine AG, Stevens G, Lane HC et al: Treatment of cytomegalovirus retinitis with dihydroxy propoxymethyl guanine. Am J Ophthalmol 101: 95, 1986.

146 Palmer RG, Kanski JJ, Ansell BM: Chlorambucil in the treatment of intractable uveitis chronic arthritis. J Rheum 12: 967, 1985.

147 Pearson PA, Amrien JM, Baldwin LB et al: Iridoschisis associated with syphilitic interstitial keratitis. Am J Ophthalmol 107: 88, 1989.

148 Pederson O: Electron microscopic studies on the blood-aqueous barrier of prostaglandin-treated rabbit eyes: I. Iridial and ciliary processes. Acta Ophthalmol (Kbh) 53: 685, 1975.

149 Pederson O: Electron microscopic studies on the blood-aqueous barrier of prostaglandin-treated rabbit eyes: II. Iris. Acta Ophthalmol (Kbh) 53: 699, 1975.

150 Pederson JE, Kenyon KR, Green WR et al: Pathology of pars planitis. Am J Ophthalmol 86: 762, 1978.

151 Pepose JS, Holland GN, Nestor MS et al: Acquired immune deficiency syndrome: pathogenic mechanisms of ocular disease. Ophthalmology 92: 474, 1985.

152 Perkins ES: Heterochromic uveitis. Trans Ophthalmol Soc UK 81: 53, 1961.

153 Perkins ES: Prostaglandins and ocular trauma. Adv Ophthalmol 34: 149, 1977.

154 Perry HD, Yanoff M, Scheie HG: Rubeosis in Fuchs' heterochromic iridocyclitis. Arch Ophthalmol 93: 337, 1975.

155 Pertshuck LP, Silverstein E, Friedland J: Immunohistologic diagnosis of sarcoidosis. Detection of angiotensin-converting enzyme in sarcoid granulomas. Am J Clin Pathol 75: 350, 1981.

156 Pezzi PP, Tamburi SD, D'Offizi GP et al: Retinal cotton-wool-like spots: a marker for AIDS ? Ann Ophthalmol 21:13, 1989.

157 Peyman G, Schulman JA: Intravitreal surgery, principles and practices. Appleton, Century-Crofts, Norwalk, 1985.

158 Pivetti-Pezzi P: Le flogosi uveali. Masson Italia Ed, Milano, 1987.

159 Pomerantz RJ, Kuritzkes DR, de la Monte SM et al: Infection of the retina by human immunodeficiency virus type I. N Eng J Med 317: 1643, 1987.

160 Pruett RC, Brockhurst RJ, Letts NF: Fluorescein angiography of peripheral uveitis. Am J Ophthalmol 77: 448, 1974.

161 Rachelefsky GS, Terasaki PI, Katz R et al: Increased prevalence of W27 in juvenile rheumatoid arthritis. N Eng J Med 290: 892, 1974.

162 Rao NA, Marak GE: Sympathetic ophthalmia simulating Vogt-Kojanagi-Harada's disease: a clinicopathologic study of four cases. Jpn J Ophthalmol 27: 506, 1983.

163 Raviola G: Effects of paracentesis on the blood-aqueous barrier: an electron microscope study of Macaca mulatta using horseradish peroxidase as a tracer. Inv Ophthalmol 13: 828, 1974.

164 Rothova A, Meenken C, Michels RP et al: Uveitis and diabetes mellitus. Am J Ophthalmol 106: 17, 1988.

165 Ryan GB: Inflammation: mediators of inflammation. Beitr Pathol 152: 272, 1974.

166 Saari KM: Anterior segment fluorescein angiography in inflammatory diseases of the cornea. Acta Ophthalmol (Kbh) 57: 781, 1979.

167 Saari KM: The International Uveitis Study Group. Acta Ophthalmol 163 (Suppl): 21, 1984.

168 Saari M, Vuorre I, Nieminen H: Fuchs' heterochromic cyclitis. A simultaneous bilateral fluorescein angiography of the iris. Br J Ophthalmol 62: 715, 1978.

169 Sakai J, Nonaka S, Utsumi T et al: Lymphocite subsets in iris tissue of uman uveitis. In Secchi AG, Fregona IA: Modern trends in immunology and immunopathology of the eye. Masson, Milano, 1989.

170 Sandor EV, Millman A, Croxon TS et al: Herpes zoster ophthalmicus in patients at risk for the acquired immune deficiency syndrome (AIDS). Am J Ophthalmol 101: 153, 1986.

171 Schepens CL: L'inflammation de la region de l'ora serrata et ses sequelles. Bull Soc Ophtalmol Fr 73: 113, 1950.

172 Schuler JD, Engstrom ER, Holland GN et al: External ocular disease and anterior segment disorders associated with AIDS. Int Ohthalmol Clin 29: 98, 1989.

173 Schuman JS, Friedman AH: Retinal manifestations of the acquired immune deficiency syndrome. Trans Ophthalmol Soc UK 103: 177, 1983.

174 Secchi AG, Fregona IA, Corsano A et al: Immunoregulation in uveitis. In O'Connor GR, Chandler JW: Advances in immunology and immunopathology of the eye. Masson, New York, 1985.

175 Smiley WK: The eye in juvenile rheumatoid arthritis. Trans Ophthalmol Soc UK 94: 817, 1974.

176 Smith RE, Godfrey WA, Kimura SJ: Chronic cyclitis. Course and visual prognosis. Trans Am Acad Ophthalmol Otolaryngol 77: 760, 1973.

177 Smith RE, Nozik RA: Uveitis. A clinical approach to diagnosis and management. William & Wilkins, Baltimore, 1983.

178 Smith RE, O'Connor GR: Cataract extraction in Fuchs' syndrome. Arch Ophthalmol 91: 39, 1974.

179 Soubrane G, Coscas G, Binaghi M et al: Birdshot retinochoroidopathy and subretinal new vessels. Br J Ophthalmol 67: 461, 1983.

180 Stevens G Jr, Chan CC, Wetzig RP et al: Iris lymphocitic infiltration in patients with clinically quiescent uveitis. Am J Ophthalmol 104: 508, 1987.

181 Stoumbos VD, Klein ML: Syphilitic retinitis in a patient with acquired immunodeficiency syndrome-related complex. Am J Ophthalmol 103: 103, 1987.

182 Tessler HH: Classifications and symptoms and signs of uveitis. In Duane TD, Jeager EA: Clinical Ophthalmology. Harper & Row, New York, 1987.

183 Turner RG, James DG, Friedmann AI et al: Neuro-ophthalmic sarcoidosis. Br J Ophthalmol 59: 657, 1975.

184 Tutein Nolthenius PA, Deutman AF: Surgical treatment of the complications of chronic uveitis. Ophthalmologica (Basel) 186: 11, 1983.

185 Unger WG, Cole DF, Hammond B: Distruption of the blood following paracentesis in the rabbit. Exp Eye Res 20: 255, 1975.

186 Van der Gaag R, Christiaans BJ, Rothoua A et al: Lymphocite subpopulations in uveitis patients. In O'Connor GR, Chandler JW: Advances in immunology and immunopathology of the eye. Masson, New York, 1985.

187 Vannas A: Fluorescein angiography of the vessels of the iris in pseudoexfoliation of the lens capsula, capsular glaucoma and some other forms of glaucoma. Acta Ophthalmologica 105 (Suppl): 1, 1969.

188 Vergani S, Brancato R, Introni U et al: Digital indocyanine green videoangiography in AIDS retinopathies. Invest Ophathloml Vis Sci 35 (Suppl): 1304, 1994.

189 Vuorre I, Saari M, Tiilikainen A et al: Fuchs' heterochromic cyclitis associated with retinitis pigmentosa. A family study. Can J Ophthalmol 14: 10, 1979.

190 Wakefield D, Abi-Hanna D: HLA antigens and their significance in the pathogenesis of anterior uveitis: a mini review. Curr Eye Res 5: 465, 1986.

191 Wakefield D, Dunlop I, McClusky PJ: Uveitis: Aetiology and disease associations in an australian population. Aust NZ J Ophthalmol 14: 181, 1986.

192 Ward DM, Hart CT: Complicated cataract extraction in Fuchs' heterochromic uveitis. Br J Ophthalmol 51: 530, 1967.

193 Weiss A, Margo CE, Ledford DK et al: Toxoplasmic retinochoroiditis as an initial manifestation of the acquired immune deficiency syndrome. Am J Ophthalmol 101: 248, 1986.

194 Wetzig RP, Chan CC, Nussenblatt RB: Clinical and immunopathological studies of pars planitis in a family. Br J Ophthalmol 72: 5, 1988.

195 Whitelocke RAF, Eakins KE: Vascular changes in the anterior uvea of the rabbit produced by prostaglandins. Arch Ophthalmol 89: 495, 1973.

196 Wilson FW: Causes and prevention of endophthalmitis. Int Ophthalmol Clin 2: 67, 1987.

197 Wobman P: Die heterochromiecyclitis Fuchs. Elektronenmikroskopische studie von 9 irisbiopsien. Albrecht von Graefes Arch Klin Exp Ophthalmol 199: 167, 1976.

198 Wolf MD, Lichter RR, Ragsdale CG: Prognostic factors in the uveitis of juvenile rheumatoid arthritis. Ophthalmology 94: 1242, 1987.

199 Womack LW, Liesegang TJ: Complications of herpes zoster ophthalmicus. Arch Ophthalmol 101: 42, 1983.

200 Wong IG: Clinical use of iris fluorescein angiography. In Blodi FC: Current concepts in Ophthalmology. CV Mosby, St Louis, 1972.

201 Wong I: Iris angiogram in Fuchs' syndrome. Surv Ophthalmol 17: Cover photograph, 1973.

202 Woods AC: Endogenous inflammation of the uveal tract. William & Wilkins, Baltimore, 1961.

203 Yoshikawa K, Takahashi Y, Ohsone T et al: Fluorescein iris angiography and anterior segment fluorophotometry in patients with Behçet's disease. Jpn J Ophthalmol 31: 425, 1987.

204 Zimmerman LE, Maumenee AE: Ocular aspects of sarcoidosis. Am Rev Resp Dis 84: 38, 1961.

205 Zollinger R: Veber das vorkommen von Gefässneubildungen auf der iris. Ophthalmologica (Basel) 123: 216, 1952.

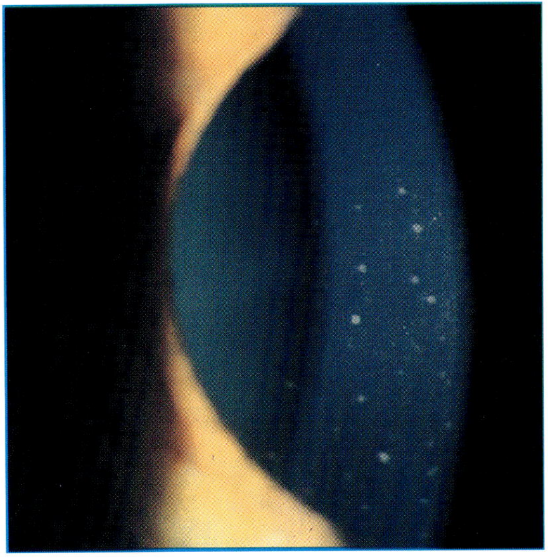

Fig. ***4.7**,1 - Endothelial precipitates in a case of anterior uveitis (biomicroscopic view).*

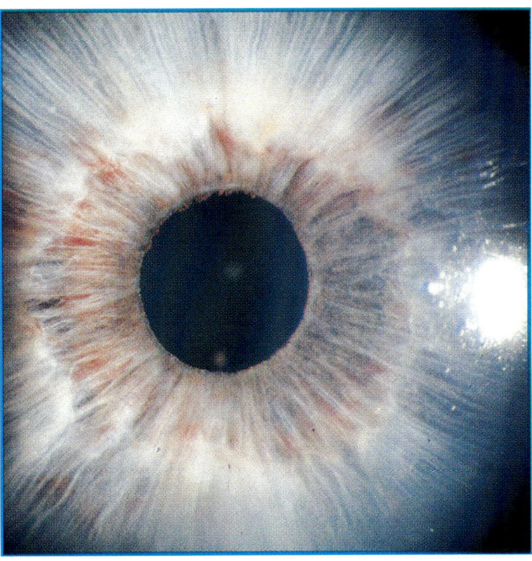

Fig. ***4.7**,2 - Hemorrhagic suffusion in iridocyclitis (biomicroscopic view).*

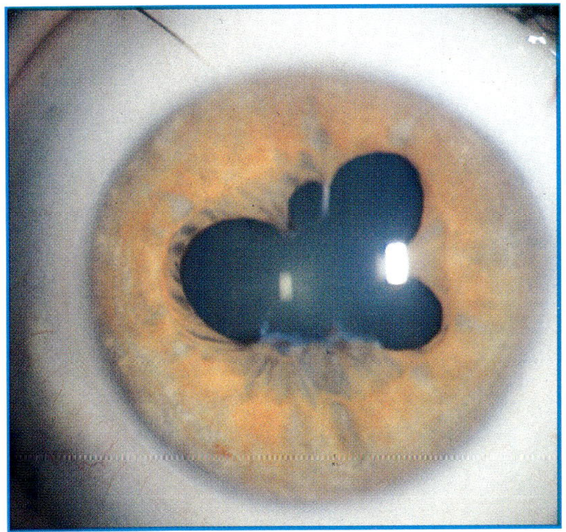

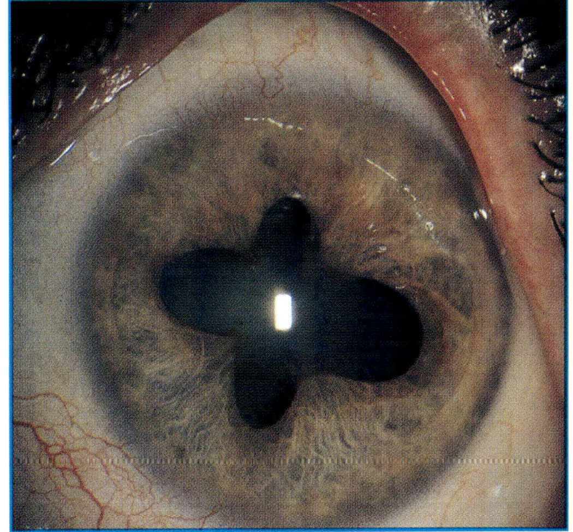

Figs. ***4.7**,3,4 - Irido-lenticular synechiae in two cases of anterior uveitis, causing pupillary deformation (biomicroscopic findings).*

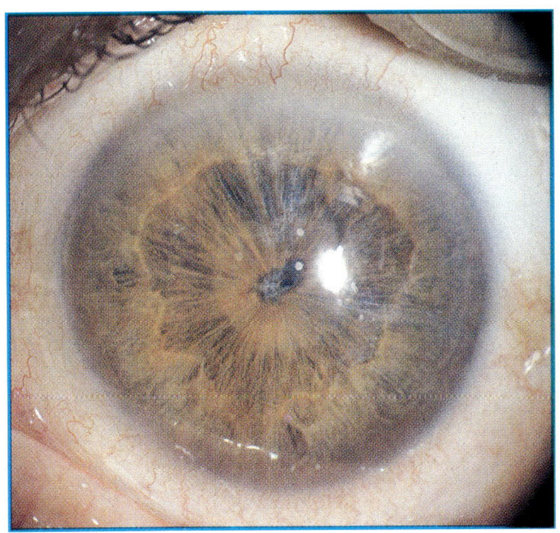

a)

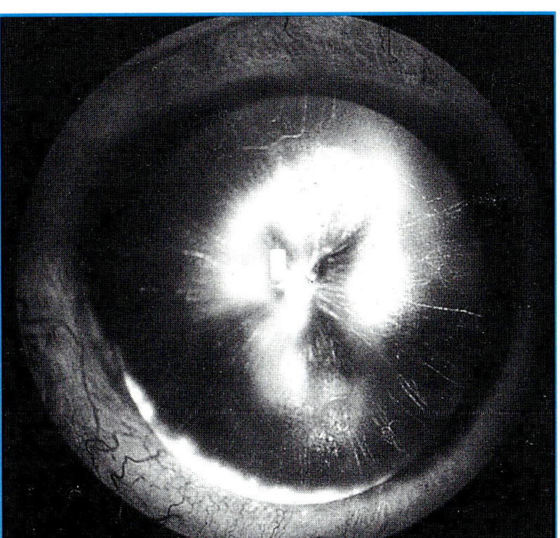

b)

Fig. ***4.7**,5 - Biomicroscopic (a) and iris fluorescein angiographic (b) findings in anterior uveitis complicated by pupillary seclusion.*

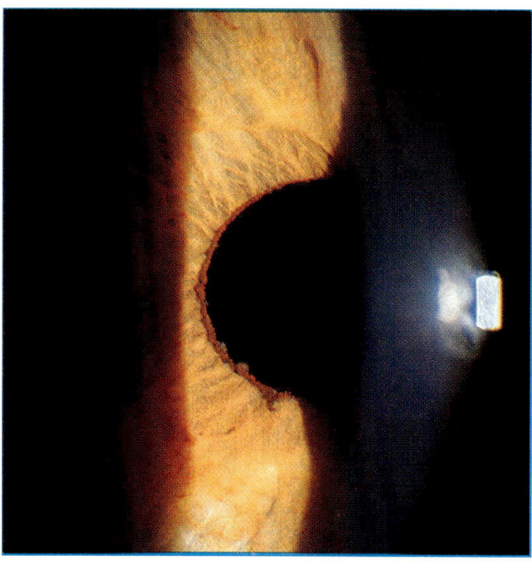

Fig. ***4.7****,6 - Biomicroscopic picture of Koëppe nodules.*

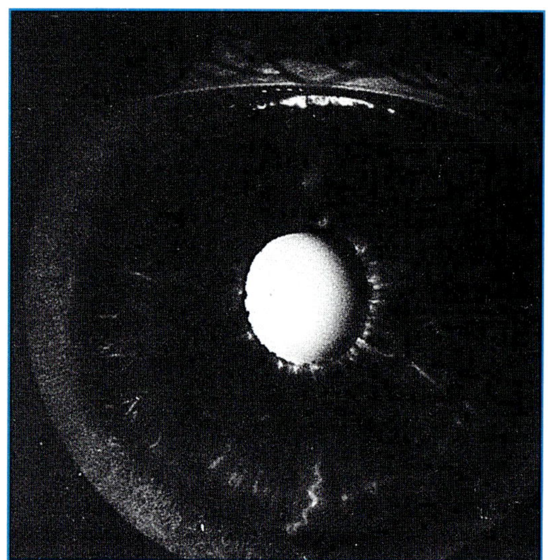

a)

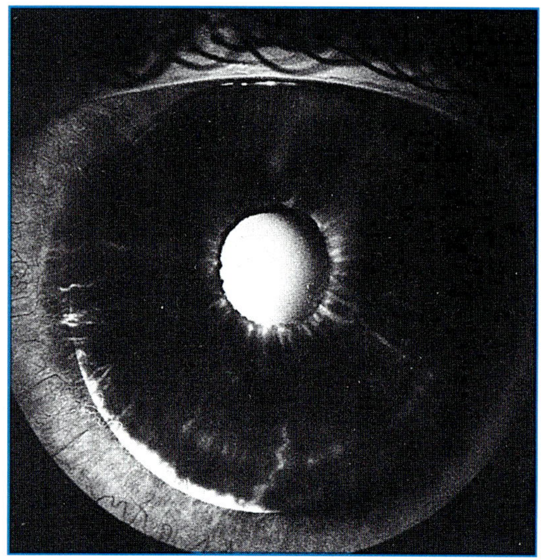

b)

Fig. ***4.7****,7 - Slight dye leakage from the pupillary border in a patient with anterior uveitis. Early (a) and late (b) iris fluorescein angiographic phases.*

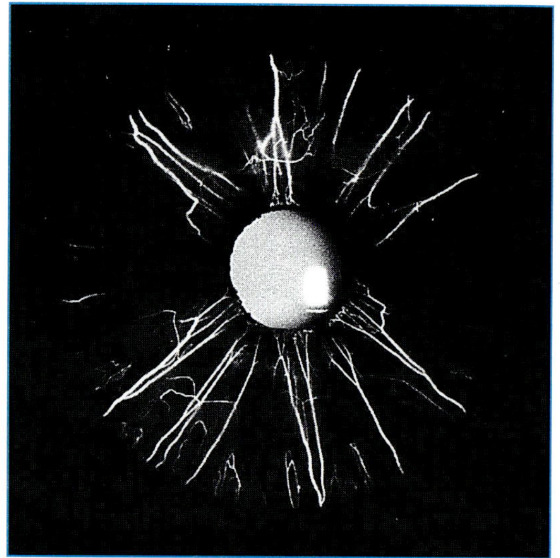

a)

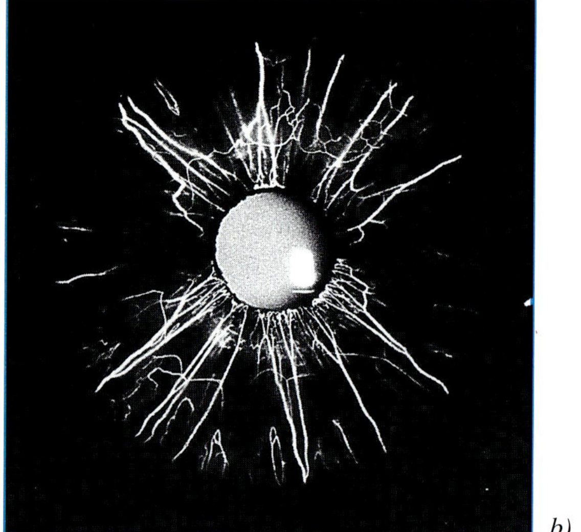

b)

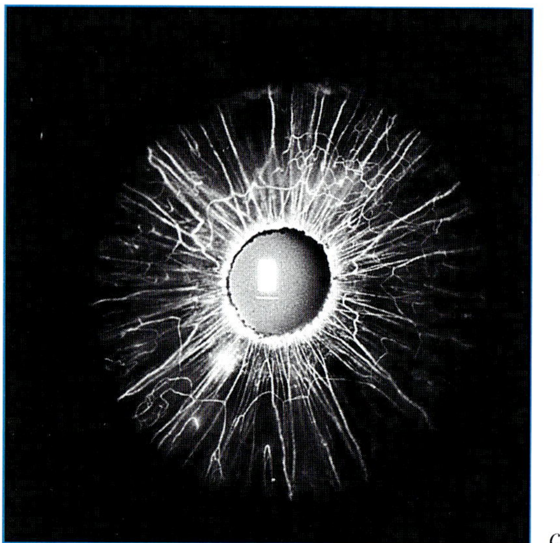

c)

Fig. ***4.7****,8 - Iris fluorescein angiographic phases (a,b,c) in a patient with iridocyclitis. Filling delays and anomalies of the radial vascular structure are visible, with dye leakage particularly at the pupillary margin.*

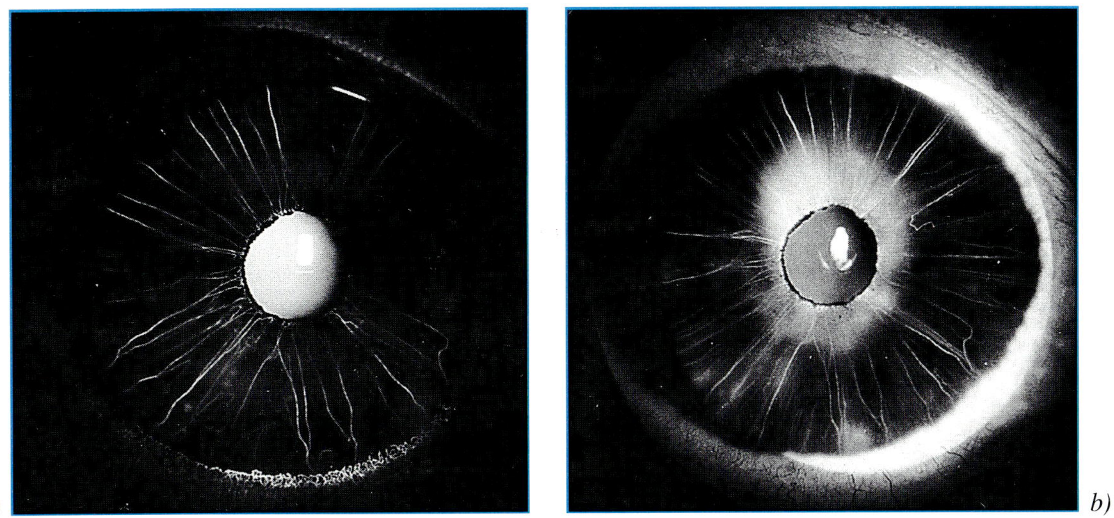

a) b)

*Fig. **4.7**,9 - Dye leakage from the pupillary border and stroma in anterior uveitis. Early (a) and late (b) iris fluorescein angiographic phases.*

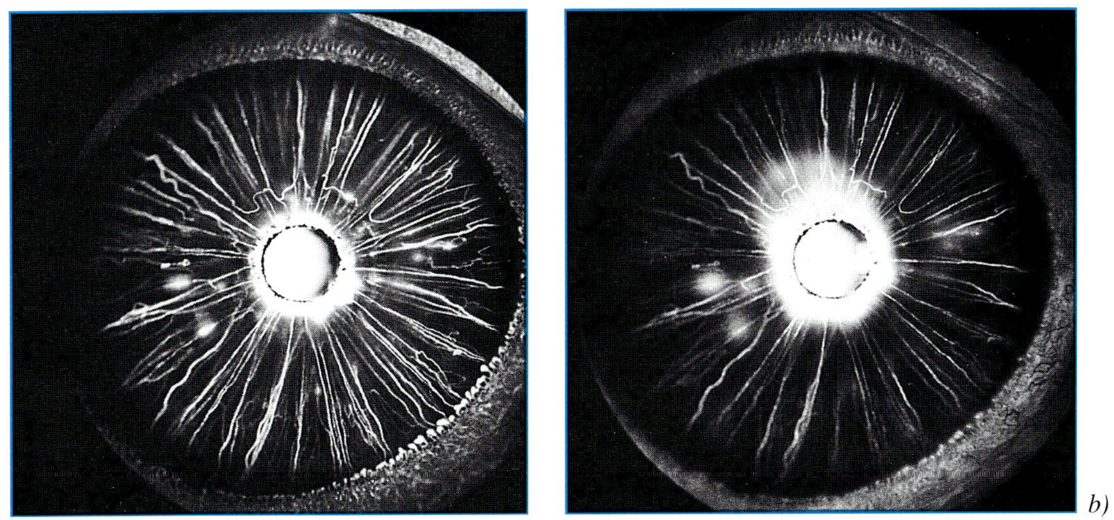

a) b)

*Fig. **4.7**,10 - Dye leakage from pupillary and radial vessels is already visible in the early (a) iris fluorescein angiographic phases, and becomes more marked in the later phases (b).*

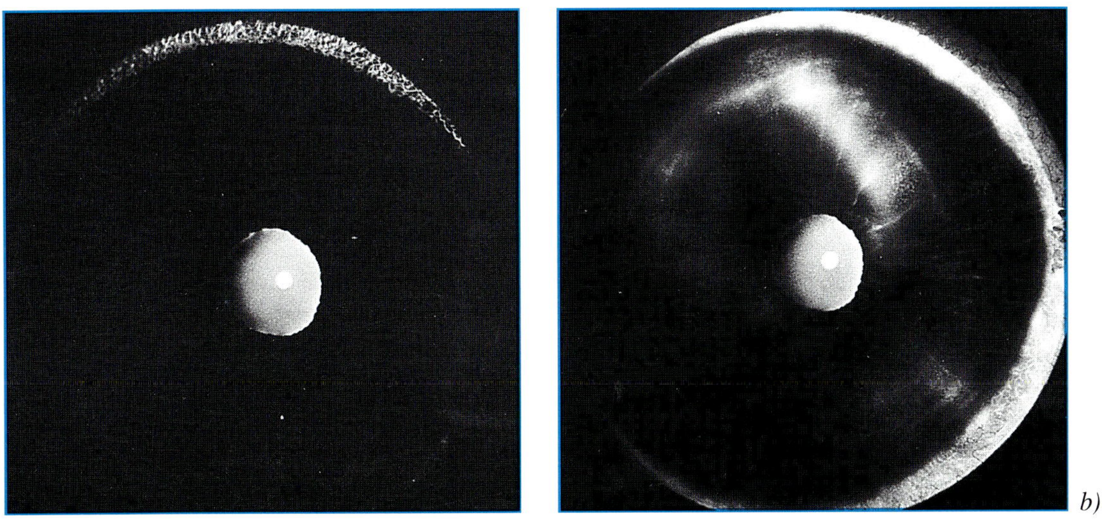

a) b)

*Fig. **4.7**,11 - Iris fluorescein angiography phases (a,b) in a patient with anterior uveitis. In the later phases (b) slight breakdown of the blood-iris barrier is evident.*

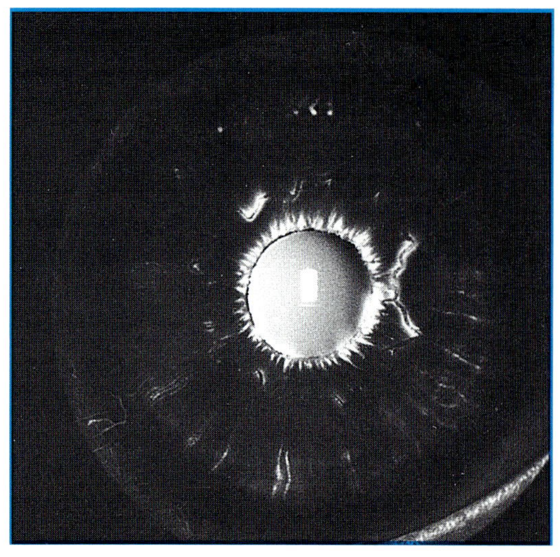
a)

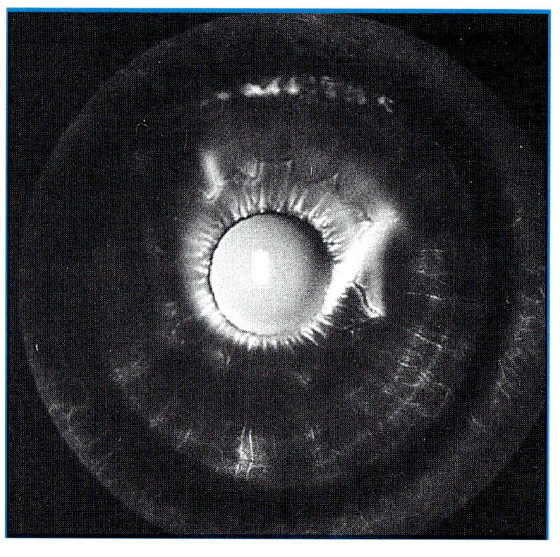
b)

*Fig. **4.7**,12 - Early (a) and late (b) iris fluorescein angiographic phases in anterior uveitis; dye leakage is more marked at the pupillary border and in the zone dividing the pupillary and ciliary sectors of the iris.*

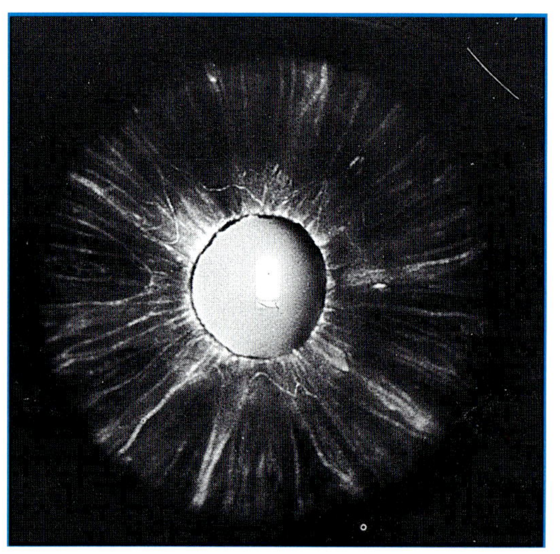
a)

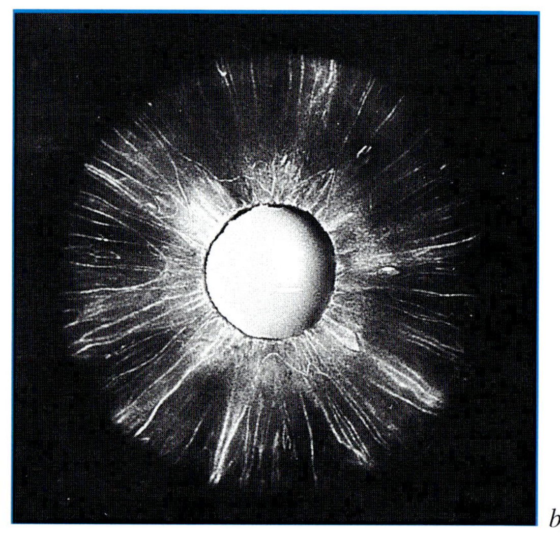
b)

*Fig. **4.7**,13 - In this case of anterior uveitis there is slight dye leakage from most of the iris vessels. Early (a) and late (b) iris fluorescein angiographic phases.*

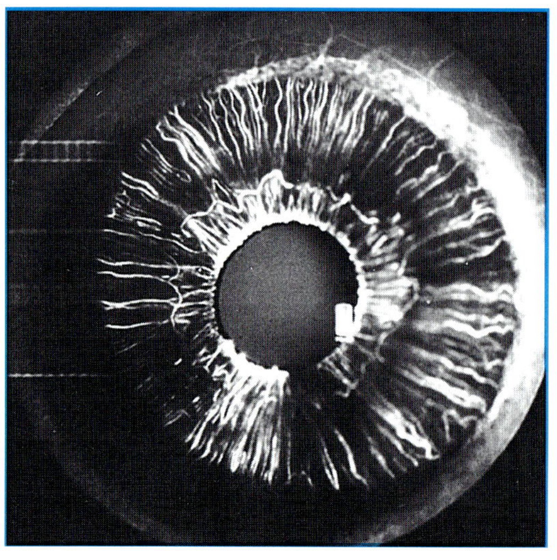
a)

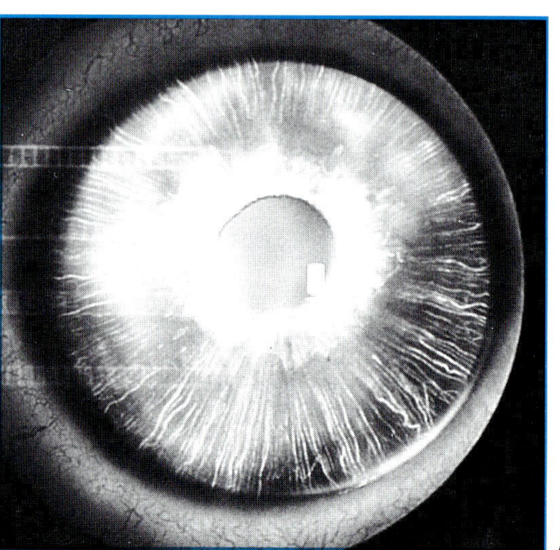
b)

*Fig. **4.7**,14 - Iris fluorescein angiographic phases (a,b) in anterior uveitis. The iris vessels are congested and tortuous and the blood-iris barrier is ruptured at many points.*

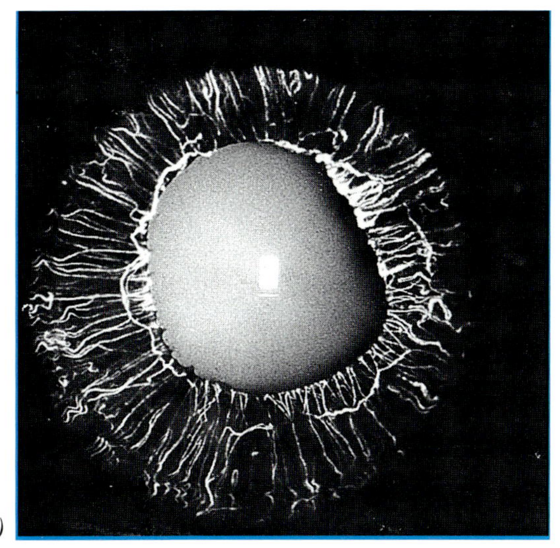

a)

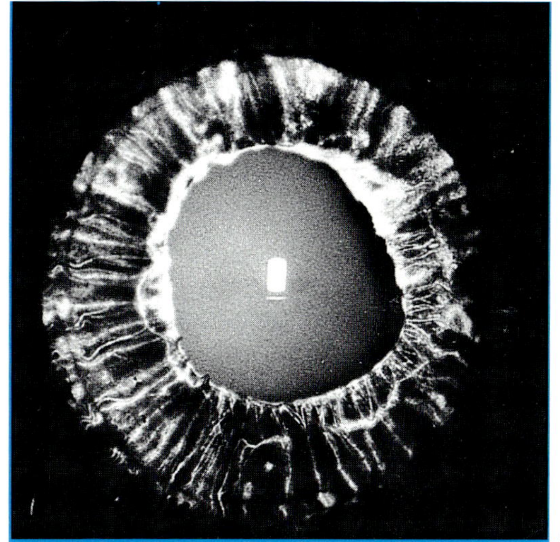

b)

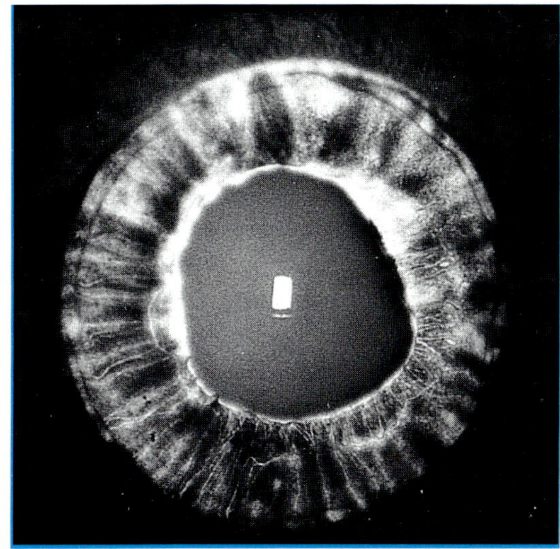

c)

Fig. ***4.7****,15 - All the iris vessels involved in the inflammatory process give early, simultaneous fluorescence (a), and the subsequent dye leakage becomes more marked in later phases (b,c).*

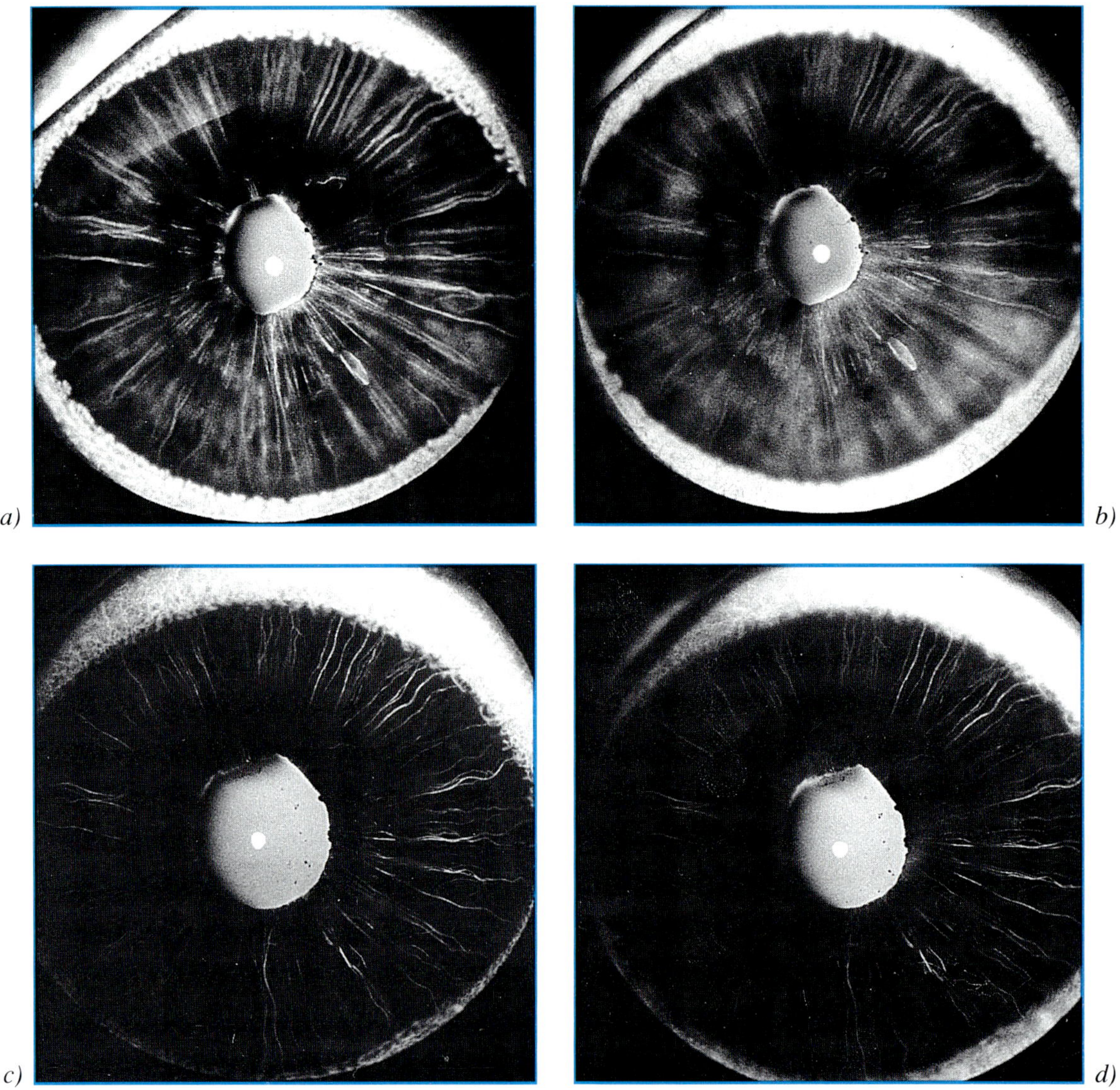

Fig. ***4.7****,16 - Iris fluorescein angiography showing rupture of the blood-iris barrier in acute anterior uveitis (a,b), and its regression (c,d).*

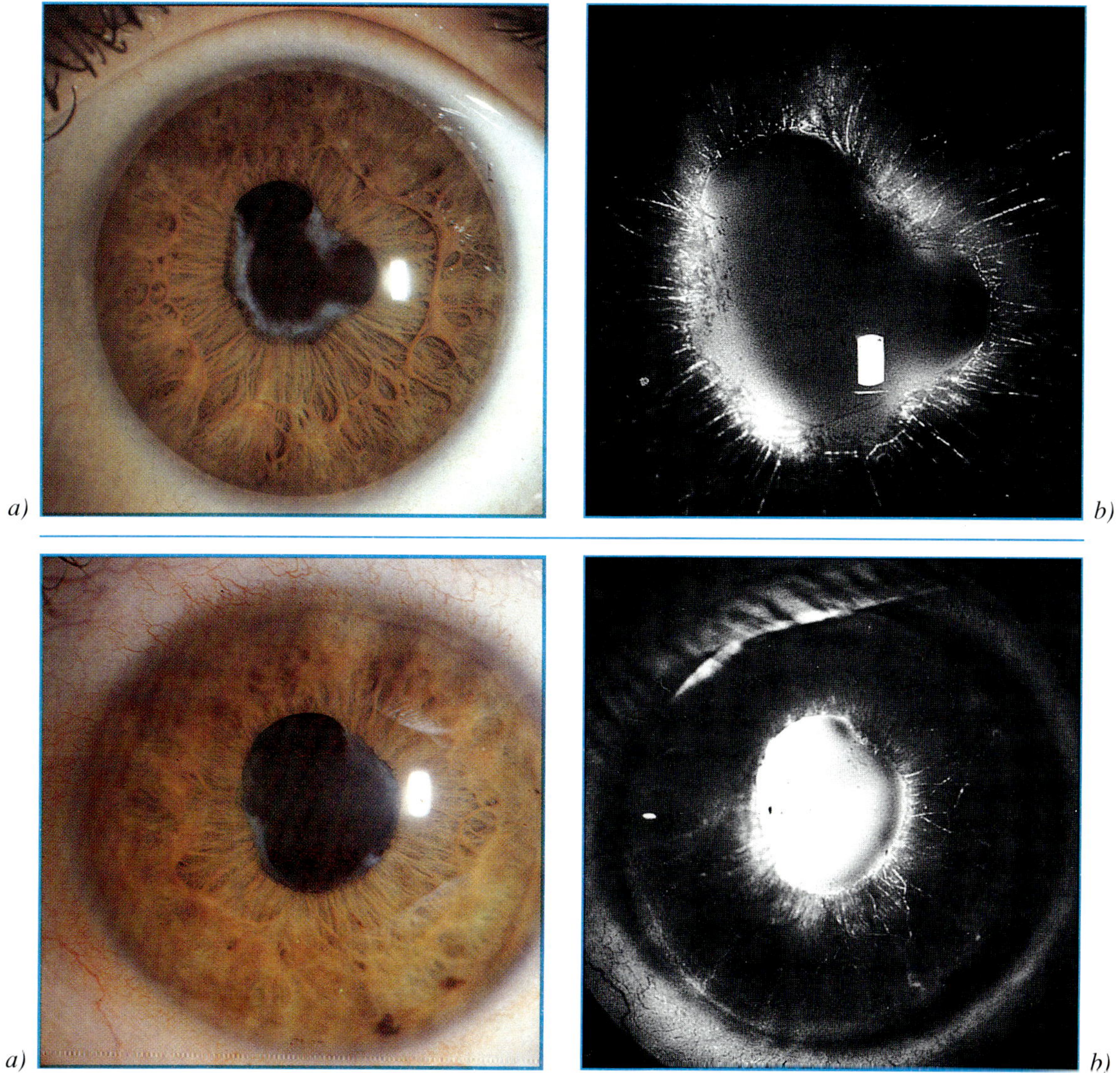

Figs. ***4.7**,17,18 - Biomicroscopic findings (a) and iris fluorescein angiography (b) in two patients after anterior uveitis. Pigment dispersion is visible on the anterior crystalline capsule, with irido-lenticular synechiae, fibrin strands, pupillary deformation and - shown up by iris fluorescein angiography - dye leakage from the pupillary border.*

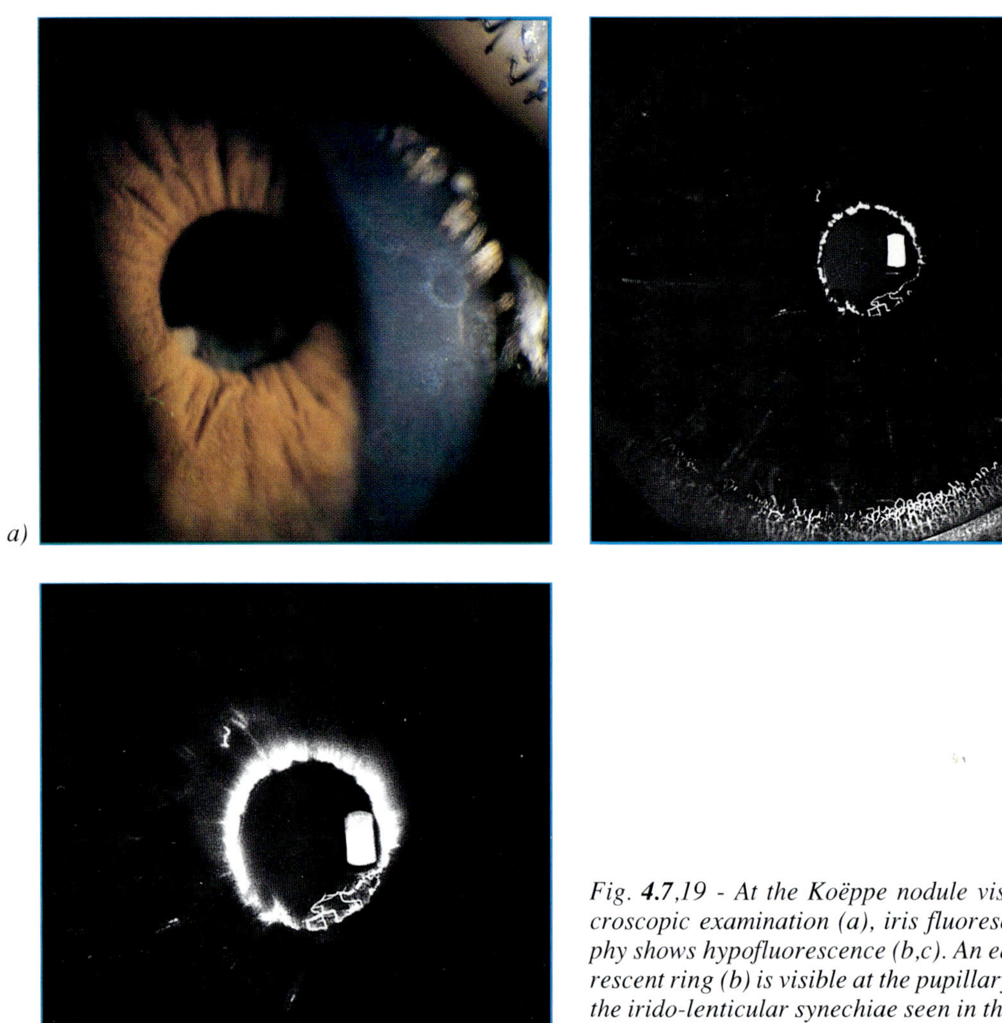

*Fig. **4.7**,19 - At the Koëppe nodule visible by biomicroscopic examination (a), iris fluorescein angiography shows hypofluorescence (b,c). An early hyperfluorescent ring (b) is visible at the pupillary margin; from the irido-lenticular synechiae seen in the lower part, it continues into a fine vascular network where dye leakage is minimal even in the later phases of the examination (c).*

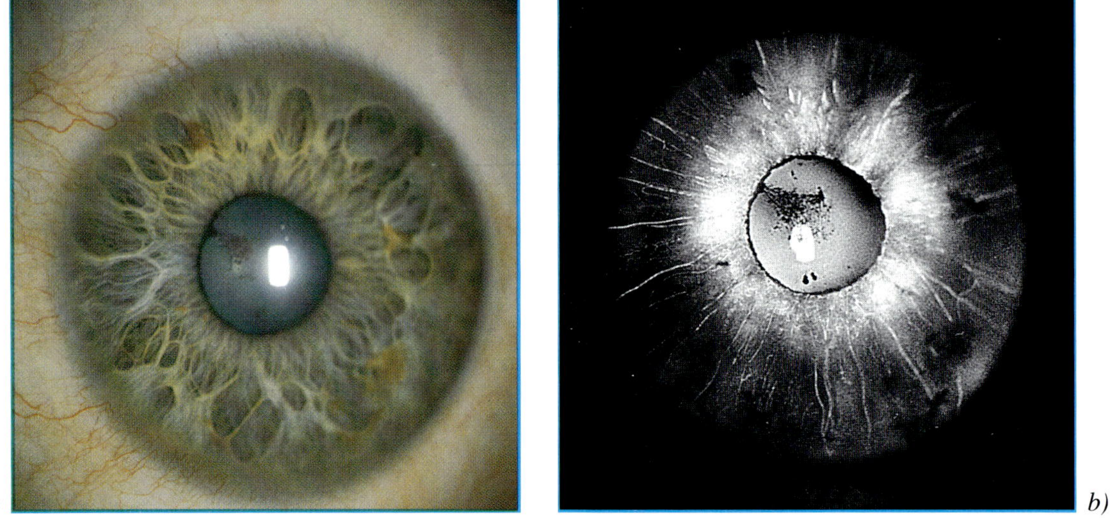

*Fig. **4.7**,20 - Biomicroscopic findings after anterior uveitis (a). Pigment dispersion is detectable and iris fluorescein angiography (b) shows rupture of the blood-iris barrier, especially in the pars pupillaris.*

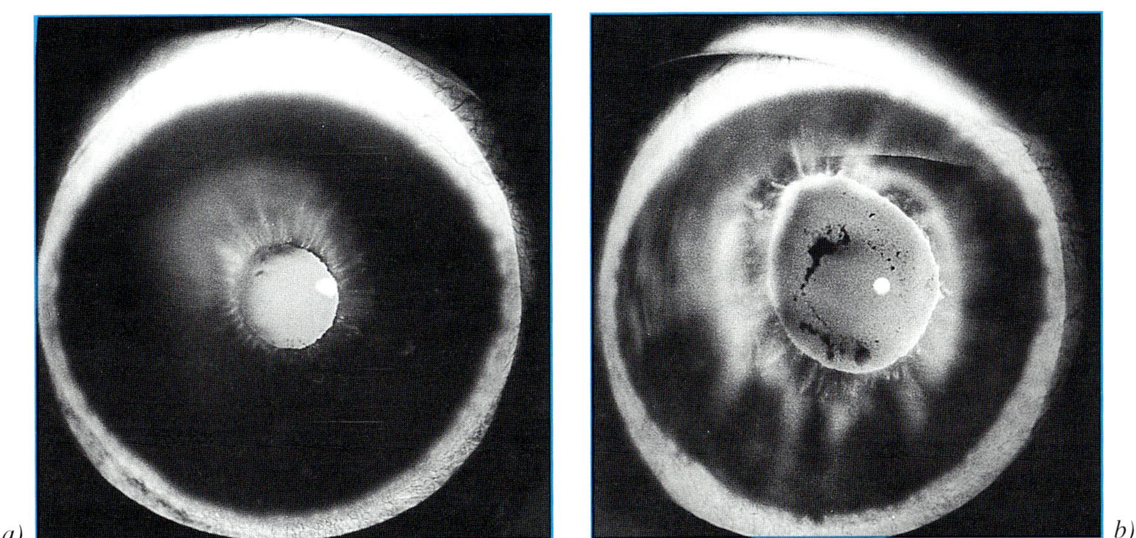

a) b)

Fig. ***4.7****,21 - Iris fluorescein angiographic findings (a) during iridocyclitis, and ten days later (b). Pigment deposits on the anterior lens capsule have increased, pupillary deformation has appeared and the blood-iris barrier can be seen to be ruptured throughout (b).*

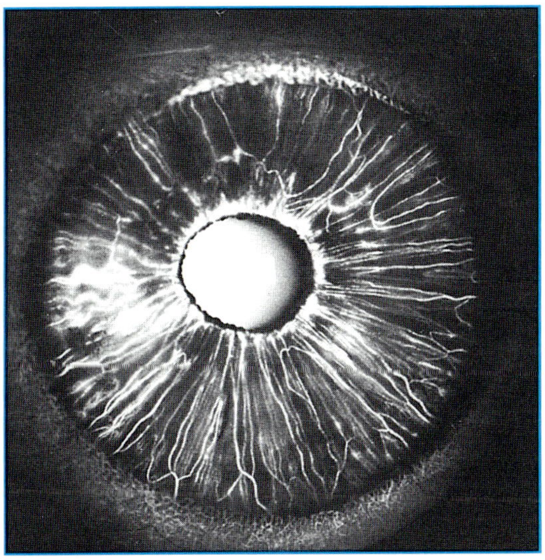

a) 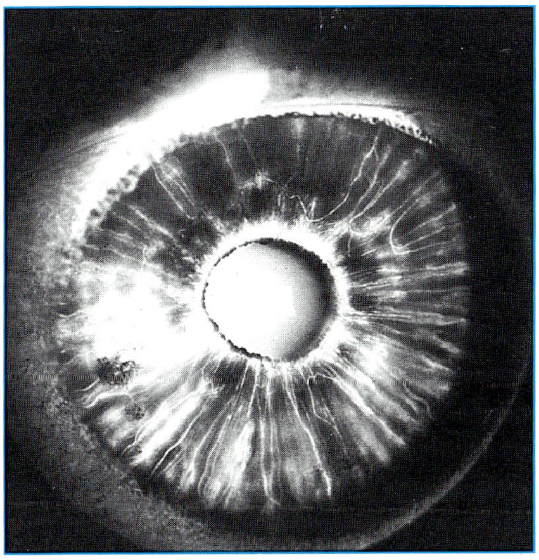 b)

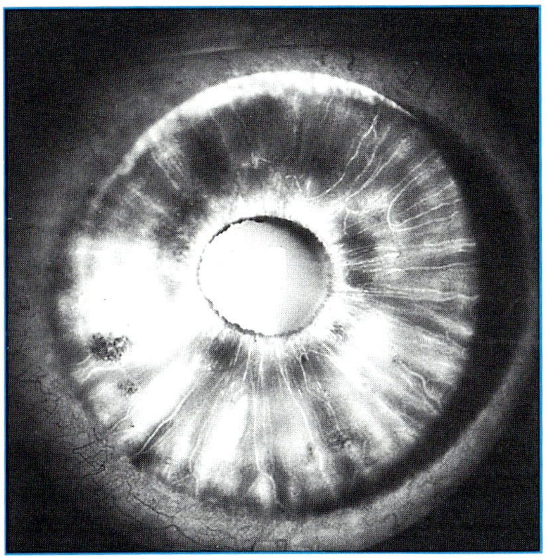

c)

Fig. ***4.7****,22 - Iris fluorescein angiographic phases (a,b,c) in anterior uveitis. The course, caliber and permeability of the iris radial vessels are altered.*

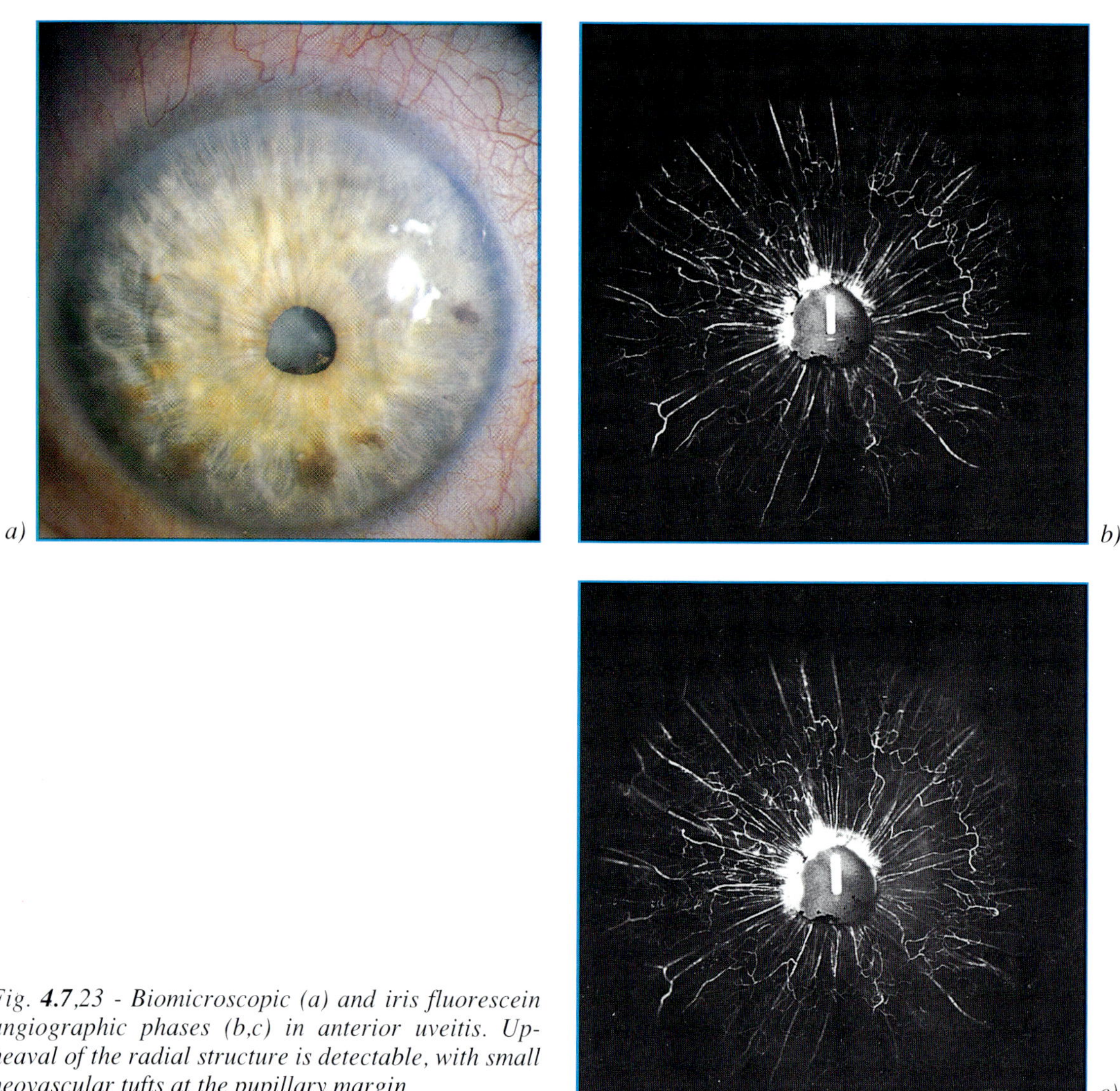

Fig. ***4.7****,23 - Biomicroscopic (a) and iris fluorescein angiographic phases (b,c) in anterior uveitis. Upheaval of the radial structure is detectable, with small neovascular tufts at the pupillary margin.*

Fig. ***4.7****,24 - Stromal vessels follow an abnormal path, taking up dye early (a) and leaking small amounts in the later (b) iris fluorescein angiographic phases. These are indicative of initial iris neovascularization.*

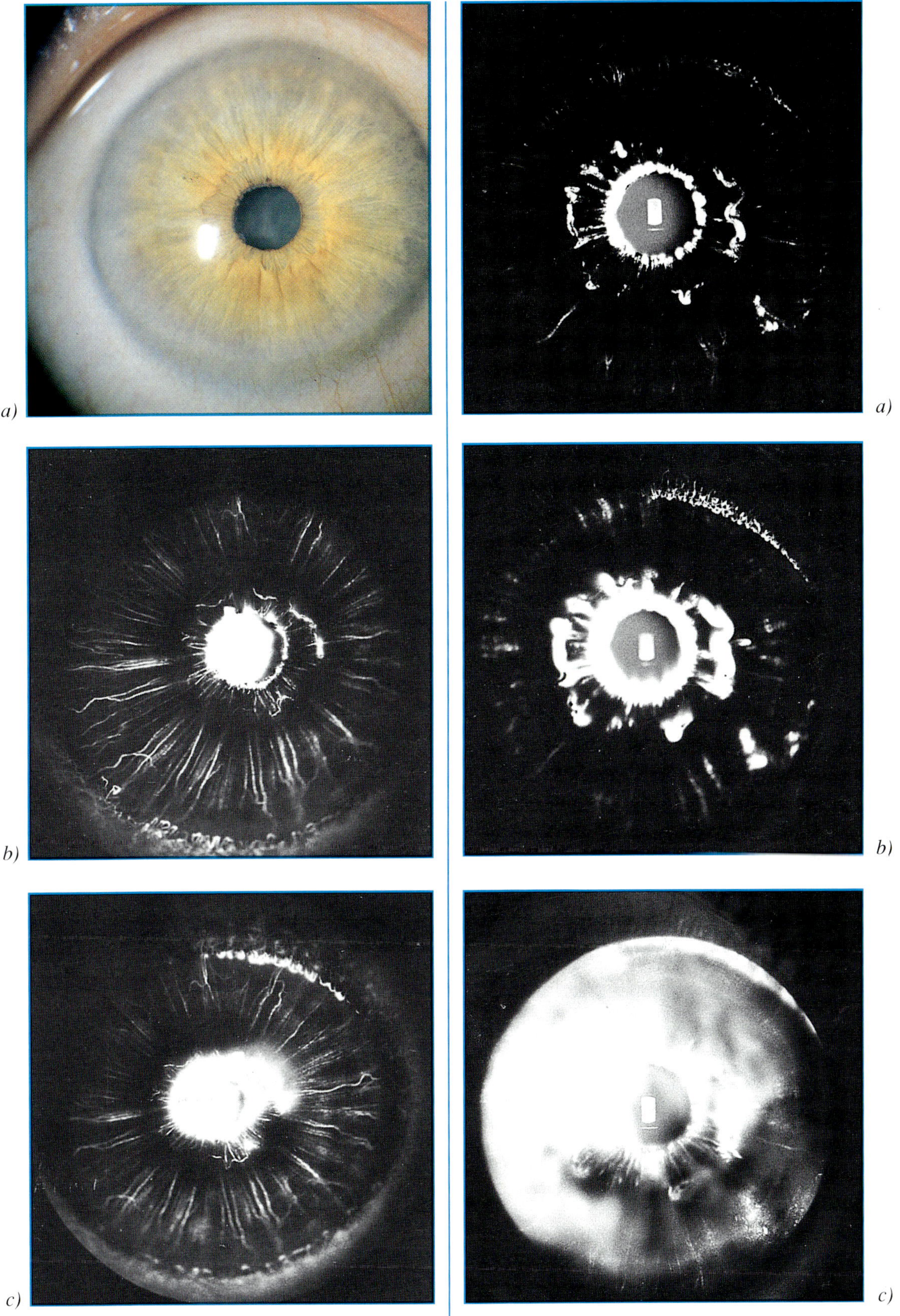

*Fig. **4.7**,25 - Initial iris neovascularization, mainly around the pupillary border, is hardly detectable by biomicroscopic examination (a) but iris fluorescein angiography shows it up clearly (b,c).*

*Fig. **4.7**,26 - Iris fluorescein angiographic phases (a,b,c) showing iris new vessels in anterior uveitis. In the late phases (c) the massive dye leakage fills the whole anterior chamber, masking the intravascular fluorescence from the iris.*

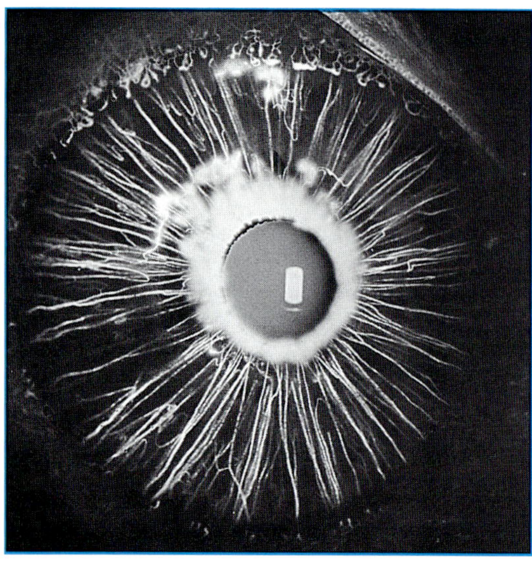

Fig. ***4.7****,27 - Neovascular tufts around the border and in the stroma in anterior uveitis (iris fluorescein angiography).*

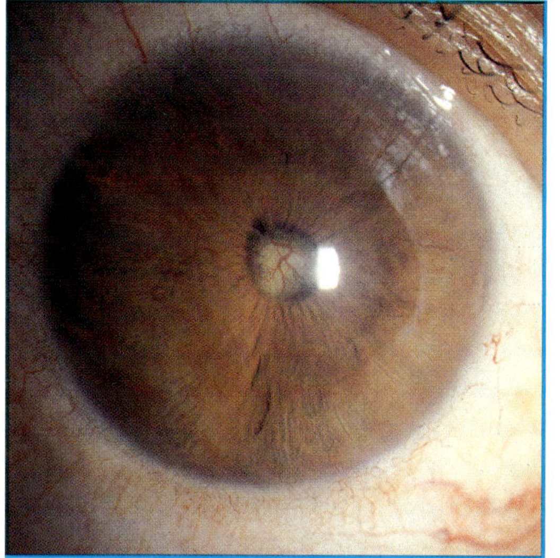

a)

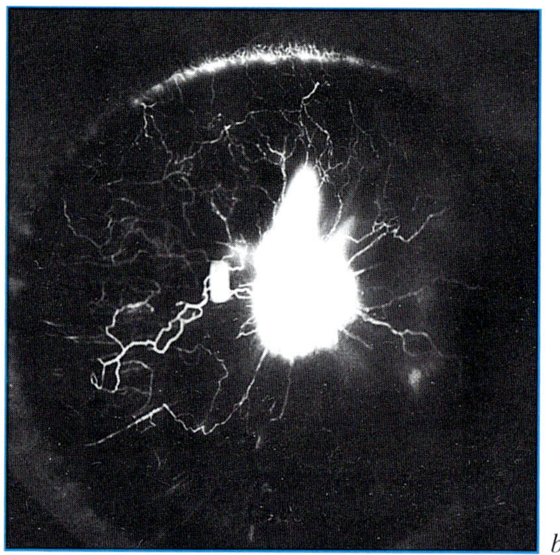

b)

Fig. ***4.7****,28 - Aftermaths of anterior uveitis complicated by a fibrovascular membrane also present in the pupillary area: biomicroscopic (a) and iris fluorescein angiographic (b) pictures.*

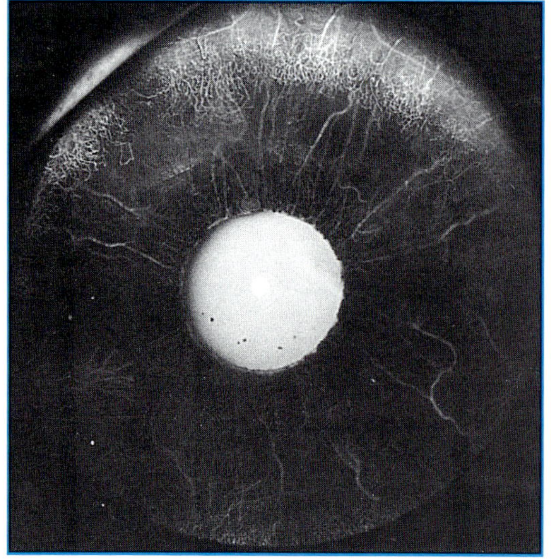

a)

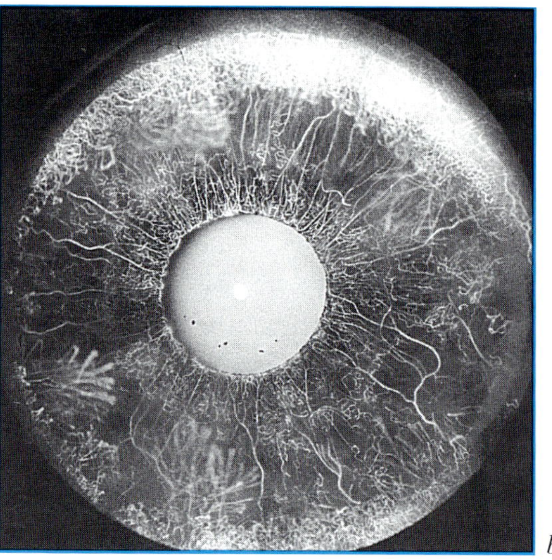

b)

Fig. ***4.7****,29 - Upheaval of the iris structures and an anarchic network of new vessels caused by anterior uveitis: early (a) and late (b) iris fluorescein angiographic pictures. The arborizing vessels that take up dye early in the periphery of the iris are an expression of corneal vascularization.*

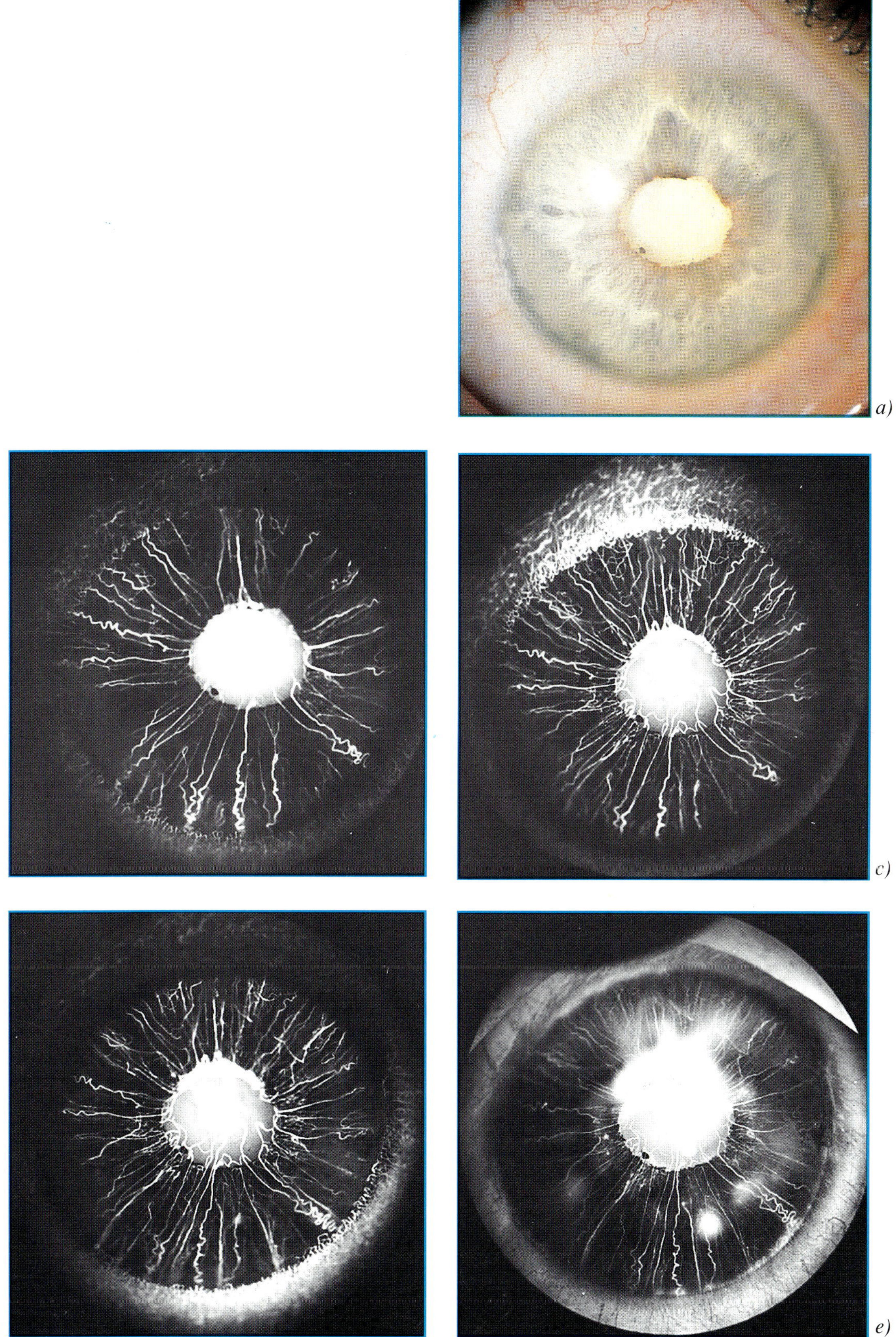

*Fig. **4.7**,30 - Biomicroscopy (a) and iris fluorescein angiographic phases (b,c,d,e) in anterior uveitis. Iris new vessels can be seen invading even the pupillary field (pupillary occlusion).*

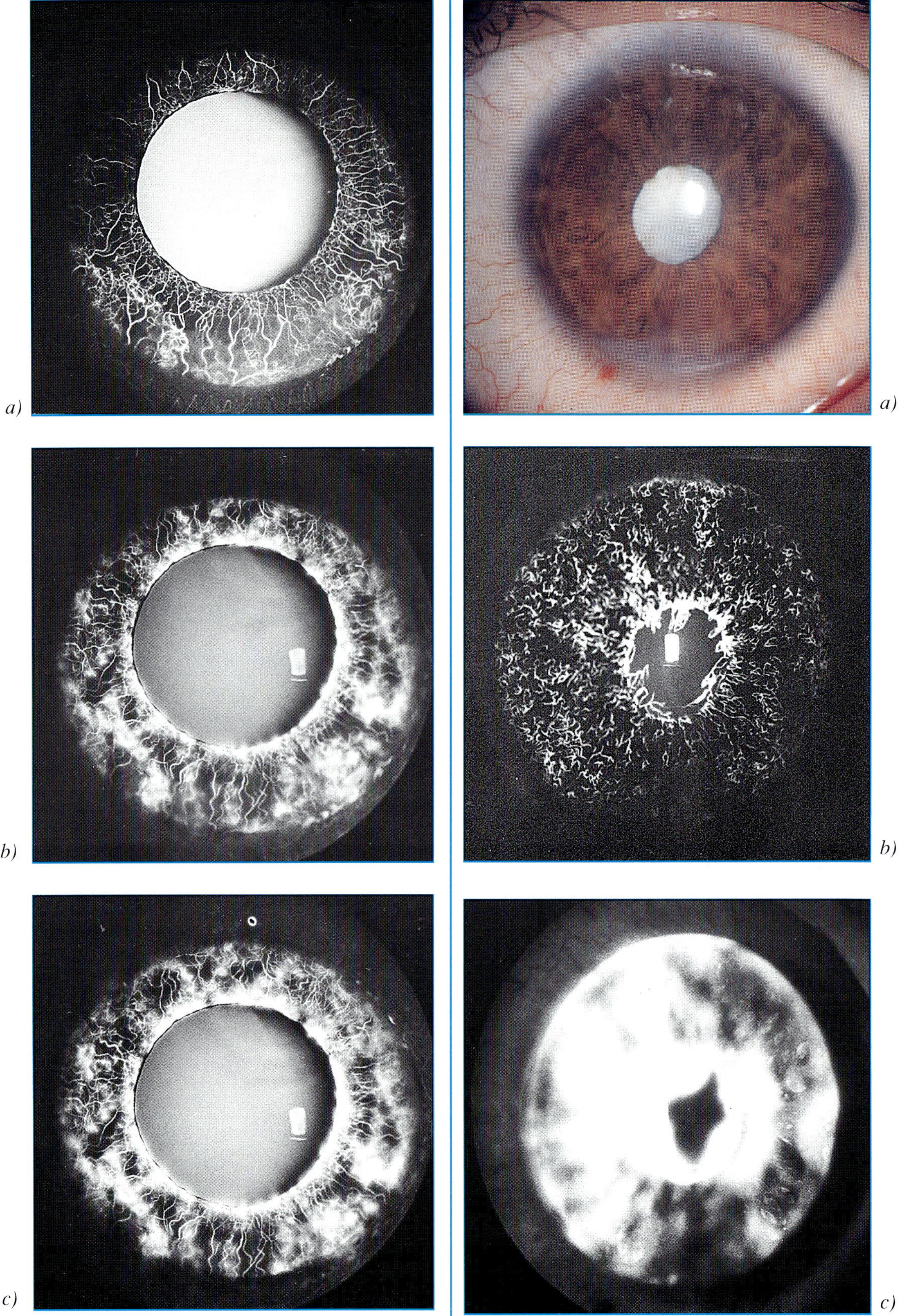

*Fig. **4.7**,31 - Diffuse neovascularization throughout the surface of the iris following anterior uveitis (a,b,c: iris fluorescein angiography phases).*

*Fig. **4.7**,32 - The dense neovascular network following uveitis (a: biomicroscopic view) is clear in the early iris fluorescein angiographic phases (b) and leaks dye profusely later (c).*

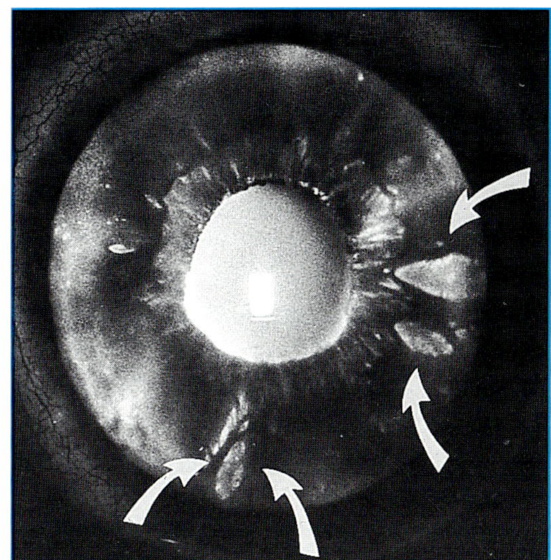

*Fig. **4.7**,33 - Iris fluorescein angiography shows the areas surrounded by pigment atrophy (see arrows) as less hypofluorescent than the rest of the iris surface, since there is less masking effect. Some degree of damage to the blood-iris barrier is evident.*

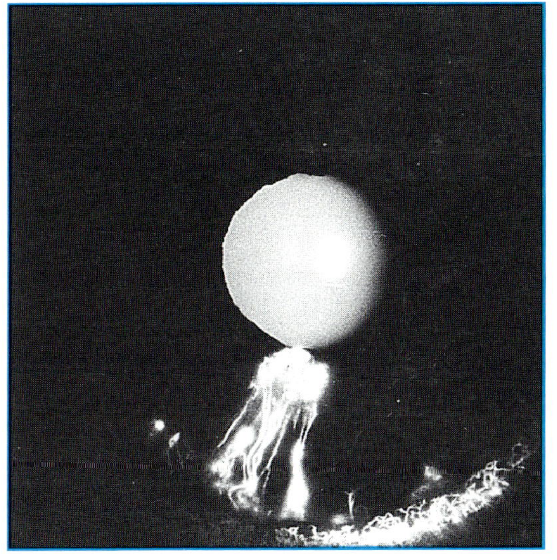

a)

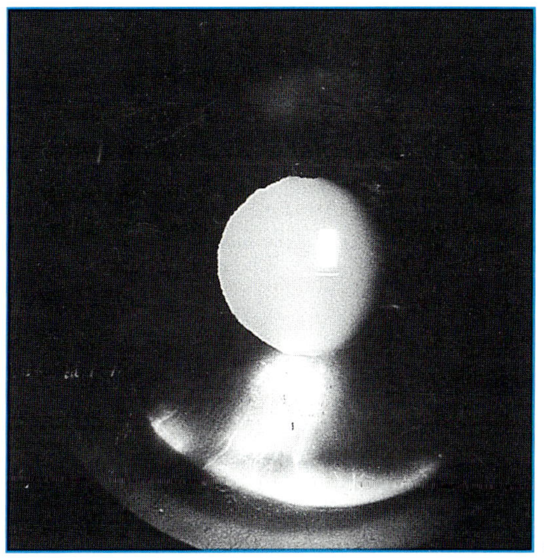

b)

*Fig. **4.7**,34 - Early (a) and late (b) iris fluorescein angiographic phases show an area of pigment atrophy in the lower sectors of the iris, where radial vessels can be seen. Their path, caliber and permeability are all altered.*

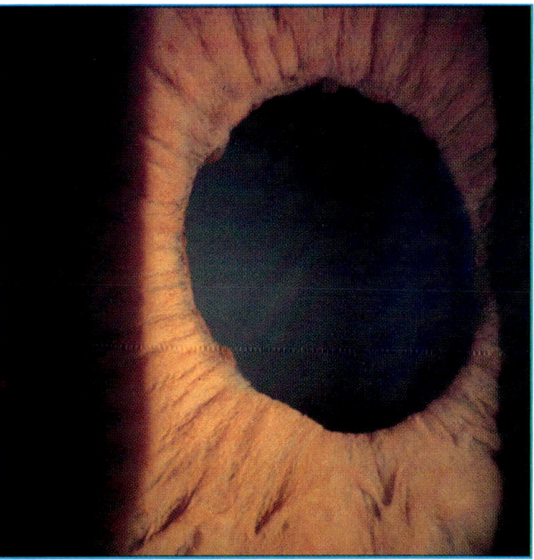

*Fig. **4.7**,35 - Iris nodules at the pupillary margin in a case of sarcoidosis (biomicroscopic findings).*

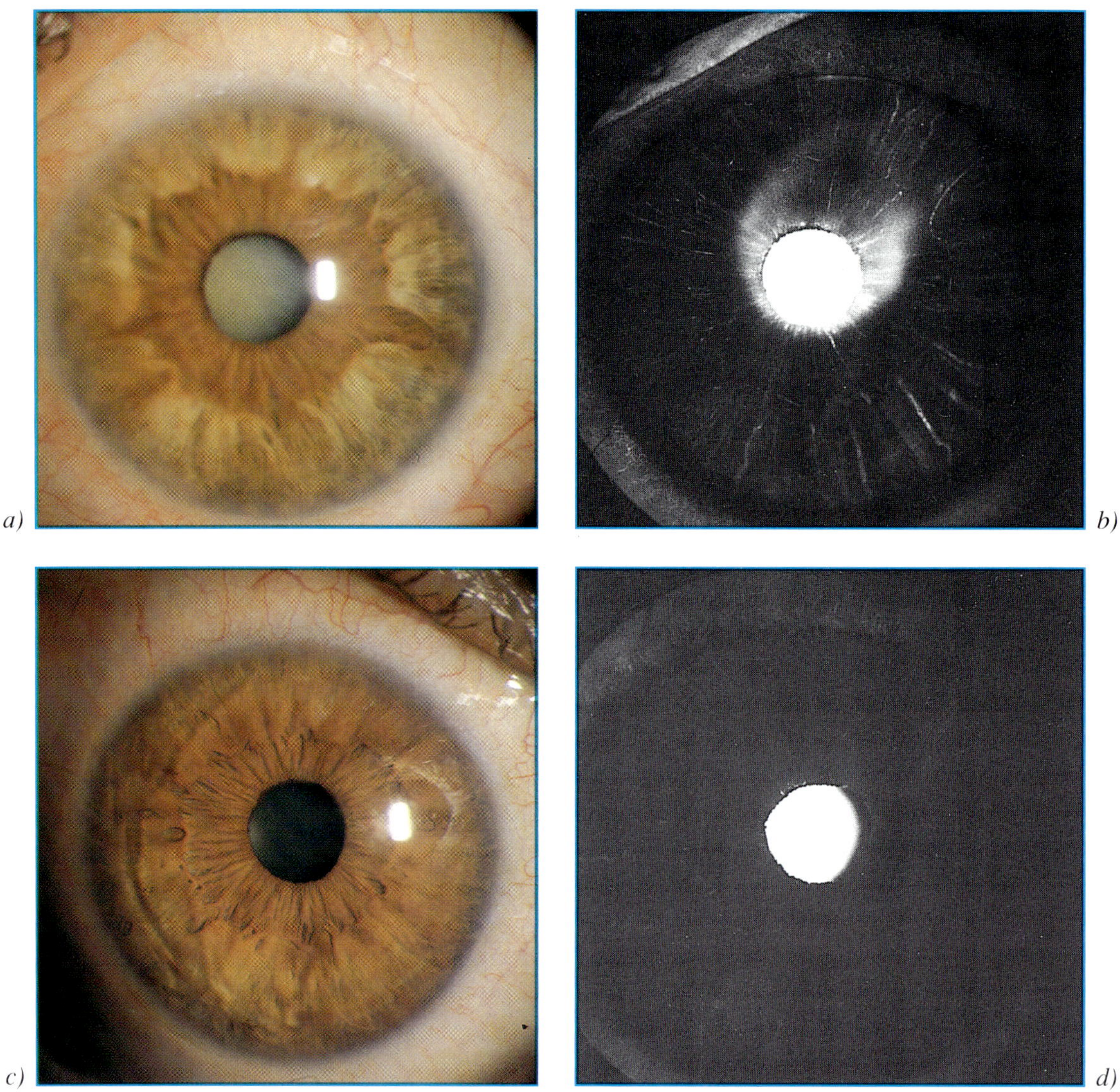

*Fig. **4.7**,36 - Biomicroscopic (a,c) and iris fluorescein angiographic findings (b,d) in an eye with Fuchs' heterochromic cyclitis (a,b) and in the contralateral eye (c,d). Angiography shows slight dye leakage at the pupillary border (b) in the affected eye, while the other one is virtually normal (d).*

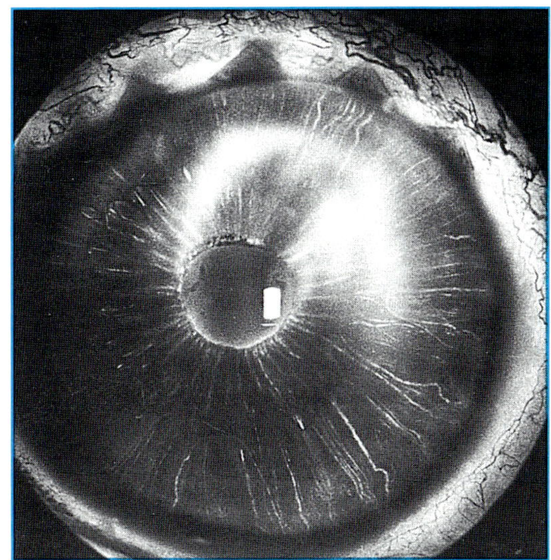

*Fig. **4.7**,37 - The same case of Fuchs' heterochromic cyclitis as above one month after cataract removal. Iris fluorescein angiography shows a slight increase in the degree of rupture of the blood-iris barrier.*

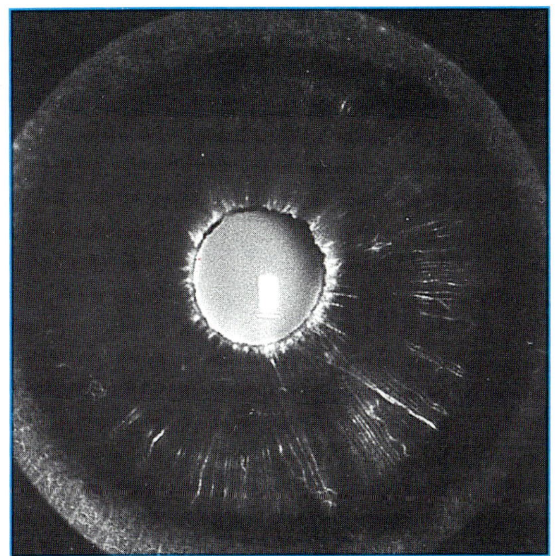

a)

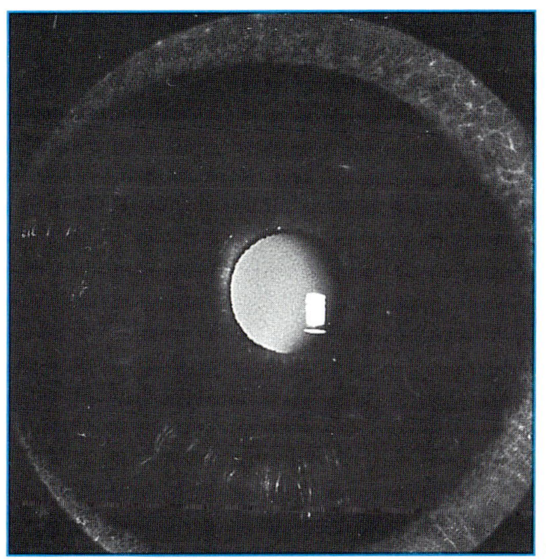

b)

*Fig. **4.7**,38 - Iris fluorangiography in another patient with Fuchs' heterochromic cyclitis (a) and in the other eye (b). Findings are comparable to those described in Fig. **4.7**,36.*

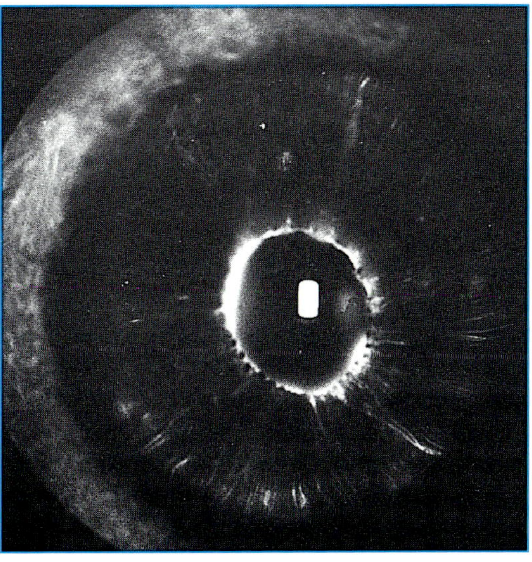

*Fig. **4.7**,39 - Same case of Fuchs' heterochromic cyclitis as above, one year after cataract removal. Iris fluorescein angiography shows no noteworthy changes.*

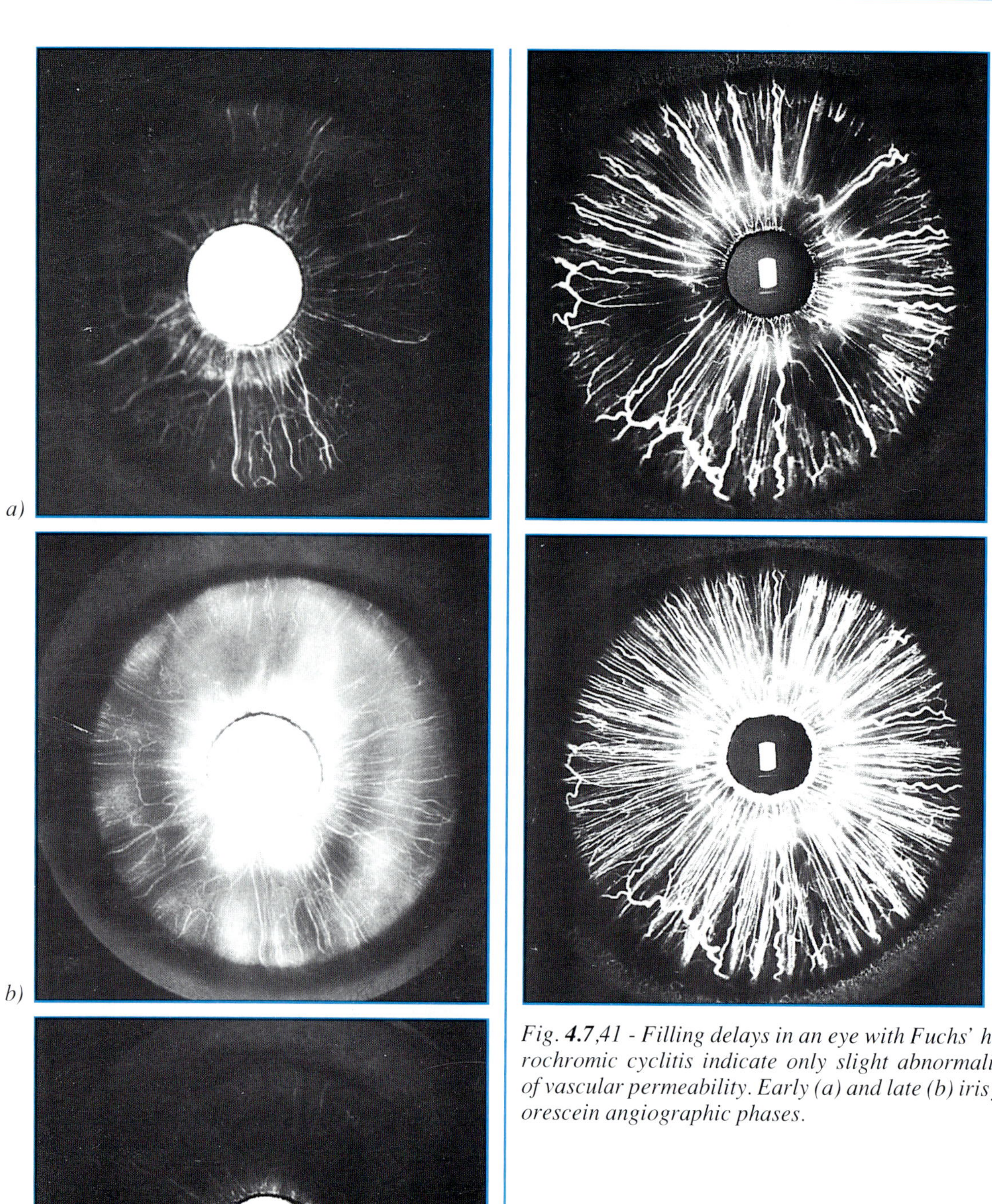

*Fig. **4.7**,40 - Iris fluorescein angiographic findings in another patient with Fuchs' heterochromic cyclitis in one eye (a,b) and the unaffected eye (c). In the affected eye the early phases of the examination (a) detect some distortion of the radial vascular structure and the later phases (b) show widespread, marked alterations to the permeability of the blood-iris barrier.*

*Fig. **4.7**,41 - Filling delays in an eye with Fuchs' heterochromic cyclitis indicate only slight abnormalities of vascular permeability. Early (a) and late (b) iris fluorescein angiographic phases.*

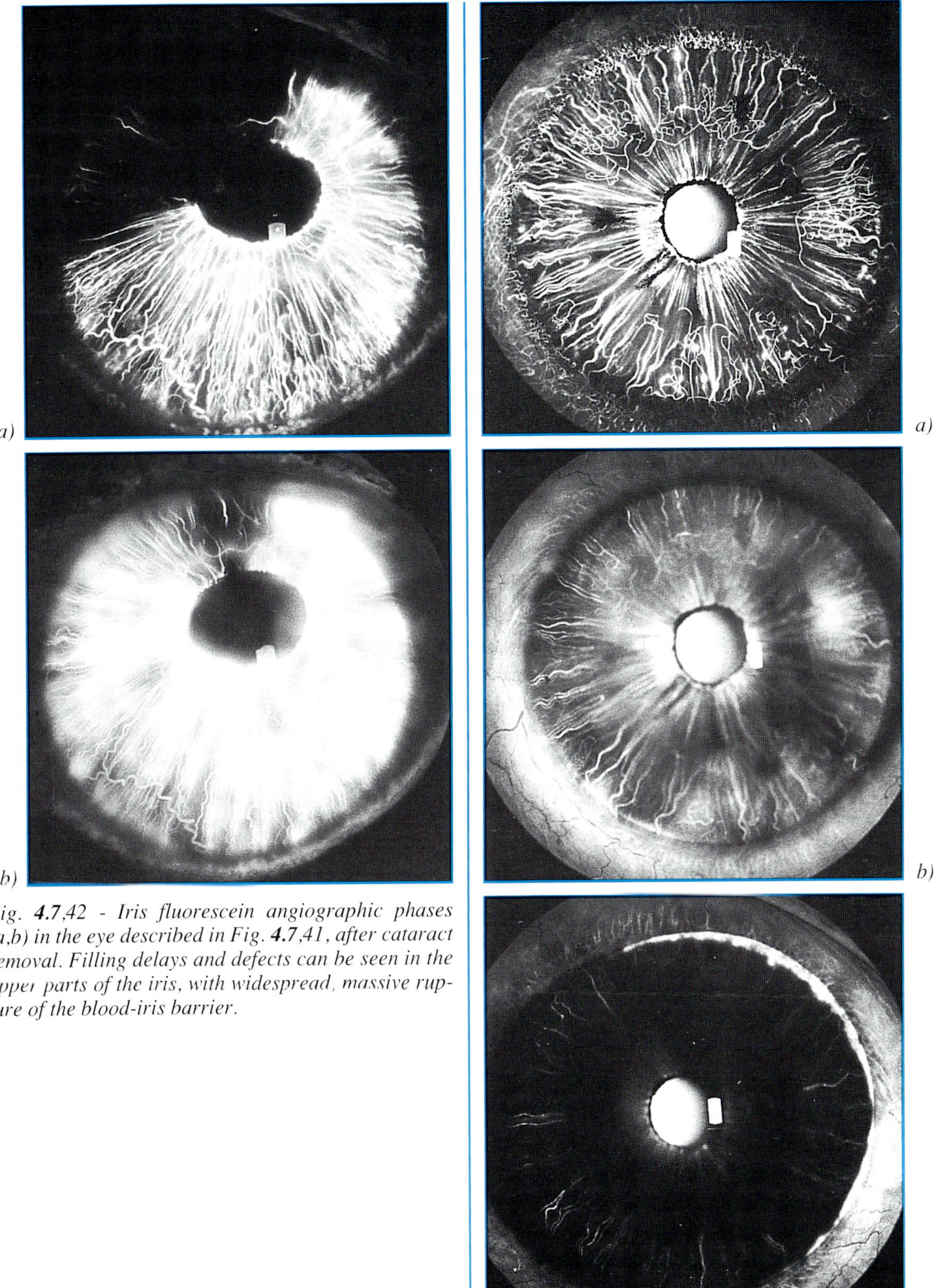

*Fig. **4.7**,42 - Iris fluorescein angiographic phases (a,b) in the eye described in Fig. **4.7**,41, after cataract removal. Filling delays and defects can be seen in the upper parts of the iris, with widespread, massive rupture of the blood-iris barrier.*

*Fig. **4.7**,43 - Early (a) and late (b) iris fluorescein angiographic phases in Fuchs' heterochromic cyclitis. Radial vessels show marked anomalies in caliber, path and permeability. The contralateral eye (c) shows virtually normal findings.*

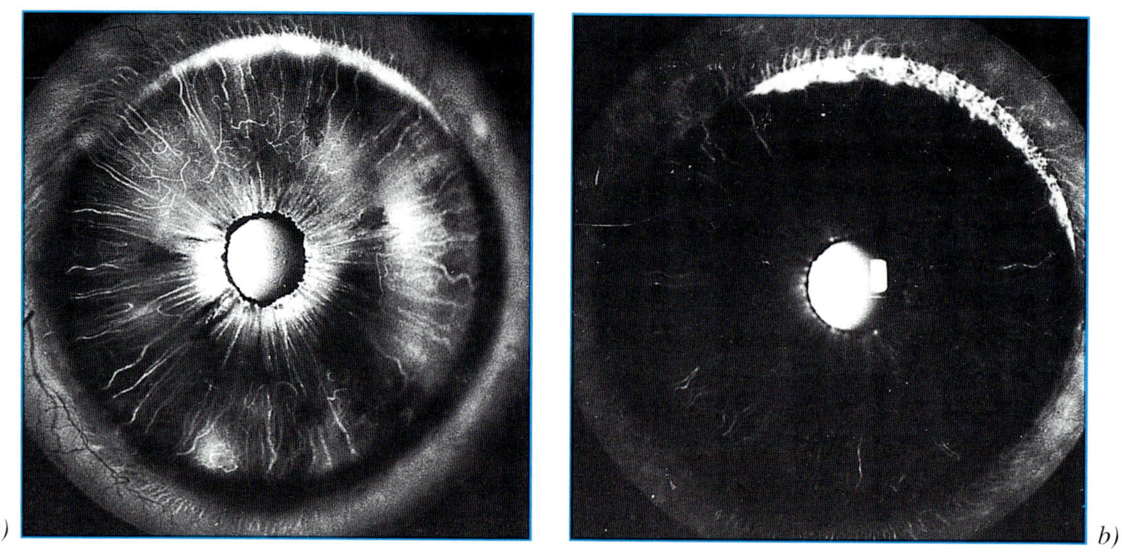

a) *b)*

*Fig. **4.7**,44 - Same case as above, one year later. The iris fluorescein angiographic pictures for the two eyes appear the same, except that there is somewhat less damage to the blood-iris barrier in the affected eye (a) (b: contralateral eye).*

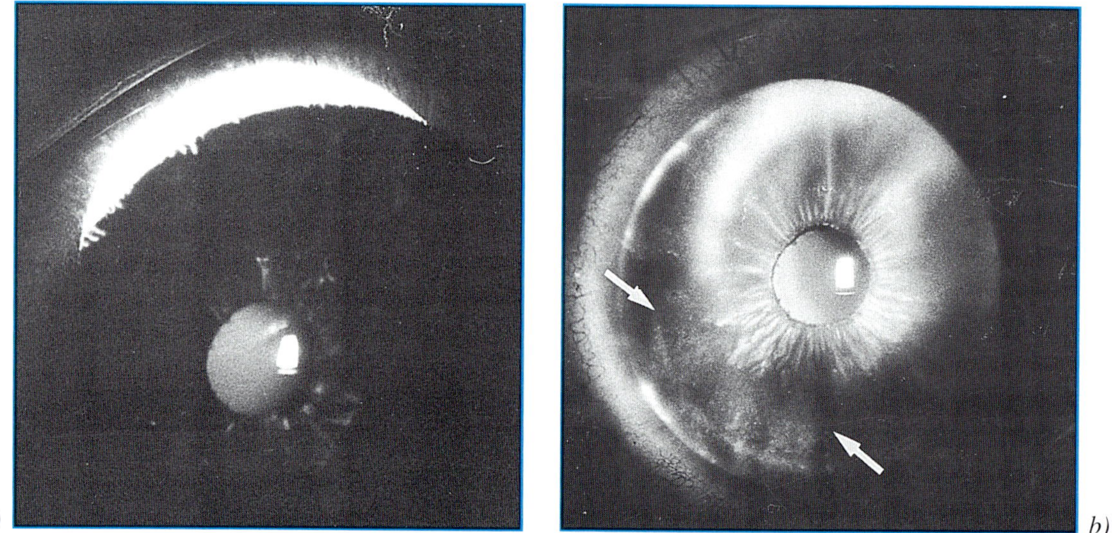

a) *b)*

*Fig. **4.7**,45 - Early (a) and late (b) iris fluorescein angiographic phases in a patient who had had the Posner-Schlossman syndrome. In the late phases diffuse hyperfluorescence is visible on account of the marked permeability of the iris vessels. In the inferior quadrants (see arrows) there is an area of uneven hyperfluorescence caused by a window effect over a zone with rarefied pigment.*

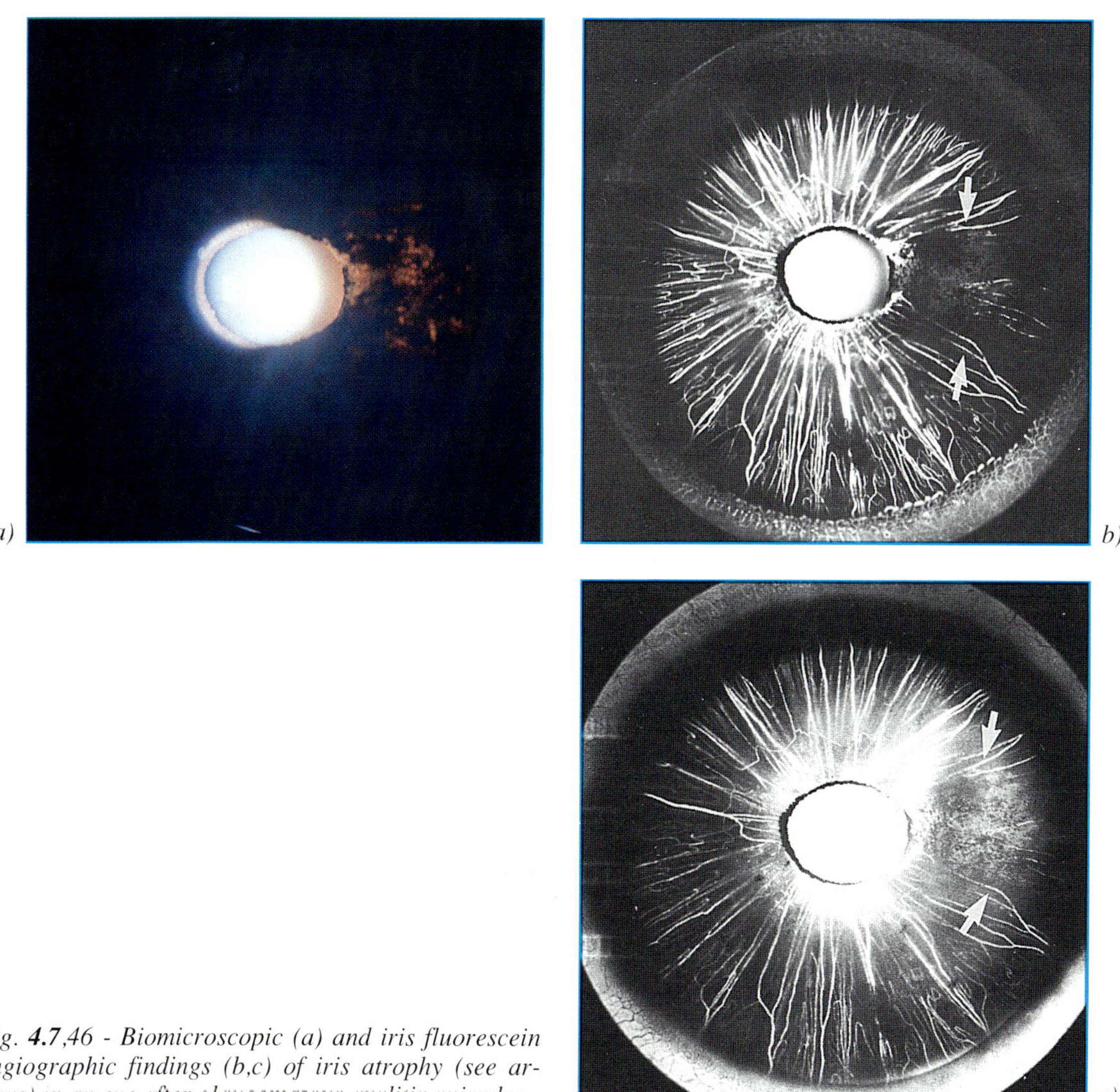

a) b) c)

*Fig. **4.7**,46 - Biomicroscopic (a) and iris fluorescein angiographic findings (b,c) of iris atrophy (see arrows) in an eye after glaucomatous-cyclitic episodes.*

a) b)

*Fig. **4.7**,47 - Same case as in the previous figure, one year later. The area of atrophy is clearly outlined and remains hypofluorescent on account of the lack of perfusion (a,b: angiographic phases).*

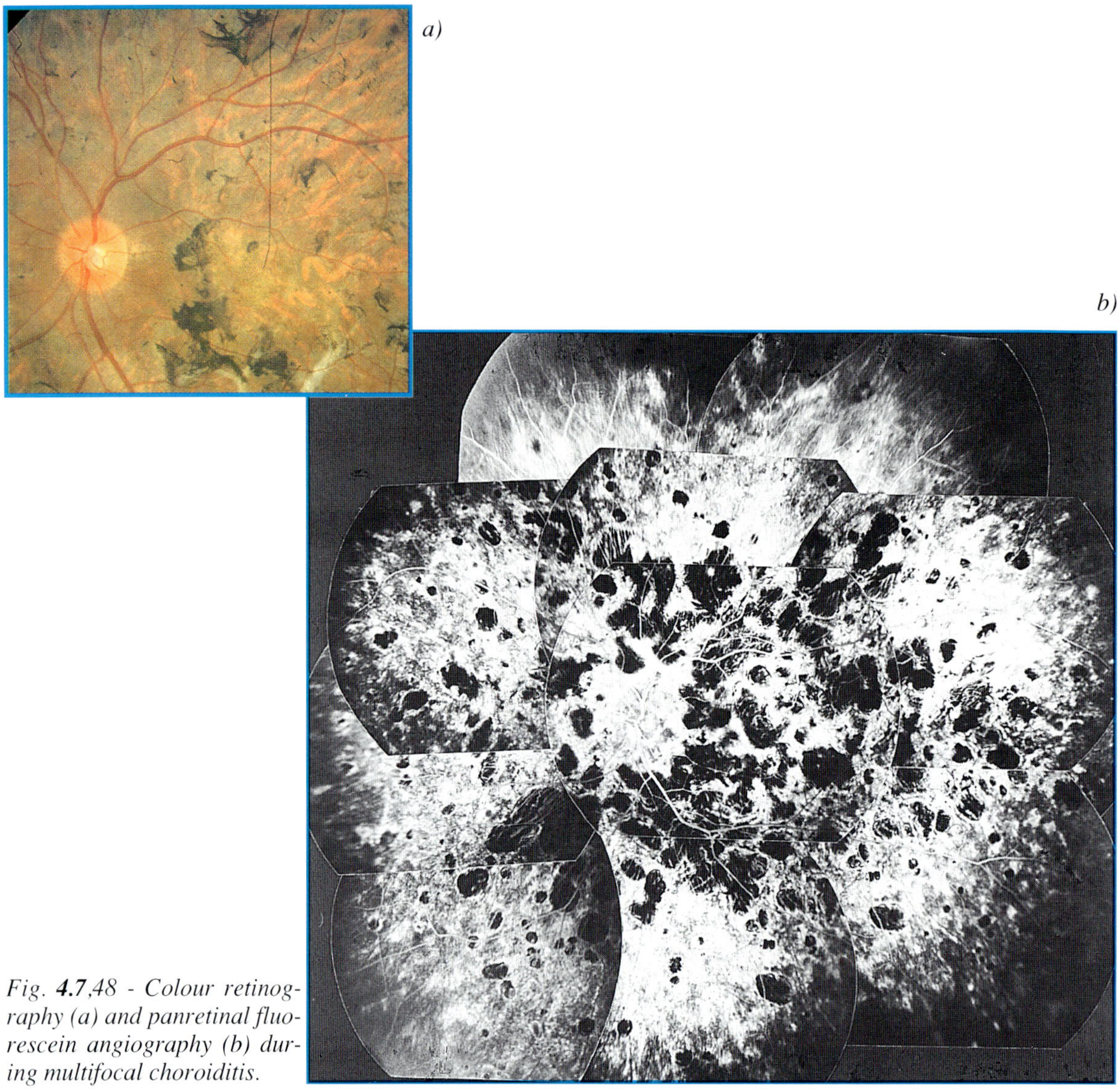

a)

b)

*Fig. **4.7**,48 - Colour retinography (a) and panretinal fluorescein angiography (b) during multifocal choroiditis.*

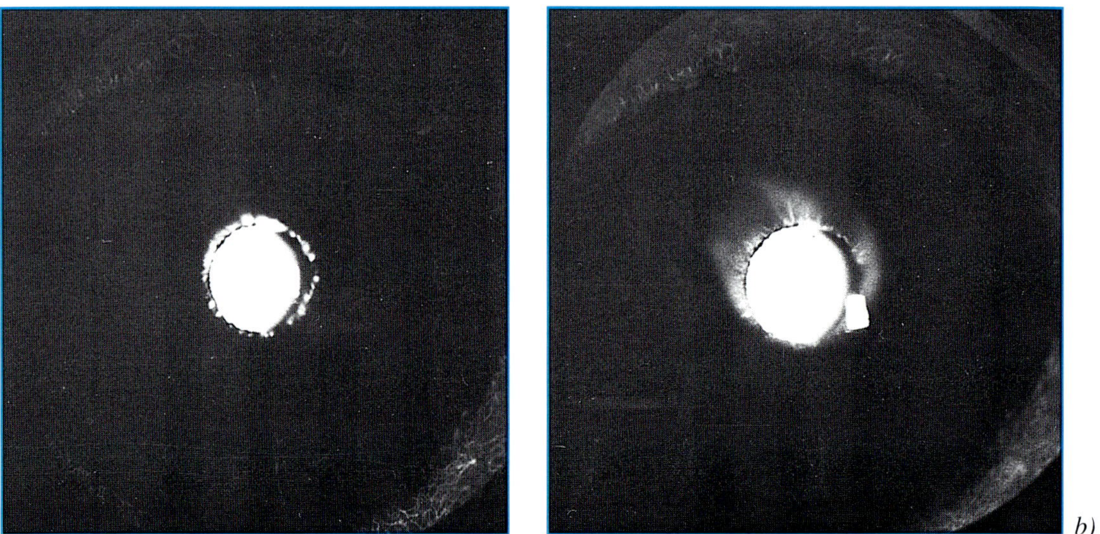

a) *b)*

*Fig. **4.7**,49 - Same case as in the previous figure: iris fluorescein angiographic findings. Initial hyperfluorescent tufts can be seen around the pupillary border (a), leaking dye in the later phases (b).*

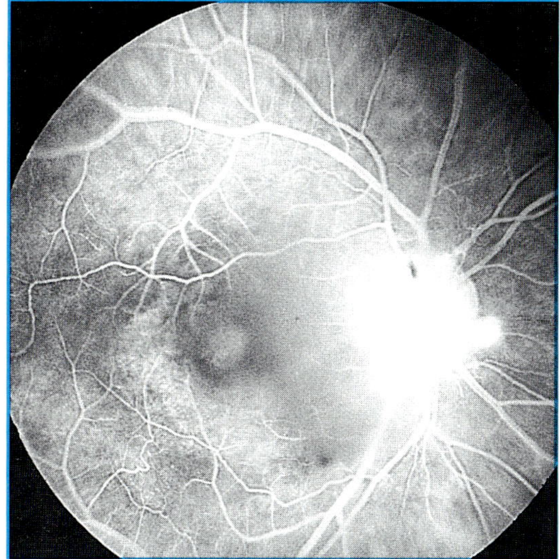

Fig. ***4.7****,50 - Posterior uveitis: retinal fluorescein angiographic picture.*

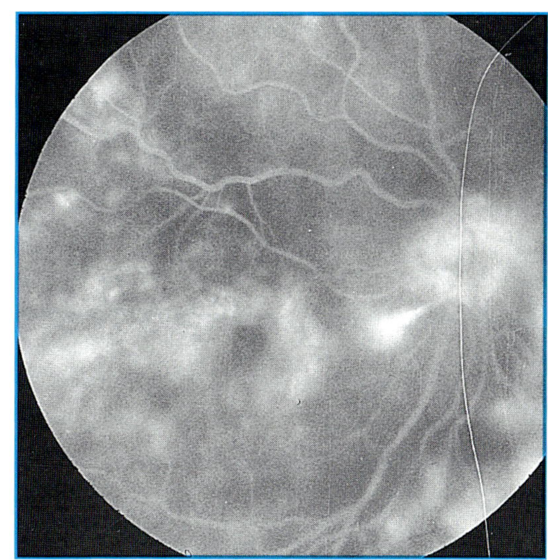

Fig. ***4.7****,52 - Another retinal fluorescein angiographic exam during posterior uveitis.*

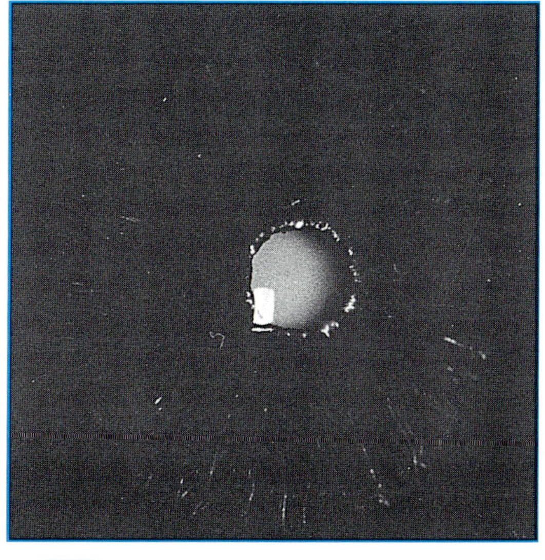

a)

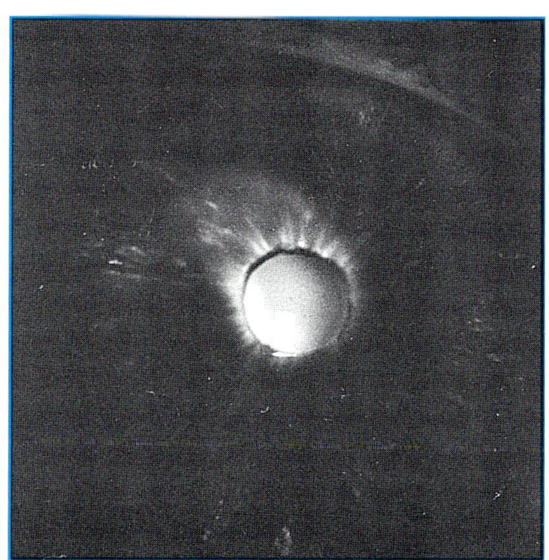

b)

Fig. ***4.7****,51 - Same case as in fig.* ***4.7****,50; iris angiography shows early hyperfluorescence around the pupillary border (a) with slight dye leakage in later phases (b).*

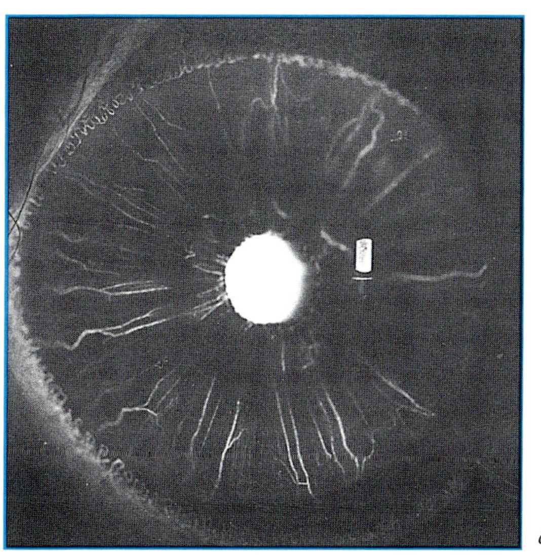

a)

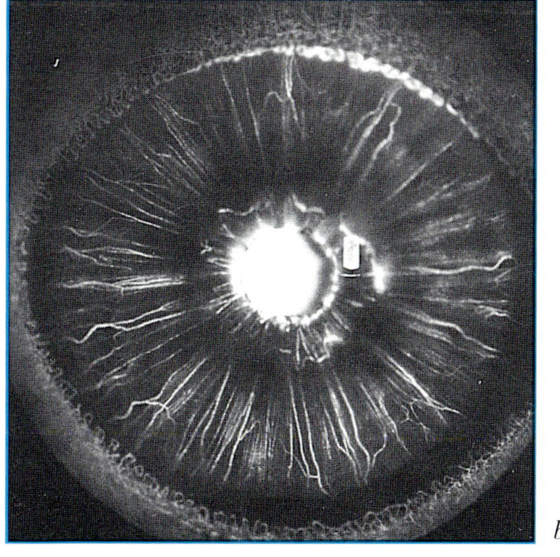

b)

Fig. ***4.7****,53 - Same case as in fig.* ***4.7****,52; early (a) and late (b) iris fluorescein angiographic phases. Permeability of the pupillary vessels of the iris is altered.*

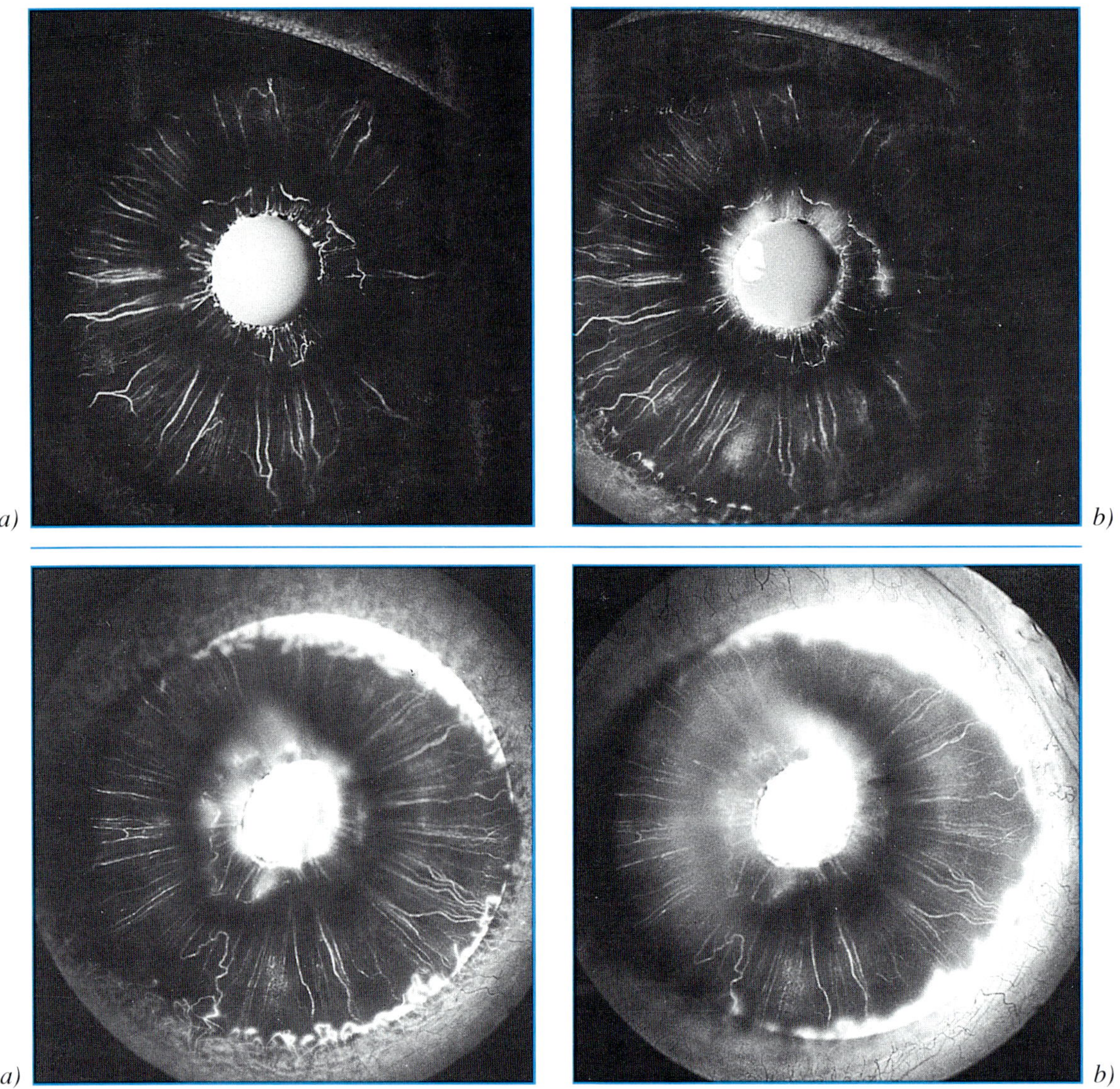

a) *b)*

a) *b)*

Figs. ***4.7****,54,55 - Early (a) and late (b) iris fluorescein angiographic findings in more cases of posterior uveitis, showing anomalies similar to those of the previous figure. Stromal vessels appear only slightly affected.*

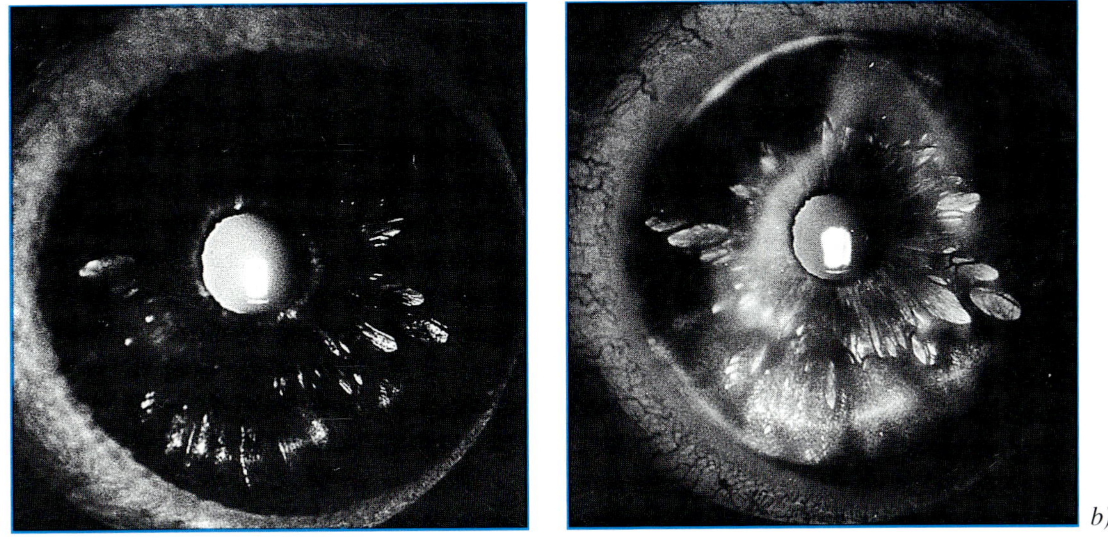

*Fig. **4.7**,56 - Early (a) and late (b) iris fluorescein findings in another instance of posterior uveitis. This case appears to have more marked concomitant anterior inflammation and the blood-iris barrier is broken in the stromal vessels too. The underlying iris vascular structure can be visualized, on account of a window effect, so the atrophic areas appear hyperfluorescent.*

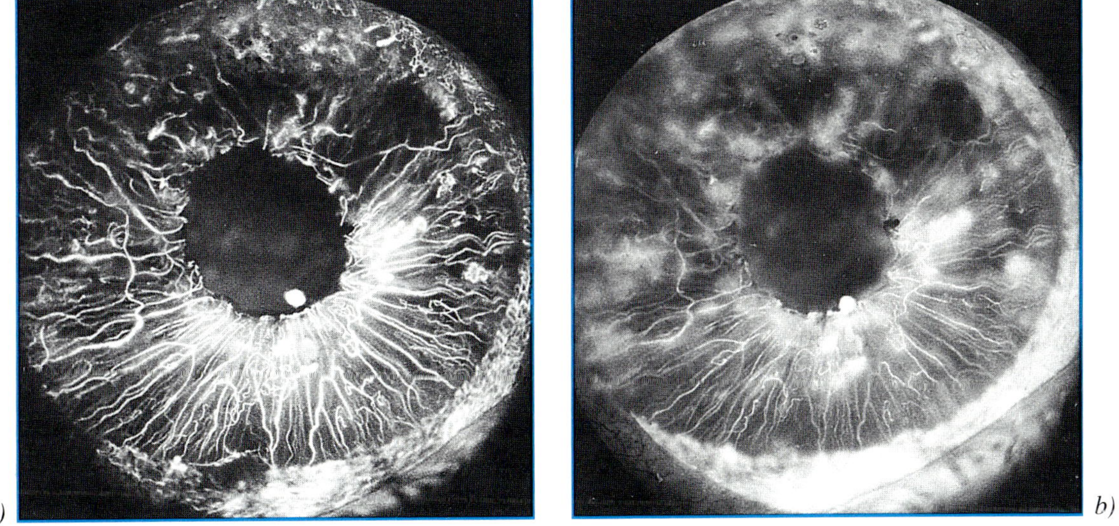

*Fig. **4.7**,57 - In posterior uveitis, the iris structure may - as in this case - be markedly distorted. Iris fluorescein angiography shows the caliber, path and permeability of all the vessels are altered and small hyperfluorescent neovascular tufts can be seen (a,b). In the superior sectors zones of ischemia remain hypofluorescent even in the late phases (b).*

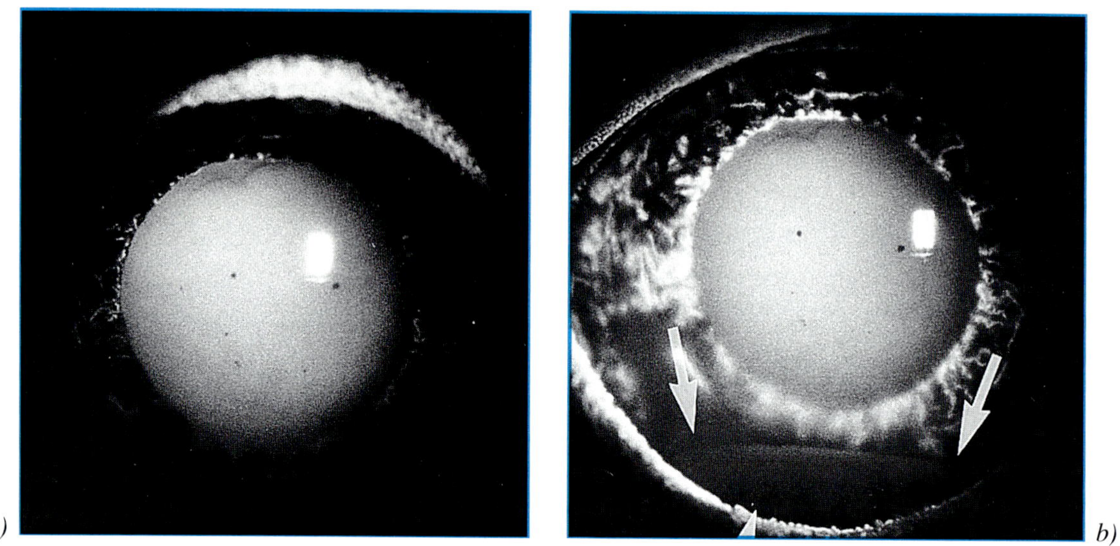

*Fig. **4.7**,58 - Early (a) and late (b) iris fluorescein angiographic pictures in neovascular glaucoma resulting from posterior uveitis. A masking effect produces hypofluorescence over the hyphema (see arrows).*

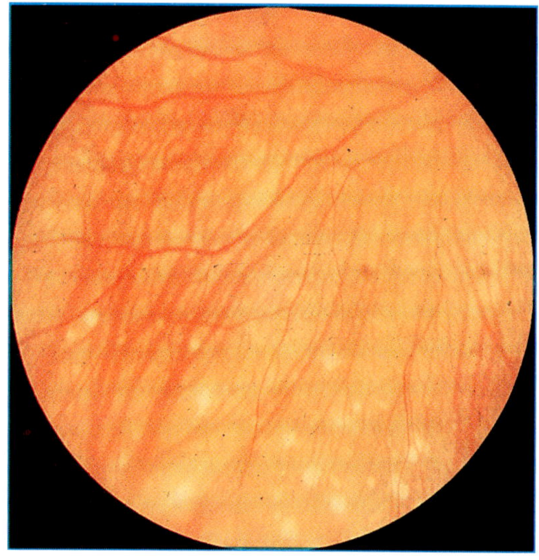

*Fig. **4.7**,59 - Birdshot retinochoroidopathy: colour retinography.*

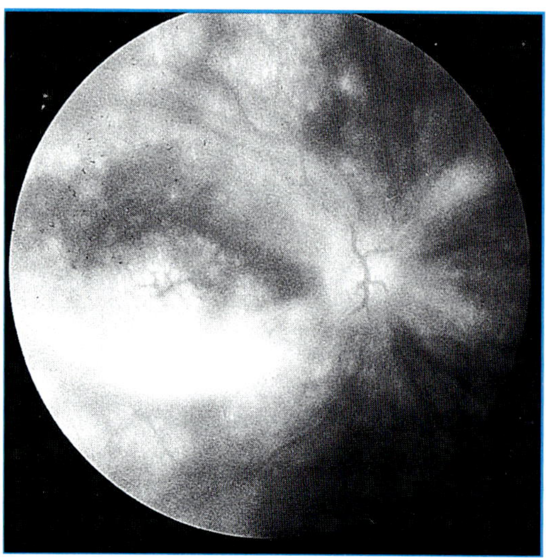

*Fig. **4.7**,60 - Retinal fluorescein angiography in Birdshot retinochoroidopathy.*

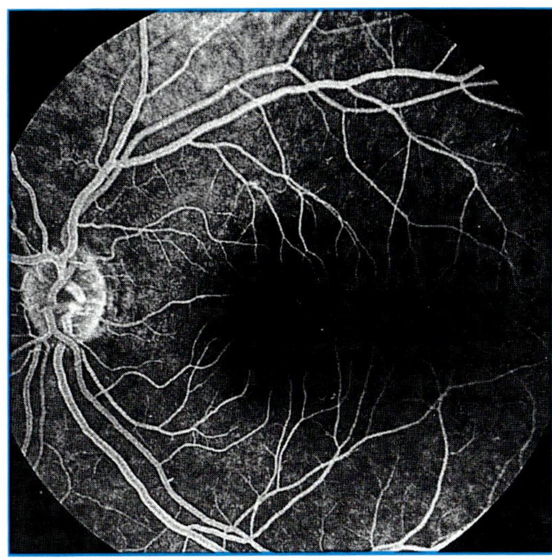

*Fig. **4.7**,61 - The other eye of the patient in the previous figure: retinal angiography is virtually normal.*

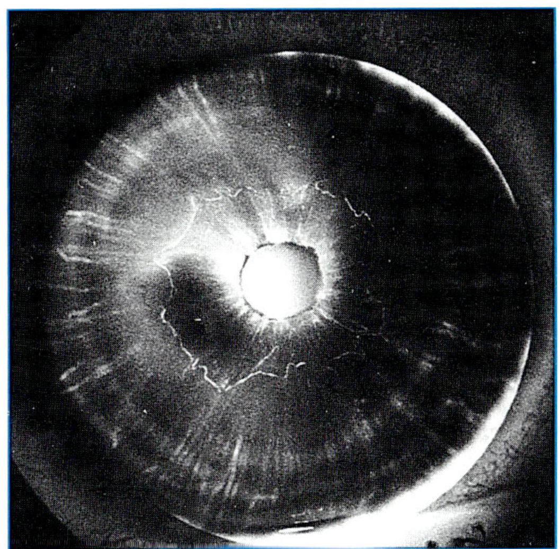

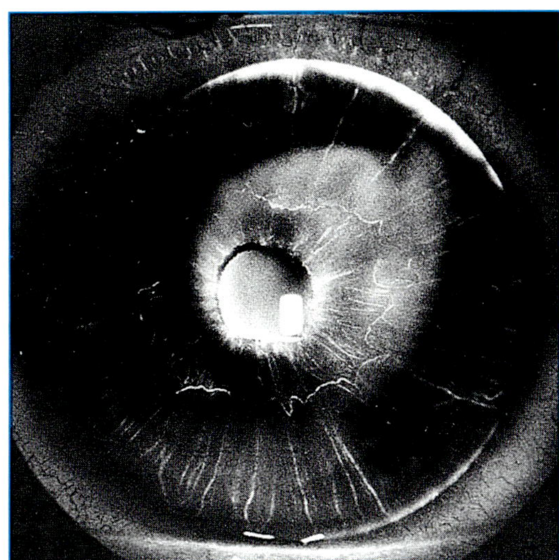

*Figs. **4.7**,62,63 - Same patient as in figures **4.7**,60,61: iris fluorescein angiographic findings are comparable in the eye with Birdshot retinochoroidopathy (Fig. **4.7**,62) and in the other eye (Fig. **4.7**,63). Both eyes present slight hyperfluorescence resulting from the altered permeability of the pupillary microvasculature.*

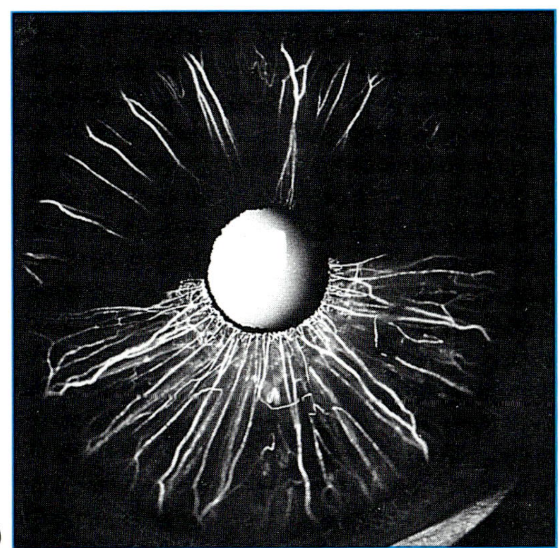

a)

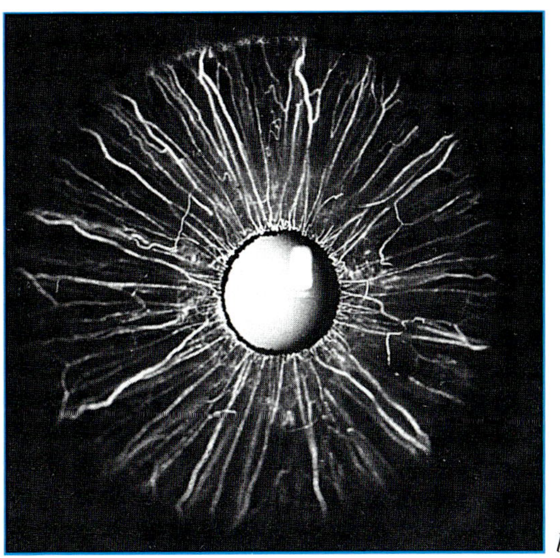

b)

*Fig. **4.7**,64 - Early (a) and late (b) iris fluorescein angiographic findings in a case of Birdshot retino-choroidopathy. The path and caliber of the radial vessels are irregular, and there are filling delays but no defects.*

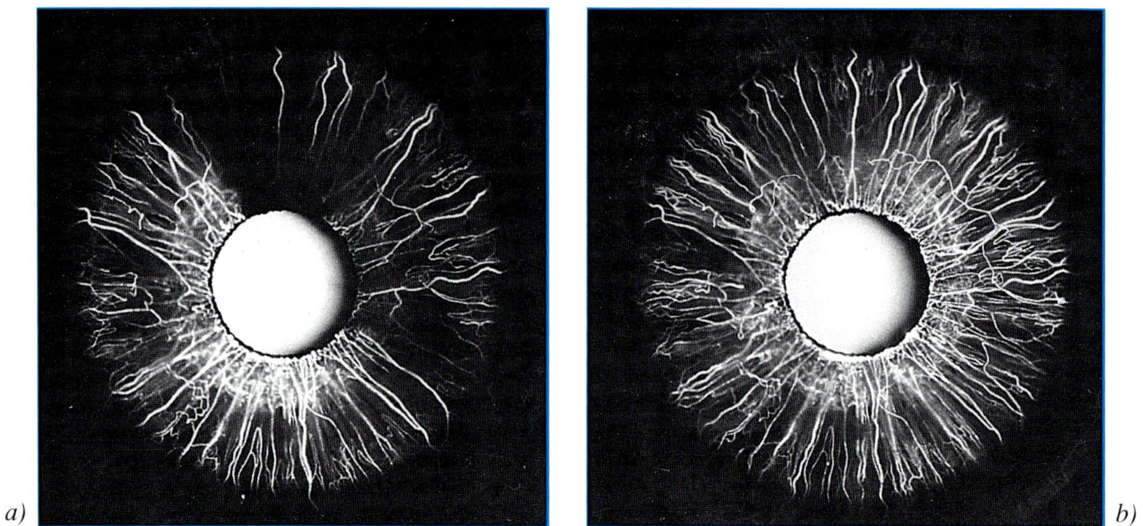

*Fig. **4.7**,65 - Early (a) and late (b) iris fluorescein angiographic findings in another case of Birdshot retinochoroidopathy with filling delays.*

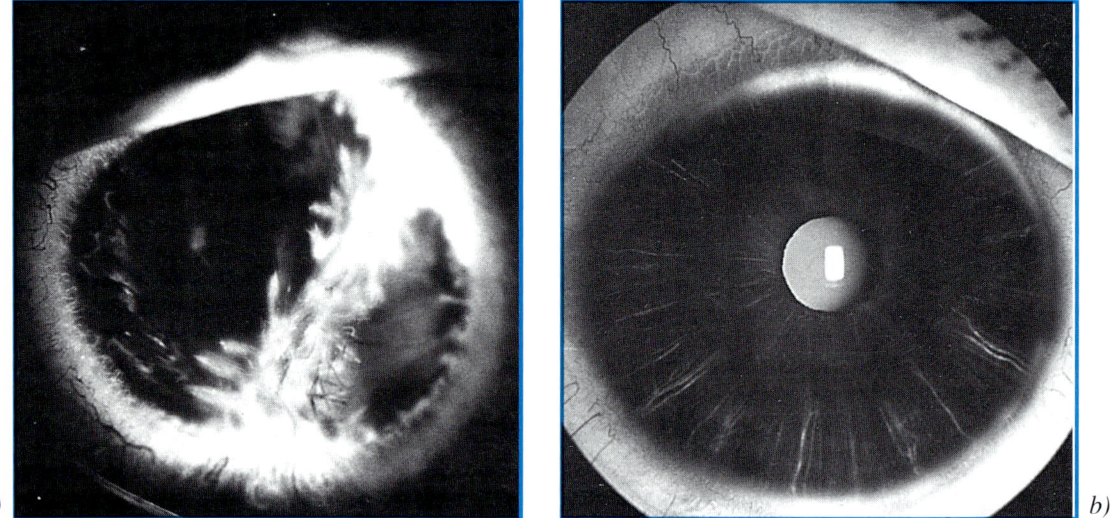

*Fig. **4.7**,66 - Iris fluorescein angiography in an eye with perforating trauma (a) and the other eye (b), which presents no noteworthy abnormalities.*

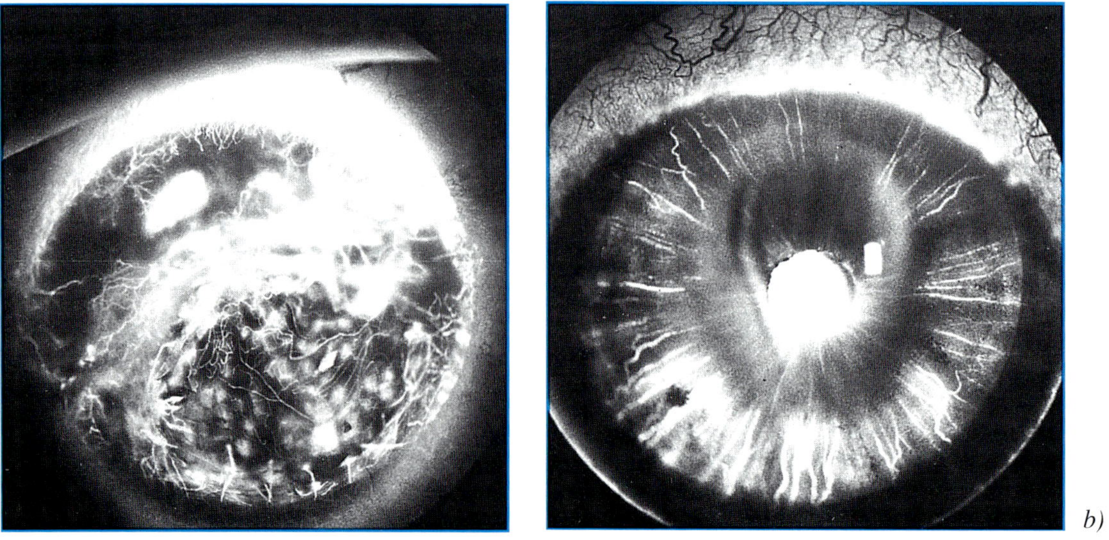

*Fig. **4.7**,67 - Trauma (a) may cause uveitis (sympathetic ophthalmia) in the contralateral eye (b) where the blood-iris barrier is markedly and extensively damaged.*

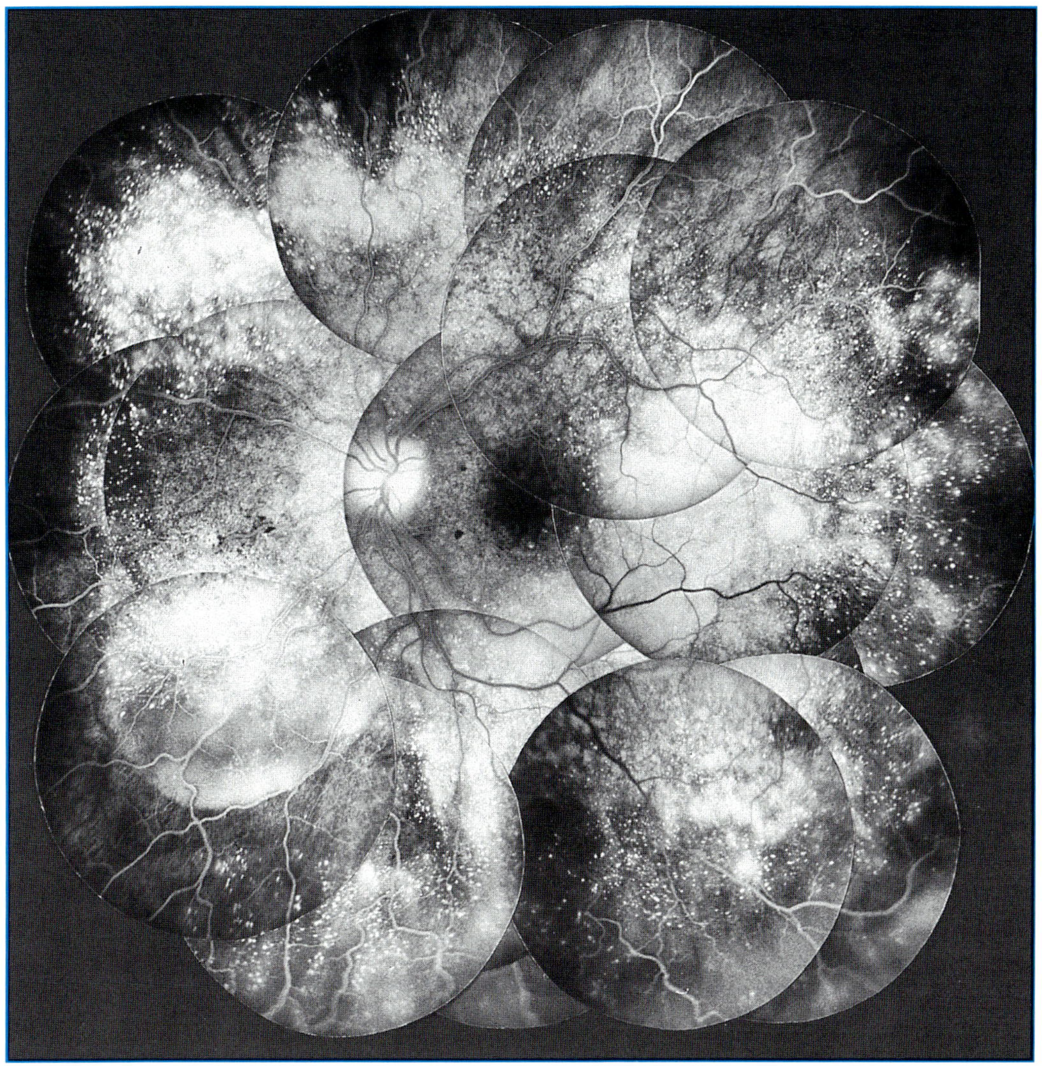

*Fig. **4.7**,68 - Vogt-Koyanagi-Harada syndrome: panretinal fluorescein angiography.*

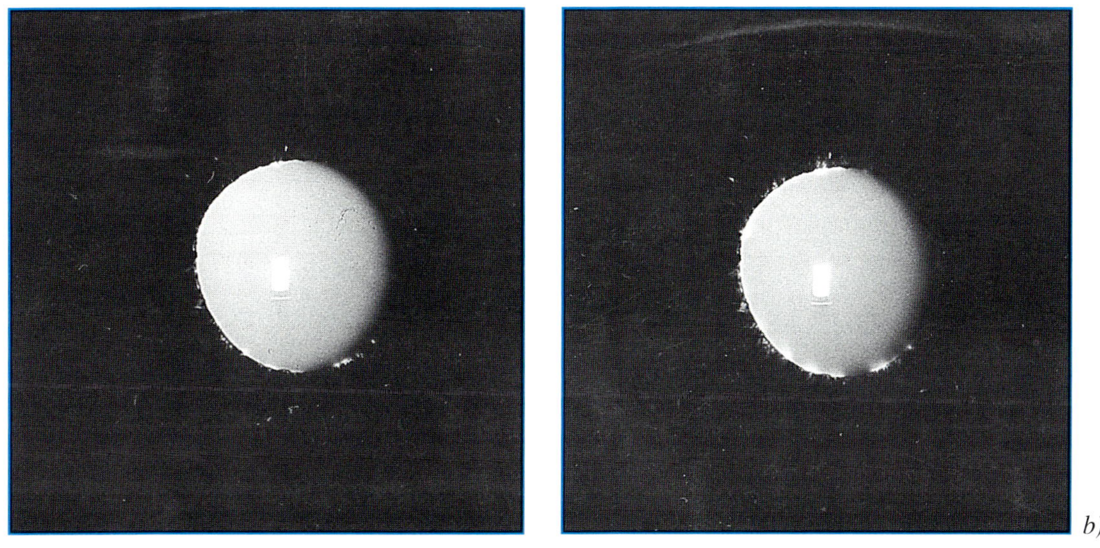

a) *b)*

*Fig. **4.7**,69 - Early (a) and late (b) iris fluorescein angiography of the same eye as in the above figure shows slight pupillary leakage.*

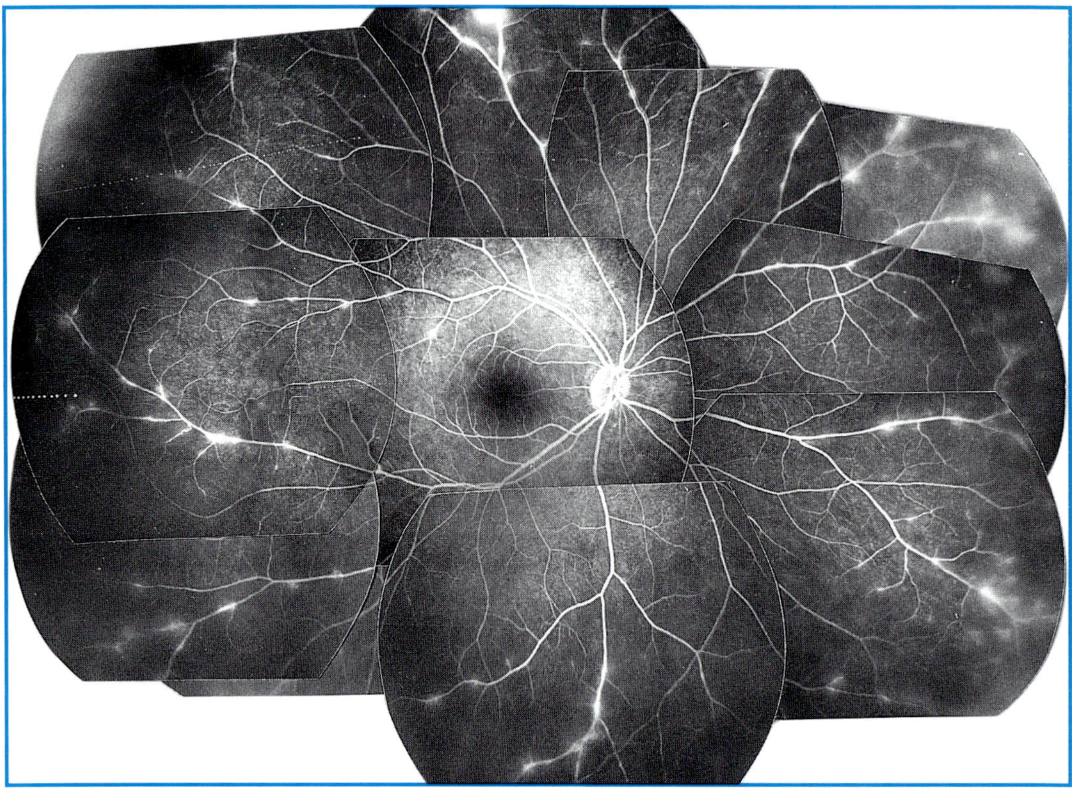

Fig. ***4.7****,70 - Panretinal fluorescein angiography in retinal vasculitis: the picture is dominated by perivascular dye leakage and large nonperfused retinal areas.*

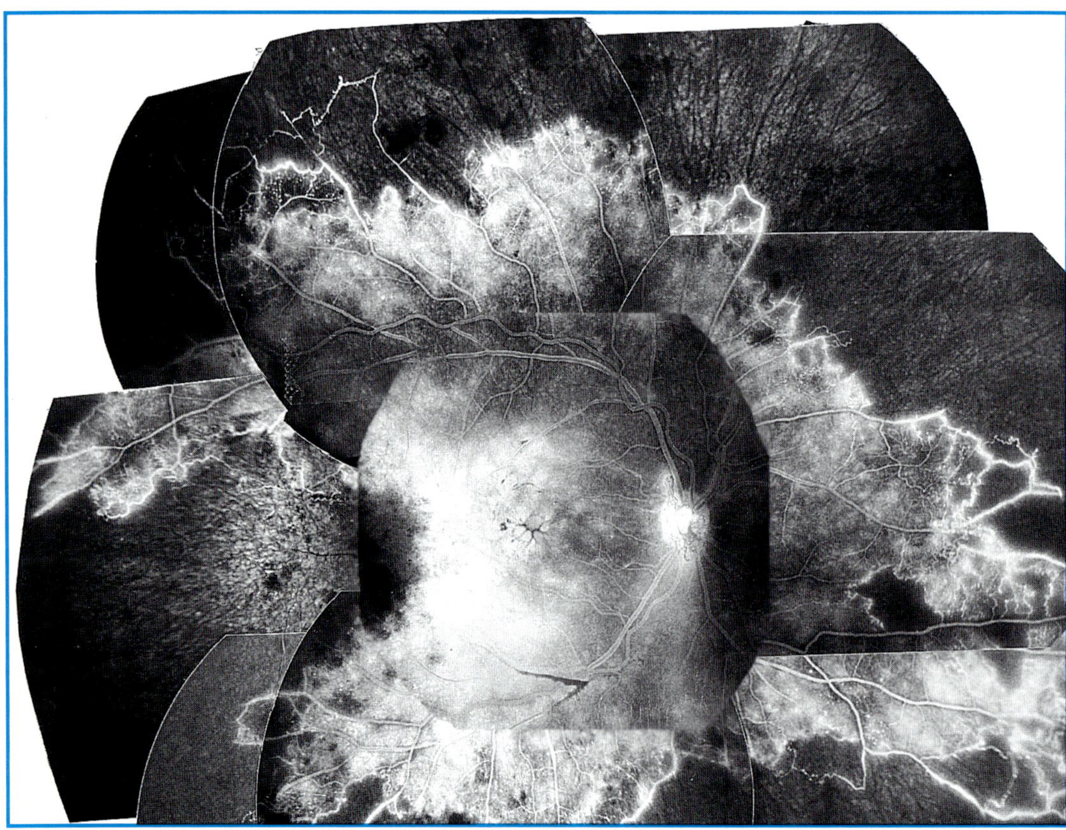

Fig. ***4.7****,71 - Another fluorescein angiographic examination in retinal vasculitis. There are wide peripheral areas with capillary nonperfusion, epipapillary new vessels and cystoid macular edema.*

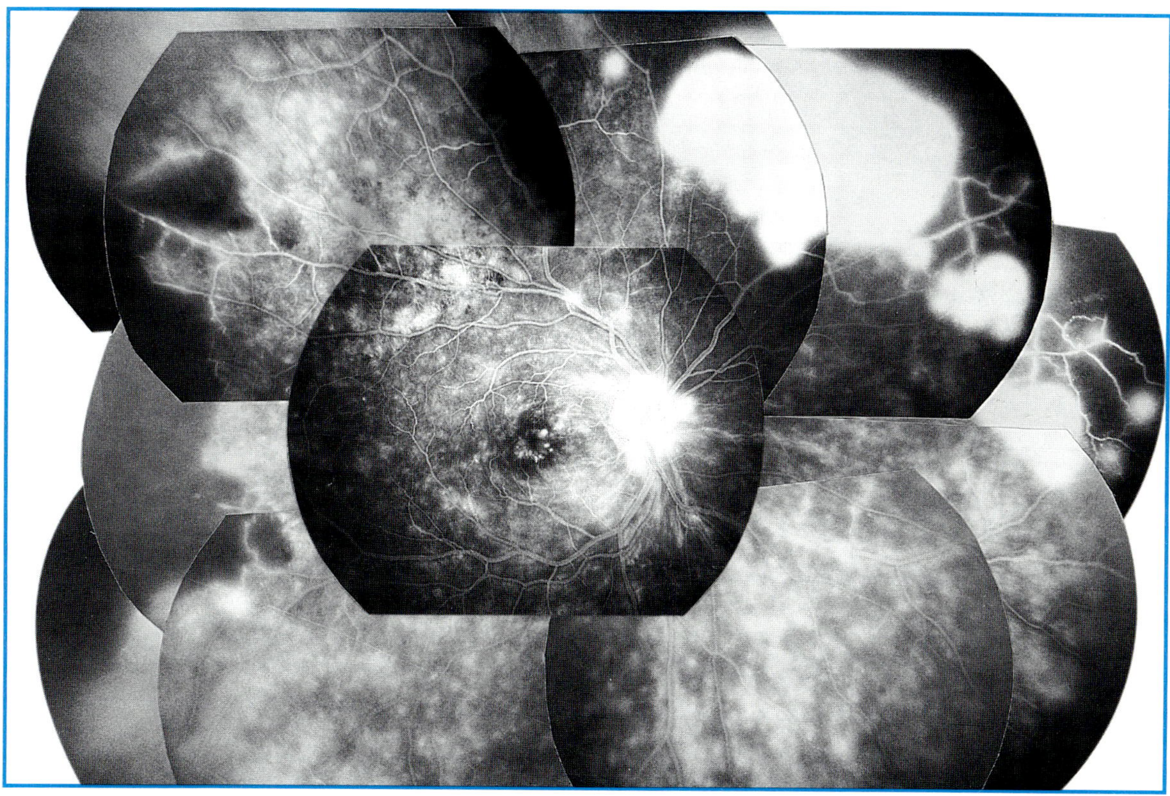

*Fig. **4.7**,72 - Retinal vasculitis complicated by large ischemic areas and imposing epiretinal and epipapillary new vessels (panretinal fluorescein angiography).*

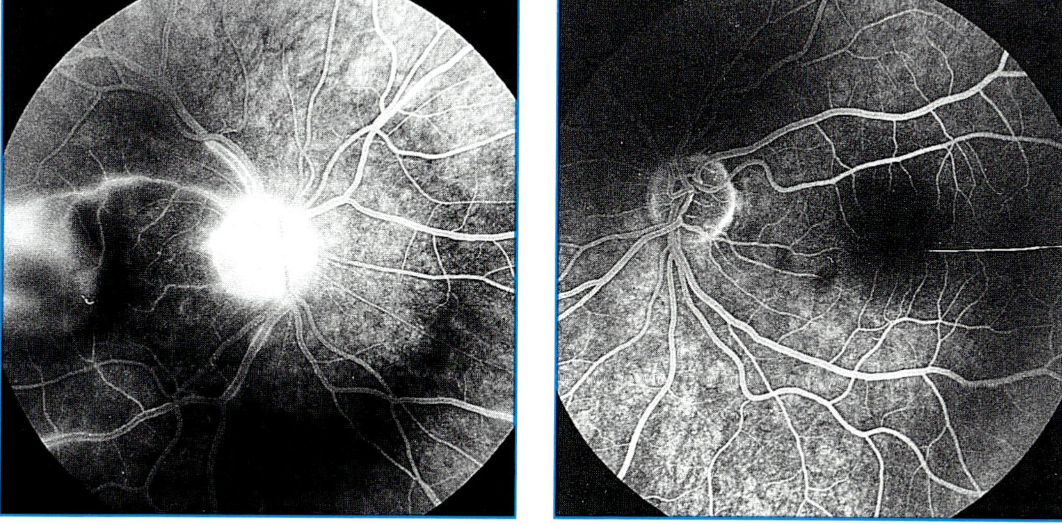

*Figs. **4.7**,73,74 - Retinal fluorescein angiography of an eye with retinal vasculitis (Fig. **4.7**,73) and the other unaffected eye (Fig. **4.7**,74).*

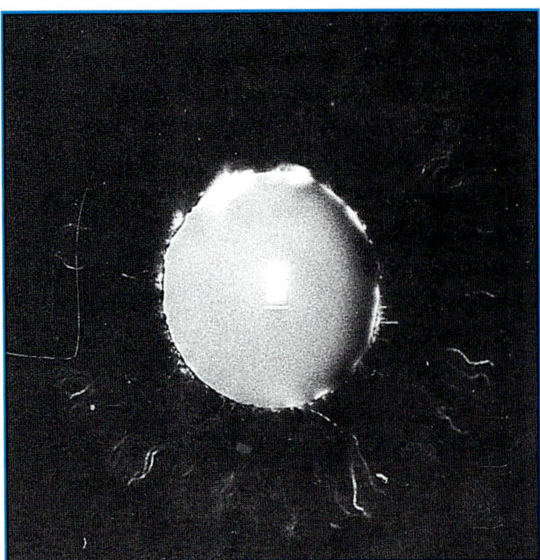

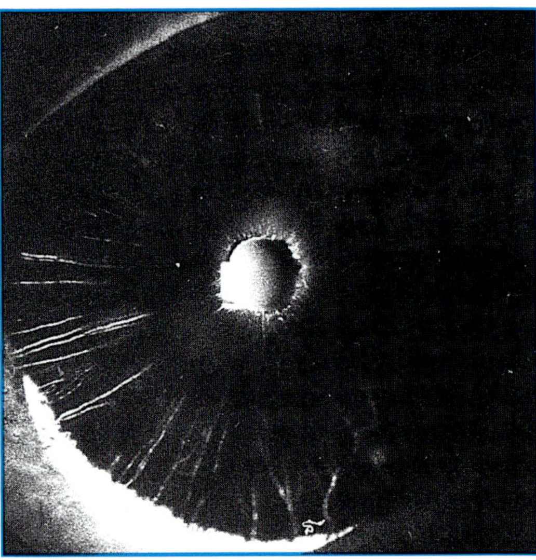

Figs. ***4.7****,75,76 - Same eyes as in figs.* ***4.7****,73,74: iris fluorescein angiography shows they differ in that pupillary dye leakage is slightly more marked in the eye with retinal vasculitis (Fig.* ***4.7****,75) than in the other one (Fig.* ***4.7****,76).*

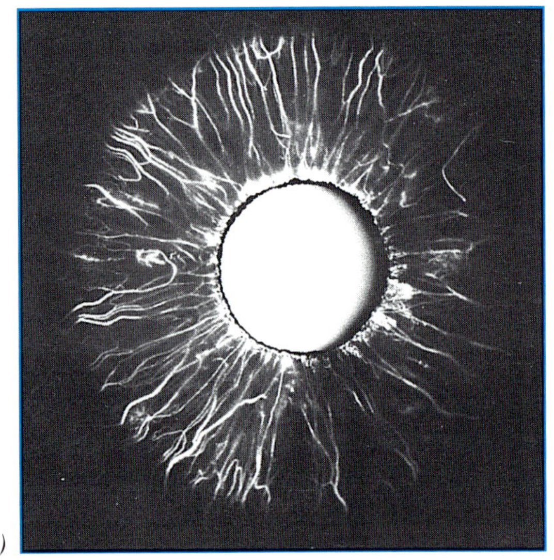

a)

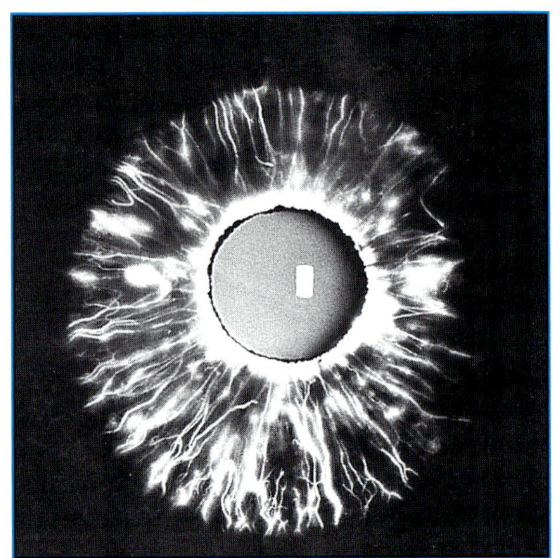

b)

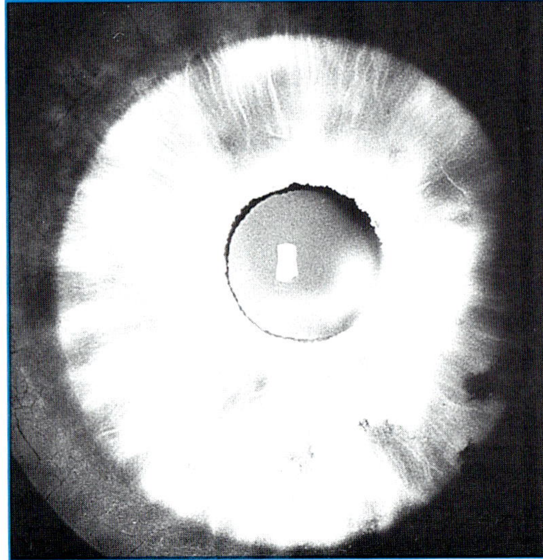

c)

Fig. ***4.7****,77 - Iris fluorescein angiography shows serious alterations in this case of retinal vasculitis. There are pupillary and extrapupillary neovascular tufts showing early hyperfluorescence (a), marked congestion of the radial vessels (b) and large-scale rupture of the entire blood-iris barrier, involving the whole anterior chamber in the later phases (c).*

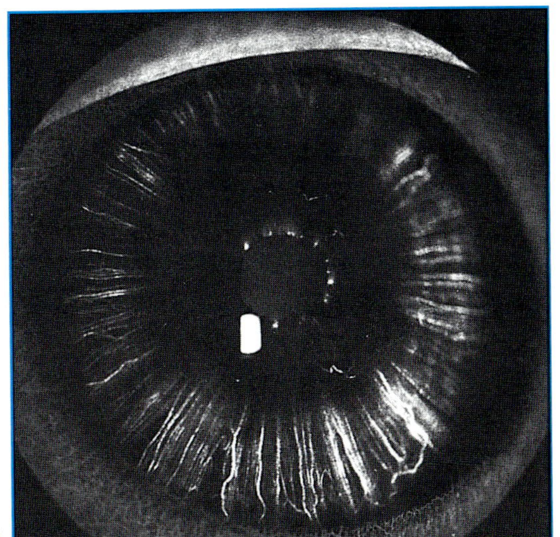
a)

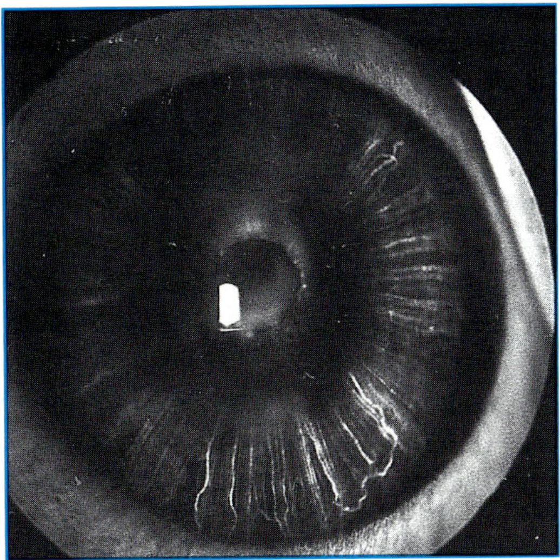
b)

*Fig. **4.7**,78 - Iris fluorescein angiographic phases (a,b) in a 40-year-old patient with Behçet's disease. The excess of pigment impedes visualization of the peripupillary vascular structure. There is slight peripupillary leakage.*

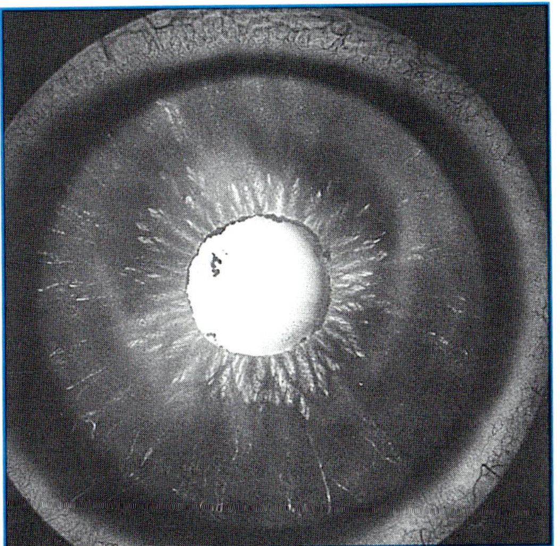

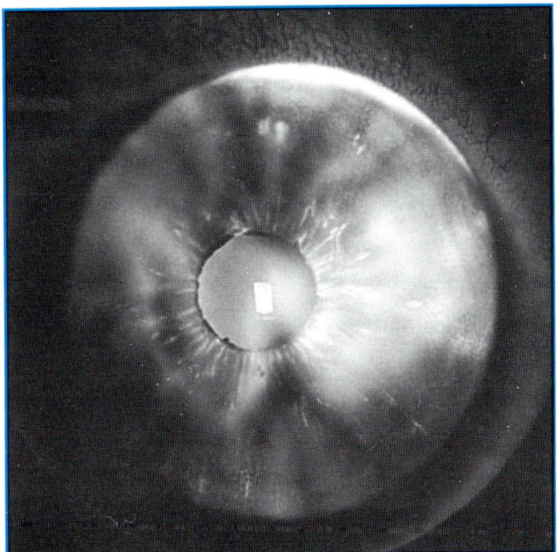

*Figs. **4.7**,79,80 - Same case of Behçet's disease before (Fig. **4.7**,79) and 12 months later (Fig. **4.7**,80). The greater amount of dye leakage is indicative of further damage to the blood-iris barrier, already ruptured at the initial visit.*

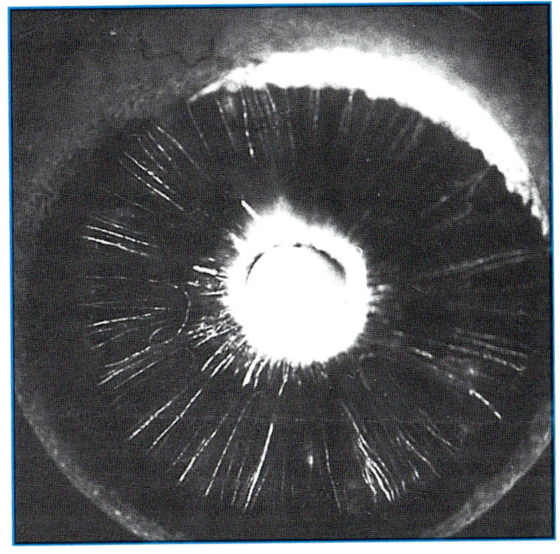
a)

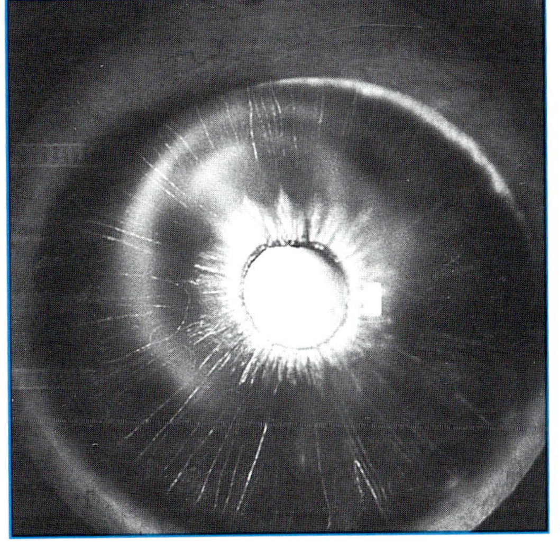
b)

*Fig. **4.7**,81 - Iris fluorescein angiographic findings (a,b) in a 34-year-old patient with Behçet's disease. The patient's age and the intensity of the hyperfluorescence are the features that suggest this peripupillary leakage is pathological, and indicative of increased vascular permeability.*

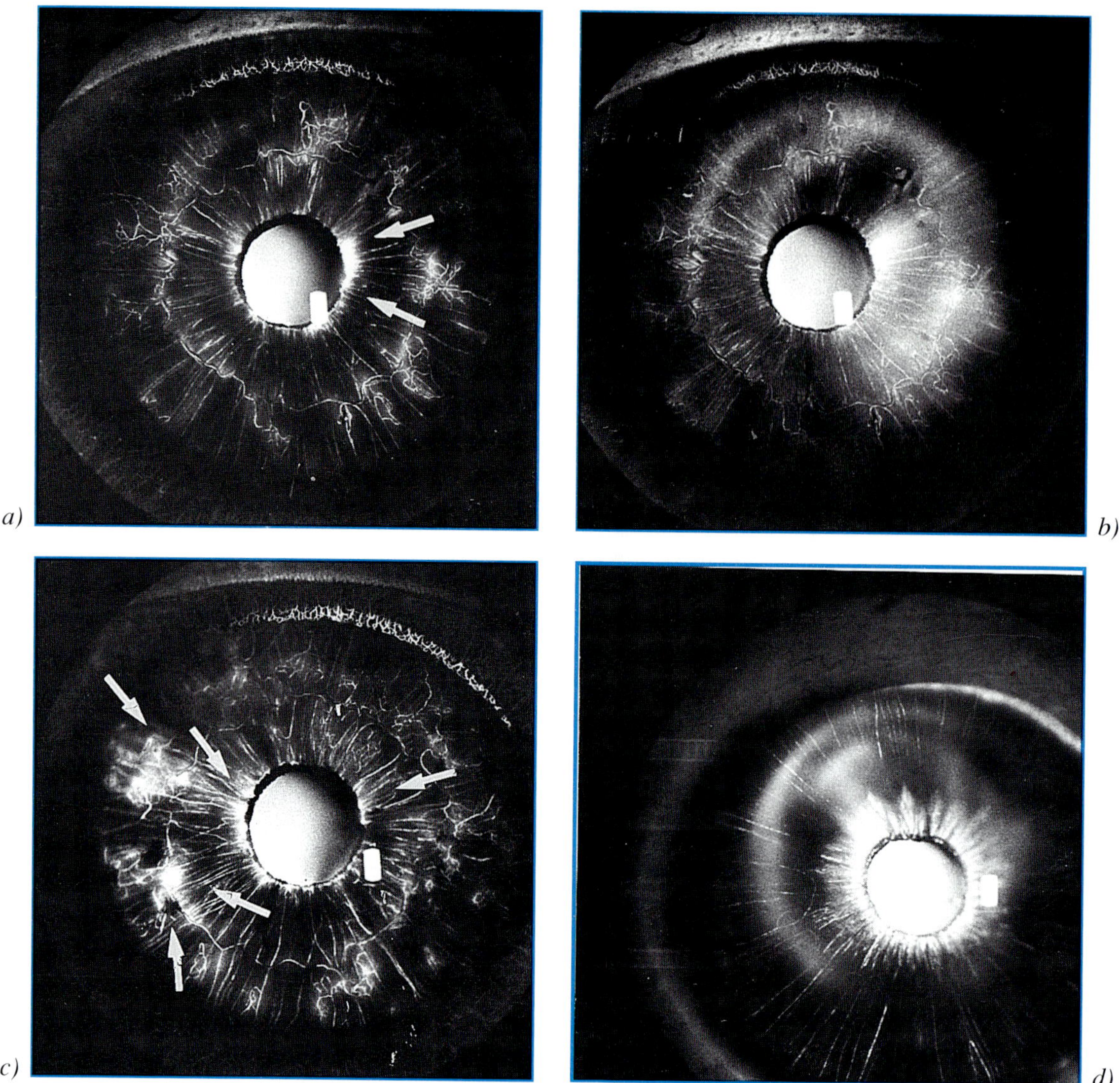

*Fig. **4.7**,82 - Marked upheaval of the radial vascular structures of both eyes (a,b: left eye; c,d: right eye), in a patient with Behçet's disease. Anomalous, tortuous vessels, taking up dye early (a,c) are visible, especially in the peripheral two thirds of the iris stroma. Leakage in the anterior chamber (b,d) starts from the areas of early hyperfluorescence in the peripupillary parts of the left eye (a) and stroma too in the right one (c) (see arrows).*

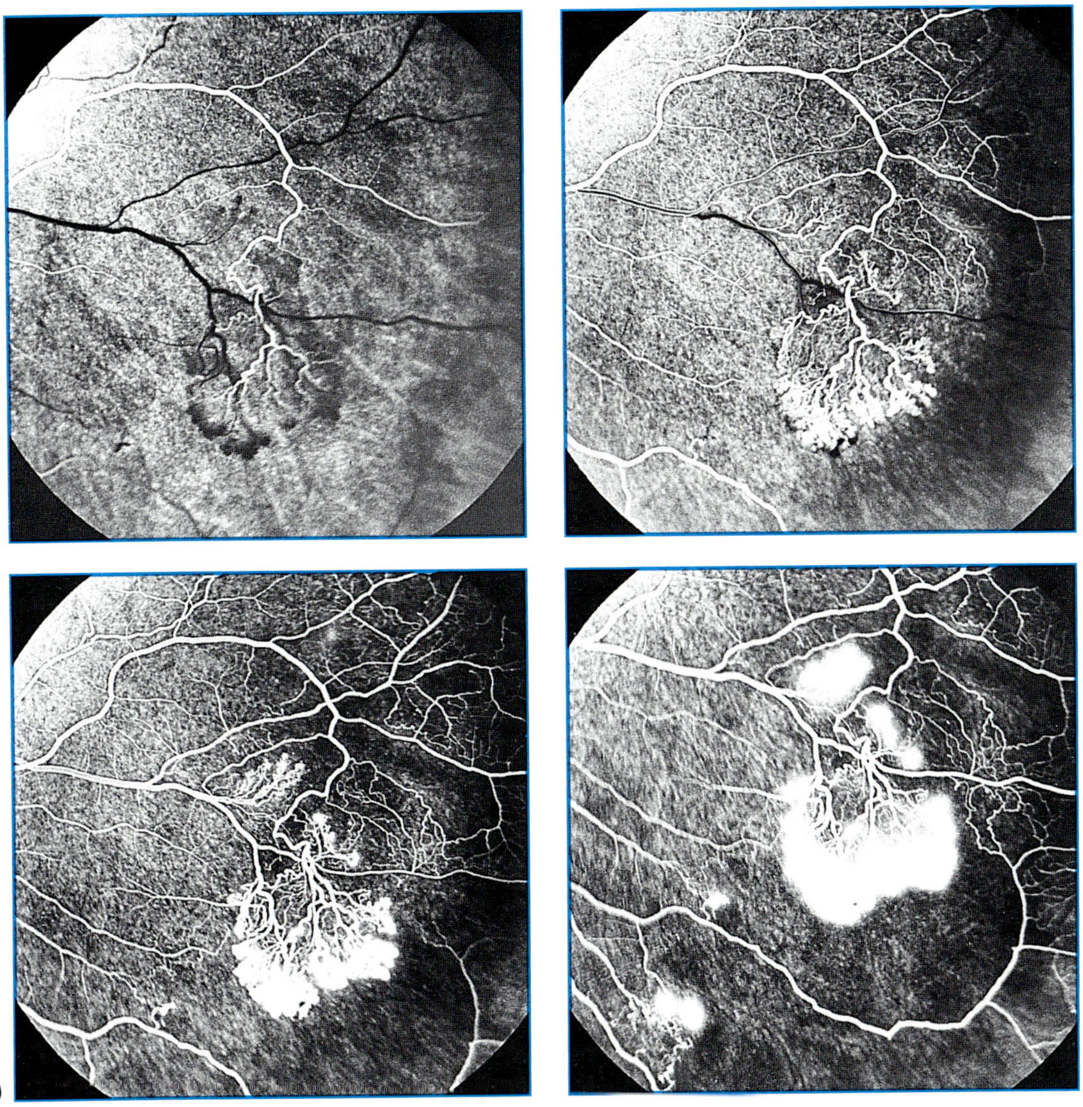

a) b)

c) d)

*Fig. **4.7**,83 - Eales' disease: retinal fluorescein angiography shows typical hyperfluorescent dendritic patterns where there are new vessels, at the edges of the nonperfused areas (a,b,c,d: fluorescein angiographic times).*

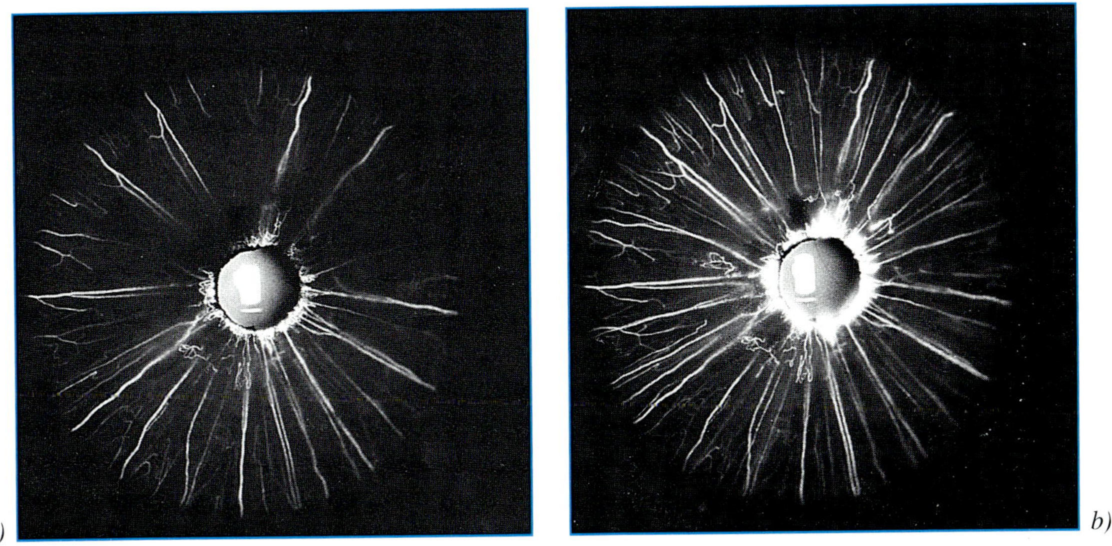

a) b)

*Fig. **4.7**,84 - Same case as in the previous figure. Initial new vessels can be seen around the pupillary border (a,b: iris fluorescein angiographic phases).*

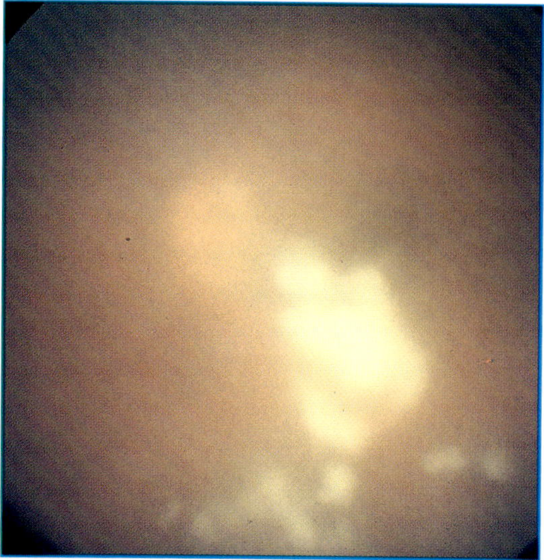

Fig. ***4.7****,85 - Candida albicans uveitis. Marked vitreal turbidity makes it difficult to see the retinal plane ophthalmoscopically. Typical cotton-wool spot exudates are visible in the lower retinal sectors and the interpapillomacular zone.*

a)

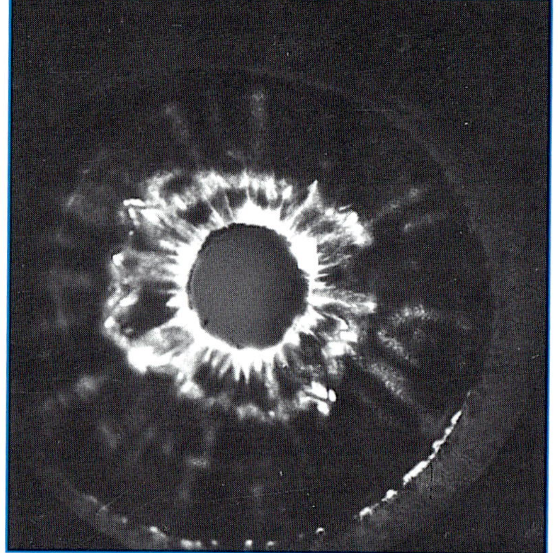

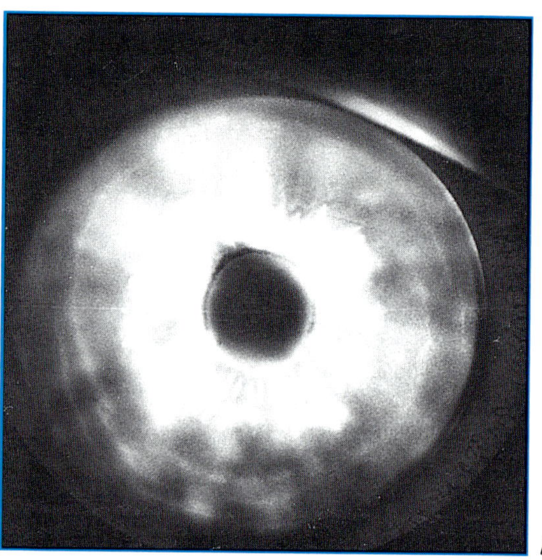

b)

Fig. ***4.7****,86 - Iris fluorescein angiography findings in Candida uveitis. Vascular congestion is generalized and profuse (a), causing dye leakage to the whole anterior chamber in the later phase (b).*

a)

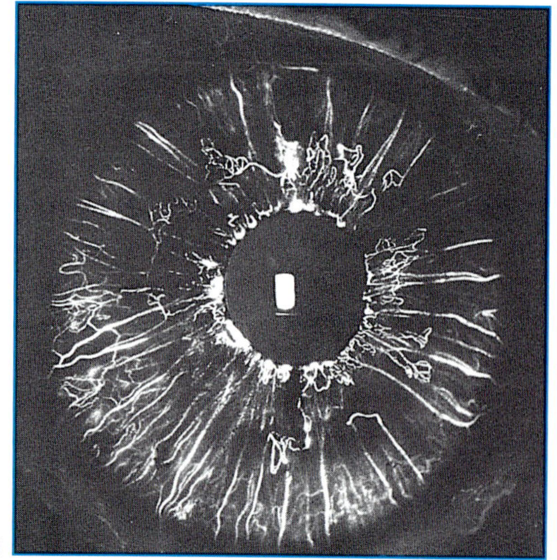

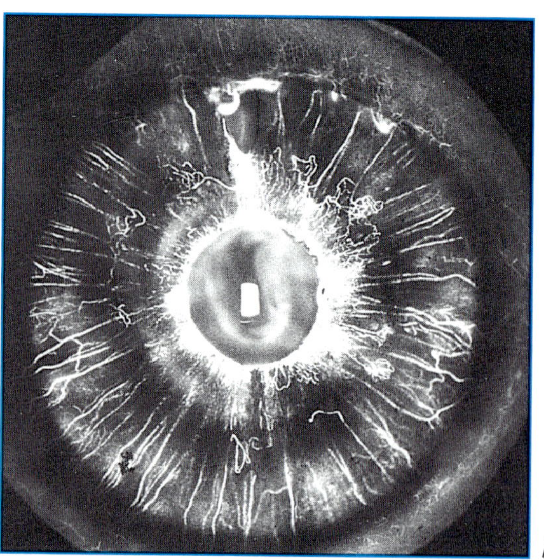

b)

Fig. ***4.7****,87 - Early (a) and late (b) phases of iris fluorescein angiography can detect mild post-surgical inflammation. In this patient cataract extraction has caused some inflammation, affecting the anatomy and increasing the permeability of iris vessels. The preoperative angiographic findings of this eye were normal.*

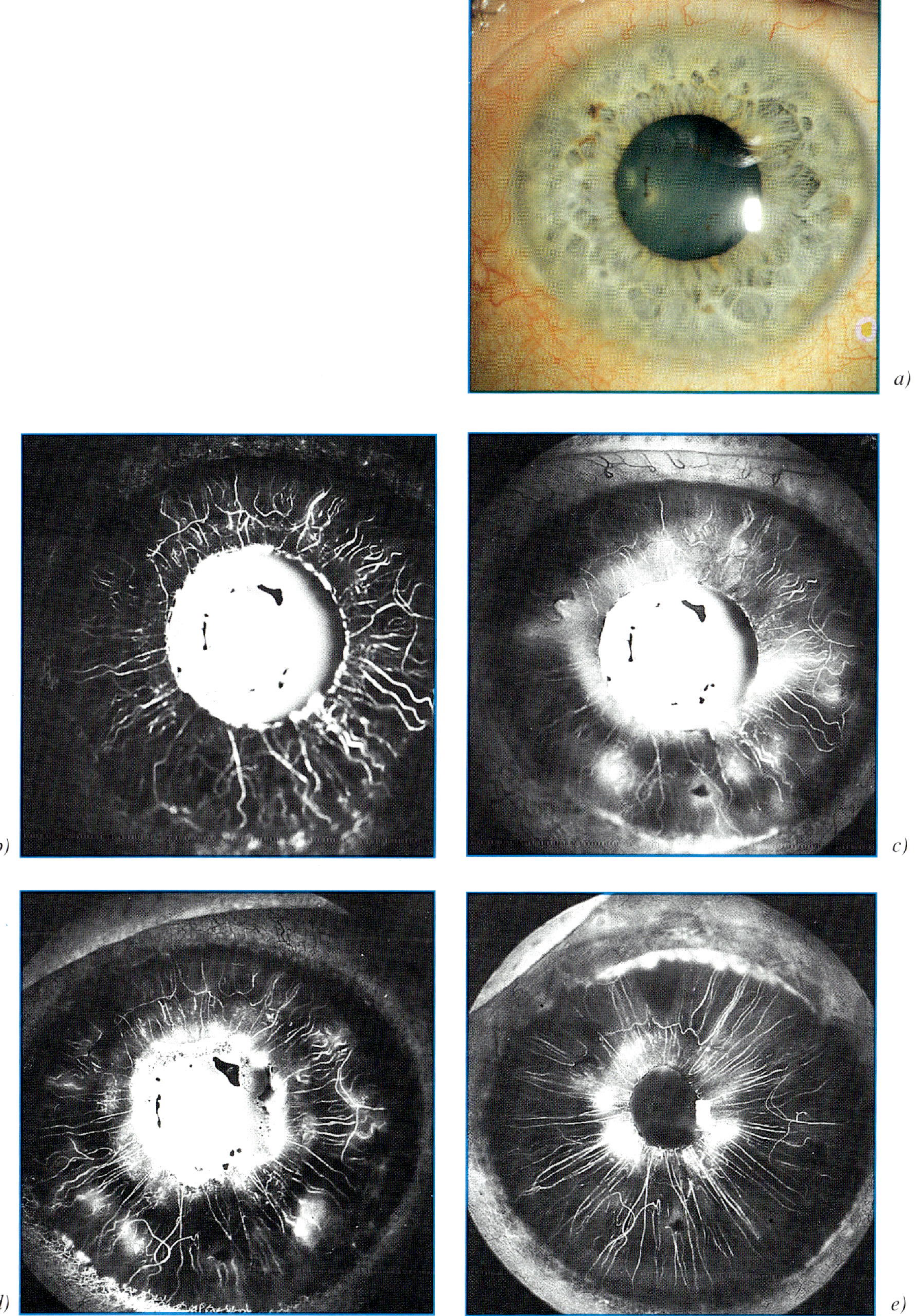

*Fig. **4.7**,88 - Biomicroscopic findings (a) and angiographic phases (b,c) in anterior uveitis. The marked rupture of the blood-iris barrier, easily detected in the late phases (c), is a contraindication to cataract removal. The same exam repeated six months later (d) showed persistent alterations to vascular permeability. Surgery was postponed until the inflammation could be reduced, and no major post-operative complications were recorded (e).*

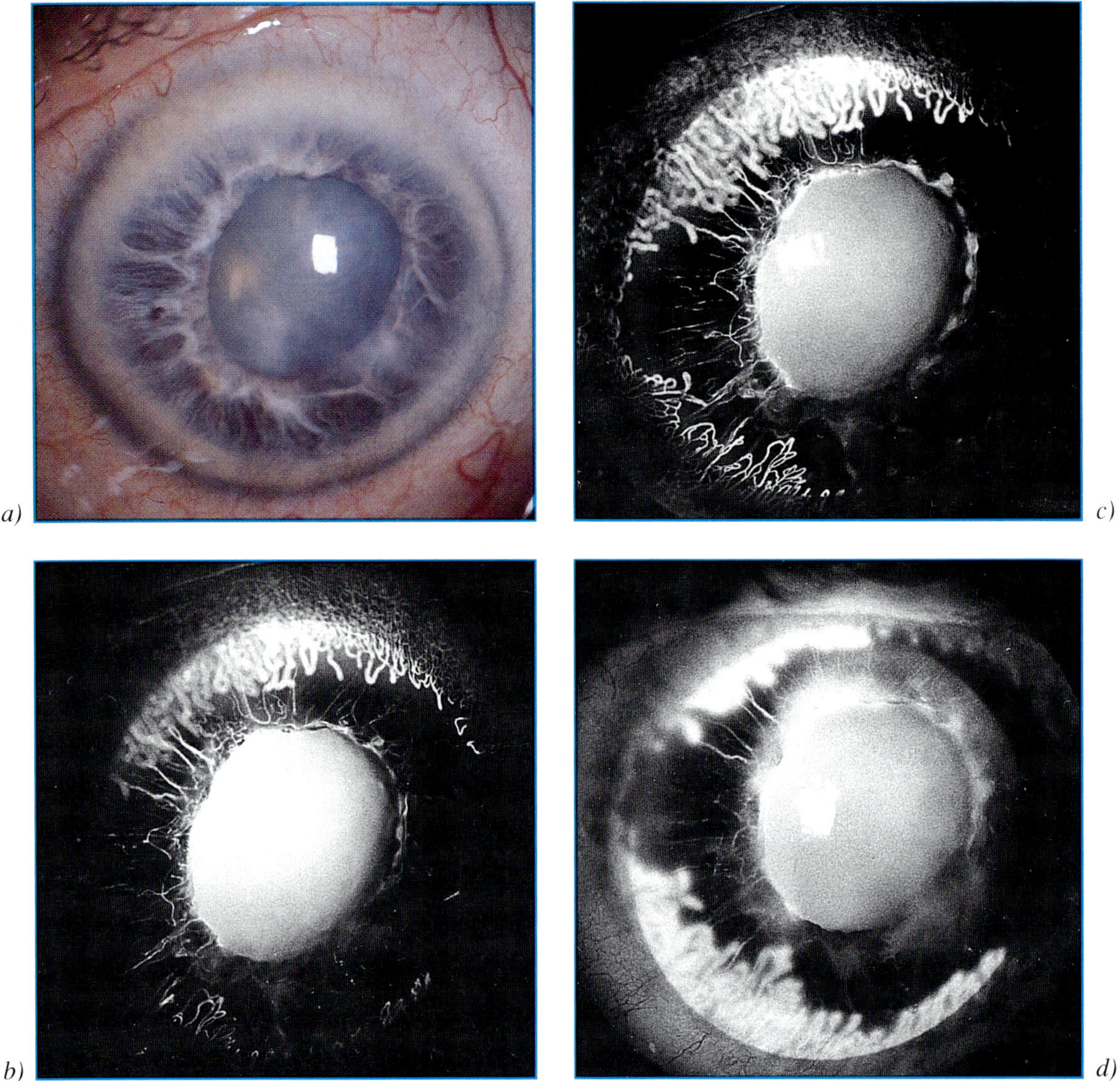

Fig. ***4.7****,89 - Biomicroscopy (a) and iris fluorescein angiographic phases (b,c,d) in a patient with Herpes zoster kerato-iritis. Two types of hyperfluorescence are visible: one in the more peripheral ring (corresponding to the limbal neovascularizations seen with the biomicroscope) and a deeper, mainly peripupillary one, corresponding to the neovascular tufts and congested iris vessels.*

R. Brancato, F. Bandello, R. Lattanzio
Atlas of Iris
Fluorescein Angiography
Kugler & Ghedini Publications 1995

Chapter 4.8

Glaucoma

High intraocular pressure, damage to the head of the optic nerve and impairment of the visual field are the three common denominators in all types of glaucoma.[76] The different forms are classified, on the basis of their etiology, as *primary*, *secondary* or *developmental*. Depending on the mechanisms causing obstruction of the aqueous outflow, and on the basis of a concept proposed by Barkan in 1938,[4] glaucoma may be further classified as *open-angle* or *angle-closure* (Tables **4.8**,I,II).

Table 4.8,I: Classification of the glaucomas based on etiology[76]

I. Open-angle glaucomas	II. Angle-closure glaucomas
A. Primary open-angle glaucoma	A. Primary angle-closure glaucoma
B. Secondary open-angle glaucomas	B. Secondary angle-closure glaucomas
1. Pre-trabecular forms	1. Anterior forms
2. Trabecular forms	2. Posterior forms
a) accumulation of material	a) with pupillary block
b) structural alterations	b) without pupillary block
3. Post-trabecular forms	C. Developmental angle-closure glaucomas
C. Developmental open-angle glaucomas	
1. Primary congenital glaucomas	
2. Developmental glaucomas with associated anomalies	

Table 4.8,II: Classification of the glaucomas based on mechanism[76]

Primary glaucomas	4. Glaucomas associated with disorders of the retina, vitreous and choroid
1. Primary open-angle glaucoma	5. Glaucomas associated with elevated episcleral venous pressure
2. Primary angle-closure glaucoma	6. Glaucomas associated with intraocular tumors
Developmental glaucomas	7. Glaucomas associated with ocular inflammation
1. Primary congenital glaucoma	8. Steroid-induced glaucoma
2. Developmental glaucomas with associated anomalies	9. Glaucomas associated with intraocular hemorrhage
Secondary glaucomas	10. Glaucomas associated with ocular trauma
1. Glaucomas associated with primary disorders of the corneal endothelium	11. Glaucomas following ocular surgery
2. Glaucomas associated with disorders of the iris	
3. Glaucomas associated with disorders of the lens	

Depending on how the hypertension arises, the damage it causes to the ocular structures is classified as *acute*, *subacute* or *chronic*.

Iris fluorescein angiography can be very valuable in assessing some of the pathogenic mechanisms in glaucoma, as it gives a direct picture of anomalies in the caliber and path of iris vessels, their filling patterns, trophism and alterations to iris tissue, the extent of breakdown of the blood-iris barrier, when present, and whether there is any neovascularization.

Abnormalities detected on iris fluorescein angiography should be assessed in relation to the following factors: the type and severity of glaucoma, how it arose, the level and duration of hypertension, and past or present drug therapy. This chapter will look at iris fluorescein angiographic findings in primary glaucoma and in some secondary forms (pseudoexfoliative, pigmentary and phakolytic). The findings in other types of secondary hypertension are described in the chapters on the pertinent primary eye diseases.

Primary open-angle glaucoma

Chronic simple glaucoma, or primary open-angle glaucoma, is the most frequent type. It is currently considered as a chronic-progressive anterior optic neuropathy and is generally accompanied by ocular hypertension, characteristic perimetric alterations, cupping and pallor of the optic disc. The hypertension is the result of an impediment to the outflow of aqueous humor and gonioscopy confirms that the iridocorneal angle is in fact open.[(75)]

The first photometric studies, by Amsler & Huber in 1946, concerned patients with simple glaucoma and showed that the concentration of fluorescein in the aqueous, after i.v. injection, was slightly higher than in normal subjects.[(2)] Such anomalies, however, were considered even then to be of no diagnostic value.[(56)]

It was only in 1969 that Vannas[(85)] first used iris fluorescein angiography to study eyes with glaucoma. In simple primary open-angle glaucoma this examination showed up only slight abnormalities - if any - compared to the findings in other forms of glaucoma (Fig. **4.8**,1). In 31 of the 33 eyes studied - all with intraocular pressure lower than 30 mmHg - Vannas reported that the iris vessels were angiographically normal in appearance and dynamics; the arteries filled quickly and, under the effect of pharmacological miosis, they were relatively straight. In 16 of these 33 eyes (48.5%) Vannas found dye leakage from the pupillary margin but in most cases this finding was age-related. In eyes with glaucoma in which the intraocular pressure was normal after pharmacological therapy or surgery, Vannas found no fluorescein angiographic abnormalities in the vascular dynamics. There was some filling delay only in the one eye in his caselist with absolute glaucoma. Only in two of the 33 eyes in that study (6.6%), both with poor intraocular pressure control and severe loss of visual field, was the fluorescein angiographic picture described as "typical neovascularization in the ciliary portion of the iris", not seen on biomicroscopy; Vannas also reported fluorescein extravasation both from the newly formed vessels and at the pupillary border (Figs. **4.8**,2-6).

Vannas sustained that these vascular anomalies in eyes with primary open-angle glaucoma , interpreted as neovascularization, might explain the hemorrhages in the anterior chamber sometimes occurring during and after filtering surgery, which tend to weaken the results of therapy.[(85)]

There are other reports too that most patients with untreated primary open-angle glaucoma do not present any noteworthy iris fluorescein angiographic alterations.[(27,38)]

Iris fluorangiographic alterations are seen after sudden intraocular pressure rises, even to less than 40 mmHg; blood flow to the iris diminishes and the resulting ischemia - especially if prolonged - gives rise to localized areas of iris atrophy mainly around the sphincter. Larger but short-lasting pressure rises (more than 70 mmHg) do not usually induce any lesions that show up with iris fluorescein angiography.[38]

The abnormal visualization and marked dye leakage from peripupillary vessels reported in 75% of the eyes with chronic glaucoma studied by Mounier[58] were interpreted as being due to the abnormal transparency of the peripupillary iris stroma resulting from degeneration, partly due to the hypertension and partly age-related (Fig.**4.8**,7).

In eyes with long-standing glaucoma, under treatment for years, the following findings were reported:[27]

1) congested, tortuous vessels;
2) dye leakage from the pupillary margin, increasing in later angiographic stages;
3) a different type of dye spread, seen in ten % of cases, which causes a fluorescent veil to swirl out from the posterior chamber, impregnating the aqueous humor.

Primary angle-closure glaucoma

In this form of glaucoma outflow of aqueous humor is impeded by angle-closure caused by the iris root becoming attached to the corneo-scleral trabecular meshwork.[5] Vannas was the first to describe the iris fluorescein angiographic findings in 20 eyes with angle-closure glaucoma, all with intraocular pressure below 24 mmHg and not in an acute phase; eight eyes had undergone filtering surgery.[85] Forty % of the cases presented vasoproliferative whorls in the ciliary part of the iris, forming a fine, dense network of new vessels in the most severe cases, covering the whole iris surface from the root to the collarette. Only one case (5%) had new-formed capillaries at the pupillary border too, although Vannas observed dye leakage in that area in 70% of the eyes studied. In 20% of the eyes with vascular proliferation Vannas noted reduced radial vascularization (Figs. **4.8**,8-12). He thus concluded that the percentage of vascular proliferation in angle-closure glaucoma (40%) was higher than in primary open-angle glaucoma (6.6%) but lower than in the pseudoexfoliation syndrome (75%) or in capsular glaucoma (98%).

Vannas also observed that the eyes that did not show vascular proliferation on iris fluorescein angiography, gave good functional results when treated by filtering surgery, with no post-operative tendency to neovascularization.[85]

In an acute attack the iris fluorescein angiographic findings are completely different. The iris shows serious damage: it becomes bloated, its vessels dilated and congested. The ischemia induced by the hypertension and the uveal congestion cause atony of the sphincter, irregular mydriasis, posterior synechiae, iris atrophy with subsequent pigment dispersion, and - later - torsion of the iris stroma.

Fluorescein angiography during the hypertensive phase of the acute attack shows the iris ischemia,[47] with the characteristic total or subtotal disappearance of the iris vascularization; only some radial vessels[27,47] or vessels in the pupillary plexus[27] may be spared (Figs. **4.8**,13,14). Another typical finding of the acute attack is prompt, marked dye leakage from the perfused vessels[47] in the iris stroma, tending to leak into the anterior chamber.[27] This heavy leakage from perfused vessels is indicative of the severe impairment to their permeability probably resulting from the ischemia.[33,47]

To investigate the effect of an acute attack on the iris circulation Vannas did iris fluorescein angiography in patients with angle-closure glaucoma 1, 3, 5, 9, 10, 11, 20 and 30 days after the attack.[85] The following abnormalities were detected one and three days after the attack: dilated radial vessels with strong fluorescence, indicating the marked increase in vascular permeability resulting from the vascular congestion; numerous hyperfluorescent spots of vascular proliferation in the pars ciliaris of the iris; circumscribed areas of nonperfusion and zones of peripupillary atrophy; heavy dye leakage from the pupillary border. Vannas did not find any arteriovenous shunts (Figs. **4.8**,15-18). Findings after the acute attack included the fluorangiographic visualization of a dense network of congested capillaries, mainly in the ciliary part of the iris. The same examination repeated nine days after the attack showed less dilatation of radial vessels, much less dye leakage and no signs of the congested capillary network that had been visible earlier. There were, however, new occlusions of radial vessels, showing up as filling defects. One month after the attack most of the eyes investigated no longer showed any leakage, but there were still filling difficulties in some parts of the iris. In these ischemic or atrophic areas, which are typical after an acute attack, the capillary network becomes completely subverted and frequently there is torsion of the iris stroma (Figs. **4.8**,19-21).

Kozlova reported focal areas of iris atrophy and marked fluorescein angiographic anomalies in eyes after an acute attack; other findings were abnormalities in diameter (stenosis and microaneurysms) of iris vessels and filling defects.[49] According to Gilson[42] these angiographic findings are the clinical expression of the iris' sensitivity to acute ocular hypertension, which itself is the cause of the ischemia of the sphincter that produces irreducible mydriasis and iris atrophy.

As Kottow stressed,[47] it is unlikely that the iris new vessels seen on angiographic examination a few days after an acute attack, disappearing within such a short time, are really new-formed vessels. Rubeosis iridis is not a frequent complication of acute glaucoma, probably because the hypoxic stimulus, though it may be strong, is too fleeting to give rise to a neovascular reaction.[33] This is in contrast with the fact that glaucoma is widely believed to be a risk factor for central retinal vein occlusion.[40] Thus in patients with neovascular glaucoma secondary to primary glaucoma, the retina should always be examined closely.[28,39] Smith[77] examined 120 eyes with rubeosis iridis in one eye and angle-closure glaucoma in the other. All the enucleated eyes with rubeosis had occlusion of either the central retinal vein or artery.

In subacute attacks, meaning glaucoma with reversible intraocular pressure spikes (in which the attachment of the iris root to the corneo-scleral trabecular meshwork may regress) the following iris fluorescein angiographic abnormalities have been reported: neovascular tufts, particularly in the mid-iris[27] or pars ciliaris,[42] and nonperfused areas in the pars ciliaris.[42] Dye leakage from the pupillary border is frequent[27,42] and hyperfluorescence in this area may be stronger than in the neovascularized areas of the ciliary part of the iris.[42]

Deodati[27] found iris fluorescein angiographic abnormalities of this type in 85% of the eyes with subacute glaucoma in his caselist. These lesions subsequently regressed or gradually diminished as the intraocular pressure returned to normal in response to medical or surgical treatment.

Iris fluorescein angiographic findings after experimental changes in intraocular pressure

The morphological and dynamic abnormalities of iris vessels detected by iris fluorescein angiography in patients with ocular hypertension are related to the effect of changes in intraocular pressure on blood flow in the eye. Intraocular pressure influences not only the perfusion of the ocular vessels, but also the integrity and efficiency of the blood-aqueous barrier. Ocular perfusion pressure and flow rate diminish in response to hypertension; and the arteries dilate to keep blood flow constant. This homeostatic mechanism works well as long as intraocular pressure remains below 60 mmHg, and there are no sudden pressure rises.

Rutowski,[72] in a study of the perfusion of iris vessels in relation to intraocular pressure, induced ocular hypertension artificially in healthy subjects and examined their eyes by iris fluorescein angiography. When intraocular pressure was raised to below the diastolic pressure in the ophthalmic artery, there was some delay in the appearance of dye in iris vessels and in their complete filling (respectively 26 and 38 seconds compared with 20 and 28 seconds in normal eyes). When intraocular pressure was raised to higher than the diastolic pressure in the ophthalmic artery, iris vessels remained nonperfused as long as the hypertension lasted (50 seconds). Dye appeared in these vessels three seconds after the pressure was allowed to drop steeply.

Angiographic findings were the same when intraocular pressure was raised to above the systolic pressure in the ophthalmic artery. When intraocular pressure was held above this level for 35 seconds, then lowered to the diastolic pressure in the artery, Rutowski[72] could see dye in the iris vessels three seconds after the lowering. During the next ten seconds, intraocular pressure was held at the diastolic pressure of the ophthalmic artery, and dye slowly filled peripheral iris vessels, without ever properly filling those in the region of the sphincter; intraocular pressure was then brought down to normal 55 seconds after fluorescein injection, and within ten seconds all the vessels filled completely. Using fluorescein to analyse the blood flow, Rutowski was thus the first to describe iris perfusion in response to ocular hypertension in man.

Similar morphological and dynamic anomalies of iris vessels in response to experimental changes in intraocular pressure have been reported in the rat and in the rabbit examined by iris-carotid fluorangiography. In the rat Castenholz[20] reported that as intraocular pressure rose, circulation was interrupted in the venous system and was segmentary in the arteries which, however, collapsed when pressure was raised further.

In the rabbit Latinovic[51] found the responses to artificial ocular hypertension of 40 and 60 mmHg were respectively a filling delay and the total lack of fluorescence. Hypertension causes compression of the iris vessels, leading to partial or total hypofluorescence. Intraocular hypotony, on the other hand, with its diminished compression of the vessels, leads to passive vasodilatation and breakdown of the blood-aqueous barrier, reflected in strong, prolonged dye leakage.

Other studies using experimental models of ocular hypotension[3,19,25,73] also reported anomalies of the ciliary structures and damage to the blood-aqueous barrier.

Glaucoma in pseudoexfoliation and pigment dispersion syndromes

The pseudoexfoliation syndrome and the pigment dispersion syndrome are two clinically distinct disorders but some anomalies are common to both. Examples are pigment dispersion throughout the anterior segment, pigment liberation upon pupillary dilatation, marked trabecular pigmentation and iris transillumination defects.[52,64,65] When correlated with an age corrected population, there is a higher incidence of open angle glaucoma in both syndromes.[43,48,55]

The pigment dispersion syndrome is more frequent in young or adult males, is associated with myopia and is typically bilateral.[7,61,79] The pseudoexfoliative syndrome is observed in elderly patients, is generally unilateral and is characterized by flecks of whitish material deposited on the surface of the lenses, on the zonular fibres, the ciliary body, pigment epithelium of the iris or in the crypts, around the pupillary border, on the trabecular meshwork and sometimes on the corneal endothelial surface.[65,80]

Since both these syndromes are fairly common and appear in different age groups, the pseudoexfoliative syndrome is quite often seen in a patient who had the pigment dispersion syndrome earlier.[52]

Pseudoexfoliation syndrome

Although this disorder was already identified at the beginning of this century, its pathogenesis is still not clear, and its interpretation is still being worked out. In 1926 Vogt interpreted the fibril-like material as a "senile exfoliation of the lens capsule" and introduced the concept of capsular glaucoma to explain the associated ocular hypertension. Later, Busacca suggested that the material found on the lens surface might in actual fact not originate from the lens capsule. This was subsequently confirmed by the histochemical studies of Dvorak-Theobald[32] who suggested the term *pseudoexfoliation*.

Ultrastructural investigations subsequently found this material underneath the capsule, closely associated with the lens epithelium. Further research also found the fibrillar material in the epithelium of the iris and ciliary body, and led to the current theory that this fibrillo-granular substance is the outcome of abnormal production and accumulation of matter like the basement membrane[67], defined as an amyloid-like substance embedded in a ground substance.[26,71] The real origin of the pseudoexfoliative material, however, remains unclear.

Iris fluorescein angiography has proved valuable in this syndrome for detecting characteristic iris abnormalities that cannot be seen with the biomicroscope. There are numerous descriptions of the iris fluorescein angiographic findings in eyes with pseudoexfoliation of the lens capsule together with ocular hypertension.[14,17,24,27,58,70,84,85] These findings always include varying degrees of vasoproliferation, mainly in the ciliary part.[14,17,24,27,58,70,85] Vannas was the first to describe this vascular proliferation - not detectable by biomicroscopy - which he defined "vascular whorls",[85] but there is general agreement that it is a typical part of the syndrome,[70] and can be considered virtually diagnostic.[24]

The new-formed vessels in the ciliary part, seen on iris fluorescein angiography, are very fine and tortuous (Fig. **4.8**,22). They fill up well with fluorescein, becoming brightly visible for a long time,[85] and the dye spreads slightly, causing a patchy leakage.[24] Fluorescence may be particularly marked where there are neovascular tufts and the new vessels in these areas may bulge like a microaneurysm or turn in a sharp bend (Figs. **4.8**,23,24).[85] The new-formed vessels look like distinct and separate superficial capillary networks, irregular in size and shape. They seem more like numerous separate networks than a vast interconnecting vascular bed (Fig. **4.8**,25).[24]

It has been calculated that new vessels are seen in the ciliary part in 75% of cases.[14,85] In the remaining 25% with no vascular whorls, Vannas found that dye leaked profusely and sooner than in the other healthy eye.[85] Neovascularization of the ciliary part is not always parallelled by new-vessel formation at the pupillary border. In cases with such new vessels, however, angiography in its early phases showed a bright, dense capillary network in the area of the sphincter; in later phases this joined up to form a fluorescent ring with blurred edges.[85]

Another frequent iris fluorescein angiographic anomaly associated with new vessels in this syndrome is a reduced amount of radial vessels, detectable especially in the venous phase of the examination. Radial arteries show a virtually normal filling pattern although radial vascularization was also said to show up poorly[85] with loss or partial closing off of iris vessels with sectorial filling defects (Fig.**4.8**,22).[14]

The characteristic alterations found only by iris fluorescein angiographic examination in the pseudoexfoliation syndrome are correlated, according to Cobb & Smith[24] with the deposition of exfoliative material demonstrated by electron microscopy; although this could be a process of primary capillary dilation, it is likely that superficial venous obstruction occurs during the exfoliation, and that the irregular capillary network serves to provide collateral drainage.

Electron microscopy studies by Ringvold[70] sought to clear up the question of the pathogenesis of the new vessels. This investigator found four types of histological alterations:

1) deposition of pseudoexfoliative material near the endothelial wall;
2) thinning and sometimes breakage of the basement membrane;
3) reduction of the vascular lumen because of enlargement of the endothelial cells;
4) fenestrated endothelium.

Ringvold suggested that the iris new vessels found on fluorangiography in the pseudoexfoliation syndrome might therefore be a response to obstruction of the iris vessels resulting from the histological changes found and that this, in turn, would lead to tissue hypoxia. Brooks[14] also believed that the neovascular reaction in pseudoexfoliation was associated with patchy occlusion of the normal iris vasculature. In a later study Brooks[17] classified the iris angiogram findings in eyes with pseudoexfoliation as follows:

1) hypoperfusion of the iris (reduced radial arterioles, sectorial filling defects, attenuated arterioles);
2) microneovascularization (stromal tufts, more complex plexuses, peripupillary neovascularization and leaking pupillary tufts);
3) anastomotic vessels (peripheral loops, lesser circle, oblique vessels).

Brooks found these anomalies in all the eyes he studied, regardless of whether intraocular pressure was elevated or not. He underlined that iris hypoperfusion was not the primary cause of pseudoexfoliation, but was more likely a consequence.

Iris fluorescein angiographic studies have also been done in the forms of pseudoexfoliation associated with ocular hypertension, sometimes referred to as capsular glaucoma.[27,84,85] The anomalies described are similar to but more severe than those in the pseudoexfoliative syndrome: varying degrees of new-vessel formation, marked dye leakage[27,85] and reduced radial vascularization.[85] However, some studies found the iris vascularization was more marked than normal[27] rather than less visible.

In some instances the iris vessels were abnormal in diameter and presented microaneurysm-like buds; sometimes there was venous congestion.[85] In other cases the new vessels themselves looked like microaneurysmic dilatations.[27] In most of the eyes analysed with capsular glaucoma, iris fluorescein angiographic abnormalities were seen in the ciliary and pupillary parts. In the severest cases it was impossible to distinguish the individual vasoproliferative whorls or clusters, since the whole iris was covered by a fine vascular mesh, from the root to the collarette) (Fig. **4.8**,26).(85

The bright fluorescence and the sharp visualization of new vessels indicates, in Vannas' opinion,[85] that they lie on the surface of the iris; stereoangiography, however, shows up tortuous new vessels deeper inside the stroma too, and close to the pigment epithelium. Even in eyes with the pseudoexfoliative syndrome associated with ocular hypertension, the abnormalities described can only be detected by iris fluorescein angiographic examination, and are not visible with the biomicroscope.

Anterior segment pigment dispersion syndrome

Much controversy still surrounds the epidemiology of this syndrome, also known as pigment glaucoma even though most patients with pigment dispersion never do develop glaucoma. The etiology, however, is still not altogether clear. It is generally held to be correlated to a mechanical obstruction of the outflow of aqueous humor in the trabecular meshwork, by pigment elements originating in the iris tissue.

Fine(36) sustained it was a developmental defect with idiopathic dysplasia of the iris epithelium; according to Kupfer too(50) it is a congenital or developmental abnormality mainly affecting the internal and external epithelial layers of the iris. Gillies(41) suggests that the anterior segment pigment dispersion syndrome is caused by a congenital defect of the mesodermal supporting tissue, resulting in a reduction of iris vascularization with shedding of pigment granules, particularly in the region where the dilator muscle is attached to the pigment epithelium. The syndrome can certainly be inherited and Scheie(74) considered a multifactorial inheritance pattern.

Perkins(61) proposed that pigment glaucoma was due to a developmental defect in the outflow channels, with pigment deposit contributing to the obstruction but not its primary cause. Campbell(18) considered the pigment release a consequence of mechanical trauma to the pigment epithelium of the posterior surface of the iris, caused by the zonular fibres of the lens suspensory apparatus. Others have suggested that pigment glaucoma is in fact a normal primary open-angle glaucoma, occasionally arising in patients with the pigment dispersion syndrome.

Clinically the syndrome presents areas of focal atrophy of the pigment epithelium (particularly marked in the mid-periphery as seen by biomicroscopy with retroillumination), the typical Krukenberg spindle and a strongly pigmented trabecular meshwork. This characteristic triad is frequently combined with iridodonesis and a higher than normal incidence of retinal detachment.

Mounier,(58) in a fluorescein angiography study, found no dye leakage in the peripheral areas of iris atrophy. Leakage in the anterior chamber from peripupillary vessels was also infrequent. This investigator found that the colour of the iris and the absence of transillumination had no effect on the frequency and strength of the angiographic signs. Similarly, Valles & Vannas(84) obtained virtually normal angiograms for two eyes with pigment glaucoma that they examined.

Gillies(41) obtained biomicroscopic evidence of atrophy of the iris stroma in six of 11 eyes studied. The architecture of the iris was subverted and the stroma was thinned to the point that the pigment epithelium could be seen. Iris fluorescein angiographic examination of the eyes in Gillies' caselist showed hypoperfusion of the iris with scant, attenuated vessels. In certain cases the radial arteries were missing in some quadrants; in others the arteries appeared to be fewer and of smaller caliber. Gillies found that all eyes had fine neovascularization at the pupillary border and in the peripupillary portion, with marked dye leakage in the late phases of the examination. This was taken as the basis for interpreting the lesions as actual new vessels and not as the normal capillary network abnormally visible because of the iris atrophy. Gillies reported finding aberrant vessels, loops in the peripheral iris stroma and a mild leakage from neovascular tufts only in two cases. Elderly and younger patients presented these anomalies. Additionally, the patients with virtually unilateral involvement also showed these vascular anomalies - though less marked - in the relatively unaffected eye. Gillies therefore stresses that neovascularization in the pigment dispersion syndrome is not as serious as in pseudoexfoliation, nor as marked as in chronic cyclitis or iritis.

Phakolytic glaucoma

This form of secondary glaucoma develops in eyes with generally hypermature cataract, and an open anterior chamber angle. A certain amount of denatured lenticular matter is released into the anterior chamber through the lens capsule which is generally either intact but thin, or with areas of degeneration and focal rupture.

Phakolytic glaucoma sometimes manifests with a gradual rise of intraocular pressure because of the inflammatory reaction in the anterior chamber. In most cases, however, it presents as an acute attack, with marked hypertension. Clinically, such cases have an inflamed eye with a hypermature cataract, intense pain, corneal edema, a normal-depth anterior chamber, cloudy aqueous humor and sometimes hypopion. The angle is open and voluminous whitish precipitates, consisting of accumulated denatured lenticular protein matter phagocytized by macrophages, can be seen on the anterior surface of the lens, on the iris and - more rarely - on the corneal endothelium.

In the presence of this clinical picture it is usually simple to diagnose phakolytic glaucoma. A differential diagnosis must, however, be made between this form and glaucoma secondary to anterior uveitis. The diagnosis is confirmed by the absence of mutton-fat precipitates on the corneal endothelium, the hypermature cataract and the finding of a considerable amount of a soluble, high-molecular-weight protein, of lenticular origin, in the anterior chamber.

The sudden rise in intraocular pressure, the intense pain, the perikeratic injection and corneal edema may sometimes simulate an attack of acute angle-closure glaucoma. However, close biomicroscopic examination and gonioscopy should detect the hypermature cataract and open angle, pathognomonic of phakolytic glaucoma.

On iris fluorescein angiography the inflammation accompanying phakolytic glaucoma causes evident breakdown of the blood-iris barrier, involving stromal vessels too (Figs. **4.8**,27,28). Breakdown of the barrier is angiographically less evident in cases with hypermature cataract but no ocular hypertension (Figs. **4.8**,29,30).

References

1 Airaksinen PJ, Alanko HI: Vascular effects of timolol and pilocarpine in the iris. A simultaneous bilateral fluorescein angiography study. Acta Ophthalmol (Kbh) 61: 195, 1983.

2 Amsler M, Huber A: Methodik und erste klinische Ergebnisse einer Funktionsprüfung der Blut-Kammerwasser-Schranke. Ophthalmologica (Basel) 111: 155, 1946.

3 Ashton N, Cunha-Vaz JG: Effect of histamine on the permeability of the ocular vessels. Arch Ophthalmol 73: 211, 1965.

4 Barkan O: Glaucoma: classification, causes and surgical control. Results of microgonioscopic research. Am J Ophthalmol 21: 1099, 1938.

5 Béchetoille A: Glaucomes primitifs par fermeture de l'angle. Encycl Méd Chir Ophtalmol 21280 A 10: 4, 1989.

6 Benedikt O: Fluorescein angiographic studies of the effect of Harms' and Dannheim's trabeculectomia ab externo. Klin Monatsbl Augenheilkd 174: 442, 1979.

7 Berger A, Ritch R, McDermott JA et al: Pigmentary dispersion, refraction, and glaucoma. Invest Ophthalmol Vis Sci 28 (Suppl): 134, 1987.

8 Blumenthal M, Gitter KA, Best M et al: Fluorescein angiography during induced ocular hypertension in man. Am J Ophthalmol 69: 39, 1970.

9 Blumenthal M, Best M, Galin A: Ocular circulation: analysis of the effect of induced ocular hypertension on retinal and choroidal blood flow in man. Am J Ophthalmol 71: 820, 1971.

10 Boguszakova J, Dubska Z: Fluorescein angiography of the iris in open-angle glaucoma. Cesk Oftalmol 40: 79, 1984.

11 Boguszakova J, Dubska Z, Dientsbier E Jr et al: The effect of long term administration of beta-blockers and pilocarpine on the permeability of blood vessels in the iris as seen in fluoroangiography. Cesk Oftalmol 41: 299, 1985.

12 Boguszakova J, Dubska Z: The fluorangiograophic picture of the iris in pseudoexfoliative glaucoma. Cesk Oftalmol 43: 237, 1987.

13 Brancato R, Menchini U, Carnevalini A: Atlante di iridografia a fluorescenza. C.I.C. Ed Int Gruppo Ed Medico, Roma, 1981.

14 Brooks AMV, Gillies WE: Fluorescein angiography and fluorophotometry of the iris in pseudoexfoliation of the lens capsule. Br J Ophthalmol 67: 249, 1983.

15 Brooks AMV, Gillies WE: Fluorescein angiography of the iris and specular microscopy of the corneal endothelium in some cases of glaucoma secondary to chronic cyclitis. Ophthalmology 95: 1624, 1988.

16 Brooks AMV, Gillies WE: The development and management of neovascular glaucoma. Aust NZ J Ophthalmol 18: 179, 1990.

17 Brooks AMV, Gillies WE: The development of microneovascular changes in the iris in pseudoexfoliation of the lens capsula. Ophthalmology 94: 1090, 1987.

18 Campbell DG: Pigmentary dispersion and glaucoma. Arch Ophthalmol 97: 1667, 1979.

19 Carlini V: Die Veränderungen des Iris und Ciliarepithels nach Punktion der Vorderkammer: Beitrag zum Studium des Productions mechanismus des Humor aqueus. Albrecht von Graefes Arch Klin Ophthalmol 77: 96, 1910.

20 Castenholz A: Morphologische und funktionelle Studien am Iriskreislauf der Ratte: Vitalmikroskopische Beobachtungen. Albrecht von Graefes Arch Klin Ophthalmol 169: 109, 1966.

21 Charles ST, Hamasaki DI: The effect of intraocular pressure on the pupil size. Arch Ophthalmol 83: 729, 1970.

22 Chew EY, Deutman AF: Pigment dispersion syndrome and pigmented pattern dystrophy of retinal pigment epithelium. Br J Ophthalmol 67: 538, 1983.

23 Clements DH, Oberman AE: Iris fluorescein angiography in iris atrophy with glaucoma. Trans Pac Coast Oto-Ophthalmol Soc Annual Meeting 53: 187, 1972.

24 Cobb B, Smith ME: Fluorescein studies of the iris in pseudoexfoliation of the lens capsule, heterochromic cyclitis and central and branch retinal vein occlusion. Proc XXIth International Congress Ophthalmology, Mexico, 1970. Excerpta Medica International Congress Series 222: 953, 1971.

25 Cole DF: The site of breakdown of the blood-aqueous barrier under the influence of vaso-dilator drugs. Exp Eye Res 19: 591, 1974.

26 Davanger M: On the molecular composition and physico-chemical properties of the pseudo-exfoliation material. Acta Ophthalmol (Kbh) 55: 621, 1977.

27 Deodati F, Bec P, Labro JB et al: Angiographie fluoresceinique du segment anteriour dans les hypertensions oculaires. Bull Mem Soc Ophtalmol Fr 83: 561, 1971.

28 Detry-Morel M: Les glaucomes vasculaires. J Fr Ophtalmol 4: 177, 1981.

29 Dollery CT, Henkind P, Konher EM et al: Effect of raised intraocular pressure on the retinal and choroidal circulation. Invest Ophthalmol 7: 191, 1968.

30 Dollery CT, Hodge JV, Engel M: Studies of the retinal circulation with fluorescein. Br Med J 11: 1210, 1962.

31 Dollery CT, Hodge JV, Engel M: Retinal photography using fluorescein. Med Biol Illus 13: 4, 1963.

32 Dvorak-Theobald G: Pseudo-exfoliation of the lens capsule. Am J Ophthalmol 37: 1, 1954.

33 Easty DL, Chignell AH: Fluorescein angiography in anterior segment ischaemia. Br J Ophthalmol 57: 18, 1973.

34 Ernest JT, Archer D, Krill AE: Ocular hypertension induced by scleral suction cup. Invest Ophthalmol 11: 29, 1972.

35 Feller DB, Weinreb RN: Breakdown and reestablishment of blood-aqueous barrier with laser trabeculoplasty. Arch Ophthalmol 102: 537, 1984.

36 Fine BS, Janoff M, Scheie RG: Pigmentary glaucoma. Ophthalmology (Rochester) 78: 314, 1974.

37 Friedburg D, Aegenheyster U: Irisveranderungen beim Glaukom. Ber Dtsch Ophthalmol Ges 73: 276, 1973.

38 Friedburg D: Fluoreszenzangiographie der Iris bei Primar-Glaukom. Buch Augenarzt 69: 79, 1976.

39 Gartner S, Henkind P: Neovascularization of the iris (Rubeosis iridis). Surv Ophthalmol 22: 291, 1978.

40 Gaudric C, Coscas G: Rubeose de l'iris et glaucome néovasculaire. J Fr Ophtalmol 2: 653, 1979.

41 Gillies WE, Tangas C: Fluorescein angiography of the iris in anterior segment pigment dispersal syndrome. Br J Ophthalmol 70: 284, 1986.

42 Gilson M: Angle-closure glaucoma. Semeiology. J Fr Ophtalmol 3: 139, 1980.

43 Henry JC, Krupin T, Schmitt M et al: Long-term follow-up of pseudoexfoliation and the development of elevated intraocular pressure. Ophthalmology 94: 545, 1987.

44 Kiskina VI, Semenov AD, Nersensov I: Fluorescent iridoangiography in patients with compensated open-angle glaucoma with artiphakia. Vestn Oftalmol 101: 14, 1985.

45 Kluzen G, Roeseler K: Irisangiogramme vor Glaukomanfall. Fortschr Ophthalmol 80: 298, 1983.

46 Kodejszko J, Kornacki B, Stefaniak T: Use of the interference filter for fluorescein angiography of the anterior eye segment. Klin Oczna 46: 269, 1976.

47 Kottow MH: Anterior segment fluorescein angiography. Williams & Wilkins, Baltimore, 1978.

48 Kozart DM, Yanoff M: Intraocular pressure status in 100 consecutive patients with exfoliation syndrome. Ophthalmology 89: 214, 1982.

49 Kozlova LP, Katsnellson LA, Boleshanskaia TI: Fluorescence iridoangiography in primary glaucoma. Vestn Oftalmol 2: 3, 1978.

50 Kupfer C, Kuwabara T, Kaiser-Kupfer M: The histopathology of pigmentary dispersion syndrome with glaucoma. Am J Ophthalmol 80: 857, 1975.

51 Latinovic S, Virno M, Pecori-Giraldi J: Morphodynamics of the iris circulation in experimentally-induced changes in intraocular pressure. Ophtalmologie 2 : 419, 1988.

52 Layden WE: Exfoliation syndrome. In Ritch R, Shields MB, Krupin T: The glaucomas. CV Mosby, St Louis, 1989.

53 Lewis ML: Iris fluorescein angiography. Dev Ophthalmol 2: 282, 1981.

54 Lichter PR: Pigmentary glaucoma. Current concepts. Ophthalmology (Rochester) 78: 309, 1974.

55 Migliazzo CV, Shaffer RN, Nykin R et al: Long-term analysis of pigmentary dispersion syndrome and pigmentary glaucoma. Ophthalmology 93: 1528, 1986.

56 Miller SJH, Swaliung H: Appearance of fluorescein in the aqueous of glaucomatous eyes. Br J Ophthalmol 35: 356, 1951.

57 Mondelski S, Bartkowska-Orlowska M: Fluorescein contrast in assessment of patency of filtrating fistula following surgery in cases of cataract combined with glaucoma. Klin Oczna 43: 435, 1973.

58 Mounier G, Plane C, Heydel P: L'angiographie fluorescéinique du segment anterieur dans les glaucomes chroniques a angle ouvert. Bull Soc Ophtalmol Fr 81: 331, 1981.

59 Nicholson DH: Occult iris erosion. A treatable cause of recurrent hyphema in iris-supported intraocular lenses. Ophthalmology 89: 113, 1982.

60 Olander KW, Mandelkorn, Hoffmann ME: Pigment dispersion syndrome and open-angle glaucoma. Ann Ophthalmol 14: 809, 1982.

61 Perkins ES, Jay BS: Pigmentary glaucoma. Trans Ophtalmol Soc UK 80: 153, 1960.

62 Pham-Duy T, Becker HU, Wollensak J et al: Tonography and fluorophotometry in the clinical study of aqueous humor dynamics. Fortschr Ophthalmol 86: 210, 1989.

63 Podgornaia NN, Litvinova GG, Drozdova NM et al: Fluorescence iridoangiography in assessing microcirculatory function of the iris after laser iridectomy. Vestn Oftalmol 101: 17, 1985.

64 Prince AM, Ritch R: Clinical signs of the pseudoexfoliation syndrome. Ophthalmology 93: 803, 1986.

65 Richardson TM: Pigmentary glaucoma. In Ritch R, Shields MB, Krupin T: The glaucomas. CV Mosby, St Louis, 1989.

66 Riddel WJB: Tangential displacement of the iris in chronic glaucoma. Br J Ophthalmol 30: 74, 1946.

67 Ringvold A: Electron microscopy of the wall of iris vessels in eyes with and without exfoliation syndrome (pseudoexfoliation of the lens capsule). Virchows Arch Pathol Anat 348: 328, 1969.

68 Ringvold A: The distribution of the exfoliation material in the iris from eyes with exfoliation syndrome (pseudoexfoliation of the lens capsule). Virchows Arch Pathol Anat 351: 168, 1970.

69 Ringvold A: Light and electron microscopy of the anterior iris surface in eyes with and without pseudo-exfoliation syndrome. Albrecht von Graefes Arch Klin Ophthalmol 188: 131, 1973.

70 Ringvold A, Davanger M: Iris neovascularisation in eyes with psudoexfoliation syndrome. Br J Ophthalmol 65: 138, 1981.

71 Ringvold A, Husby G: Pseudoexfoliation material: an amyloid-like substance. Exp Eye Res 17: 289, 1973.

72 Rutkowski PC, Thompson S: Midriasis and increased intraocular pressure. II. Iris fluorescein studies. Arch Ophthalmol 87: 25, 1972.

73 Samojloff AJ: Über die Oxydationsprozesse in den Ciliarepithelzellen und die reaktive Hypertonie des Auges. Albrecht von Graefes Arch Klin Ophthalmol 118: 391, 1927.

74 Scheie HG, Cameron JD: Pigment dispersion syndrome: a clinical study. Br J Ophthalmol 65: 264, 1981.

75 Sellem E: Glaucome primitif à angle ouvert. Editions Techniques, Encycl Méd Chir Ophtalmol 21275 A10: 6, 1990.

76 Shields MB: Textbook of glaucoma. Williams & Wilkins, Baltimore, 1987.

77 Smith ME, Ott FT: Rubeosis iridis and primary angle-closure glaucoma. Int Ophthalmol Clin 2: 161, 1971.

78 Sugar HS: Pigmantary glaucoma and the glaucoma associated with the exfoliation-pseudoexfoliation syndrome. Ophthalmology 91: 307, 1984.

79 Sugar HS, Harding C, Barsky D: The exfoliation syndrome. Ann Ophthalmol 8: 1165, 1976.

80 Sunde OA: Senile exfoliation of the anterior lens capsule. Acta Ophthalmol 45 (Suppl): 1, 1956.

81 Tarkkannen A: Pseudoexfoliation of the lens capsule. Acta Ophthalmol (Kbh) 71 (Suppl): 1, 1962.

82 Tuovinen E: Therapeutic results in primary glaucoma with special reference to tonographic observations. Acta Ophthalmol (Kbh) 67 (Suppl): 1, 1961.

83 Unger WG, Brown NA, Edwards J: Response of the human eye to laser irradiation of the iris. Br J Ophthalmol 61: 148, 1977.

84 Valles O, Vannas A: The cyclopentolate provocative test in suspected or untreated open-angle glaucoma. IV. Fluorescein angiography of the vessels of the iris in open-angle glaucoma eyes with a positive cyclopentolate response. Acta Ophthalmol (Kbh) 54: 783, 1976.

85 Vannas A: Fluorescein angiography of the vessels of the iris in pseudoexfoliation of the lens capsula, capsular glaucoma and some other forms of glaucoma. Acta Ophthalmol (Kbh) 105 (Suppl): 1, 1969.

86 Vannas S, Raitta C: Microcirculatory disturbances of occlusive diseases of the eye. Doc Ophthalmol 33: 345, 1972.

87 Winstanley J: Iris atrophy in primary glaucoma. Trans Ophthalmol Soc UK 81: 23, 1961.

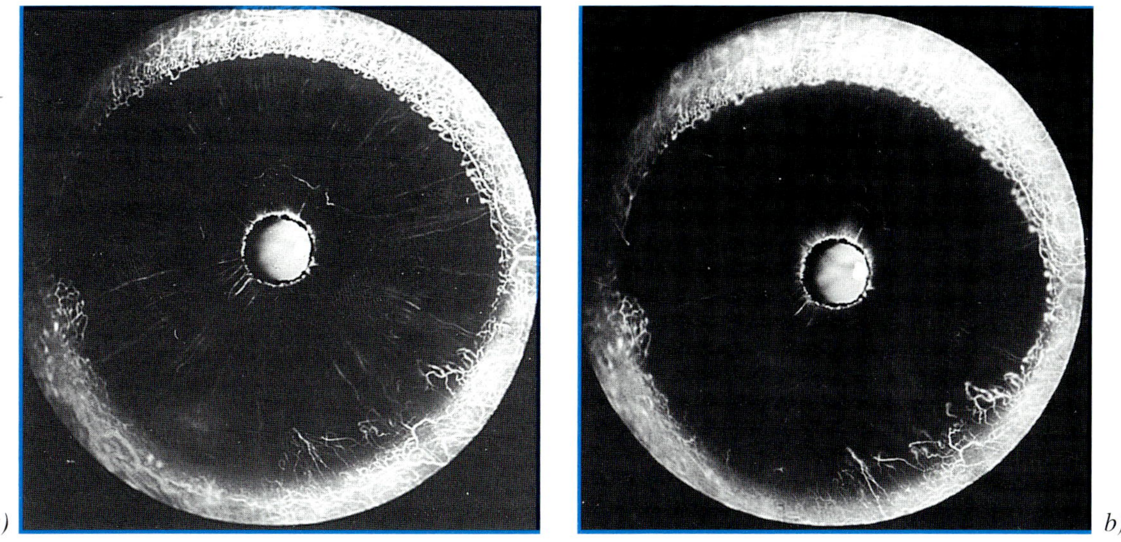

*Fig. **4.8**,1 - Iris fluorescein angiographic phases (a,b) in a patient with primary open-angle glaucoma. The situation looks virtually normal.*

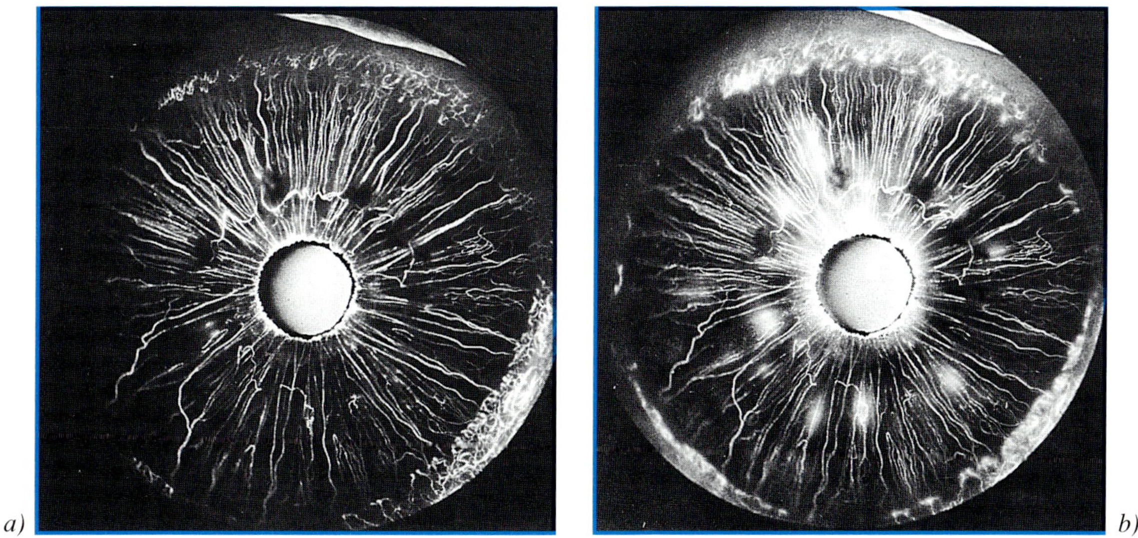

*Fig. **4.8**,2 - Iris fluorescein angiography in a patient with chronic open-angle glaucoma. In the early phases (a) no real neovascularization can be seen. The hyperfluorescence seen in the later phases (b) is mainly from the congested radial vessels which are abnormally permeable.*

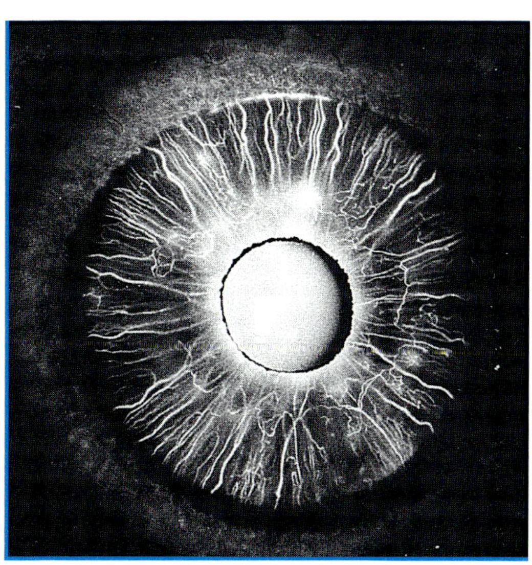

*Fig. **4.8**,3 - Initial neovascularization in the pars ciliaris in a patient with primary open-angle glaucoma: fluorescein angiographic picture.*

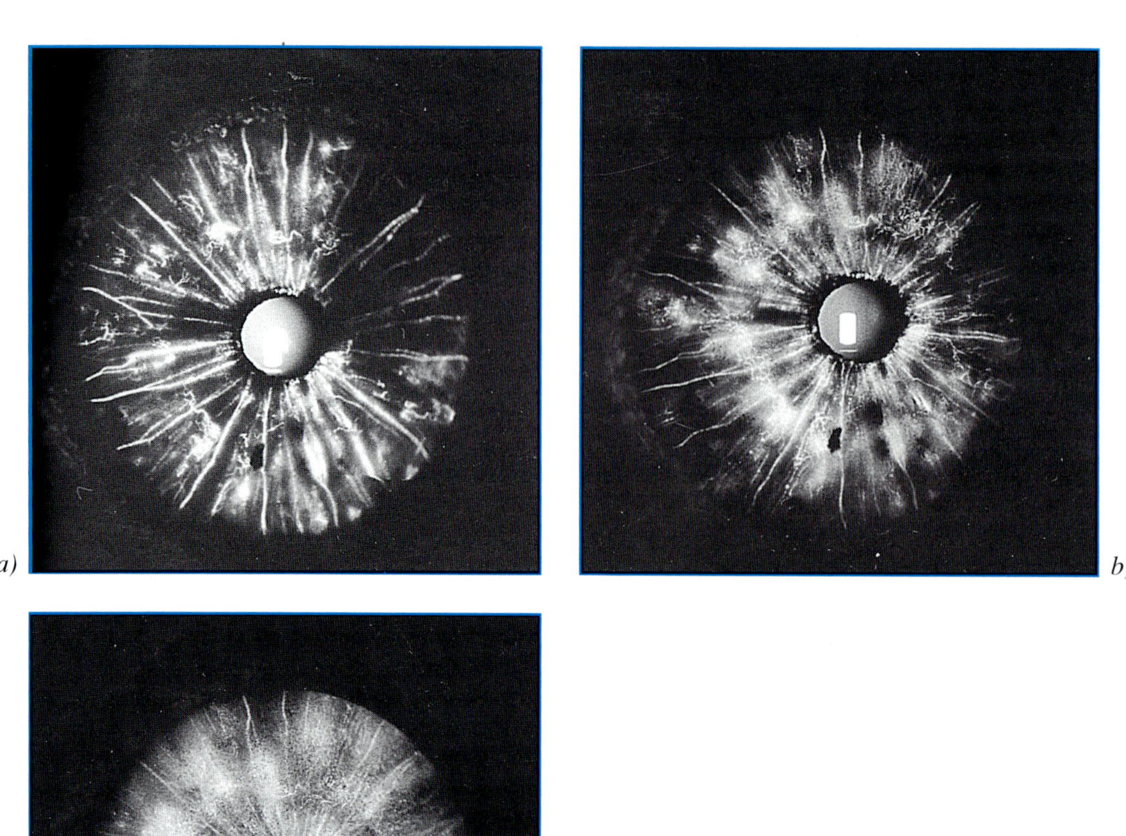

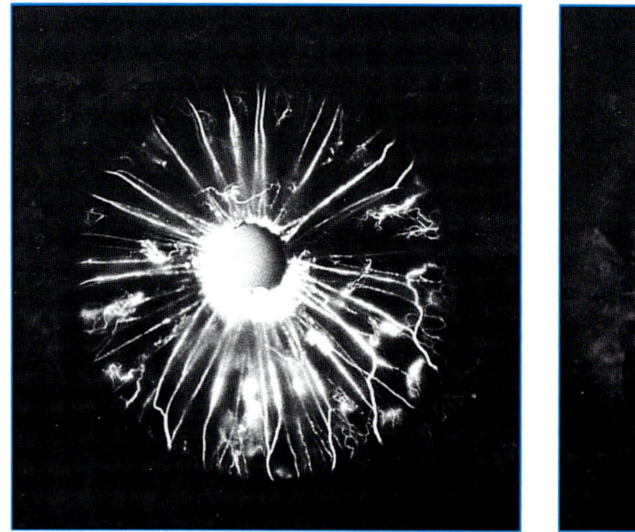

Fig. ***4.8****,4 - In this case of primary open-angle glaucoma the neovascularization is typically located in the pars ciliaris (a,b,c: iris fluorescein angiographic phases).*

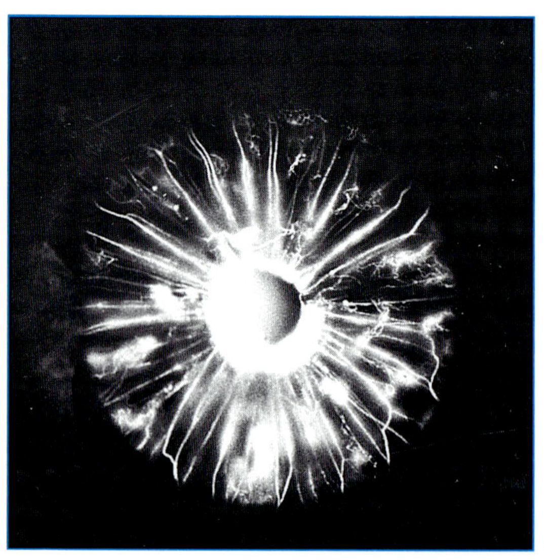

Fig. ***4.8****,5 - Neovascularization at the pupillary border and in the stroma in another case with primary open-angle glaucoma: early (a) and late (b) iris fluorescein angiographic phases. There is marked congestion of radial vessels and some iris districts do not fill.*

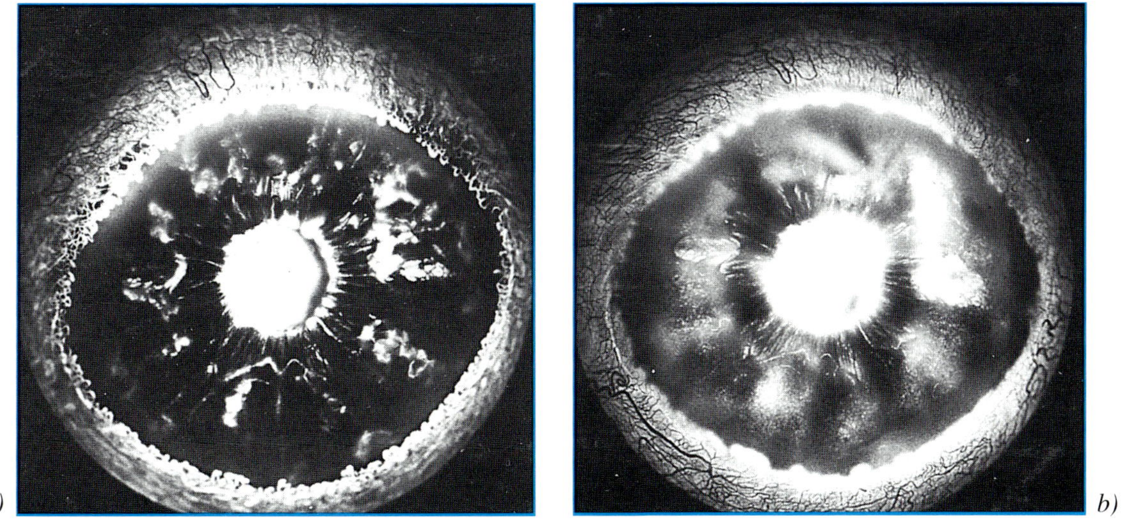
a) b)

*Fig. **4.8**,6 - Proliferative iridopathy from open-angle glaucoma: early (a) and late (b) iris fluorescein angiographic phases.*

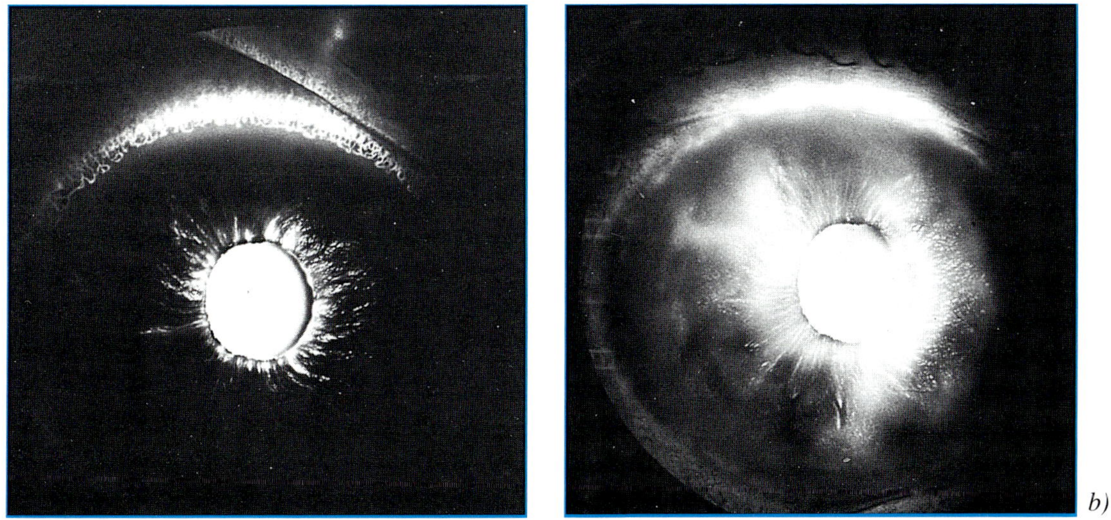
a) b)

*Fig. **4.8**,7 - Open-angle glaucoma: iris fluorescein angiography. Vessels in the pupillary plexus take up dye early (a) and are abnormally visualized, leaking dye markedly throughout the whole anterior chamber in the later phase (b).*

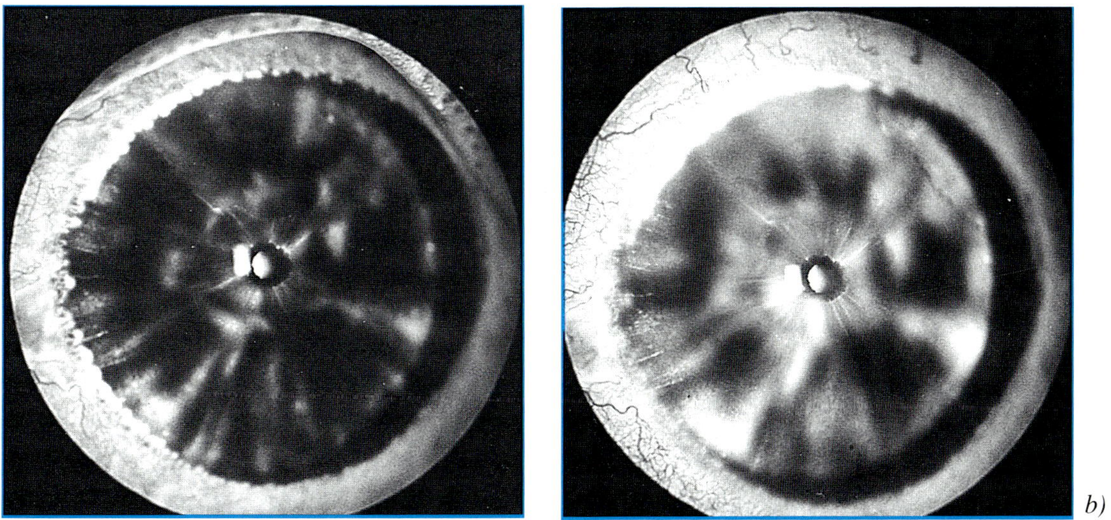
a) b)

*Fig. **4.8**,8 - Diffuse breakdown of the blood-iris barrier in angle-closure glaucoma (a,b: iris fluorescein angiographic phases).*

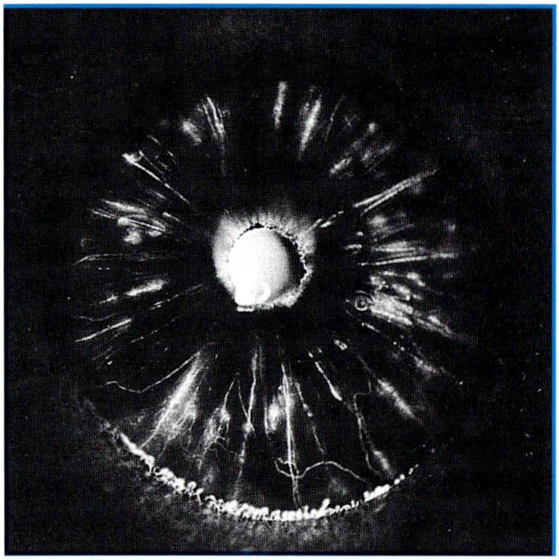

a)

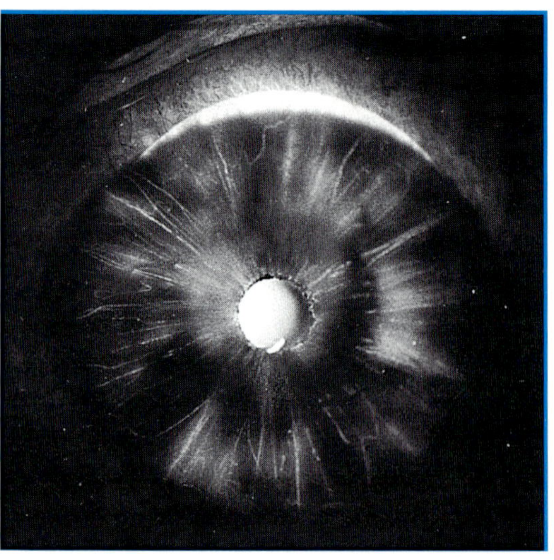

b)

Fig. ***4.8****,9 - Dye leakage from the pupillary border and radial vessels in a patient with angle-closure glaucoma complicated by central retinal vein occlusion. Stromal vessels in the sectors of the iris show microvascular ectasia and amputations along their paths: early (a) and late (b) iris fluorescein angiographic phases.*

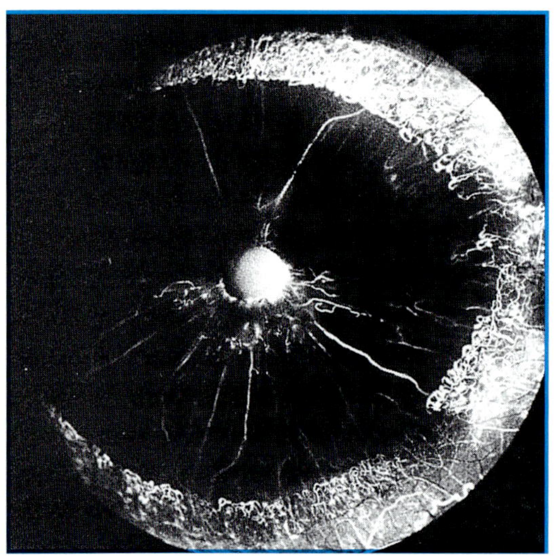

a)

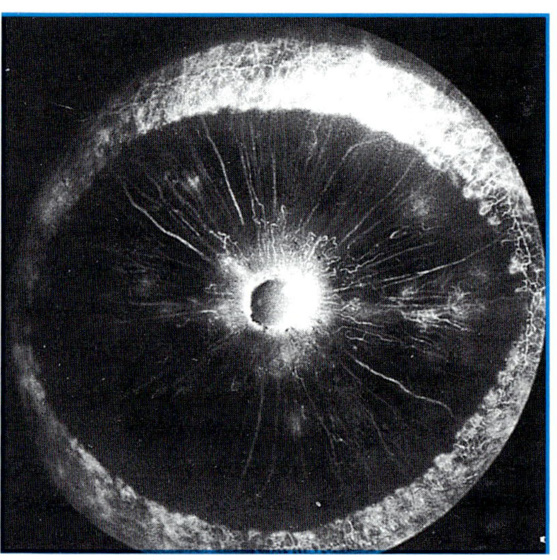

b)

Fig. ***4.8****,10 - Filling delays and loss of vascular architecture in a patient with long-standing angle-closure glaucoma (early (a) and late (b) iris fluorescein angiographic phases).*

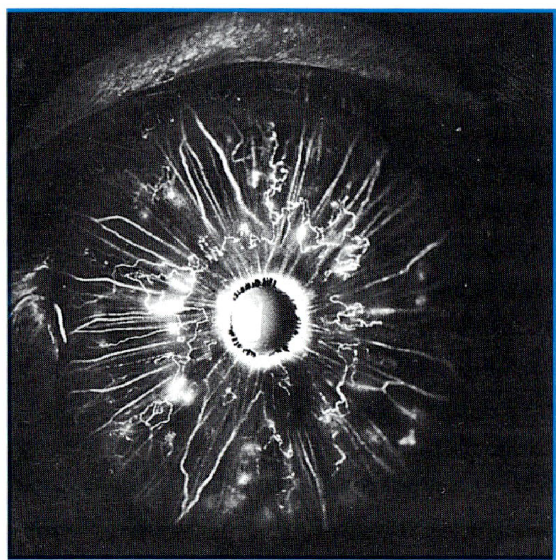

a)

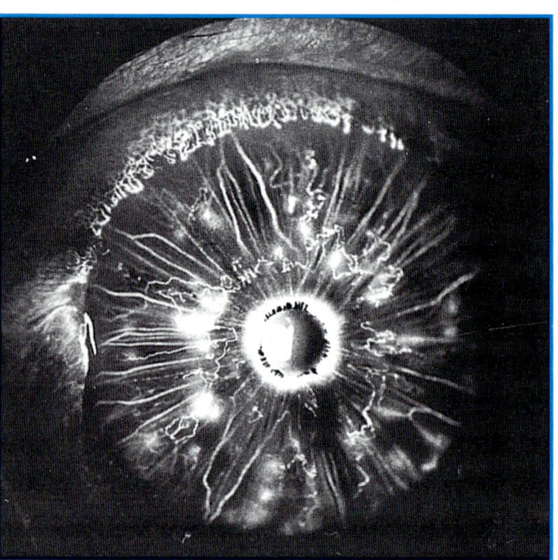

b)

Fig. ***4.8****,11 - Early (a) and late (b) iris fluorescein angiographic phases show iris neovascularization mainly in the pars ciliaris in primary angle-closure glaucoma.*

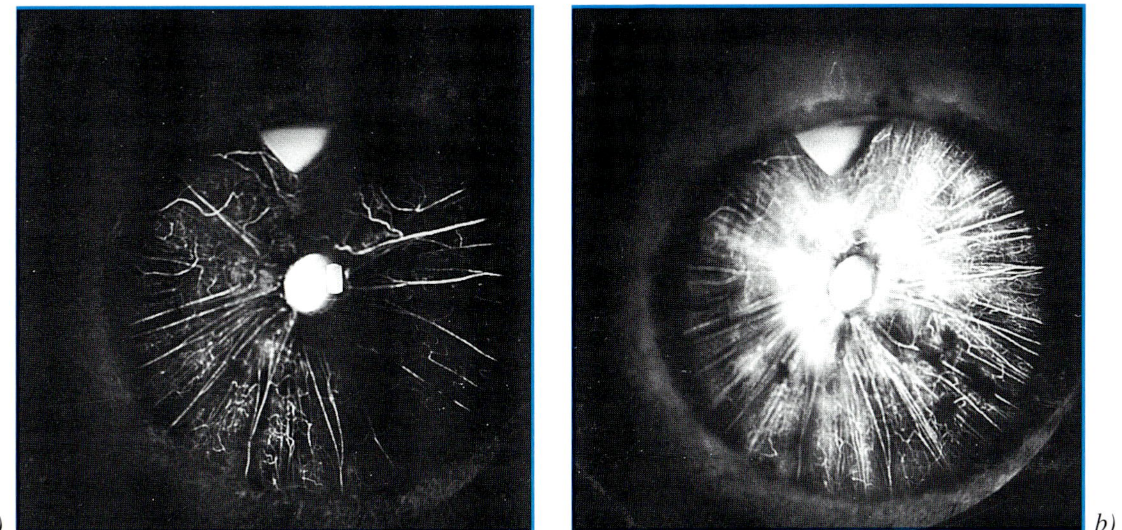

*Fig. **4.8**,12 - Abnormal vascular network covering most the surface of the iris (a), with heavy dye leakage in the late phases (b) in a patient with angle-closure glaucoma.*

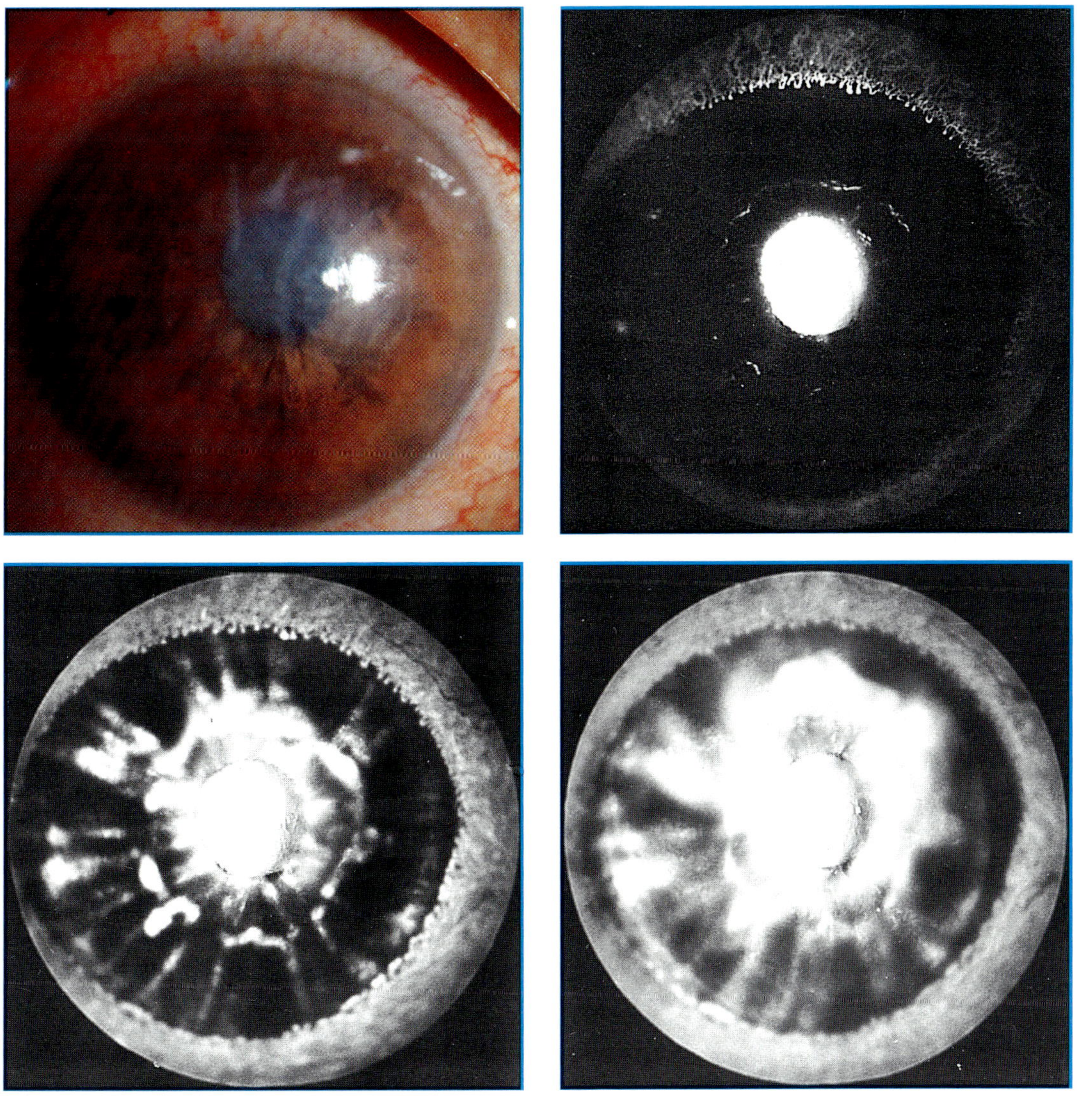

*Fig. **4.8**,13 - Biomicroscopy (a) and iris fluorescein angiographic phases (b,c,d) in an eye with angle-closure glaucoma three days after the acute attack. Despite the corneal edema, diffuse ischemia of the iris can still be seen, with marked congestion of the perfused vessels, causing heavy dye leakage, increasing in later angiographic phases.*

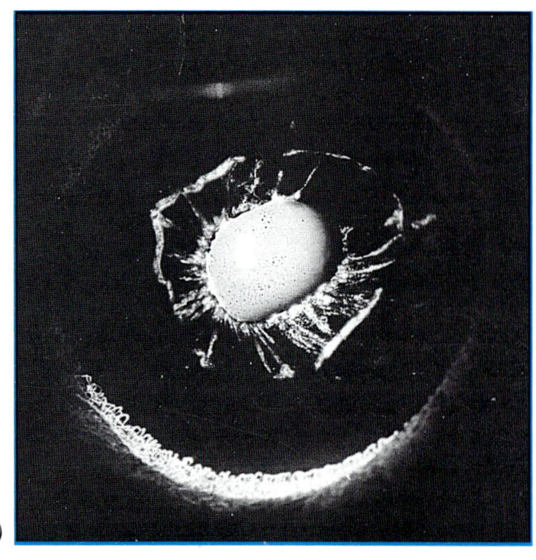

a)

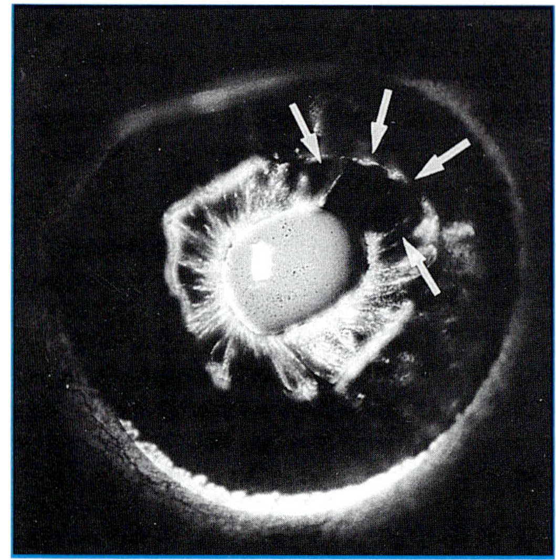

b)

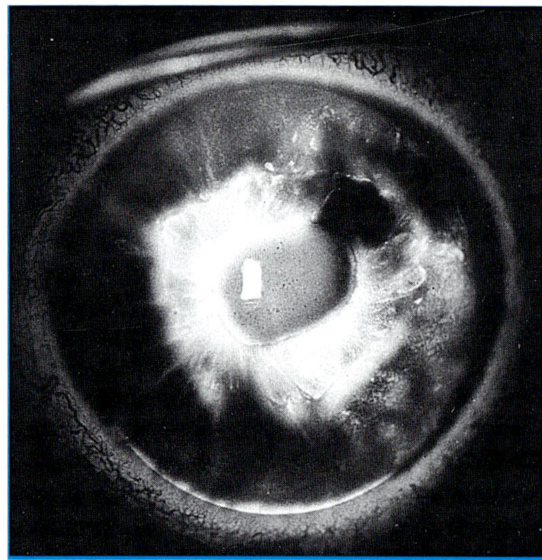

c)

Fig. ***4.8****,14 - Angle-closure glaucoma five days after the acute attack: iris fluorescein angiographic phases (a,b,c). The area remaining hypofluorescent (arrows) is the result of a circumscribed filling defect. Fluorescing vessels in the pupillary plexus are congested. There is some pigment loss with dispersion into the pupillary field.*

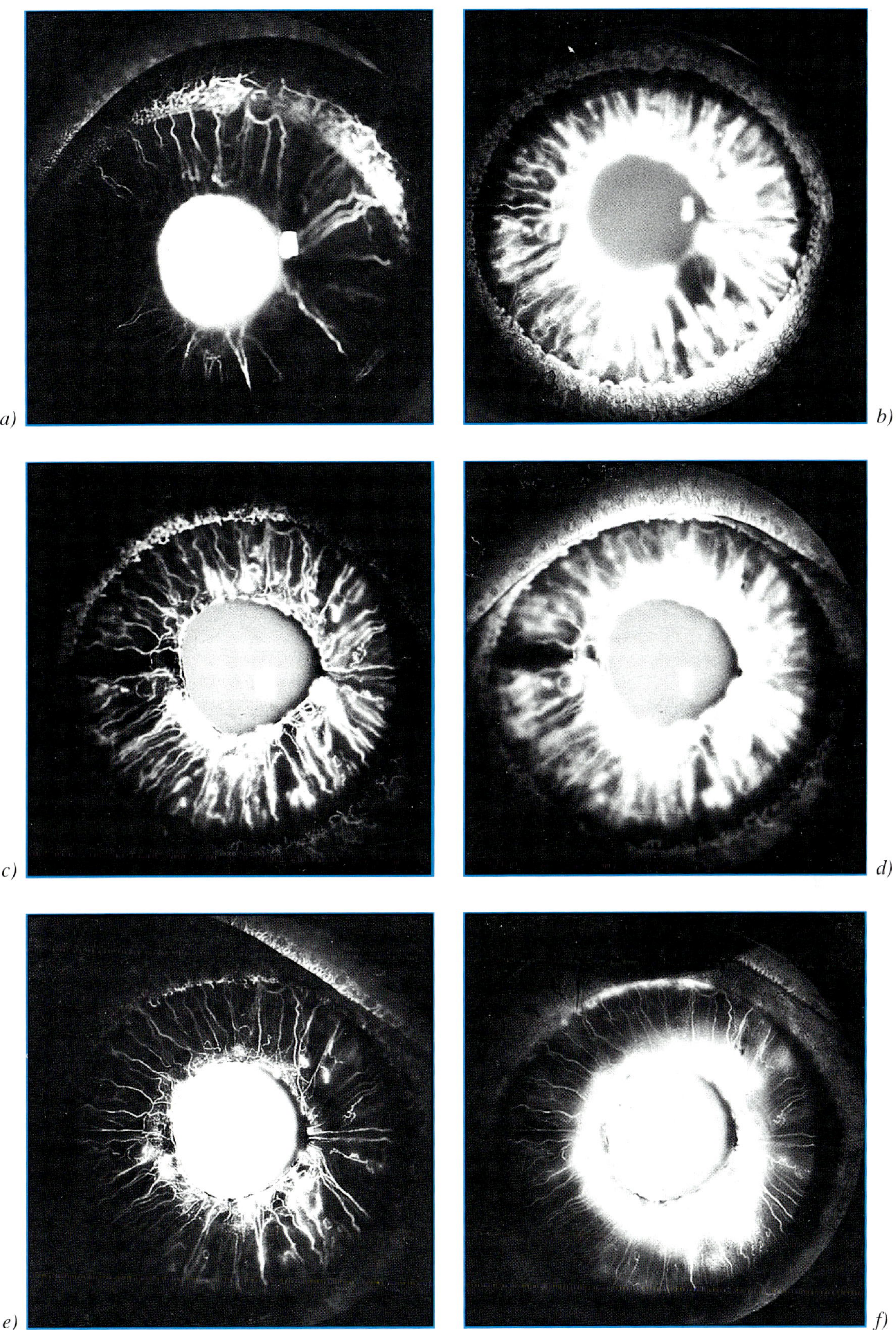

*Fig. **4.8**,15 - Early and late iris fluorescein angiographic phases in a case of angle-closure glaucoma three (a,b), eight (c,d) and 30 days (e,f) after the acute attack. Filling delays and defects are predominant, and there is marked vascular congestion, tending to diminish with time, leaving circumscribed areas of ischemia and neovascularization, especially in the pupillary portion.*

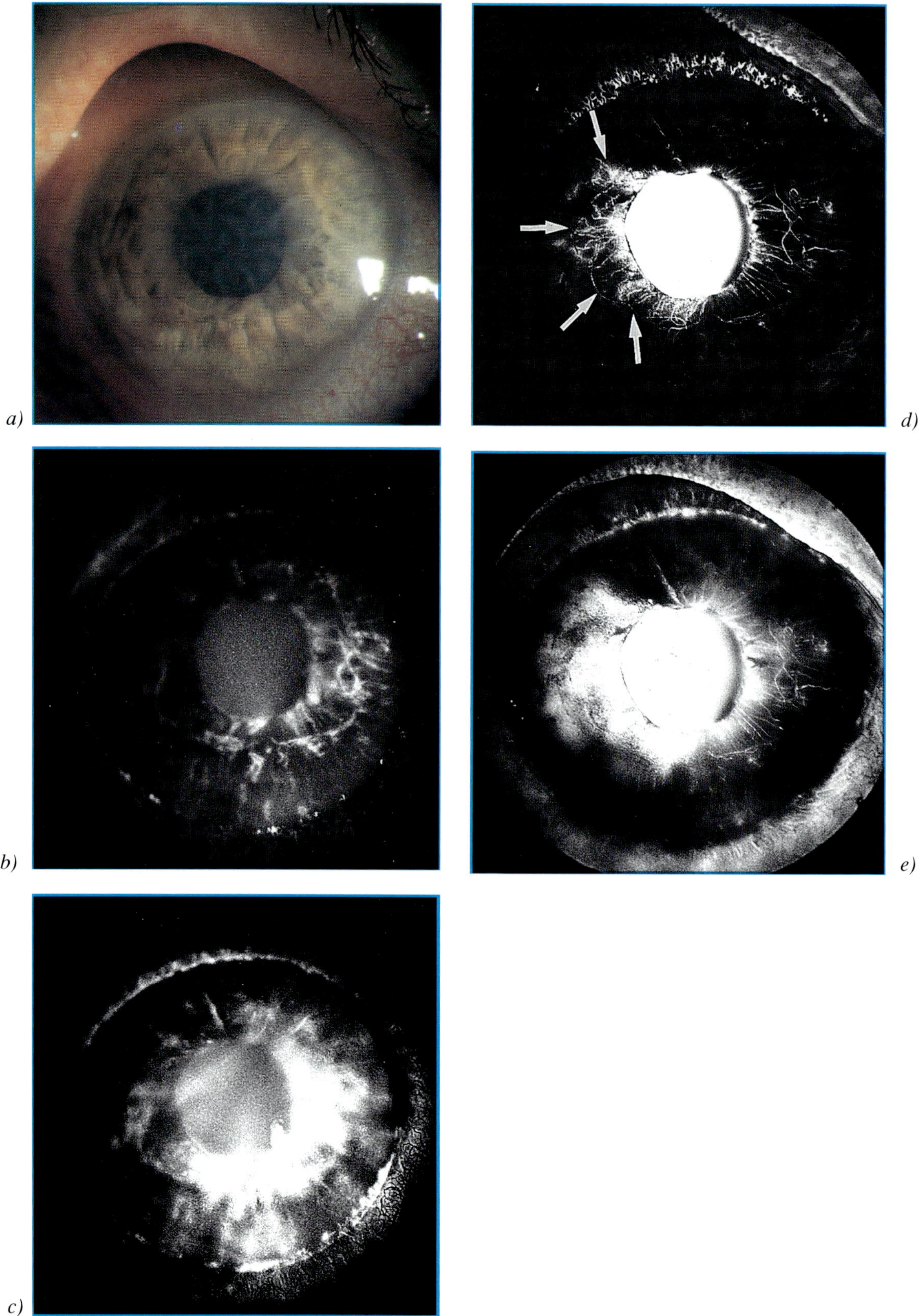

*Fig. **4.8**,16 - Another case of angle-closure glaucoma. Three days after the acute attack the corneal edema seen with the biomicroscope (a) interferes with the good resolution of the iris fluorescein angiographic images (b,c). Iris vascularization, however, is noticeably reduced, with marked congestion in the vessels that fill (mainly in the capillary plexus), and dye leakage in the later phases. By twelve days (d,e) in the areas that presented filling difficulties earlier (arrows) iris atrophy is setting in, making it possible to visualize the iris vessels. These are dis-*

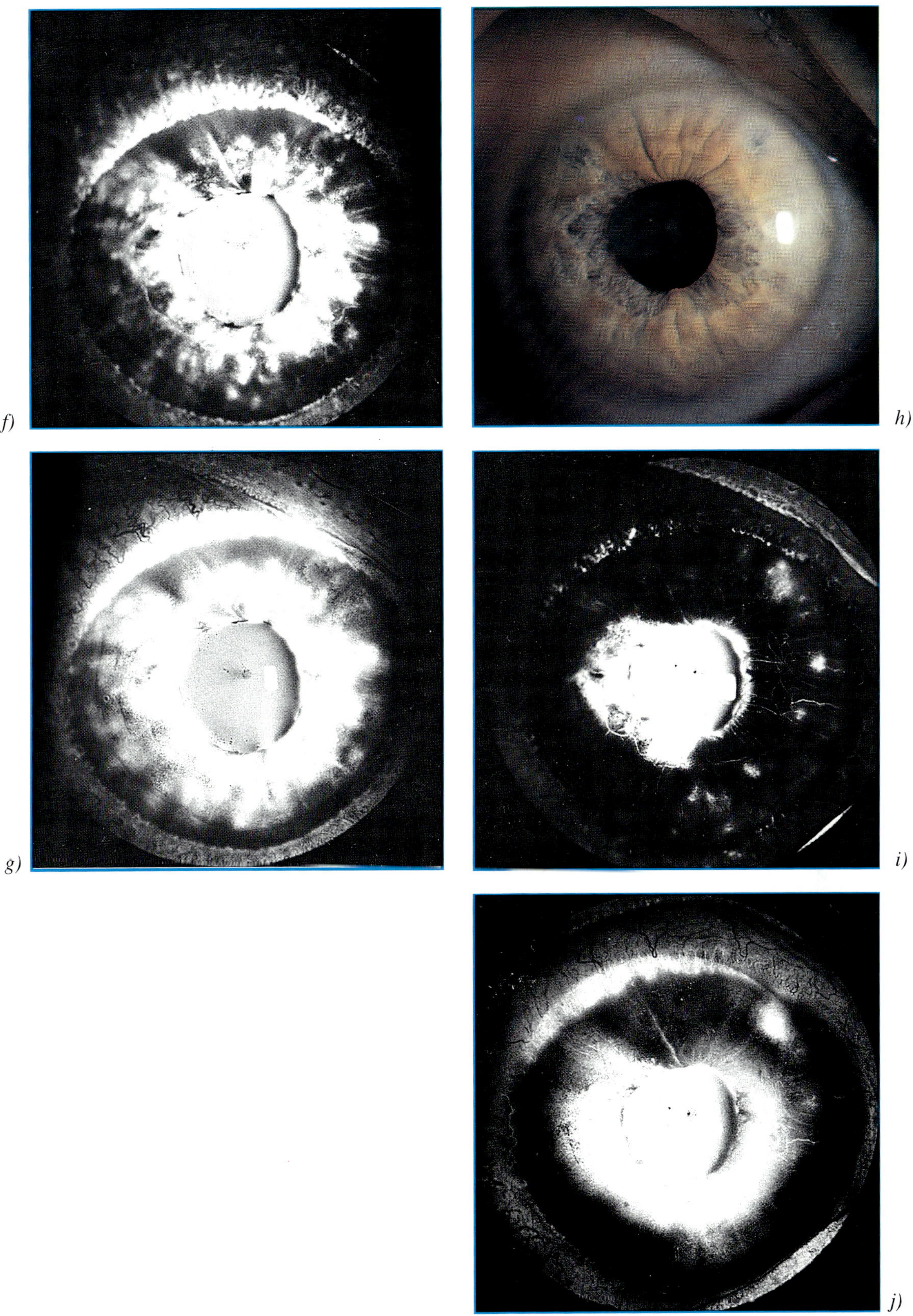

f) h) g) i) j)

orderly and leak dye. Small hyperfluorescent foci of vascular proliferation can be seen in the ciliary part. After three weeks (f,g) the whole iris vascular network appears congested, its permeability increased. In the later phases of the examination dye leaks from all over the iris surface. Biomicroscopy at two months (h) shows the iris atrophy is well defined. Iris fluorescein angiography shows there is less damage to the blood-iris barrier but there are persistent neovascular tufts in the stroma too, with filling defects (i,j).

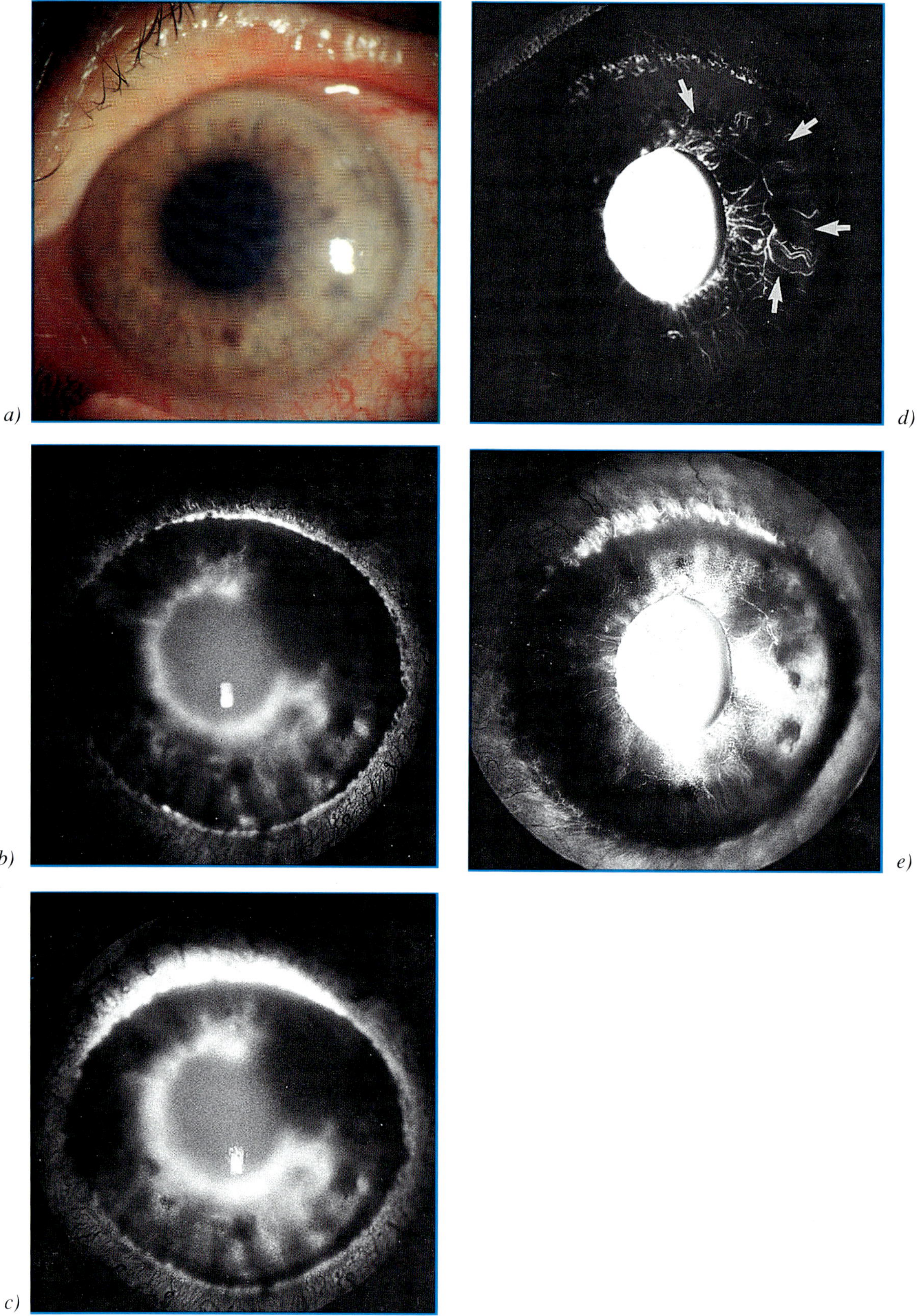
a)
b)
c)
d)
e)

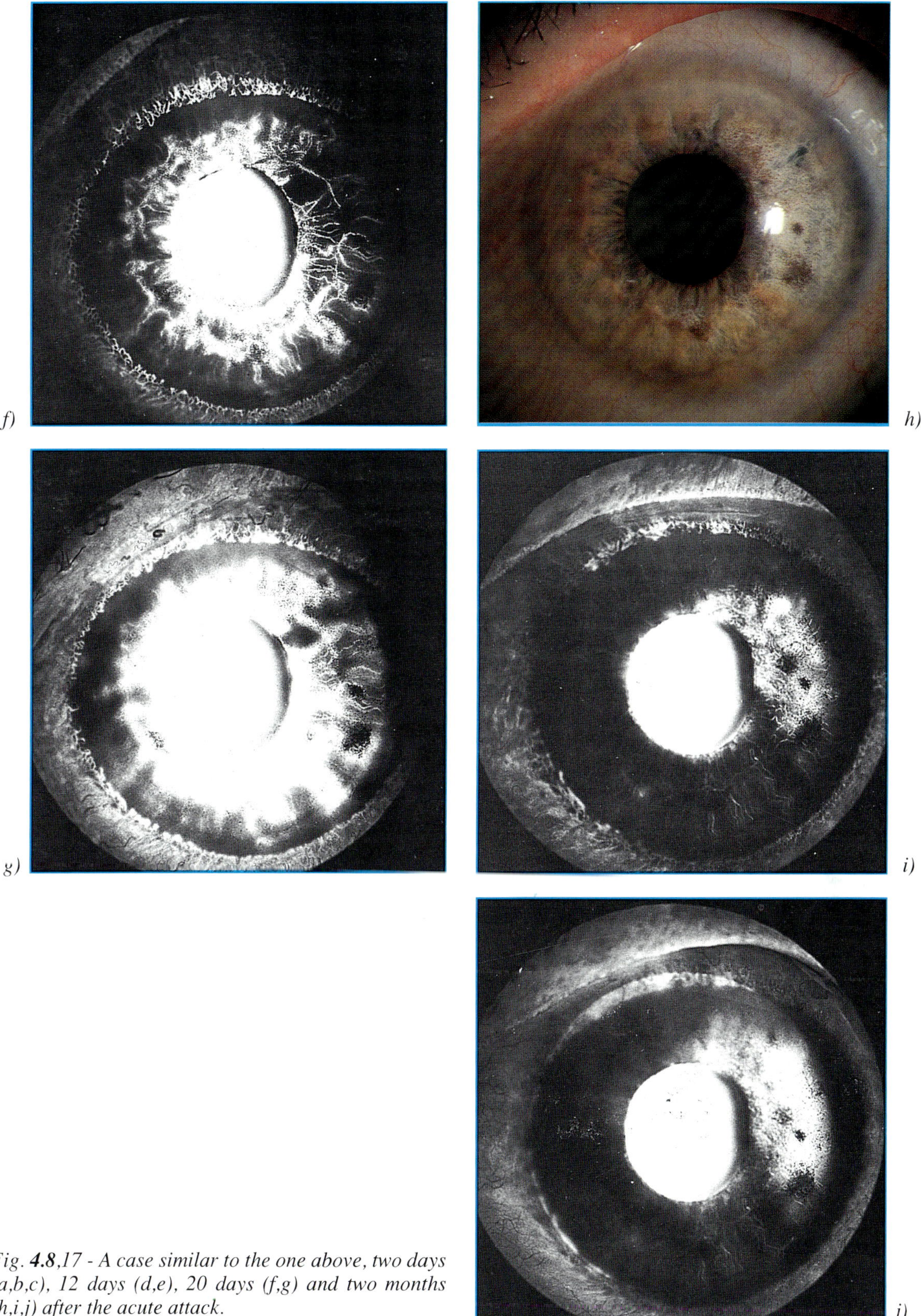

*Fig. **4.8**,17 - A case similar to the one above, two days (a,b,c), 12 days (d,e), 20 days (f,g) and two months (h,i,j) after the acute attack.*

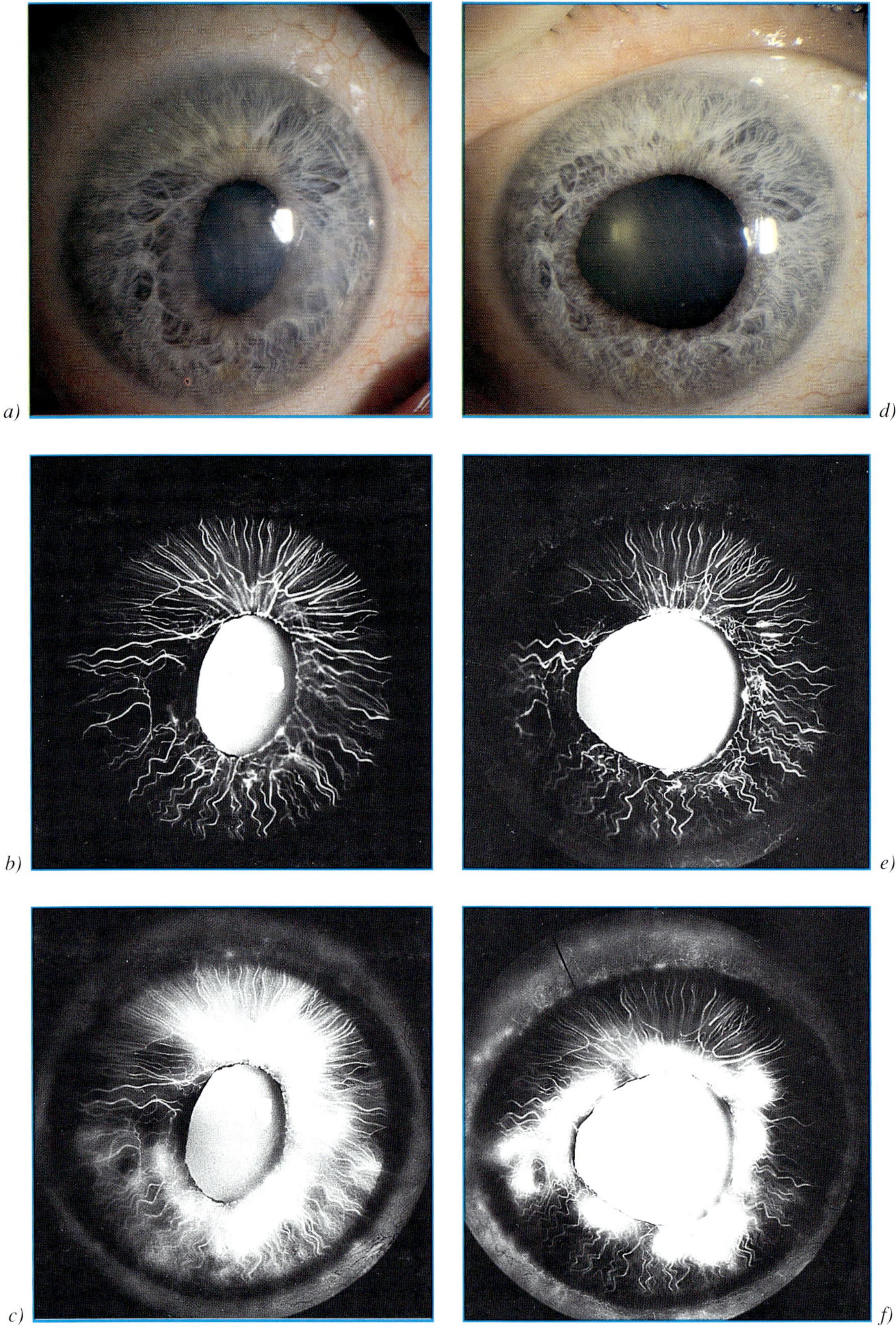
a)
d)
b)
e)
c)
f)

g) 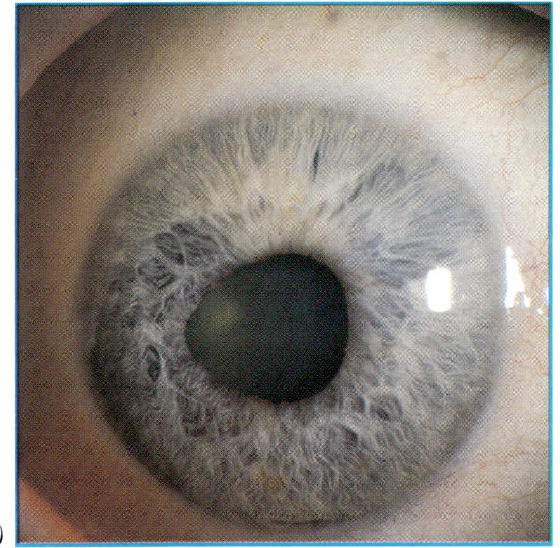

h) 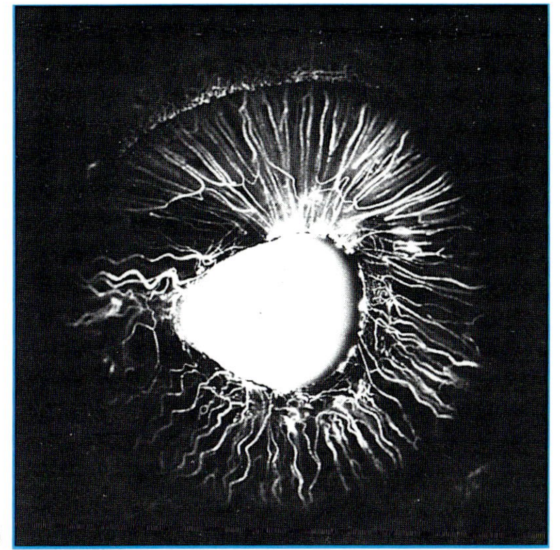

i) 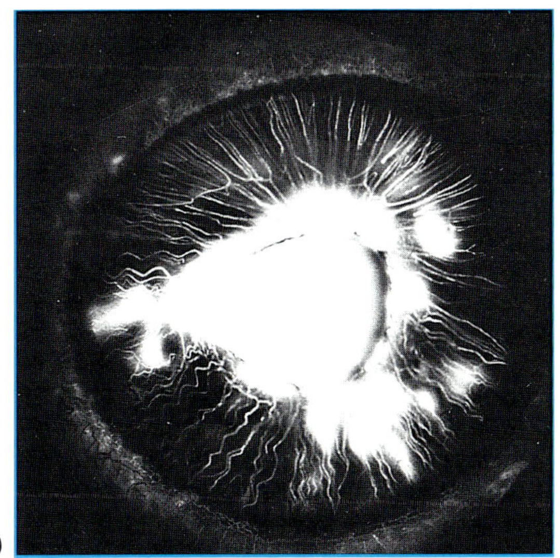

*Fig. **4.8**,18 - Biomicroscopy and early and late iris fluorescein angiographic phases in a case of angle-closure one (a,b,c), ten (d,e,f) and 30 days (g,h,i) from the acute attack (right eye). Filling delays and defects can be seen immediately after the attack in the temporal segment, with slight torsion of the stroma; later angiographic phases show marked rupture of the blood-iris barrier. By ten days persisting circumscribed areas of iris ischemia can be seen, most of the radial vessels are more tortuous, and neovascularization is starting at the pupillary border and in the stroma. These findings persist at 30 days, by which time the pupil is much more deformed.*

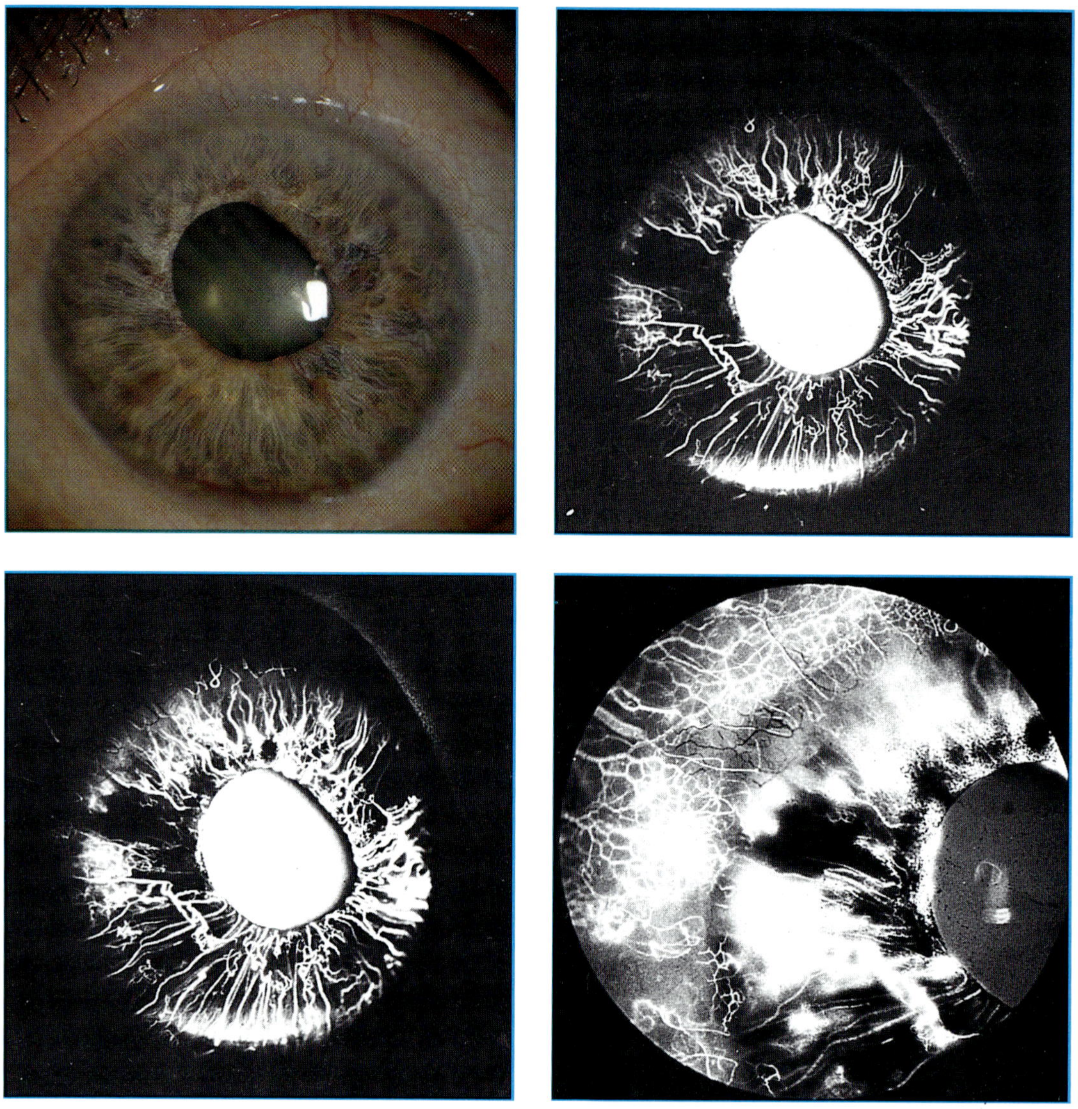

a) *b)*

c) *d)*

*Fig. **4.8**,19 - Diffuse ischemia, congested perfused radial vessels, abnormally increased permeability and initial vascular tufts, mainly in the pupillary plexus, mark the iris fluorescein angiographic images after this acute attack of angle-closure glaucoma (b,c,d). Biomicroscopy (a) shows areas of pigment atrophy where there is ischemia. There is also very mild hyphema.*

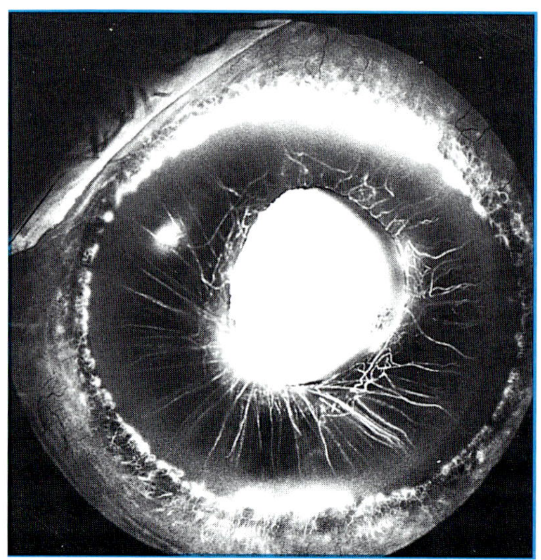

*Fig. **4.8**,20 - Limited neovascularization at the pupillary border and in the stroma subsequent to an acute attack of glaucoma (fluorescein angiography). Marked torsion of the iris stroma, altering the path of the radial vessels and causing irregular mydriasis can be seen.*

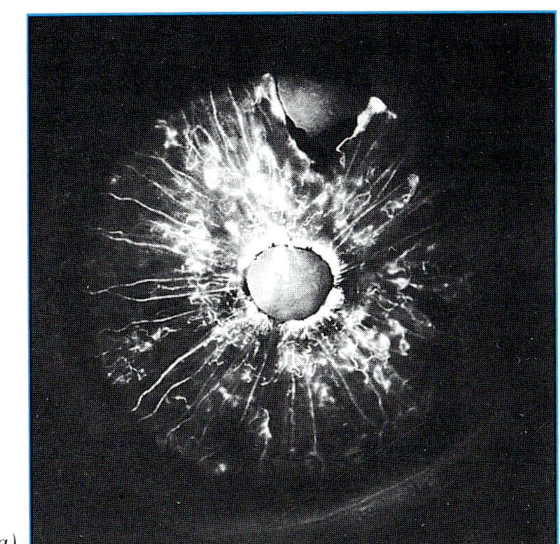

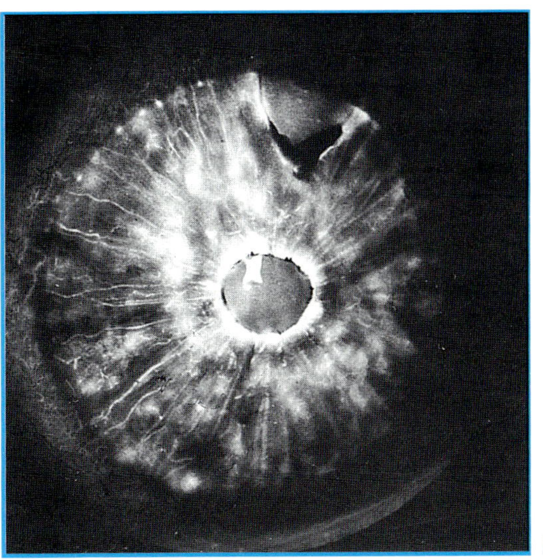

a) b)

*Fig. **4.8**,21 - Iris fluorescein angiography (a,b) in a case of angle-closure glaucoma, after an acute attack. The ocular hypertension has caused occlusion of some iris vessels, resulting in ischemic areas; the permeability of the vessels that fluoresce is altered and there are numerous hyperfluorescent foci of microvascular proliferation in the ciliary and pupillary parts.*

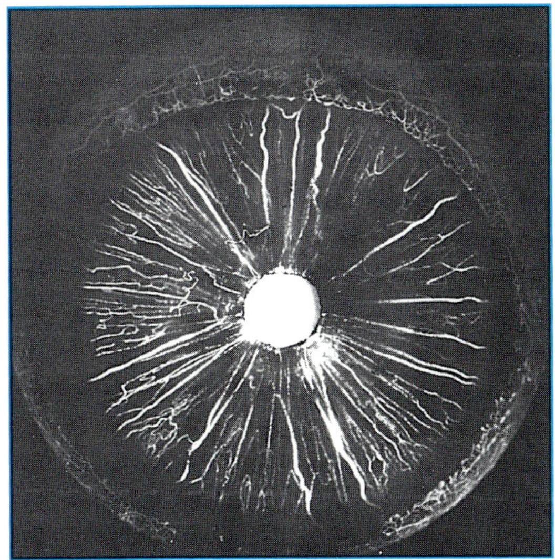

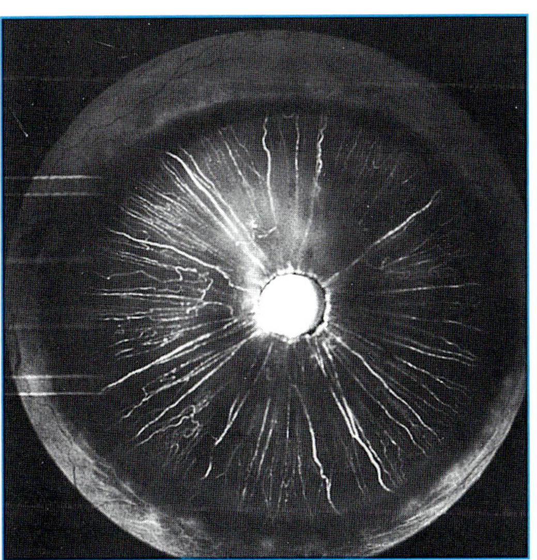

a) b)

*Fig. **4.8**,22 - Early (a) and late (b) iris fluorescein angiographic phases in a right eye with pseudoexfoliation syndrome. Initial distortion of radial vessels is detectable, with thinning and tortuosity mainly in the temporal ciliary part. In the nasal-superior sector there is a reduced amount of radial vessels, giving rise to a sectorial filling defect. Dye leakage in the late phase (b) comes mainly from the pupillary margin.*

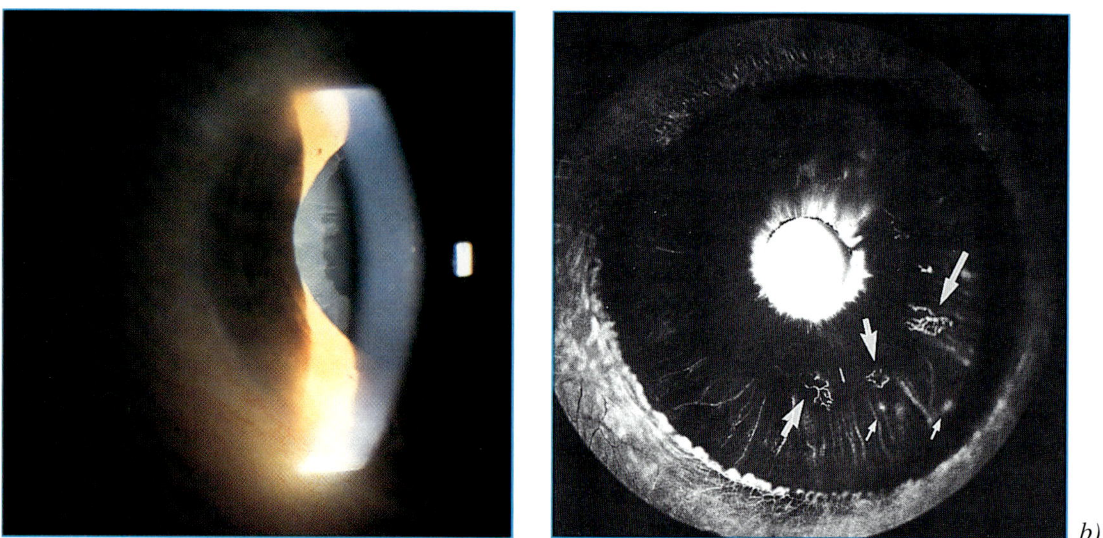

*Fig. **4.8**,23 - Biomicroscopy in mid-mydriasis (a) and iris fluorescein angiography (b) in a case of pseudoexfoliation syndrome. Angiography shows the typical anarchic tufts of new-formed vessels in the pars ciliaris (large arrows); radial vessels present microaneurysmatic dilatations (small arrows) and there is marked pupillary leakage.*

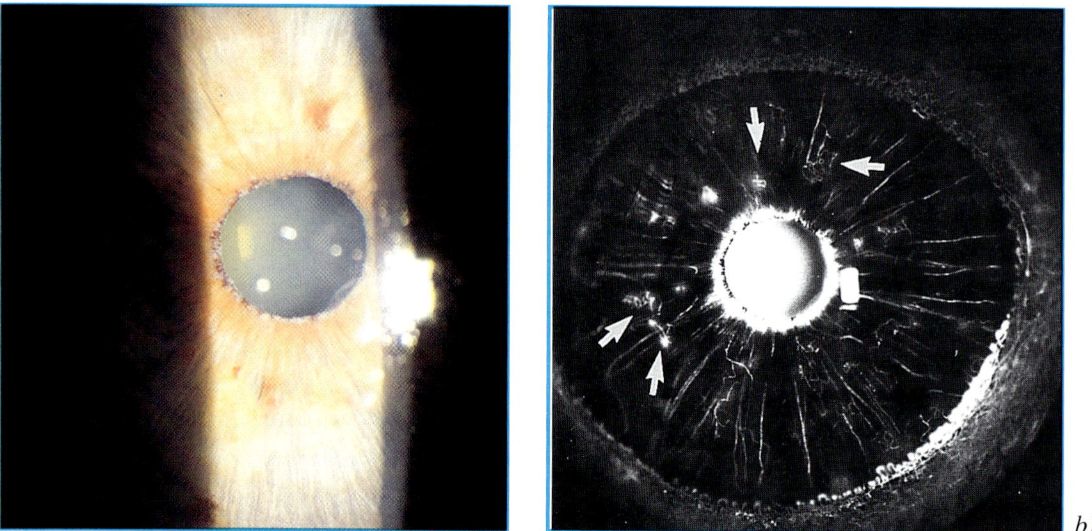

*Fig. **4.8**,24 - A case similar to the one above (a, biomicroscopy; b, iris fluorescein angiography). Radial vessels in the pars ciliaris follow an abnormal path, their size is altered and they show up poorly. Microneovascular tufts can be seen, leaking dye and becoming brightly visible (arrows).*

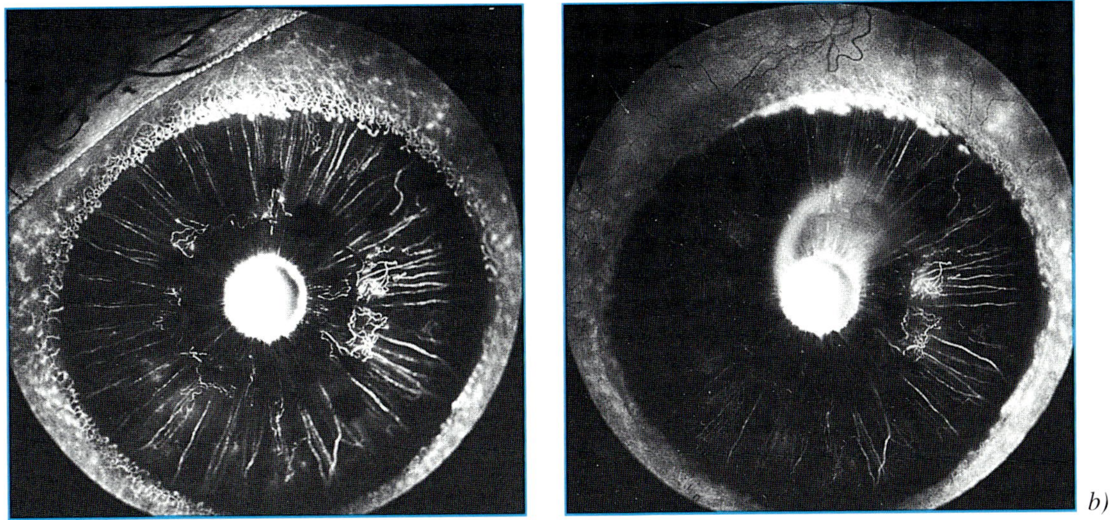

a) *b)*

Fig. ***4.8****,25 - Pseudoexfoliation syndrome; a, b) angiographic phases. In the pars ciliaris new-formed capillary networks can be seen, irregular in size and shape, taking up dye well and causing patchy leakage.*

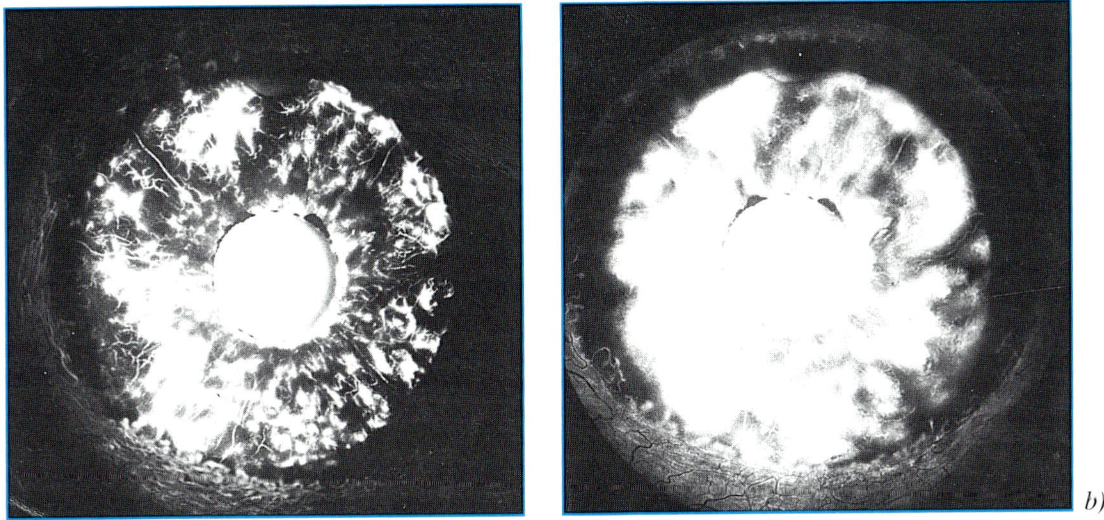

a) *b)*

Fig. ***4.8****,26 - Pseudoexfoliation syndrome with ocular hypertension. The whole vascular structure of the iris has been taken over by a dense neovascular network, clearly visible in the early phase (a) and leaking large amounts of dye in the later phase (b), finally covering the whole surface of the iris. Iridectomy is visible in the 12 o'clock position.*

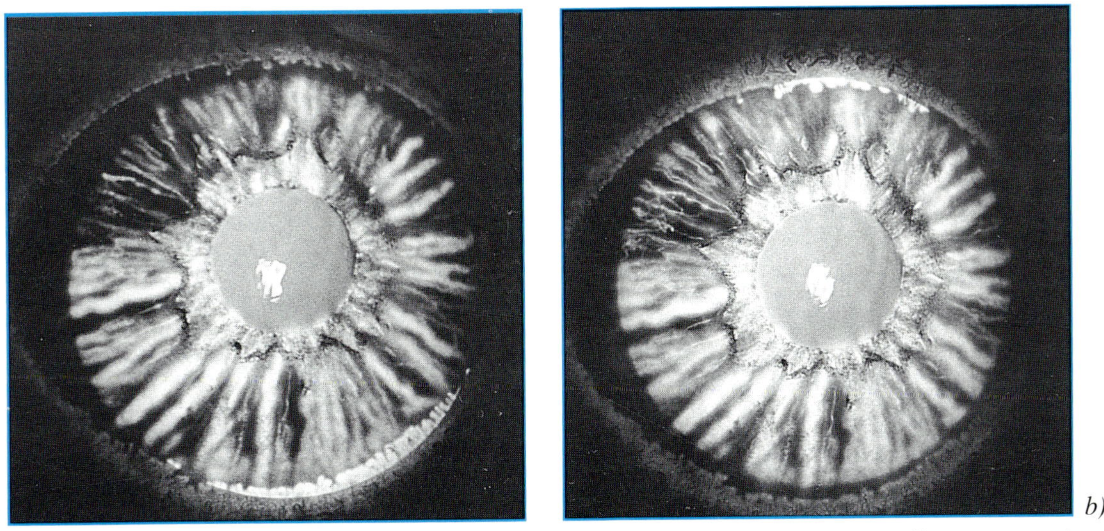

a) *b)*

Fig. ***4.8****,27 - Marked breakdown of the blood-iris barrier in a case of phakolytic glaucoma. Severe congestion of radial vessels and paravascular leakage are the dominant findings: a, b) iris fluorescein angiographic phases.*

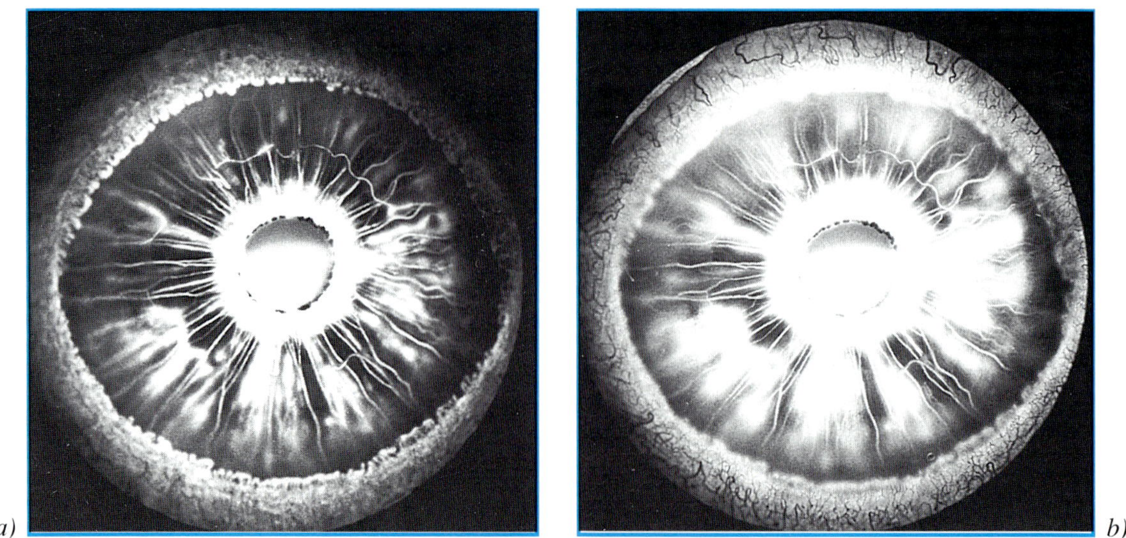

a) b)

*Fig. **4.8**,28 - Another case of phakolytic glaucoma seen in two angiographic phases (a,b). The darker half-moon in the top part of the pupillary field is caused by downwards subluxation of the hypermature lens. The resulting inflammation can be seen from the marked pupillary and stromal dye leakage, starting mainly from congested radial vessels.*

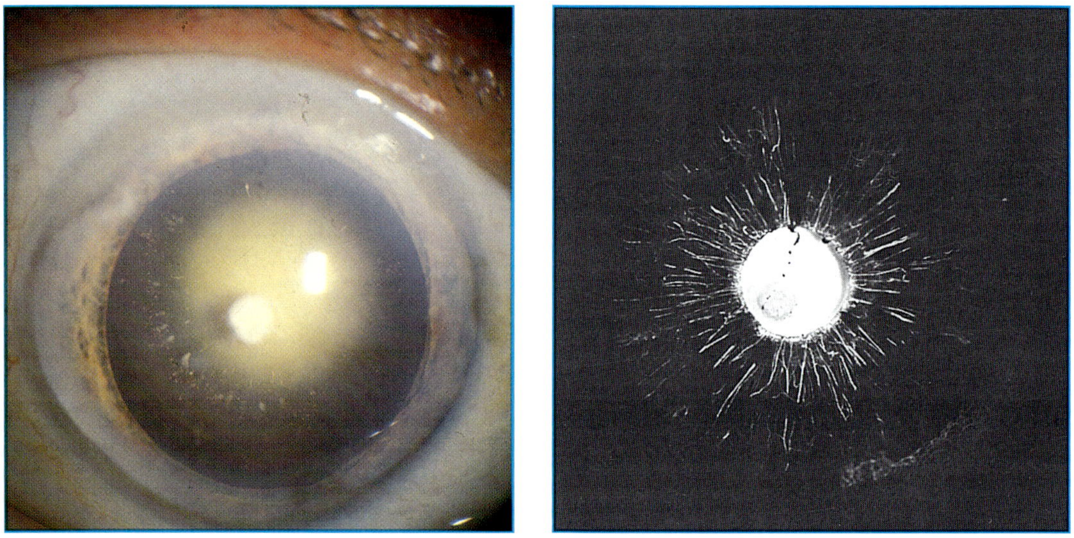

a) b)

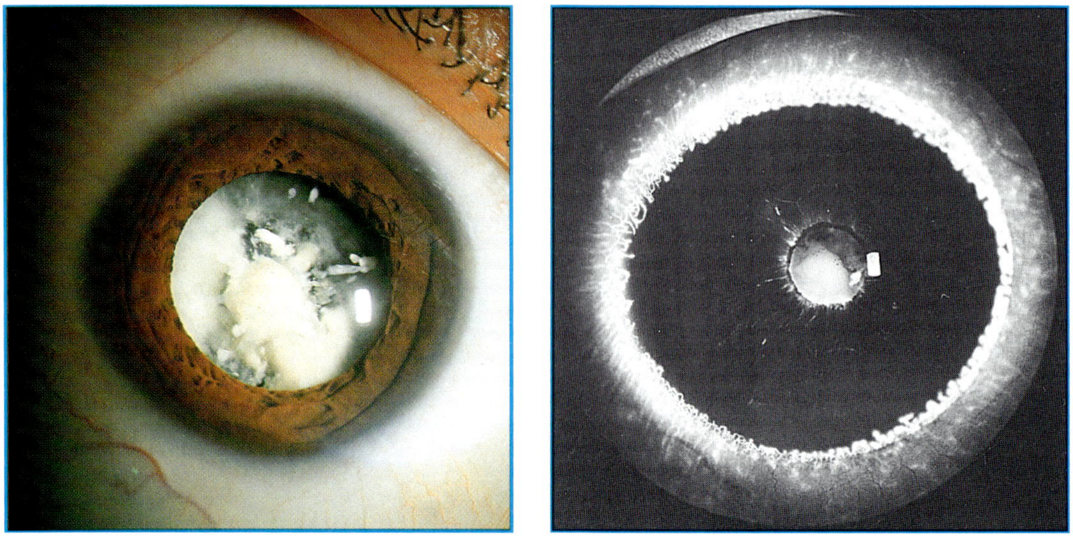

a) b)

*Figs. **4.8**,29,30 - Two cases of hypermature cataract: biomicroscopy in mydriasis (a) and angiographic (b) findings.*

R. Brancato, F. Bandello, R. Lattanzio
Atlas of Iris
Fluorescein Angiography
Kugler & Ghedini Publications 1995

Chapter 4.9

Surgical diseases

Iris fluorescein angiography is a useful means of detecting or quantifying iris abnormalities that cannot be assessed by other methods that might constitute either absolute or relative contraindications to surgery. Postponing an operation and taking therapeutic measures to facilitate the regression of the abnormality may help avoid serious complications in certain cases.

Many surgical procedures cause direct or indirect damage to the iris and in such cases iris fluorescein angiography can be employed after the operation to check on the effects on the hemato-aqueous barrier, and to monitor recovery of the iris circulation.

Cataract extraction

Iris fluorescein angiography serves to assess the vascular situation in the iris and the state of the hemato-aqueous barrier, besides providing indirect information on lesions to the fundus. It can be very useful, therefore, in patients with opacities in general and in those with cataract in particular.

Iris fluorescein angiography before cataract extraction

This examination should be done before cataract extraction in patients with:

1) current or past uveitis;
2) current or past vascular diseases (diabetes mellitus, retinal vein occlusion, etc.);
3) retinal vascular diseases (Eales' disease, etc.);
4) aftermaths of bulbar trauma.

Cataract in patients with current or past uveitis

In these patients iris fluorescein angiography plays an essential part in assessing the state of quiet of the globe before surgery for cataract extraction. This is valid for true cyclitic cataract, where the opacity of the lens is due to uveal inflammation, and for cases in which the cataract is associated with anterior, intermediate or posterior uveitis. This is the only investigation that will show up mild inflammation that is biomicroscopically silent or causes few symptoms.

Alterations detectable on iris fluorescein angiography that should cause surgery to be postponed are almost all associated with rupture of the blood-iris barrier, which leads, depending on the severity of the damage, to fluorescein leakage in the whole iris or parts of it (pars pupillaris and pars ciliaris). Occasionally new vessels are seen, or sectorial filling defects. Surgery done when iris fluorescein angiography shows these signs exposes the patient to the risk of intra- and post-operative complications. It is therefore wise to postpone cataract extraction and prescribe antiinflammatory drugs until the activity in the eye has died down.

Angiography of the iris is valuable in that it gives a precise picture of vascularization of the irido-lenticular membrane in patients with pupillary seclusion and/or occlusion caused by uveitis, and for scheduling the most appropriate surgical tactics. When the investigation shows none of these alterations, cataract surgery may be planned, with or without implantation of an intraocular lens, as this does not normally involve extra complications.

Cataract with current or past vascular diseases

In diabetic patients the presence of diabetic microangiopathy, which involves both the retina and iris, raises certain problems when they require cataract extraction. It is thus essential to obtain information on the type and severity of this disorder so as to avoid the risk of serious complications in these patients. If not adequately treated, diabetic retinopathy may progress after cataract extraction, as has been amply documented.[5,8,49,84,102,130,134,141,150] Studies on the course of diabetic iridopathy are far fewer.

A thorough preoperative evaluation including fluorescein angiography of the anterior segment is essential therefore for diabetic patients with cataract. This investigation, giving a detailed view of the iris vessels, shows up abnormalities that may not be visible on biomicroscopy, but that could be aggravated by surgery (Figs. **4.9**,1-5). Additionally, since retinal and iris vascular lesions are so closely related, iris fluorescein angiography gives indirect information on the type and degree of diabetic retinopathy in cases where a cataract makes it impossible to explore the fundus.

As mentioned in the chapter on Diabetic Microangiopathy, the size of the ischemic area of the retina is also closely correlated with alterations to the iris and advanced diabetic iridopathies are generally associated with extensive areas of retinal ischemia.[39] In a study on 225 eyes we ourselves found that angiographic detection of diabetic iridopathy in any form - non-proliferative, proliferative and neovascular glaucoma - was associated with diabetic retinopathy in no less than 93% of cases. We have also noticed that any case presenting proliferative iridopathy is sure to have serious forms of diabetic retinopathy too (pre-proliferative or proliferative).[16] This illustrates the importance of iris fluorescein angiographic examination before surgery in patients with diabetes requiring cataract extraction. If the examination shows active diabetic iridopathy, surgery must wait.

There are two main forms of active diabetic iridopathy that will show up on iris fluorescein angiography:

1) non-proliferative diabetic iridopathy with marked rupture of the blood-iris barrier in the pars stromalis;
2) proliferative diabetic iridopathy, grades 1, 2 and 3 (see chapter on Diabetic Microangiopathy) (Figs. **4.9**,6-8).

Cataract extraction in such cases must always be preceded by Krypton-laser retinal photocoagulation or, if the lens is too opaque to permit this, by cryocoagulation,[34] trans-scleral coagulation by continuous-wave Nd:YAG laser[36] or diode laser (Fig. **4.9**,9). Clearly these treatments must be selected, case by case, on the basis of careful ultrasound investigation of the conditions of the retina. If partial or total secondary retinal detachment is found, or even simply vitreoretinal traction, the indication to cryotreatment, for example, must be very carefully weighed up, as it may worsen the situation on account of the contraction of fibrovascular tissue it causes. If at follow-up three months after the photocoagulation, cryocoagulation, or whatever therapy was decided on, the iris fluorescein angiographic picture looks normal, then cataract extraction can be scheduled.

This whole procedure is based on the widely accepted pathogenic theory that iris neovascularization is a consequence of a vasoformative factor from ischemic areas of the retina spreading to the iris. Destruction of these areas by photocoagulation, cryocoagulation, trans-scleral continuous-wave Nd:YAG or diode lasers reduces the production of this presumed factor, permitting regression of the iridopathy (Figs. **4.9**,10-13).

If cataract surgery is done without these precautionary measures, there is the risk of rubeosis in a high percentage of patients presenting marked dye leakage from stromal vessels, or of existing neovascularization, when present, developing into the much more serious neovascular glaucoma.[5,34,110,127,129,134] The incidence of these complications is lower with extracapsular extraction than with the intracapsular technique.[34,102,129,134,174] This is largely interpreted as being due to the fact that the capsular diaphragm acts as a barrier to the spread of vasoformative factor from ischemic areas to the iris.[24,25,34,117,171] There is still much debate on whether this is the result of an active or passive mechanism in the posterior capsule of the lens (Fig. **4.9**,14).

Insertion of an artificial lens used to be contraindicated in diabetic patients but it is now considered possible as long as these patients have no retinopathy, or have exudative retinopathy, preferably already treated by laser photocoagulation, or even ischemic and/or proliferative retinopathy if it has been successfully treated with photocoagulation.[9,34,37,130,132,141] Thus diabetic retinopathy need no longer be considered a contraindication to intraocular lens implantation.[49,150]

Iris fluorescein angiography is useful in other vascular disorders too, such as *central retinal vein occlusion* or *branch occlusion*. As mentioned earlier, like diabetes mellitus these occlusions may cause ischemia of the retinal capillaries, leading to iris neovascularization. Once again, iris fluorescein angiography gives important indirect information on the situation in the retinal circulation (Fig.**4.9**,15).

Cataract associated with retinal vasculitis

These disorders involve both inflammatory and ischemic lesions, causing various degrees of retinal damage depending on the severity of the pathology. Iris fluorescein angiography supplies information on both these aspects of the disease, and is therefore useful as a diagnostic tool in assessing patients with cataract, giving indirect information on the retinal circulation.

Cataract and aftermaths of bulbar trauma

In all cases of traumatic cataract iris fluorescein angiography can help in checking for vascular structures inside any strands or synechiae and for assessing the extent of inflammation and degree of rupture of the blood-iris barrier. This investigation gives information that serves as a basis for scheduling extraction of the lens at the best time, and deciding on intraocular lens insertion, so as to prevent or at least limit the likelihood of intra- and post-operative complications.

Iris fluorescein angiography after cataract extraction with implantation of an intraocular lens

There is virtually a consensus among surgeons today that extracapsular extraction of a cataract, with insertion of an intraocular lens (IOL), is the most effective way of keeping down the number of complications and ensuring the best possible anatomical and functional results. This situation is the result of several developments:

1) the introduction of the operating microscope which, together with today's increasingly sophisticated instruments, has made the technique much more precise and reliable;

2) detailed study of post-operative complications, which are understood to be less frequent with extra- than intra-capsular extraction;
3) the implantation of artificial IOL in the posterior chamber, as an optimal optical solution to aphakia.

The last two points together have resulted in enormous gains over the intracapsular extraction and here, once more, iris fluorescein angiography has played a role in showing up the lesions caused by IOL in the anterior chamber.

Iris fluorescein angiographic studies[38,104,120] in patients with IOL in the anterior chamber showed up different types of pathological reactions in the iris:

1) dilated, compressed and displaced vessels;
2) abnormal vessel leakage, especially in the stroma;
3) focal leakage adjacent to the loops and in the zone where the implanted lens comes into contact with the surface of the iris;
4) incomplete vascular filling and areas of nonperfusion;
5) neovascularization.

When the lens is implanted in the anterior chamber and fixed to the iris in this point there may be compression of the vessels, resulting in areas of nonperfusion. With a pathogenic mechanism similar to that in the retina, these areas then become responsible for neovascularization. Demeler and Buhr-Ungher, however, could not confirm this (Figs. **4.9**,16-20).[52]

The iris fluorescein angiographic abnormalities described are rarely seen after implantation of the new anterior chamber intraocular lenses now on the market, which cause less damage to the iris architecture and less vascular irritation (Figs. **4.9**,21-23).

Iris fluorescein angiographic findings were as follows in patients operated for cataract with IOL implants in the posterior chamber:[91,104,111-113,120,161,162]

1) dye spread from the pupillary border, not always apparently age-related;
2) capillary dilatation with marked, circumscribed or diffuse dye leakage (from stroma too);
3) localized areas of dye leakage around the loops, correlated with hidden areas of iris erosion;
4) increased permeability of the iris at the points where the lens rests on the iris (Figs. **4.9**,24-27).

Rupture of the blood-iris barrier, observed in half the patients one month after surgery,[111] tends to diminish with time, disappearing generally by six months or a year.[52,55,136,146] Presumably the iris alterations noted in patients with an IOL implant are the result of microtrauma produced by the lens loops.[7,100,116] However, it has been suggested[7,18,46] that these lesions are due not only to mechanical factors but also to humoral transport of substances such as prostaglandins, or to activation of the complement system,[163] which cause rupture of the blood-iris barrier and inflammation in the anterior segment (Figs. **4.9**,28,29).

There is less risk of the "rubbing syndrome" when the implant is made in the capsular bag instead of the ciliary sulcus. There is also less likelihood of complications such as erosion and inflammation as the bag is in an area with less metabolic activity, and the anatomical position is more physiological. Iris angiography confirms that implant sin the capsular bag are better tolerated - there was a lower incidence of stromal dye leakage in patients with this implant than in those with a lens in the ciliary sulcus (Figs. **4.9**,30,31).

In an iris fluorescein angiographic study[62] comparing patients with silicone and PMMA lenses, the former had less rupture of the blood-iris barrier, probably reflecting the weaker mechanical impact of the silicone lens ion the local microvascular system. We ourselves found that Hydrogel IOL gave rise to less edematous iridopathy (Fig. **4.9**,32).

The increase in permeability observed with iris angiography and taken as an expression of the mild post-operative cyclitis, that is not detectable with the biomicroscope, could in some situations be reduced by post-operative administration of local or general anti-inflammatory agents.[58,162] Pre-operative instillation of indomethacin enhances the integrity of the blood-iris barrier.[6,13,15,17,18,162] Atropine has no effect on the hemato-ocular barrier but it does appear that preoperative miosis leads to greater dye leakage.[15,17]

Appropriate therapy must be started if iris angiography shows a marked and lasting increase in the permeability of iris vessels.[52,57]

In cases of post-aphakic cystoid macular edema (the *Irvine-Gass syndrome*),[71,72,82] iris fluorescein angiography shows a considerable increase in the permeability of iris vessels (edematous iridopathy), indicative of chronic iridocyclitis due to irritation from the IOL.[14,94,97,99] Pathological rupture of the blood-iris barrier corresponds to rupture of the blood-retinal barrier that gives rise to cystoid macular edema.[35,37,95,97] The abnormal permeability of the iris vessels manifests itself in dye leakage from radial vessels - which may be moderate, or else so massive and active as to mask the iris vessels and completely fill the anterior chamber.[32,33,35,57,95,97] As the cystoid edema regresses there is a parallel reduction and eventual disappearance of the iris leakage (Figs. **4.9**,33-36).

Cystoid macular edema with simultaneous edematous iridopathy is seen not only in pseudophakic eyes but also occurs as a late complication in patients operated for cataract removal without IOL implantation. Although it cannot be stated with certainty that implants themselves either cause the increased iris permeability or induce the macular edema, IOL must be viewed as an additional hazard in eyes that are already at risk. Iris fluorescein angiography may be a useful diagnostic aid in patients in whom macular edema is suspected. Any lasting increase in the permeability of iris vessels, combined with any degree of visual loss, should serve as a warning sign for possible further visual loss and eventual cystoid macular degeneration.[57]

Anterior segment ischemia

Anterior segment ischemia is a well-established complication that may arise after certain surgical maneuvers and/or after treatment that may affect the anterior chamber blood supply. Varying degrees of damage to the cornea, iris, ciliary body and lens are all features of ischemia.[116] The anterior segment perfusion deficiencies described in previous chapters as resulting from vascular insufficiencies at the posterior retinal areas or in the whole eye do not generally give rise to sudden massive ischemia of the anterior segment. Either they start slowly, allowing for neovascular compensation or reaction, or they are sudden but only limited in duration and extent, and therefore cause sectorial filling defects that are not drastic enough to induce total ischemia.

In anterior segment ischemia, however, the basic lesion is tissue death, with consequent atrophy and scar formation. There is no new vessel formation, and the atrophic areas of the iris generally remain avascular, without developing rubeosis.[95] In mild cases, the vascular damage to the pupillary sphincter results in a slight defect in the pupil's response to light stimulus, in the ischemic sector. More severe cases present the classic clinical appearance of an oval, semi-dilated pupil with distortion and bunching of radial stromal fibres. The iris stroma is visibly altered only after the more severe attacks.[56]

Simple sit-lamp examination of the iris may not show up the real extent of the underlying vascular disorder. Iris fluorescein angiography is then a useful diagnostic aid, and quantifies the impairment in blood supply to the atrophic areas. Signs in the anterior segment may in fact be very similar to those resulting from other stimuli such as operative trauma, infections or acute increases in intraocular pressure, and this may easily lead to misdiagnosis and wrong therapy.

Fluorangiographic findings in patients with anterior segment ischemia can be summarized as follows:[44,56,95,109]

- leakage from the affected iris segment, either localized (generally at the pupillary border), or generalized, from pupillary and stromal vessels. The severity of this leakage is proportional to the severity of ischemia;
- filling delays;
- filling defects (iris ischemia), especially when biomicroscopy shows marked iris stromal atrophy;
- patches of diffuse fluorescence in the ischemic area (rare);
- loss of iris vascular architecture;
- radial vessels amputated where they enter the ischemic area, with heaviest dye leakage from this distal stump;
- abnormal vascular patterns;
- limited neovascularization around the nonperfused areas (rare) (Figs. **4.9**,37-42).

Experimental studies on anterior segment ischemic have found iris angiographic findings similar to those set out above.[10,69,76,96,98,142,167,168]

Ischemia of the anterior segment may also be induced by surgery, as in the following cases:

1) *interruption of blood flow in the anterior ciliary arteries by temporary disinsertion of the rectus muscles.*[73,77,78,153,169] This has been reported after extensive extraocular muscle surgery in patients with strabismus, when three or four recti are simultaneously disinserted.[20,56,63-65,68,73,77,83,95,101,125,126,137,147,148,154,157,169,170] Currently, when three rectus muscles need operating, some surgeons[68,147,148,154] prefer to divide the procedure into two operations at an interval of three to five months, or else botulin toxin is used,[22,66] so that no more than two muscles are operated at the same time. This appears to reduce the risk of anterior segment ischemia. In the interval between operations the blood flow to the anterior uvea should have time to become re-established through collateral circulation. The major risk of damage is thus after the first operation on the rectus muscles, and more risk is attached to detachment of vertical recti muscles than in cutting the horizontal muscles.[77,125,126]

   Hayreh & Scott,[77] the first to report iris fluorescein angiographic studies in strabismus surgery, analysed post-operative patterns in relation to the different types of tenotomy of the recti. They found that tenotomy of one or both horizontal recti induced no appreciable circulatory disturbance in the iris; however, tenotomy of the superior or inferior rectus caused circulatory delay in the respective temporal sectors of the iris. Combined tenotomies of a horizontal and one or two vertical recti resulted in lesions only in the region of the vertical rectus. The blood supply to the nasal half of the iris was not normally deranged by tenotomy of the vertical and/or medial rectus.[77]

   In another fluorescein angiographic study of the iris, Olver & Lee[126] reported characteristic iris sectorial perfusion defects in 89% of the eyes operated by primary vertical muscle surgery. They used iris angiography to quantify the degree of anterior segment ischemia, measuring the filling delay and the size of the iris sector that presented filling defects.
2) *diathermy or cryotherapy damage to the long posterior ciliary arteries;*[29,153,175]
3) *use of too tight or badly placed encircling scleral band or buckles;*[44,54,78,140,143]

4) *compression of the vortex veins, cutting uveal blood flow because of reduced drainage.*[75,76,78]

All these maneuvers, which reduce blood flow to the iris, may result in anterior segment ischemia in eyes operated for retinal detachment.[28,29,44,47,53,56,74,95,175] Placing tight encircling polyethylene tubes or bands has often been shown to cause the most serious complications.[28] Reactions to these procedures may even include iridocyclitis, hyphema, hypotony and cataract formation. Affected eyes may become blind and so painful that enucleation is the only solution. Nevertheless, the lesions may not be easily visible and iris fluorescein angiography may be the only method that detects them. Treatment for severe anterior segment ischemia involves promptly cutting or loosening the encircling band in cases with a high encircling scleral buckle. In other cases the scleral buckle may be adapted so as to cause less compression of the vortex veins.

The iris neovascularization observed after surgery in patients with rhegmatogenous retinal detachment is a different type of complication from anterior segment ischemia. It has been suggested that two factors are important in the pathogenesis of iris neovascularization in this type of detachment. Persistent retinal detachment is an essential factor since it reduces retinal circulation, and the reduction of choroidal circulation caused by severe myopia, increased intraocular pressure or surgical complications may act as a second contributory factor.[27,31,41,48,78,155,158,159,165,177,178]

Neovascularization of the iris is an ominous prognostic sign of rhegmatogenous retinal detachment and it can only be prevented by prompt reattachment of the retina and constructive efforts to prevent the reduction in choroidal circulation (Figs. **4.9**,43-45).

Vitrectomy for complications of diabetic retinopathy

Neovascular glaucoma is one of the most common and dangerous complications following vitrectomy for severe proliferative diabetic retinopathy.[1-4,23,26,106,114,115] The pathogenesis of iris neovascularization and neovascular glaucoma in these patients remains a question for debate. There are several putative predisposing high-risk factors:

1) active proliferative diabetic retinopathy at the time of vitrectomy;
2) persistent retinal ischemia after vitrectomy in patients who have not undergone panretinal photocoagulation;
3) retinal detachment persisting after surgery;[4,27,114,115,172]
4) aphakia, since the lens as well as the anterior and posterior capsules and the anterior hyaloid are all believed to act as barriers to anterior diffusion of vasoproliferative agents released by the retina, and to posterior diffusion of oxygen from the anterior segment;[2,25]
5) post-operative inflammation. Here, low-molecular-weight volatile components and any impurities in the silicone oil are also believed to play a role.[51,61,87,155]

Controversy still surrounds the question whether silicone oil tamponade influences the development of rubeosis iridis in diabetic vitrectomized eyes. The oil is widely considered important in preventing the onset or aggravation of rubeosis iridis[40,43,61,79,107] or may even reduce the frequency of neovascular glaucoma.[105,139] Some Authors do not consider it to influence the evolution of iris microangiopathy.[17] However, there is still no clear-cut demonstration of how and whether silicone oil influences post-operative iris neovascularization.[50,108,176]

In the diabetic eye neovascular glaucoma tends to become manifest within six months of vitrectomy[26,114] although iris fluorescein angiography may show up early alterations in the first few weeks.

The incidence of neovascular glaucoma after vitrectomy in diabetic patients varies widely, from 9-25% in different studies.[3,4,26,59,74,106,114,115,119,124] It appears to be higher if vitrectomy and lens extraction are combined. Although rubeosis can develop de novo after vitrectomy, numerous studies have found that the incidence of neovascular glaucoma is higher in eyes presenting this condition preoperatively (Figs. **4.9**,46-52).[1-4,23,59,103,106,119,124,128,173,179]

Iris fluorescein angiography, giving a better picture than biomicroscopy of initial iris new vessels, is thus very useful for preoperative assessment of diabetic patients scheduled for vitrectomy.

In some studies this investigational method was employed to assess rubeosis iridis in diabetic patients after vitrectomy. Ehrenberg[58] found a significant correlation between the degree of preoperative leakage and post-operative rubeosis: rubeosis was detected after surgery in 39% of the eyes that had shown marked preoperative dye leakage from the pupillary margin, in 73% of the eyes with diffuse pupillary margin leakage and circumscribed stromal leakage, and in all the cases with diffuse pupillary and stromal leakage. Ehrenberg[58] also investigated whether post-operative topical steroid therapy reduced the risk of iris new vessels developing but iris fluorescein angiography showed no difference in the degree of rubeosis in treated and untreated eyes. However, neovascular glaucoma, which occurred post-operatively in 9% of the eyes considered, was statistically more frequent in the non-steroid group.

Moyenin & Bonnet[118] found rubeosis was unchanged in 82% of eyes after vitrectomy and therefore concluded that surgery did not aggravate iris neovascularization; however, in their study two thirds of the eyes already had advanced rubeosis preoperatively. Zakow & Lewis[179] reported a 63% incidence of post-operative neovascular glaucoma in patients with preoperative rubeosis, graded 3 or 4 by their iris fluorangiographic classification system (see chapter on Diabetic Microangiopathy). Blankenship[23] found that neovascular glaucoma developed during the six-month follow-up after surgery in 33% of eyes with preoperative neovascularization, compared to 17% of those without rubeosis before surgery.

It thus appears that the incidence and characteristics of rubeosis iridis after surgery are directly proportional to the severity of preoperative damage to the iris.

Summarizing the state of today's knowledge, therefore, there are several measures the surgeon can and should take with the aim of reducing the risk of rubeosis iridis:

- all possible efforts to ensure the quiescence of proliferative diabetic microangiopathy in the retina and iris, before vitrectomy, ideally by ablating retinal ischemia through both laser photocoagulation and trans-scleral cryoapplication before surgery. In cases in which the vitreoretinal conditions do not permit this, panretinal photocoagulation is mandatory either at the time of surgery or immediately thereafter (Figs. **4.9**,53,54);
- surgical repair of retinal detachment at the time of vitrectomy;
- leaving the lens intact whenever possible;
- prompt, vigorous treatment of inflammation;
- to use iridography to monitor the small peripheral retinal detachments usually remaining in eyes filled with silicone, which often do not affect the final outcome of surgery but might cause worsening of diabetic iridopathy.[12]

In diabetic patients needing vitrectomy iris fluorescein angiography can provide useful predictive parameters and is a valuable aid in establishing the exact effects of the surgical procedure on the course of iris microangiopathy (Fig. **4.9**,55).

Microsurgery of the anterior segment using the Nd:YAG laser

The oftalmologist has now had access to the therapeutic possibilities of the Nd:YAG laser for about ten years and is fully familiar with the many advantages it offers over traditional surgical approaches, especially in capsulotomies, iridotomies and synechiotomies. However, its use calls for constant vigilance on account of the large amount of energy released by this instrument and the resulting shock wave inside the globe. Iris fluorescein angiography provides a convenient means of investigating its side effects and complications.

Menchini[109] investigated the changes to the blood-iris barrier before and one month after treatment of the anterior segment with the Nd:YAG laser in 89 patients. The findings can be summarized as follows:

- in 22 out of 24 capsulotomies, the iris angiographic findings were substantially the same after treatment. The two exceptions both presented rupture of the blood-iris barrier before and after treatment (Figs. **4.9**,56-59);
- in 8 out of 16 photoresections of retropupillary membranes, the iris fluorescein angiographic picture showed virtually no activity. In the other eight there was an increase in the extent of rupture of the blood-iris barrier, which was already damaged before surgery;
- in 16 cases of anterior vitreolysis, there was always a clear-cut improvement of the damage to the blood-iris barrier. The greater the traction of vitreal strands on the iris before treatment, the more striking was the beneficial effect on stromal dye leakage;
- in 20 cases of iridotomy, postoperative iris fluorescein angiography showed circumscribed leakage from radial vessels around the incision, with little involvement of other iris sectors (Figs. **4.9**,60,61);
- in 13 cases of coreoplasty and coreopraxy postoperative iris fluorescein angiography showed extensive rupture of the blood-iris barrier, with marked dye leakage from all the stromal vessels (Fig. **4.9**,62).

Nd:YAG laser treatments thus appear to have a negative effect on the blood-iris barrier only when it is already damaged by trauma or surgery. When photoresection eliminates the source of irritation, angiographic findings show considerable improvement. However, it is advisable before treatment to examine any eyes suspected of not being quiet by iris fluorescein angiography, as the findings provide useful guidelines on when and how to conduct Nd:YAG photoresection (Fig. **4.9**,63).

References

1 Aaberg TM: Vitrectomy for diabetic retinopathy. In Freeman HM, Hirose T, Schepens CL: Vitreous surgery and advances in fundus diagnosis and treatment. Appleton Century Croft, New York, 1977.

2 Aaberg TM: Clinical results in vitrectomy for diabetic traction retinal detachment. Am J Ophthalmol 88: 246, 1979.

3 Aaberg TM: Advanced diabetic retinopathy: surgical treatment of complications. Ann Int Med 99: 562, 1983.

4 Aaberg TM, VanHorn DL: Late complications of pars plana vitreous surgery. Ophthalmology 85: 126, 1978.

5 Aiello LM, Wand M, Liang G: Neovascular glaucoma and vitreous hemorrhage following cataract surgery in patients with diabetes mellitus. Ophthalmology 90: 814, 1983.

6 Albertini G, Montard M, Entraygues H et al: Implants et iris: etude angiographique. Bull Soc Ophtalmol Fr 5: 663, 1982.

7 Alpar JJ: Progressive iris pigment loss following cataract operation. Part III. Contribution to Binkhorst-Norddlohne barrier deprivation syndrome. Contact Intraocul Lens Med J 5: 81, 1979.

8 Alpar JJ: Cataract extraction and diabetic retinopathy. J Am Intraocul Implant Soc 10: 433, 1984.

9 Alpar JJ: Diabetes, cataract extraction and intraocular lenses. J Cataract Refract Surg 13: 43, 1987.

10 Anderson DM, Morin JD: Experimental anterior segment necrosis and rubeosis iridis. Can J Ophthalmol 6: 196, 1971.

11 Apple DJ, Craythorn JM, Olsen RJ et al: Anterior segment complications and neovascular glaucoma following implantation of a posterior chamber intraocular lens. Ophthalmology 91: 403, 1984.

12 Azzolini C, Brancato R, Camesasca F et al: Influence of silicone oil on iris microangiopathy in diabetic vitrectomized eyes. Ophthalmology 100: 1152, 1993.

13 Baikoff G, Bechetoille A, Colin J et al: Implants "Médaillon" et fluorographie de la chambre antérieure. J Fr Ophtalmol 3:165, 1980.

14 Baikoff G, Dallas N, O'Malley R: Aphakic macular oedema following prosthetic lens implantation. Br J Ophthalmol 61: 321, 1977.

15 Baikoff G, Drouan P, Colin J: Fluorographie du segment anterieur apres implantation intraoculaire. Bull Soc Ophtalmol Fr 4-5: 451, 1980.

16 Bandello F, Brancato R, Lattanzio R et al: Relation between iridopathy and retinopathy in diabetes. Br J Ophthalmol 78: 542, 1994.

17 Bechetoille A, Baikoff G, Drouan P et al: Fluorographie du segment anterieur et chirurgie intraoculaire. Bull Soc Ophtalmol Fr 10: 897, 1979.

18 Bechetoille A, Chabanais JL, Jallet G et al: Contusion et perméabilité de la barrière hémato-aqueuse à la fluorescéine. J Fr Ophtalmol 1-2: 139, 1978.

19 Bengtsson E: Studies on the mechanism of the breakdown of the blood. Aqueous barrier in the rabbit eye. Acta Ophthalmologica 130 (Suppl): 7, 1977.

20 Beran V, Vydrova J: Fluorescencni angiografie duhovky po operaci silhani a po operaci odchlipene sitnice. Cesk Oftalmol 39: 255, 1983.

21 Berens C, Girard LJ: Transplantation of the superior and inferior rectus muscles for paralysis of the lateral rectus. Am J Ophthalmol 33: 1041, 1950.

22 Biglan AW, Burnstine RA, Rogers GL et al: Management of strabismus with botulinim A toxin. Ophthalmology 96: 935, 1989.

23 Blankenship GW: Preoperative iris rubeosis and diabetic vitrectomy results. Ophthalmology 87: 176, 1980.

24 Blankenship GW: Posterior chamber intraocular lens implantation during pars plana lensectomy and vitrectomy for diabetic complications. Graefe's Arch Clin Exp Ophthalmol 227: 136, 1989.

25 Blankenship GW, Cortez R, Machemer R: The lens and pars plana vitrectomy for diabetic retinopathy complications. Arch Ophthalmol 97: 1263, 1979.

26 Blankenship GW, Machemer R: Long-term diabetic vitrectomy results: report of 10 years follow-up. Ophthalmology 92: 503, 1985.

27 Blumenkranz MS, Hernandez E: Rubeosis iridis and vitrectomy. Invest Ophthalmol Vis Sci 22 (Suppl): 234, 1982.

28 Boniuk M, Zimmerman LE: Necrosis of the iris, ciliary body, lens and retina following scleral buckling operations with circling polyethylene tubes. Trans Am Acad Ophthalmol Otolaryngol 65: 671, 1961.

29 Boniuk M, Zimmerman LE: Necrosis of uvea, sclera and retina following operations for retinal detachment. Arch Ophthalmol 66: 318, 1961.

30 Bonnet M: Les facteurs de pronostic du Syndrome d'Irvine-Gass. Ann Ocul 208: 275, 1975.

31 Bonnet M: Peripheral neovascularization complicating rhegmatogenous retinal detachments of long duration. Graefe's Arch Clin Exp Ophthalmol 225: 59, 1987.

32 Bonnet M, Bievelez B: Iris fluorescein angiography and Irvine Gass' syndrome. Albrecht von Graefes Arch Klin Exp Ophthalmol 194: 217, 1980.

33 Bonnet M, Bievelez B: Angiographie fluoresceinique de l'iris et syndrome d'Irvine-Gass. Bull Soc Ophtalmol Fr 11: 1001, 1981.

34 Brancato R, Bandello F, Carnevalini A et al: Intraocular lens and diabetes. In Maumenee AE, Stark WJ, Esente I: Cataract and refractive microsurgery. Proc 4th International Congress, 1987. Fogliazza Ed, Milano, 1988.

35 Brancato R, Bandello F, Lattanzio R et al: La fluoroiridografia e la fluorofotometria nell'impianto di cristallino artificiale. Atti Congresso "IOL nel solco o nel sacco: perchè e quando?", Trieste, 1987. Maccari Ed, Parma, 1988.

36 Brancato R, Leoni G, Trabucchi G: Contact trans-scleral irradiation of human chorioretina with continuous-wave Nd:YAG laser. Ophthalmic Res 21:1, 1989.

37 Brancato R, Menchini U, Carnevalini A: Atlante di iridografia a fluorescenza. C.I.C. Ed Int Gruppo Ed Medico, Roma, 1981.

38 Brancato R, Menchini U, Carnevalini A: Iris fluorescein angiography in the anterior chamber lens implantation. In Maumenee AE, Esente I: Cataract surgery and visual rehabilitation. Libreria Scientifica Ghedini, Milano, 1982.

39 Brancato R, Menchini U, Carnevalini A et al: Rubeosis iridis et rétinopathie diabétique. Proc Symposium International sur la Rétinopathie Diabétique, Paris, 1984. Rev Int Chibret 105: 287, 1985.

40 Brourman ND, Blumenkranz MS, Cox MS et al: Silicone oil for the treatment of severe proliferative diabetic retinopathy. Ophthalmology 96: 759, 1989.

41 Brown GC, Magargal LE, Simeone FA et al: Arterial obstruction and ocular neovascularization. Ophthalmology 89: 139, 1982.

42 Chabanais JL: Traumatisme et perméabilité de la barrière hémato oculaire. Thèse Médicine, Angers, 1977.

43 Charles S: Vitreous microsurgery. Williams & Wilkins, Baltimore, 1989.

44 Chignell AH: Complications after retinal detachment surgery. Trans Ophthalmol Soc UK 95: 134, 1975.

45 Clayman HM, Jaffe NS, Light DS: Lens implantation and diabetes mellitus. Am J Ophthalmol 88: 990, 1979.

46 Cole DF, Unger WG: Prostaglandins as mediators for the responses of the eye to trauma. Exp Eye Res 17: 357, 1973.

47 Crock G: Clinical syndromes of anterior segment ischaemia. Trans Ophthalmol Soc UK 87: 513, 1967.

48 Cunha-Vaz JG, Fonseca JR, Vieira R: Retinal blood flow in retinal detachment. Mod Probl Ophthalmol 20: 89, 1979.

49 Cunliffe IA, Flanagan DW, George NDL et al: Extracapsular surgery with lens implantation in diabetics with and without proliferative retinopathy. Br J Ophthalmol 75: 9, 1991.

50 deCorral LR, Peyman GA: Pars plana vitrectomy and intravitreal silicone oil injection in eyes with rubeosis iridis. Can J Ophthalmol 21: 10, 1986.

51 deJuan E, Hardy M, Hatchell DL et al: The effect of intraocular silicone oil on anterior chamber oxygen pressure in cats. Arch Ophthalmol 104: 1063, 1986.

52 Demeler U, Buhr-Unger H: Irisangiographische Befunde nach intra und extrakapsularer Kataraktextraktion und implantation einer Binkhorst-4- Schlingen-Linse. Fortschr Ophthalmol 80: 244, 1983.

53 Duguid IM: Anterior segment necrosis following retinal detachment surgery. Trans Ophthalmol Soc UK 87: 171, 1967.

54 Eagle RC Jr, Yanoff M, Morse PH: Anterior segment necrosis following scleral buckling in hemoglobin SC disease. Am J Ophthalmol 75: 426, 1973.

55 Easty DL: Anterior segment fluorescein angiography following lens implantation. Proc Roy Soc Med 69: 911, 1976.

56 Easty DL, Chignell AH: Fluorescein angiography in anterior segment ischaemia. Br J Ophthalmol 57: 18, 1973.

57 Easty DL, Dallas N, O'Malley R: Aphakic macular oedema following prosthetic lens implantation. Br J Ophthalmol 61: 321, 1977.

58 Ehrenberg M, Brooks W, McCuen BW: Rubeosis iridis: preoperative iris fluorescein angiography and periocular steroids. Ophthalmology 91: 321, 1984.

59 Eichenbaum DM: Iris neovascularization after pars plana vitrectomy. In Freeman HM, Hirose T, Schepens CL: Vitreous surgery and advances in fundus diagnosis and treatment. Appleton Century Croft, New York, 1977.

60 Ellingson FT: The uveitis-glaucoma-hyphaema syndrome associated with the mark VIII anterior chamber lens implant. Am Intraocul Implant Soc J 4: 50, 1978.

61 Federman JL, Schubert HD: Complications associated with the use of silicone oil in 150 eyes after retina-vitreous surgery. Ophthalmology 95: 870, 1988.

62 Fedorov SN, Egorova EV, Kiskina VY: Fluorescent iridoangiography in assessment of the iridal micro-circulation in implantation of silicon or polymethacrylate intra-ocular lenses. Vestn Oftalmol 103: 18, 1987.

63 Fells P: Vertical rectus muscle transplantation to restore abduction. In Mein J, Bierlaagh JJM, Brummelkamp-Dons TEA: Orthoptics. Proc 2nd International Orthoptic Congress, 1971. Excerpta Medica, Amsterdam, 1972.

64 Fells P: Anterior segment ischaemia. Lens changes after strabismus surgery. Trans Ophthalmol Soc UK 100: 398, 1980.

65 Fishman PH, Repka MX, Green WR et al: A primate model of anterior ischemia after strabismus surgery. The role of the conjunctival circulation. Ophthalmology 97: 456, 1990.

66 Fitzsimons R, Lee JP, Elston J: Treatment of sixth nerve palsy in adults with combined botulinum toxin chemodenervation and surgery. Ophthalmology 95: 1535, 1988.

67 Forber SB: Muscle transplantation for external rectus paralysis: report of a case with unusual complications. Am J Ophthalmol 48: 248, 1959.

68 France TD, Simon JW: Anterior segment ischemia syndrome following muscle surgery. J Pediatric Ophthalmol Strabismus 23: 87, 1986.

69 Freeman HM, Hawkins WR, Schepens CL: Anterior segment necrosis. An experimental study. Arch Ophthalmol 75: 644, 1966.

70 Gartner S, Henkind P: Neovascularization of the iris (rubeosis iridis). Surv Ophthalmol 22: 219, 1978.

71 Gass JDM, Norton EWD: Cystoid macular edema and papilledema following cataract extraction. A fluorescein funduscopic and angiographic study. Arch Ophthalmol 76: 646, 1966.

72 Gass JDM, Norton EWD: Follow-up study of cystoid macula edema following cataract extraction. Trans Am Acad Ophthalmol Otolaryngol 73: 665, 1969.

73 Girard LJ, Beltranena F: Early and late complications of extensive muscle surgery. Arch Ophthalmol 64: 576, 1960.

74 Gitter KA, Cohen G: Complications of vitrectomy. In Gitter KA: Current concepts of the vitreous including vitrectomy. CV Mosby, St Louis, 1976.

75 Hayreh SS, Baines JAB: Occlusion of the posterior ciliary artery. I. Effects on choroidal circulation. Br J Ophthalmol 56: 719, 1972.

76 Hayreh SS, Baines JAB: Occlusion of the vortex veins: an experimental study. Br J Ophthalmol 57: 217, 1973.

77 Hayreh SS, Scott WE: Fluorescein iris angiography. II. Disturbances in iris circulation following strabismus operation on the various recti. Arch Ophthalmol 96: 1390, 1978.

78 Hayreh SS, Scott WE: Anterior segment ischemia following retinal detachment surgery. Mod Probl Ophthalmol 20: 148, 1979.

79 Heimann K, Dahl B, Dimopoulos S et al: Pars plana vitrectomy and silicone oil injection in proliferative diabetic retinopathy. Graefe's Arch Clin Exp Ophthalmol 227: 152, 1989.

80 Helvestone EM: Muscle transposition procedures. Surv Ophthalmol 16: 92, 1971.

81 Hutton WL, Pesicka GA, Fuller DG: Cataract extraction in the diabetic eye after vitrectomy. Am J Ophthalmol 104: 1, 1987.

82 Irvine SR: A newly defined vitreous syndrome following cataract surgery: interpreted according to recent concepts of the structure of vitreous. Am J Ophthalmol 36: 599, 1953.

83 Jacobs DS, Vastine DW, Urist MJ: Anterior segment ischemia and sector iris atrophy after strabismus surgery in a patient with chronic lymphocytic leukemia. Ophthalmic Surg 7: 42, 1976.

84 Jaffe GJ, Burton TC: Progression of nonproliferative diabetic retinopathy following cataract extraction. Arch Ophthalmol 106: 745, 1988.

85 Jaffe GJ, Clayman H, Jaffe M: Cystoid macular edema after intracapsular and extracapsular extraction with and without an intraocular lens. Ophthalmology 89: 25, 1982.

86 Jensen CDF: Rectus muscle union: a new operation for paralysis of the rectus muscles. Trans Pac Coast Oto Ophthalmol Soc 45: 359, 1964.

87 Johnson RN, Flynn HW, Parel JM et al: Transient hypopyon with marked anterior chamber fibrin following pars plana vitrectomy. Arch Ophthalmol 107: 683, 1989.

88 Jost BF, Olk RJ, Patz A et al: Anterior segment ischaemia following laser photocoagulation in a patient with systemic lupus erythematosus. Br J Ophthalmol 72: 11, 1988.

89 Khodadoust AA, Arkfeld DF, Caprioli J et al: Ocular effects of Neodymium:YAG laser. Am J Ophthalmol 98: 144, 1984.

90 Kishkina VY: Fluorescein angiography of the anterior segment. In Fyodorov SN: Microsurgery of the eye: main aspects. Mir Publishers, Moskow, 1987.

91 Klein S, Beer EM: Fluorescein angiography of the iris in various intraocular lenses. Fortschr Ophthalmol 82: 329, 1985.

92 Knox DL: Ischaemic ocular inflammation. Am J Ophthalmol 60: 995, 1965.

93 Knox DL, Palmer CA, English F: Iris atrophy after quinine amblyopia. Arch Ophthalmol 76: 359, 1966.

94 Kondo T: Cystoid macular oedema after lens implantation. J Ocular Ther Euro 1: 45, 1982.

95 Kottow MH: Anterior segment fluorescein angiography. Williams & Wilkins, Baltimore, 1978.

96 Kottow MH: Anterior segment reactions after experimental trauma to rabbit eyes. Albrecht von Graefes Arch Klin Exp Ophthalmol 209: 125, 1978.

97 Kottow MH, Hendrickson P: Iris angiography in cystoid macular edema after cataract extraction. Arch Ophthalmol 93: 487, 1975.

98 Kottow MH, Vassileva P, Hendrickson P: Provoked iris ischemia in the rabbit: a fluorescein angiographic study. Can J Ophthalmol 10: 255, 1975.

99 Kraff MC, Sanders DR, Peyman GA et al: Slit-lamp fluorophotometry in intraocular lens patients. Ophthalmology 87: 877, 1980.

100 Krause U: Effects of lens implants on iris fluorescein angiography and the iris pigment layer. Acta Ophthalmologica 63: 369, 1985.

101 Lee JP, Olver JM: Anterior segment ischemia. Eye 4: 1, 1990.

102 Levin ML, Kincaid MC, Eifler CW et al: Effect of cataract surgery and intraocular lenses on diabetic retinopathy. J Cataract Refract Surg 14: 642, 1988.

103 Lewis ML: Iris fluorescein angiography. In: Developments in Ophthalmology. S Karger, Basel, 1981.

104 Lieppman ME: Intermittent visual “white out”. A new intraocular lens complication. Ophthalmology 89: 109, 1982.

105 Lucke KH, Foerster MH, Laqua H: Long-term results of vitrectomy and silicone oil in 500 cases of complicated retinal detachments. Am J Ophthalmol 104: 624, 1987.

106 Mandelcorn MS, Blankenship GW, Machemer R: Pars plana vitrectomy for the management of severe diabetic retinopathy. Am J Ophthalmol 81: 561, 1976.

107 McCuen BW, Rinkoff JS: Silicone oil for progressive anterior ocular neovascularization after failed diabetic vitrectomy. Arch Ophthalmol 107: 677, 1989.

108 McLeod D: Silicone oil injection during closed microsurgery for diabetic retinal detachment. Graefe’s Arch Clin Exp Ophthalmol 224: 55, 1986.

109 Menchini U, Carnevalini A, Pece A et al: La fluoroiridografia nella microchirurgia del segmento anteriore con Nd:YAG laser. Atti I Congresso Società Italiana Laser in Oftalmologia, 1985. Verduci Ed, Roma, 1985.

110 Menchini U, Carnevalini A, Scialdone A et al: Cataract surgery and diabetic retinopathy. Proc 3rd Congress Cataract Surgery and Visual Rehabilitation, 1984. Kugler Ed, Amsterdam, 1985.

111 Menchini U, Scialdone A, Carnevalini A et al: Fluoroiridigraphy in posterior chamber implants. In Maumenee AE, Stark WJ, Esente I: Cataract and refractive microsurgery. Fogliazza Ed, Milano, 1988.

112 Menezo JL, Marin FJ, Harto M: Iris and macular angiography in intraocular implants. Am Intra-ocular Implant Soc J 10: 25, 1984.

113 Metge P, Chauvet G, Bonnefoy C: Angiographie de l’iris et fluorometrie de la chambre anterieur chez les aphaques et les implantes. Bull Soc Ophtalmol Fr 3: 415, 1982.

114 Michels RG: Vitrectomy for complications of diabetic retinopathy. Arch Ophthalmol 96: 237, 1978.

115 Michels RG, Wilkinson CP, Rice TA: Retinal detachment. CV Mosby, St Louis, 1990.

116 Miller D, Doane MG: High speed photographic evaluation of intraocular lens movements. Am J Ophthalmol 97: 752, 1984.

117 Moffat K, Blumenkranz MS, Hernandez E: The lens capsule and rubeosis iridis: an angiographic study. Can J Ophthalmol 3: 130, 1984.

118 Moyenin P, Bonnet M: Angio-fluo irienne dans les retinopathies diabetiques proliferantes traitees par vitrectomie. Bull Soc Ophtalmol Fr 5: 619, 1987.

119 Myers FL, Bresnick GH, Brightbill FS: Vitrectomy in proliferative diabetic retinopathy: an analysis of 60 consecutive cases. In McPherson A: New and controversial aspects of vitreoretinal surgery. CV Mosby, St Louis, 1977.

120 Nicholson DH: Occult iris erosion. A treatable cause of recurrent hyphema in iris-supported intraocular lenses. Ophthalmology 89: 113, 1982.

121 Norn MS: Can defects in the iris pigment layers regenerate? A postoperative examination of cataract operated patients with transpupillary transillumination according to Abrams. Acta Ophthalmol (Kbh) 46: 243, 1968.

122 O’Conner R: Transplantation of ocular muscles. Am J Ophthalmol 4: 838, 1921.

123 O’Day D, Hoyt WF, Crock G: Monocular blindness from combined internal carotid thrombosis and external carotid-cavernous fistula. Med J Austr 2: 460, 1970.

124 Okun E: Discussion. In Freeman HM, Hirose T, Schepens CL: Vitreous surgery and advances in fundus diagnosis and treatment. Appleton Century Croft, New York, 1977.

125 Olver JM, Lee JP: The effects of strabismus surgery on anterior segment circulation. Eye 3: 318, 1989.

126 Olver JM, Lee JP: Recovery of anterior segment circulation after strabismus surgery in adult patients. Ophthalmology 99: 305, 1992.

127 Pavese T, Insler MS: Effects of extracapsular cataract extraction with posterior chamber lens implantation on the development of neovascular glaucoma in diabetics. J Cataract Refract Surg 13: 197, 1987.

128 Peyman GA, Sanders D: Advances in uveal surgery, vitreous surgery, and the treatment of endophthalmitis. Appleton Century Croft, New York, 1975.

129 Poliner LS, Christianson DJ, Escoffery RF et al: Neovascular glaucoma after intracapsular and extracapsular cataract extraction in diabetic patients. Am J Ophthalmol 100: 637, 1985.

130 Pollack A, Dotan S, Oliver M: Course of diabetic retinopathy following cataract surgery. Br J Ophthalmol 75: 2, 1991.

131 Pollack A, Leiba H, Bukelman A et al: Cystoid macular oedema following cataract extraction in patients with diabetes. Br J Ophthalmol 76: 221, 1992.

132 Pollack A, Leiba H, Bukelman A et al: The course of diabetic retinopathy following cataract surgery in eyes previously treated by laser photocoagulation. Br J Ophthalmol 76: 228, 1992.

133 Pollack A, Leiba H, Oliver M: Progression of diabetic retinopathy after cataract surgery. Br J Ophthalmol 75: 547, 1991.

134 Prasad P, Setna PH, Dunne JA: Accelerated ocular neovascularization in diabetics following posterior chamber lens implantation. Br J Ophthalmol 74: 313, 1990.

135 Raitta C, Knape B: Das pra und postoperative fluoresceinangiogramm der iris bei cataracta senilis. Albrecht von Graefes Arch Klin Exp Ophthalmol 182: 283, 1971.

136 Raitta C, Knape B: Fluorescein angiography of the vessels of the iris in senile cataract before and after operation. Surv Ophthalmol 18: 318, 1974.

137 Raizman MB, Beck RW: Iris ischemia following surgery on two rectus muscles (letter). Arch Ophthalmol 103: 1783, 1985.

138 Rice TA, Michels RG, Maguire MG et al: The effect of lensectomy on the incidence of iris neovascularization and neovascular glaucoma after vitrectomy for diabetic retinopathy. Am J Ophthalmol 95: 1, 1983.

139 Rinkoff JS, de Juan E, McCuen BW: Silicone oil for retinal detachment with advanced proliferative vitreoretinopathy following failed vitrectomy for proliferative diabetic retinopathy. Am J Ophthalmol 101: 181, 1986.

140 Robertson DM: Anterior segment ischemia after segmental episcleral buckling and cryopexy. Am J Ophthalmol 79: 871, 1975.

141 Ruiz RS, Saatci OA: Posterior chamber intraocular lens implantation in eyes with inactive and active proliferative diabetic retinopathy. Am J Ophthalmol 111: 158, 1991.

142 Ruskell GL: Blood vessels of the orbit and globe. In Prince JH: The rabbit in eye research. Charles C Thomas Publisher, Springfield, 1964.

143 Ryan SJ, Goldberg MF: Anterior segment ischemia following scleral buckling in sickle cell hemoglobinopathy. Am J Ophthalmol 72: 35, 1971.

144 Saari M, Nieminen H: Fluorescein angiography and infrared transillumination stereo technique for studying the ciliary body and iris. In Francois J: Blood circulation in the uvea, the retina and the optic nerve (Physiology and pathology). Ferdinand Enke Verlag, Stuttgart, 1978.

145 Sanders MD, Hoyt WF: Hypoxic ocular sequelae of carotid-cavernous fistulae: study of the causes of visual failure before and after neurosurgical treatment in a series of 125 cases. Br J Ophthalmol 55: 82, 1969.

146 Sanders DR, Kraff MC, Lieberman HL et al: Breakdown and reestabilishment of blood-aqueous barrier with implant surgery. Arch Ophthalmol 100: 588, 1982.

147 Saunders RA, Phillips MS: Anterior segment ischemia after three rectus muscle surgery. Ophthalmology 95: 533, 1988.

148 Saunders RA, Sandall GS: Anterior segment ischemia syndrome following rectus muscle transposition. Am J Ophthalmol 93: 34, 1982.

149 Scuderi JJ, Blumenkranz MS, Blankenship GW: Regression of diabetic rubeosis iridis following successful surgical reattachment of the retina by vitrectomy. Retina 2: 193, 1982.

150 Sebestyen JG: Intraocular lenses and diabetes mellitus. Am J Ophthalmol 101: 425, 1986.

151 Sebestyen JG, Wafai MZ: Experience with intraocular lens implants in patients with diabetes. Am J Ophthalmol 96: 94, 1983.

152 Severin TD, Severin SL: Pseudophakic cystoid macular edema: a revised comparison of the incidence with intracapsular and extracapsular cataract extraction. Ophthalmic Surg 19: 116, 1988.

153 Shea M: Complications common to all surgical procedures. In Schepens CL, Regan CDJ: Controversial aspects of the management of retinal detachment. Little Brown, Boston, 1965.

154 Simon JW, Price EC, Krohel GB et al: Anterior segment ischemia following strabismus surgery. J Pediatric Ophthalmol Strabismus 21: 179, 1984.

155 Stefansson E, Landers MB, Wolbarsht ML et al: Neovascularization of the iris: an experimental model in cats. Invest Ophthalmol Vis Sci 25: 361, 1984.

156 Straatsma BR, Pettit TH, Wheeler N et al: Diabetes mellitus and intraocular lens implantation. Ophthalmology 90: 336, 1983.

157 Stucchi C, Bianchi G: Dépigmentation en secteur de l'iris consécutive à des transplantation musculaires. Ophthalmologica 133: 231, 1957.

158 Takahashi S: Studies on choroidal blood flow using the hydrogen clearance method. III. Effects of vortex vein occlusion. Folia Ophthalmol Jpn 33: 958, 1982.

159 Tanaka S, Ideta H, Yonemoto J et al: Neovascularization of the iris in rhegmatogenous retinal detachment. Am J Ophthalmol 112: 632, 1991.

160 Thompson SM, Kritzinger EE, Roper-Hall MJ: Should diabetes be a contraindication for an intraocular lens? Trans Ophthalmol Soc UK 103: 115, 1983.

161 Tremoulet O: Angiographie fluoresceinique du segment anterieur chez les porteurs de cristallins artificiels. Clin Ophtalmol 3: 53, 1978.

162 Tremoulet O, Parizot H, Mawas ED: Angiographie fluoresceinique du segment anterieur chez les porteurs de cristallins artificiels: etude de 30 cas. Bull Soc Ophtalmol Fr 4-5: 343, 1980.

163 Tuberville AW, Galin MA, Perez HD et al: Complement activation by nylon and polypropylene-looped prosthetic intraocular lenses. Invest Ophthalmol Vis Sci 22: 727, 1982.

164 Unger WG, Brown NAP, Edwards J: Response of the human eye to laser irradiation of the iris. Br J Ophthalmol 61: 148, 1977.

165 Uno T, Sato M, Danjo S et al: Rubeosis iridis following retinal detachment surgery. Jpn Rev Clin Ophthalmol 84: 196, 1990.

166 Uribe LE: Muscle transplantation in ocular paralysis. Am J Ophthalmol 65: 601, 1968.

167 Vassileva P, Kottow MH, Weigelin E: Provoked iris ischaemia in the rabbit. I. Clinical and histopathological examinations. Albrecht von Graefes Arch Klin Ophthalmol 196: 231, 1975.

168 Vassileva P, Kottow MH, Weigelin E: Provoked iris ischaemia in the rabbit. II. Histochemical localization of sodium fluorescein. Albrecht von Graefes Arch Klin Ophthalmol 197: 31, 1975.

169 Virdi PS, Hayreh SS: Anterior segment ischemia after recession of various recti. An experimental study. Ophthalmology 94: 1258, 1987.

170 von Noorden GK: Anterior segment ischemia following the Jensen procedure. Arch Ophthalmol 94: 845, 1976.

171 Wand M: Hyaloid membrane vs posterior capsule as a protective barrier (letter). Arch Ophthalmol 103: 1112, 1985.

172 Wand M, Madigan JC, Gaudio AR et al: Neovascular glaucoma following pars plana vitrectomy for complications of diabetic retinophaty. Ophthalmic Surg 21: 113, 1990.

173 Wetzig PC, Thatcher DB: Vitrectomy in proliferative diabetic retinopathy. In McPherson A: New and controversial aspects of vitreoretinal surgery. CV Mosby, St Louis, 1977.

174 Wetzig PC, Thatcher DB, Christiansen J: The intracapsular versus the extracapsular cataract technique in relationship to retinal problems. Trans Am Ophthalmol Soc 77: 339, 1979.

175 Wilson WA, Irvine SR: Pathological changes following disruption of blood supply to iris and ciliary body. Trans Am Acad Ophthalmol Otolaryngol 59: 501, 1955.

176 Yeo JH, Glaser BM, Michels RG: Silicone oil in the treatment of complicated retinal detachment. Ophthalmology 94: 1109, 1987.

177 Yoshida A, Hirokawa H, Fukui Y et al: Choroidal circulatory changes after scleral buckling procedures. Acta Soc Ophthalmol Jpn 92: 610, 1988.

178 Yoshihara M: Clinical studies on fundus changes and hemodynamics in degenerative myopes. Acta Soc Ophthalmol Jpn 82: 610, 1978.

179 Zakov ZN, Lewis ML: Iris fluorescein angiography in diabetic vitrectomy patients. Albrecht von Graefes Arch Klin Exp Ophthalmol 206: 17, 1978.

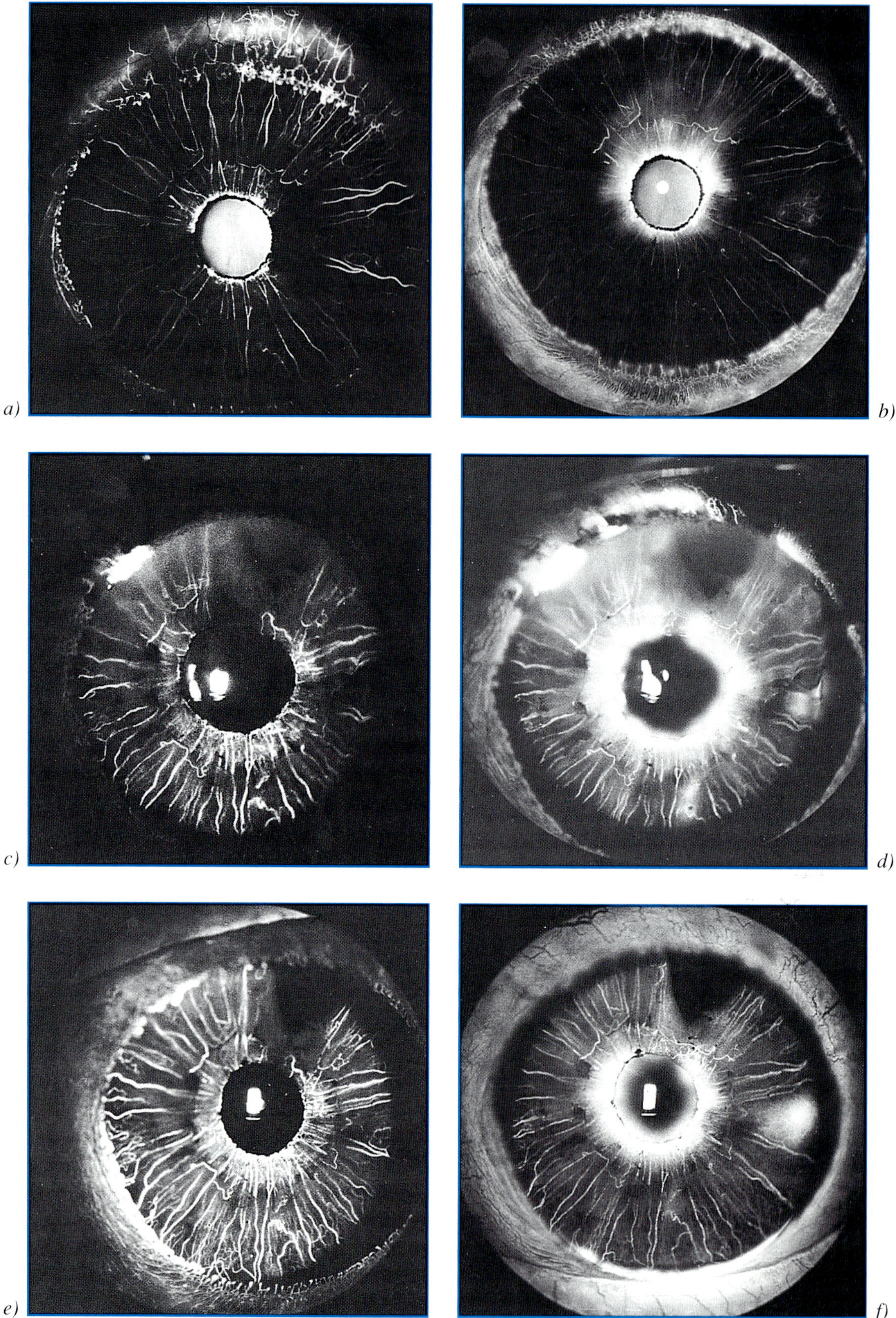

*Fig. **4.9**,1 - Iris fluorescein angiographic phases in a diabetic patient before (a,b), one month (c,d) and four months after (e,f) cataract extraction with a posterior chamber lens implant. Rupture of the blood-iris barrier in response to surgery is more marked in the pupillary part (c,d) but diminishes with time (e,f).*

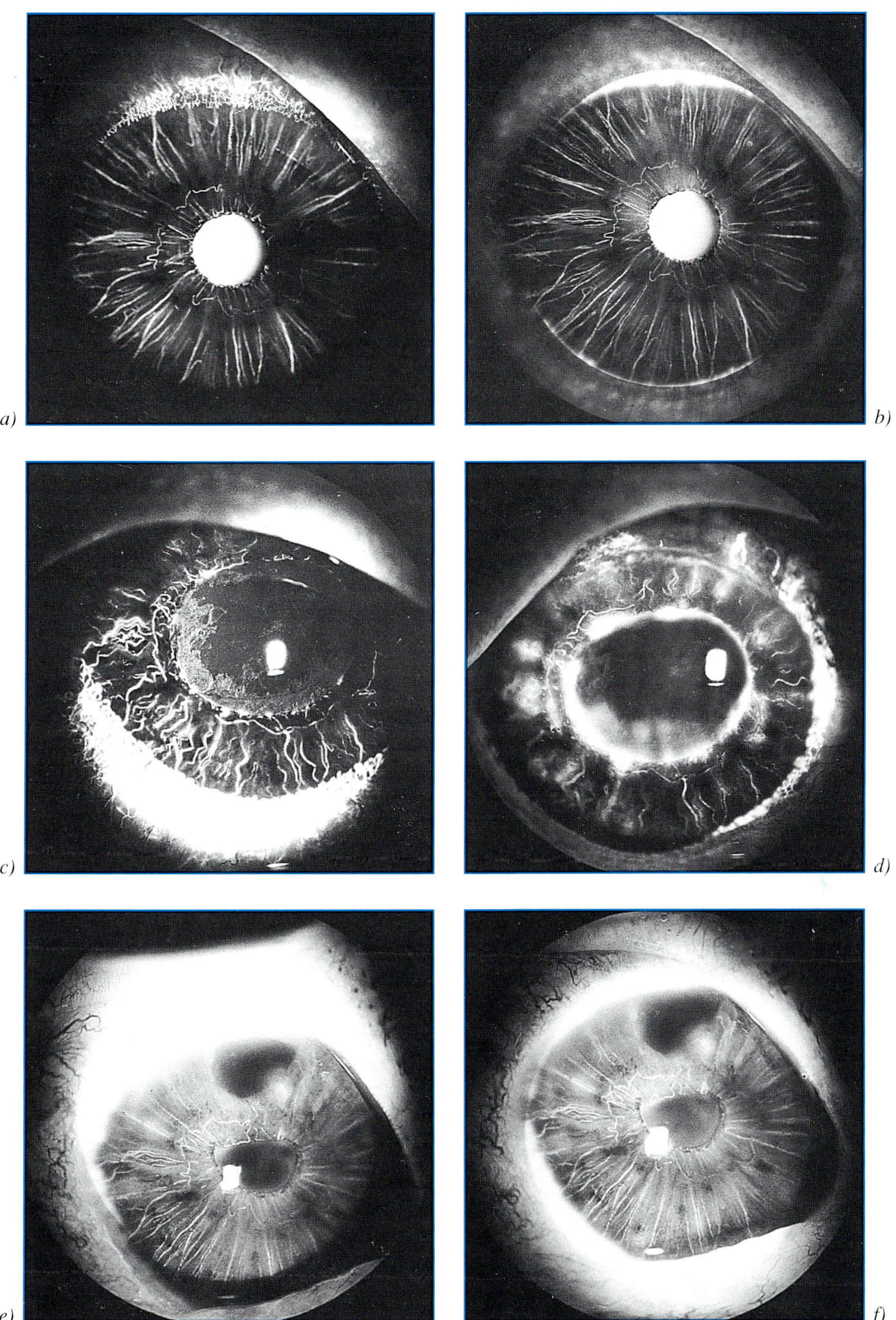

Fig. ***4.9**,2 - Iris fluorescein angiographic phases in a diabetic patient before (a,b), three weeks (c,d) and three months after (e,f) cataract extraction with a posterior chamber lens implant. Breakdown of the blood-iris is still visible several months after the surgery.*

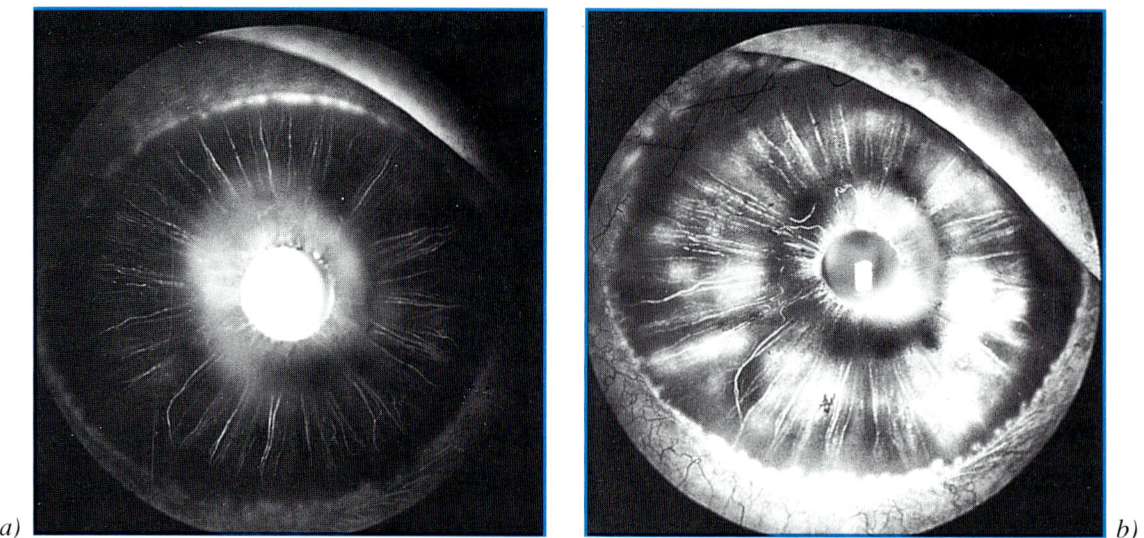

a) *b)*

*Fig. **4.9**,3 - Marked peripupillary leakage in a diabetic patient with cataract (a). One month after surgery for extraction of the cataract, with implantation of an intraocular lens in posterior chamber, diffuse rupture of the blood-iris barrier is still visible (b).*

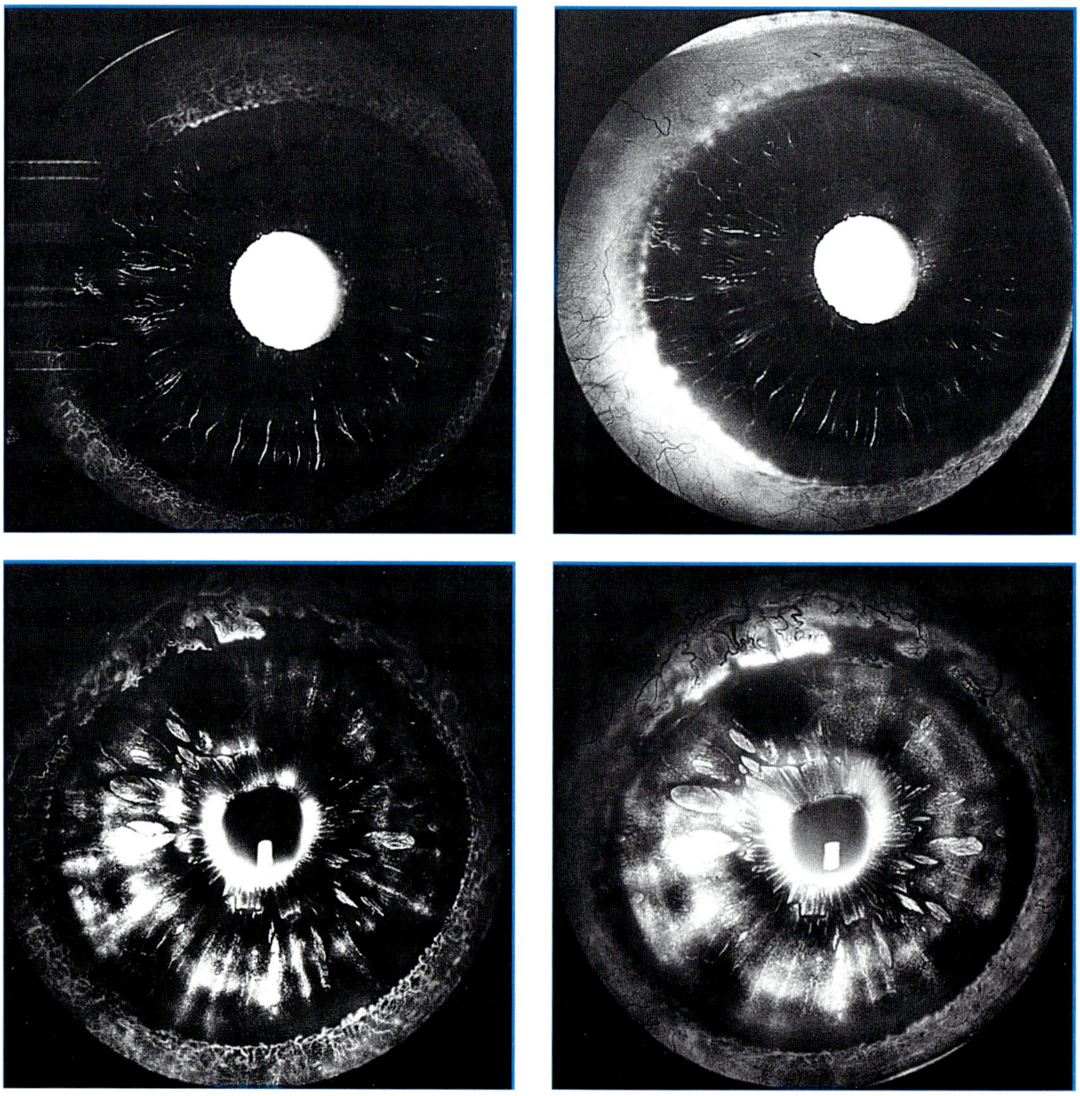

a) *b)*

c) *d)*

*Fig. **4.9**,4 - This diabetic patient presented no evident signs of diabetic iridopathy before extracapsular cataract extraction with implantation of a posterior chamber lens (a,b). However, two months after surgery there was diffuse leakage from pupillary and radial vessels (c,d).*

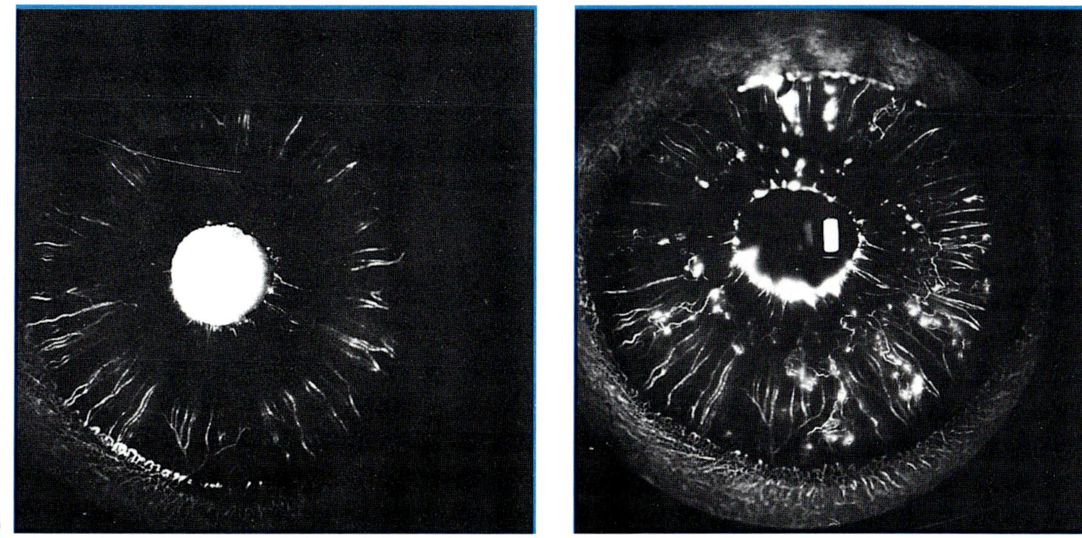

a) b)

Fig. ***4.9****,5 - Hyperfluorescent dots at the pupillary border in a diabetic patient (a). After cataract extraction neovascular tufts can be seen, especially in the ciliary part (b).*

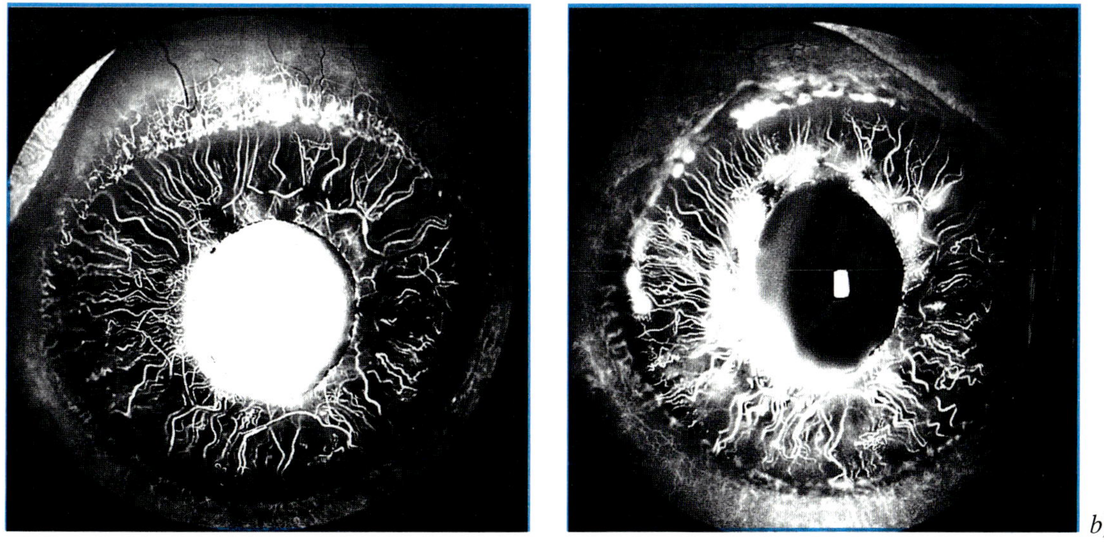

a) b)

Fig. ***4.9****,6 - Marked distortion of the vascular architecture and circumscribed filling defects in a diabetic patient with cataract (a). The iris fluorescein angiographic findings 45 days after cataract extraction (b) shows dye leakage from the congested, abnormally permeable iris vessels, and from circumscribed areas of neovascular proliferation.*

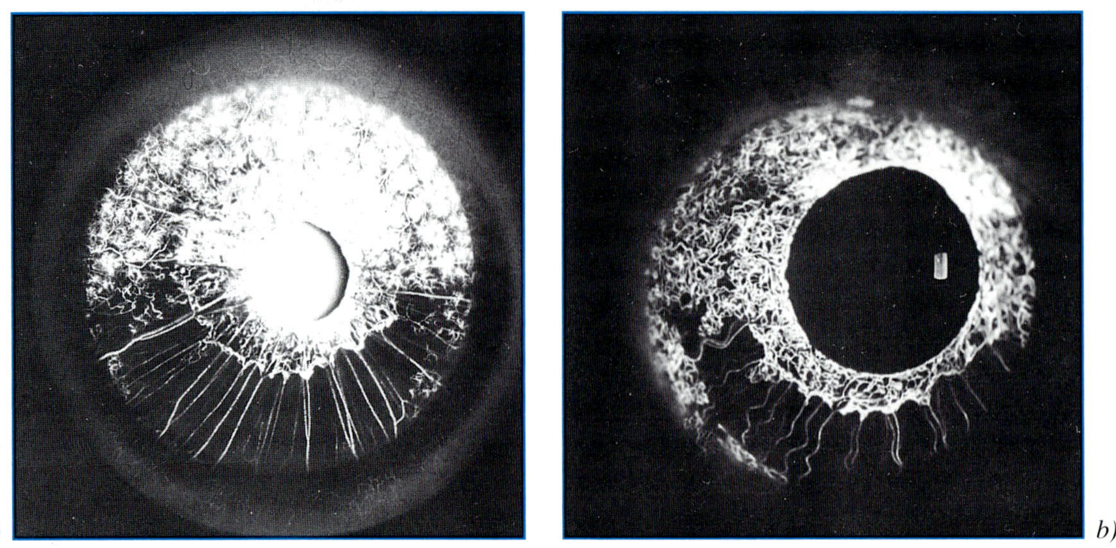

a) b)

*Fig. **4.9**,7 - Advanced proliferative iridopathy in a diabetic patient before (a) and after (b) cataract extraction. Surgery in patients presenting this type of iris microangiopathy tends to be followed by irreducible ocular hypertension if panretinal photocoagulation is not done immediately.*

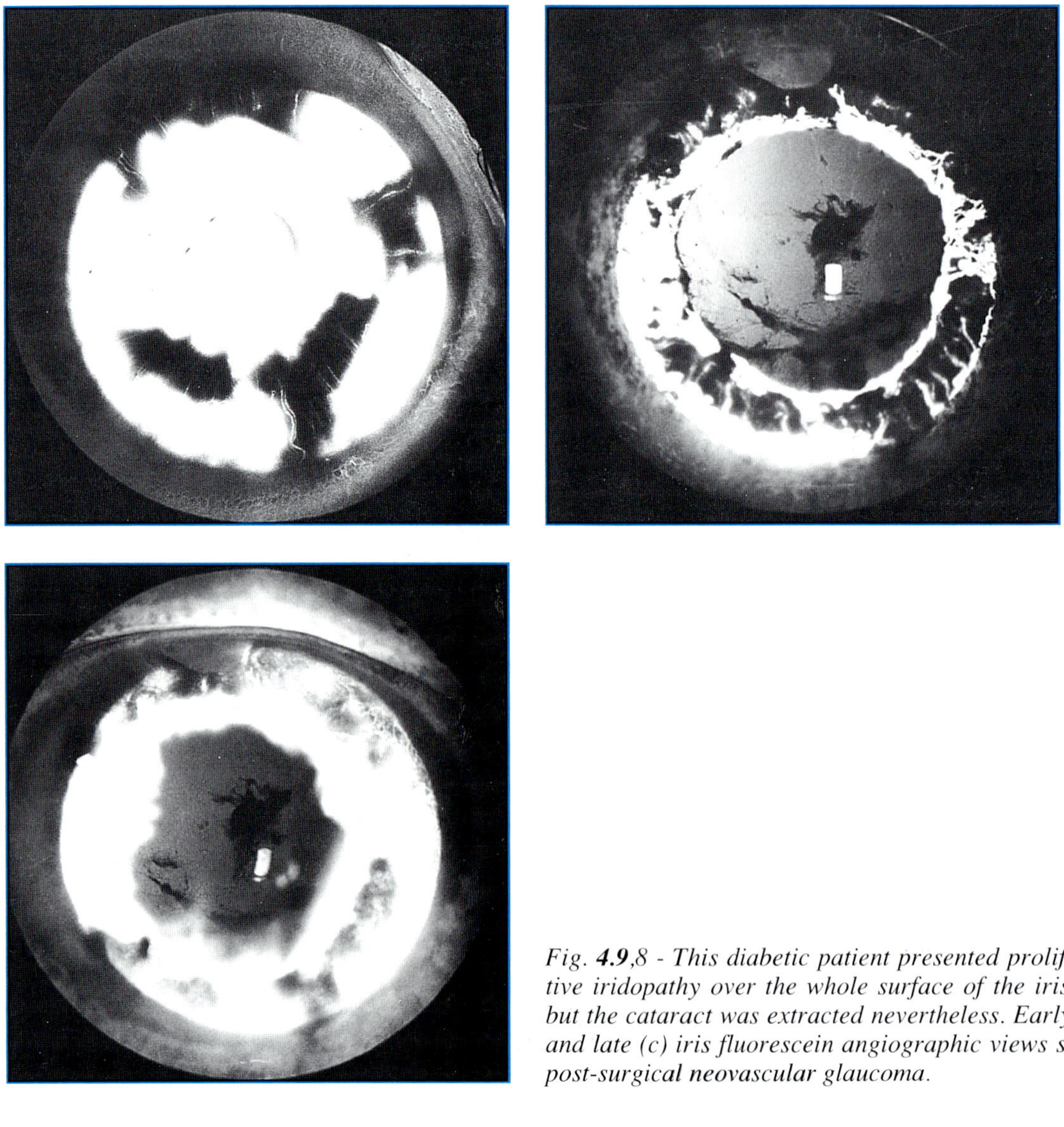

a) b)

c)

*Fig. **4.9**,8 - This diabetic patient presented proliferative iridopathy over the whole surface of the iris (a) but the cataract was extracted nevertheless. Early (b) and late (c) iris fluorescein angiographic views show post-surgical neovascular glaucoma.*

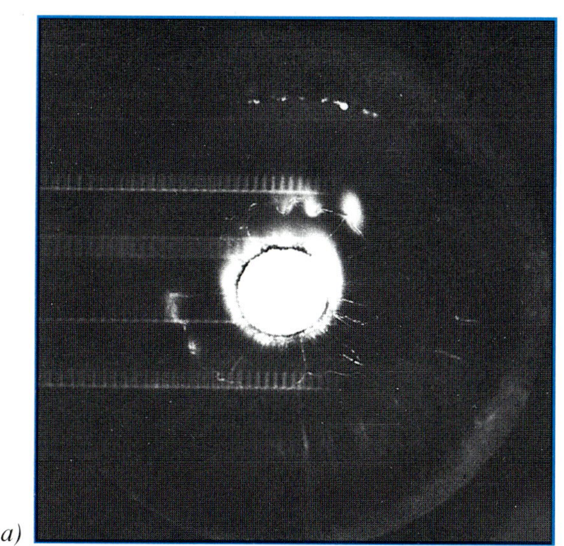
a)

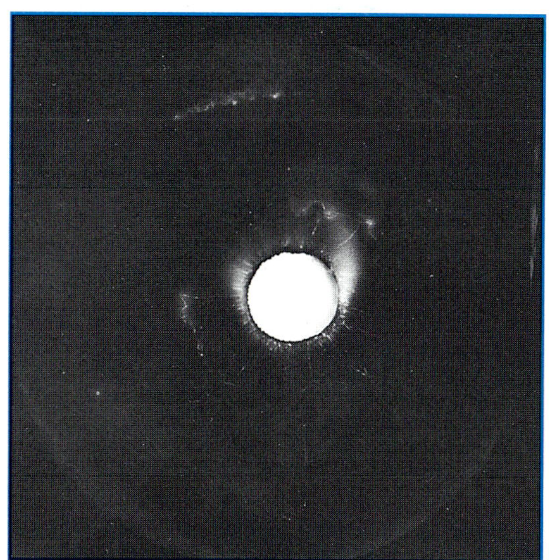
b)

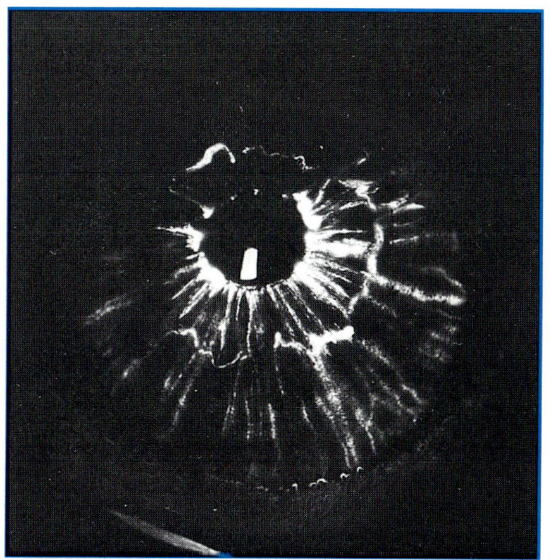
c)

*Fig. **4.9**,9 - Rubeosis iridis in a diabetic patient with cataract before (a) and after (b) retinal cryocoagulation therapy. Extraction of the cataract only after regression of the iris new vessels avoided the serious complications of post-surgical iris microangiopathy. Iris fluorescein angiography one month after surgery (c) showed filling delays and defects in the superior sectors, marked vascular congestion but no noteworthy neovascularization.*

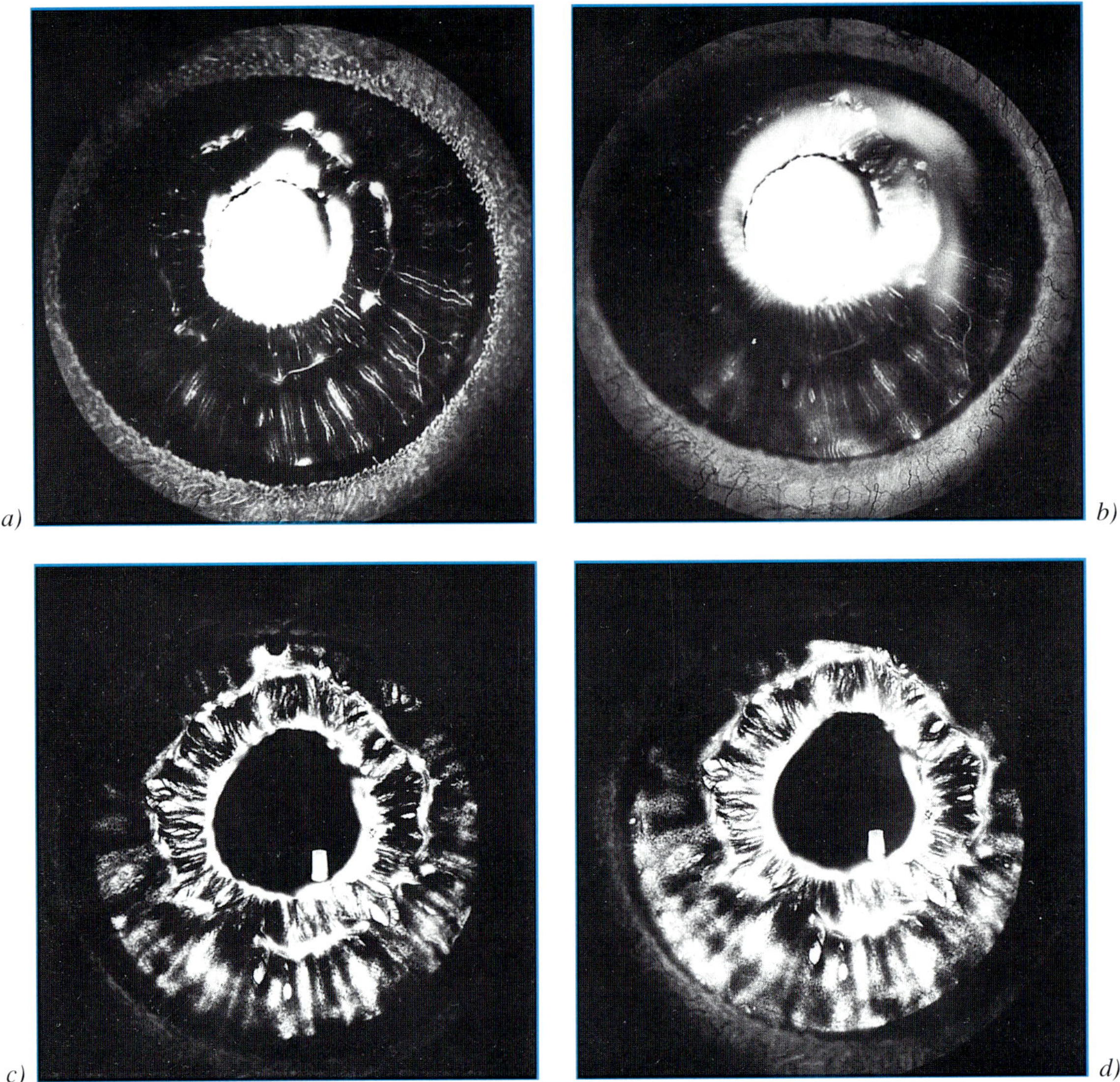

Fig. ***4.9****,10 - Iris new vessels in a diabetic patient with cataract (a,b). Iris fluorescein angiography one week after surgery for cataract extraction (c,d) showed diffuse dye leakage. The superior sectors show filling defects and in the other sectors perfused vessels are congested. Cataract extraction in this patient was followed immediately by panretinal photocoagulation therapy which prevented the iridopathy progressing to neovascular glaucoma.*

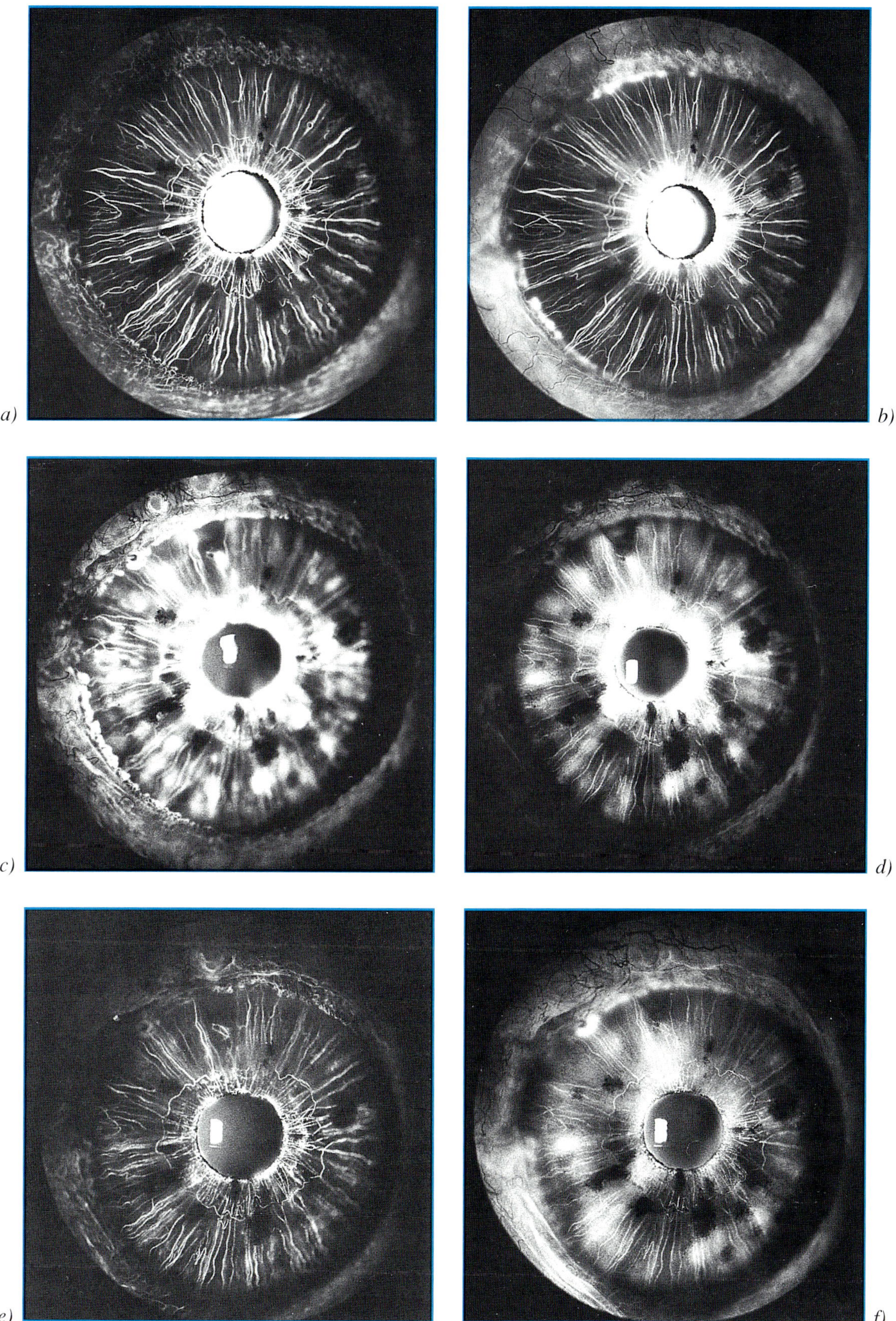

*Fig. **4.9**,11 - Cataract in a diabetic patient with slight neovascularization at the pupillary border (a,b). As the iridopathy progressed after cataract extraction (c,d) and diabetic proliferative retinopathy was present, panretinal photocoagulation was done immediately. Three months later the iris fluorescein angiographic findings are normal, and only diffuse rupture of the blood-iris barrier persists (e,f).*

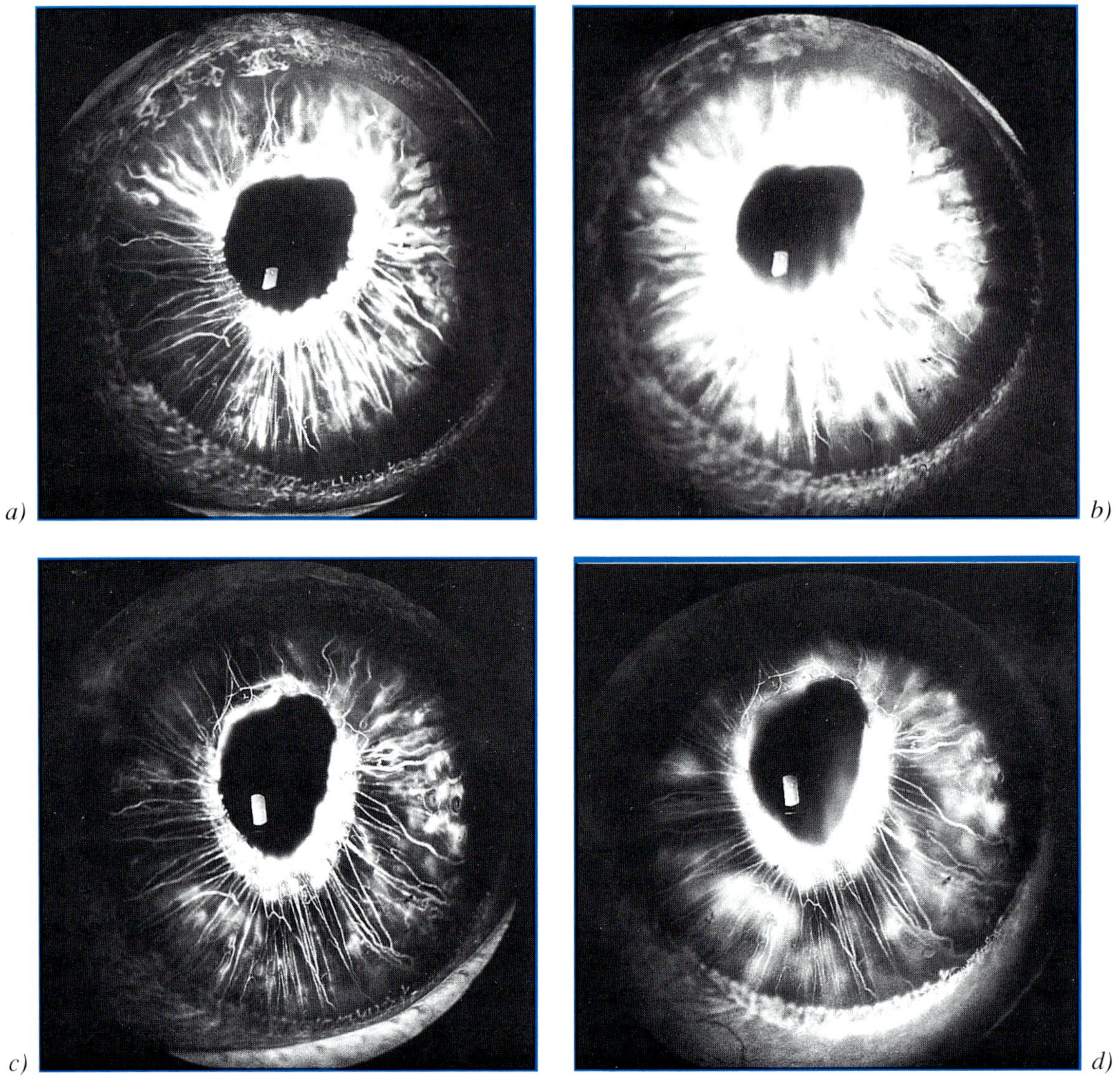

a) *b)*

c) *d)*

*Fig. **4.9**,12 - Imposing, diffuse rupture of the blood-iris barrier in a pseudophakic eye of a diabetic patient, two months after surgery (a,b) and its reduction after panretinal photocoagulation (c,d).*

*Fig. **4.9**,13 - Proliferative diabetic iridopathy (a). After cataract extraction the patient presented iris ischemia, diffuse neovascular proliferation and rupture of the blood-iris barrier where the radial vessels were perfused (b,c). Panretinal photocoagulation after surgery resulted in gradual reduction of the neovascularization. In fluorescein angiograms taken three months (d,e) and one year (f,g) after photocoagulation marked destructuring of the iris vessels persisted, however, and there was a gradual increase in the ischemia.*

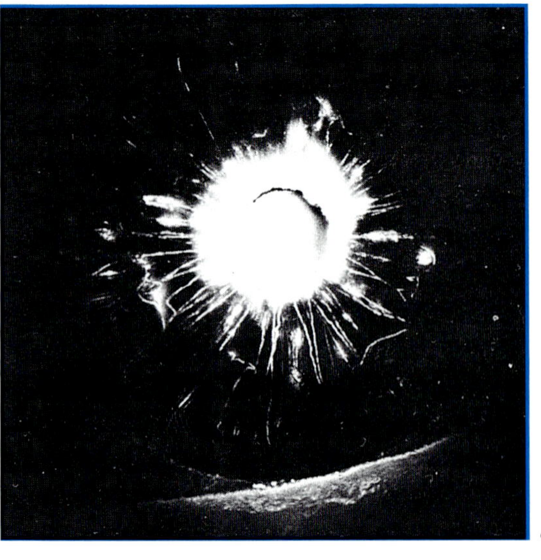

a)

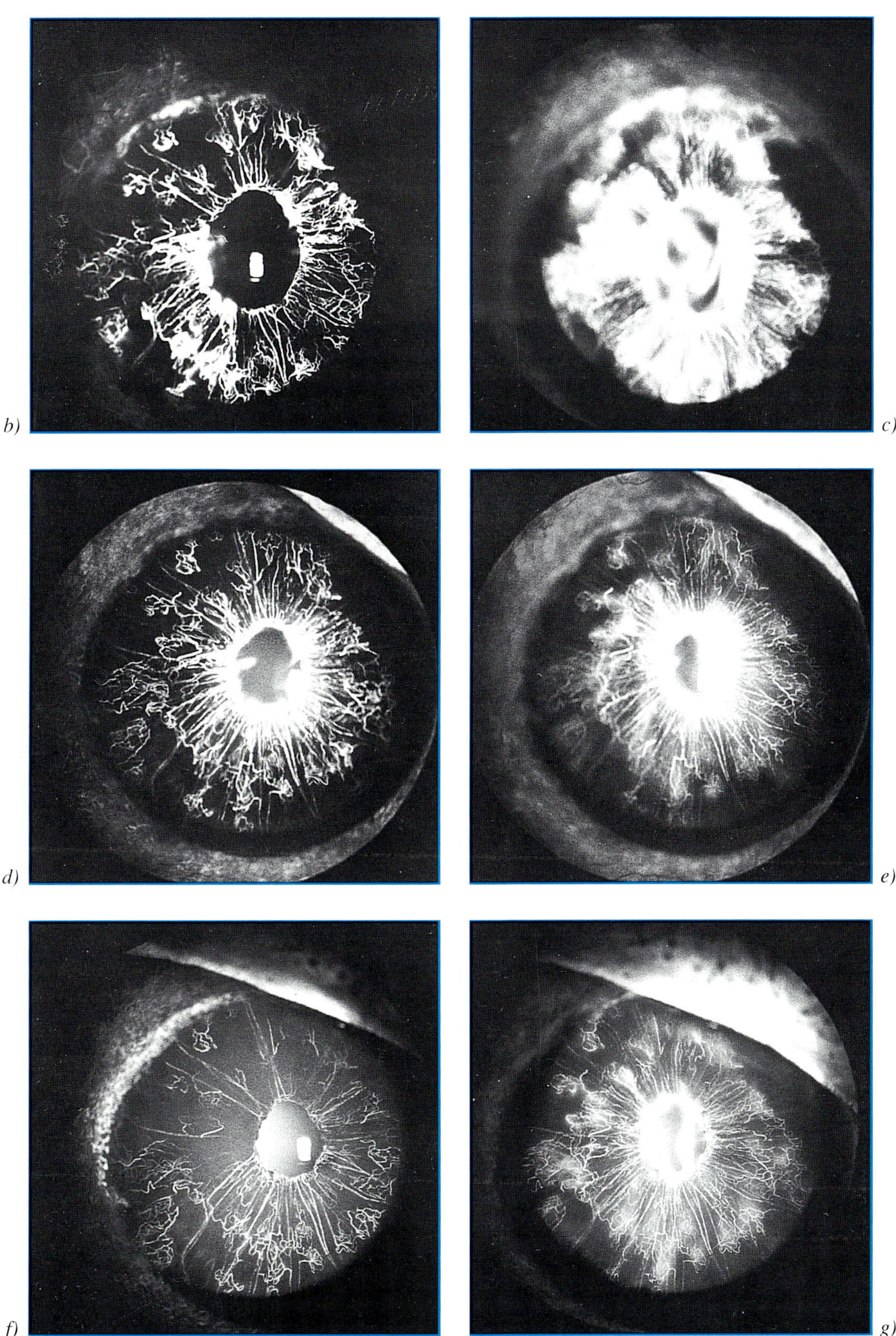
b)
c)
d)
e)
f)
g)

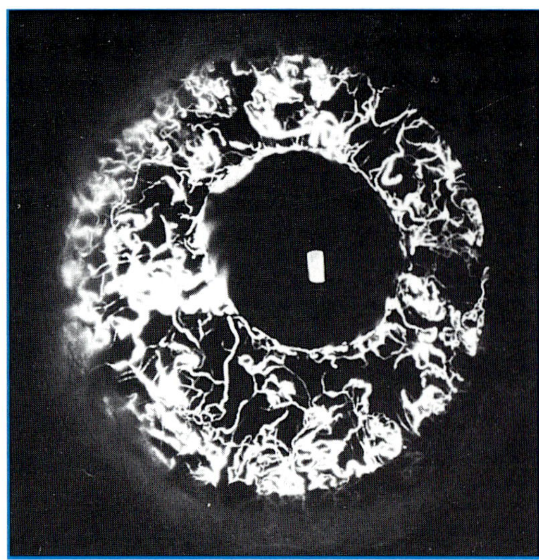

*Fig. **4.9**,14 - New vessels over the whole surface of the iris in a diabetic patient after intracapsular lens extraction (iris fluorescein angiography).*

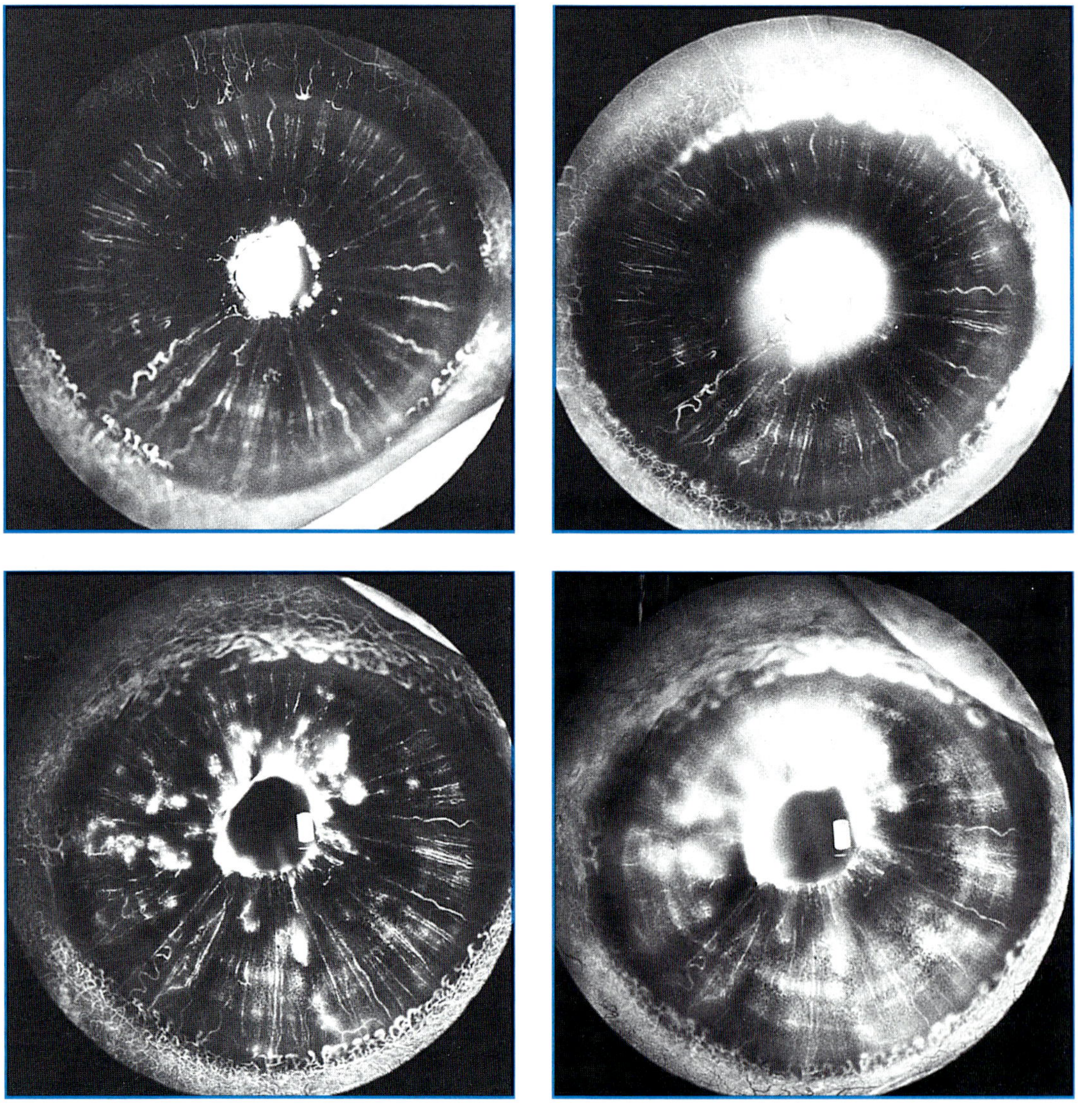

a) *b)*

c) *d)*

*Fig. **4.9**,15 - Iris fluorescein angiographic phases in a patient with central retinal vein occlusion whit ischemic capillaropathy before (a,b) and one month after (c,d) cataract extraction with implantation of a posterior chamber intraocular lens. Neovascularization was limited to the pupillary border preoperatively (a,b) but involved the ciliary part too after (c,d). Panretinal photocoagulation was completed after surgery.*

a) 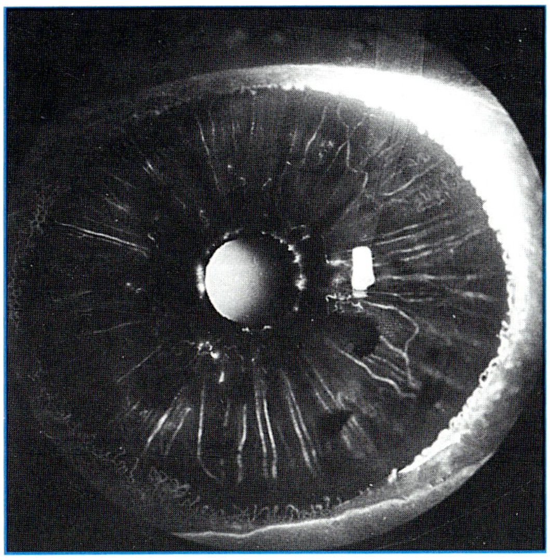 b)

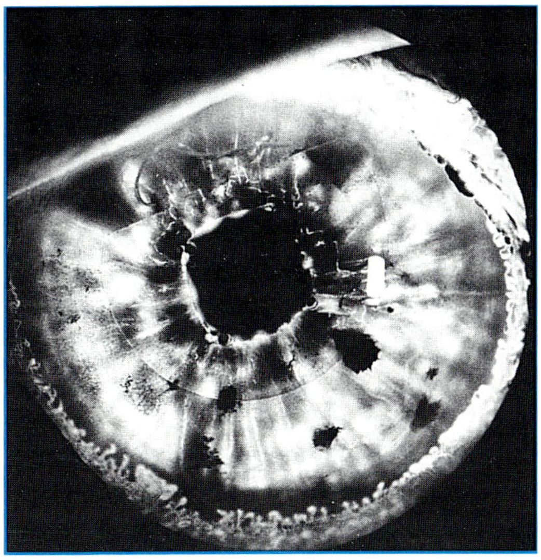

c)

*Fig. **4.9**,16 - A case before (a), two months (b) and one year (c) after cataract extraction with implantation of a Worst lens with steel wire iris fixation. Immediately after surgery (b) dot-like neovascular proliferation can be seen, with congested radial vessels and marked breakdown of the blood-iris barrier. Vascular involvement diminishes with time (c).*

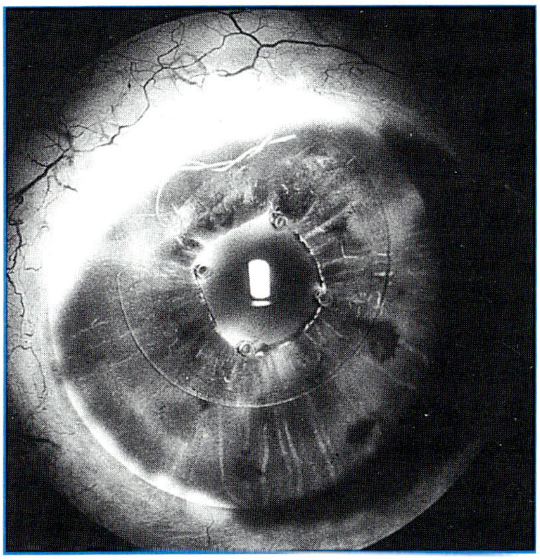

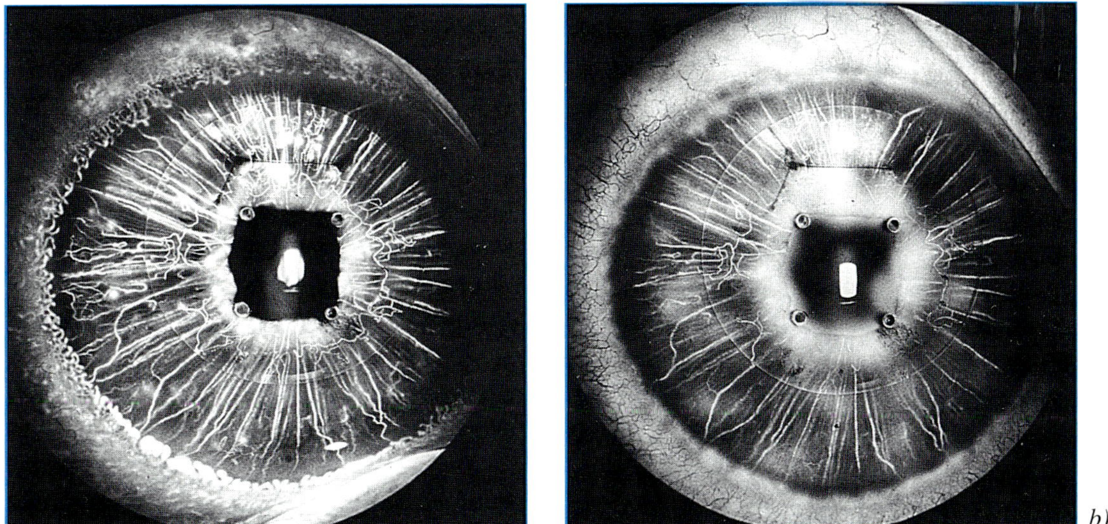

a) b)

*Fig. **4.9**,17 - Iris fluorescein angiographic phases (a,b) in a patient with a Worst lens with iris fixation. Neovascular tufts can be seen in the ciliary part of the upper hemi-iris.*

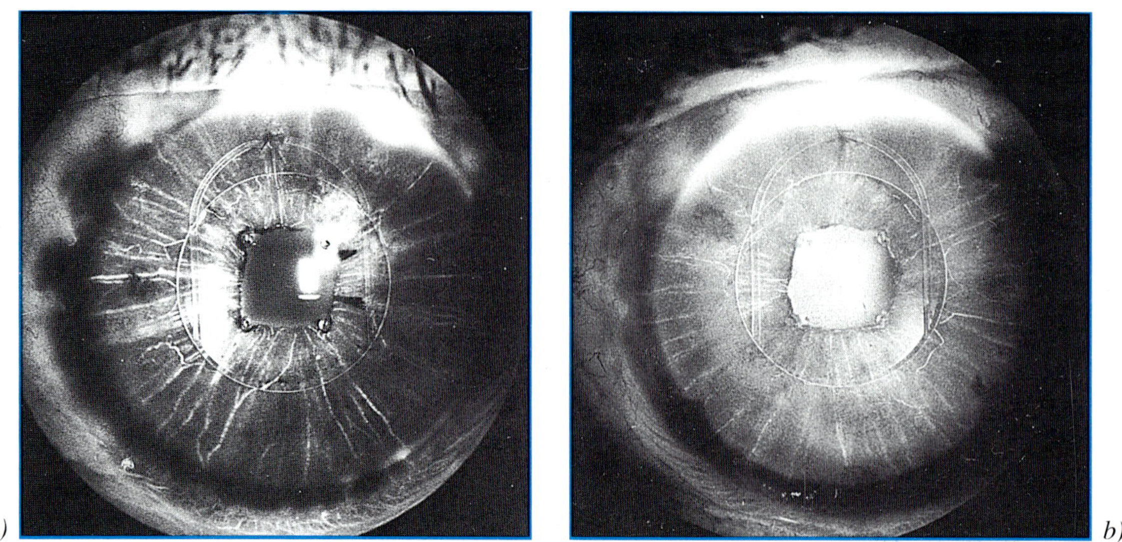

Fig. ***4.9****,18 - Early (a) and late (b) iris fluorescein angiographic phases in a pseudophakic eye with an intraocular lens with iris fixation. Dye leakage can be seen at some of the points where the lens meets the iris surface but there is no vascular proliferation.*

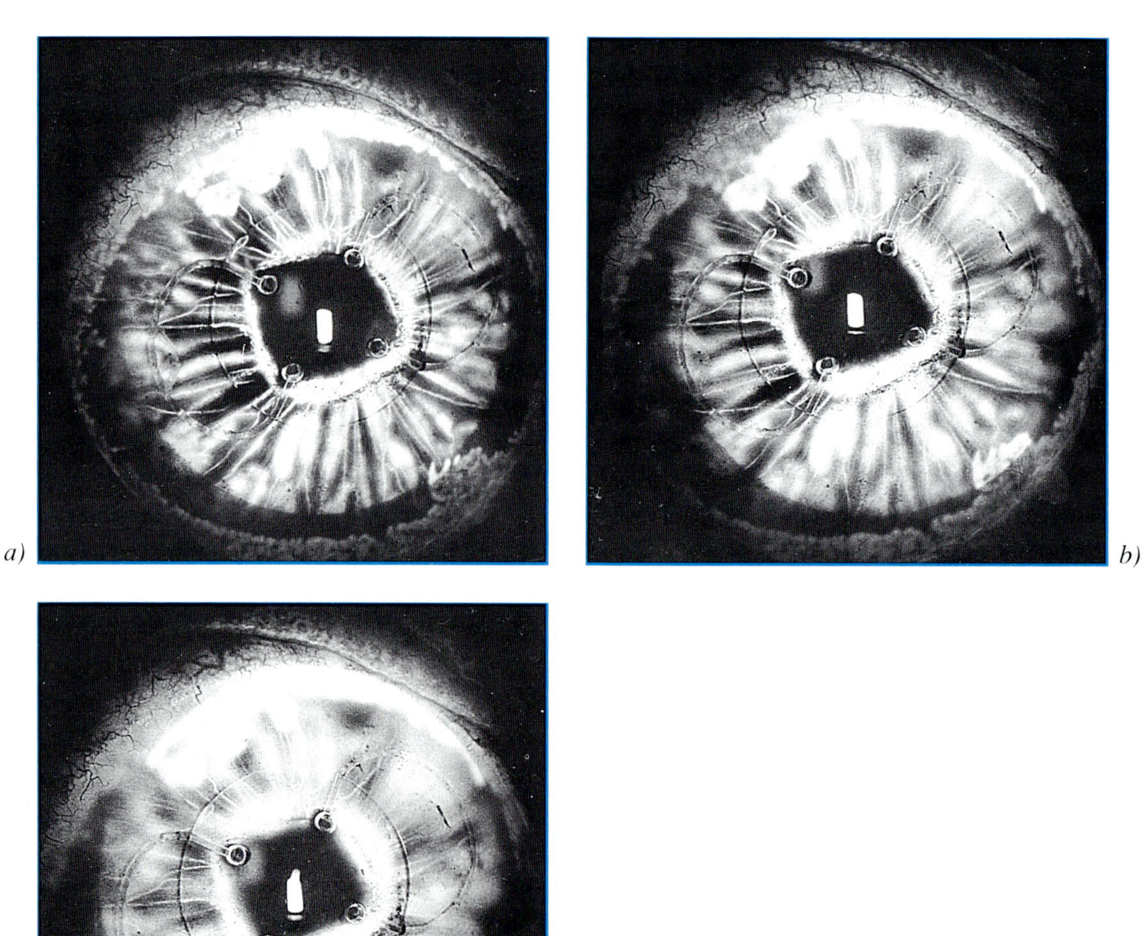

Fig. ***4.9****,19 - Iris fluorescein angiographic phases (a,b,c) in an eye after cataract extraction, with a four-loop Binkhorst intraocular lens. The marked vascular congestion gives rise to dye leakage that grows in subsequent angiographic phases. Circumscribed areas of iris ischemia can be seen.*

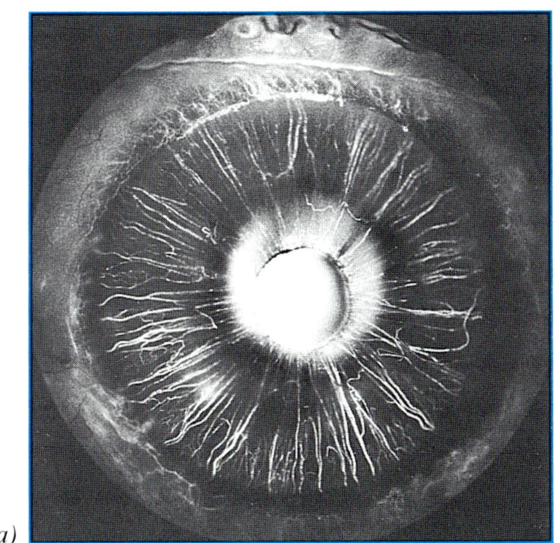
a)

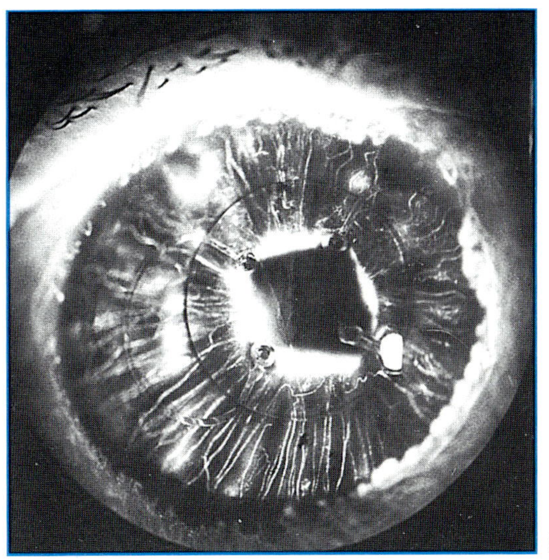
b)

*Fig. **4.9**,20 - Iris fluorescein angiographic examination of an eye with cataract and age-related pupillary margin leakage (a). After cataract extraction and implantation of a four-loop Binkhorst lens (b) congested iris vessels and focal leakage in the stroma can be seen. Dye leakage is heavy at the pupillary margin.*

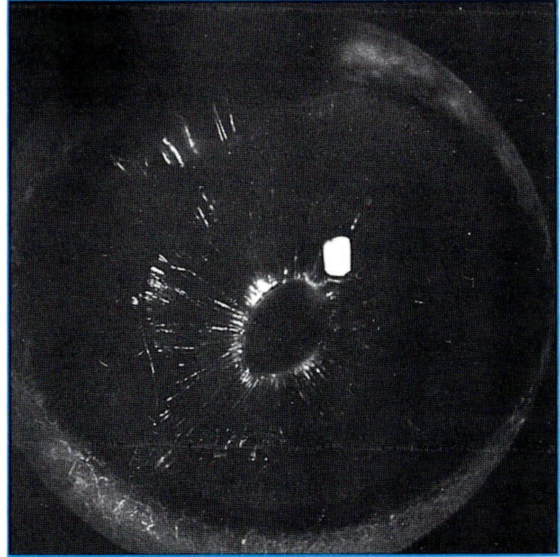
a)

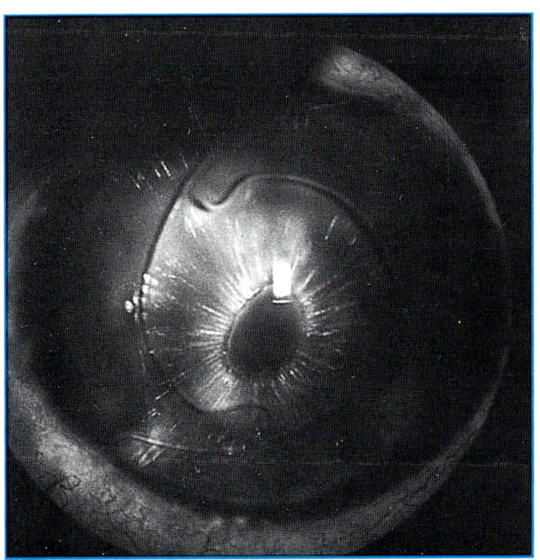
b)

*Fig. **4.9**,21 - Pseudophakic eye with a two open-loop intraocular lens in the anterior chamber: early (a) and late (b) iris fluorescein angiographic views. These anterior chamber lenses are new on the market and cause less harm to iris vessels.*

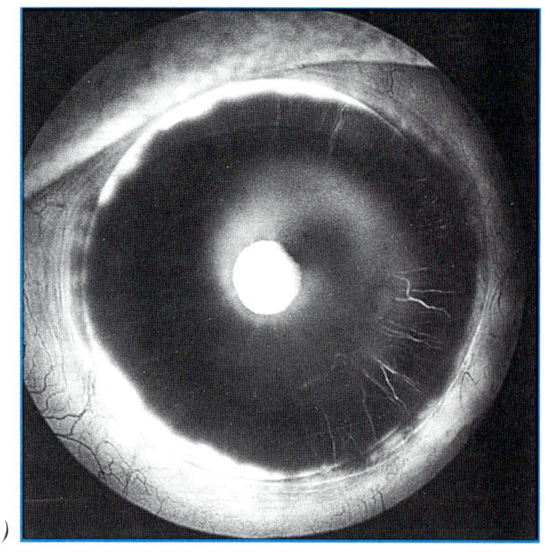
a)

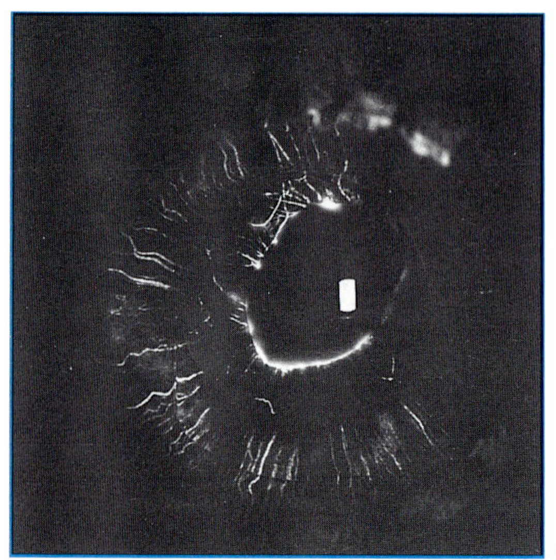
b)

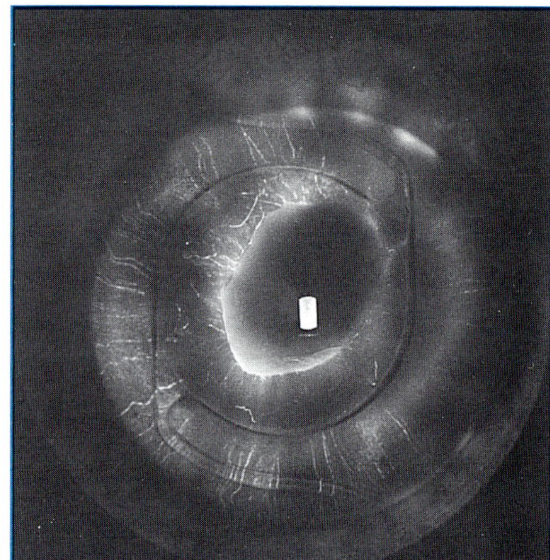
c)

*Fig. **4.9**,22 - A case before (a) and after (b,c) cataract extraction and implantation of an anterior chamber two open-loop lens. Vessels in the pupillary microcirculation show limited alterations.*

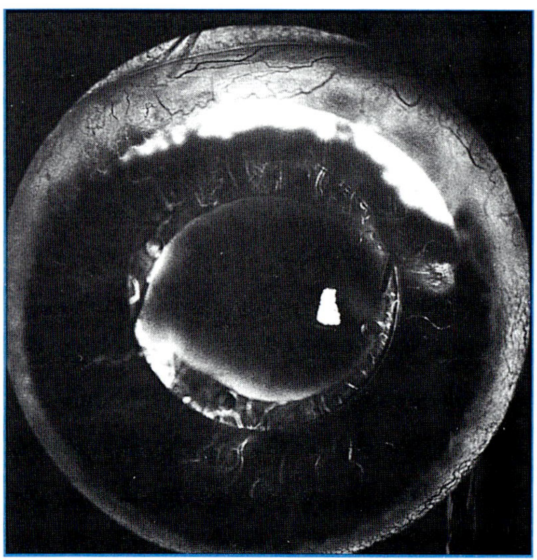

*Fig. **4.9**,23 - Posterior chamber intraocular lens dislocated into the anterior chamber. Dye leakage is marked where it touches the iris surface.*

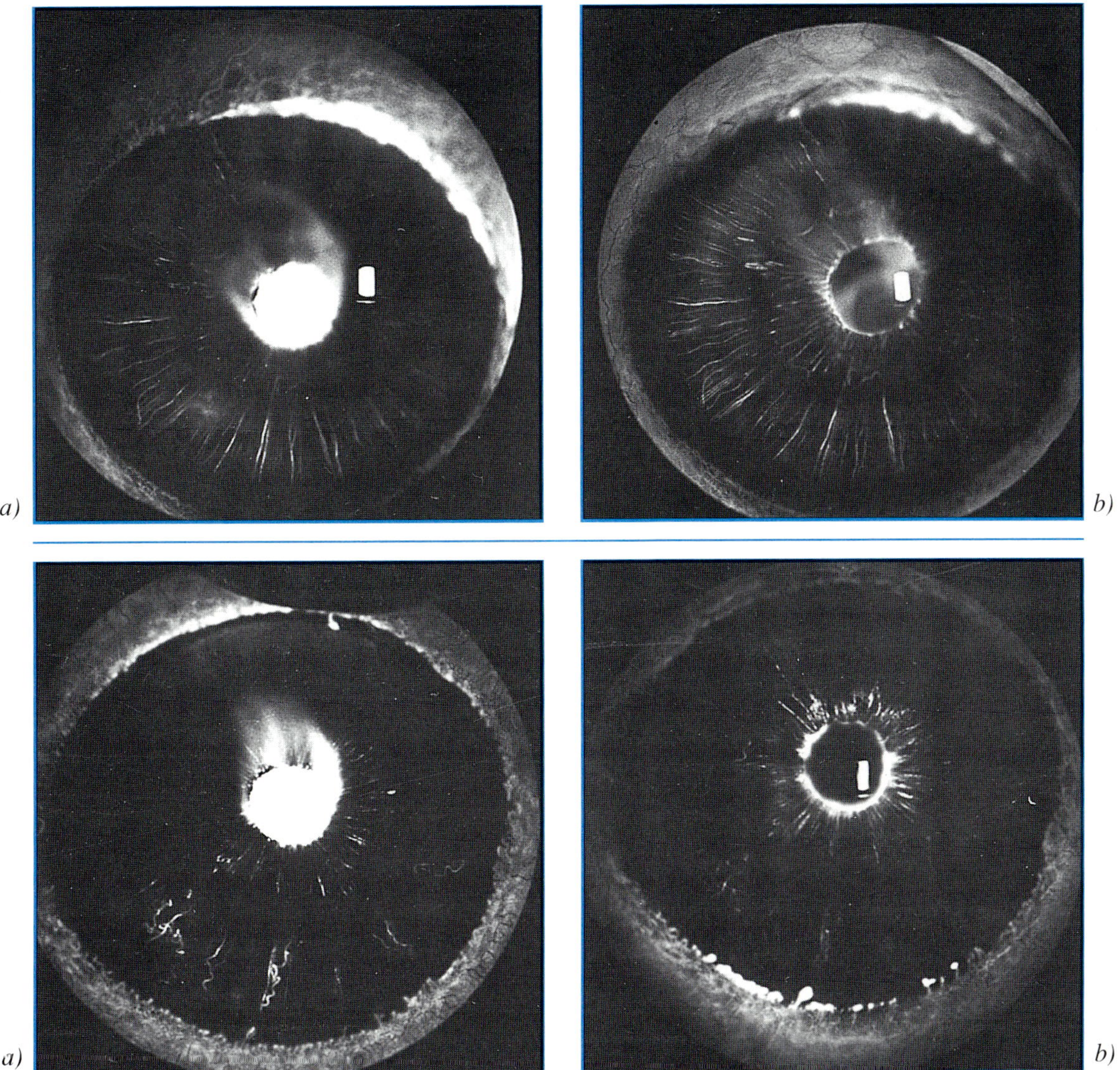

Figs. ***4.9****,24,25 - Iris fluorescein angiography in two patients before (a) and after (b) cataract extraction and implantation of a posterior chamber intraocular lens. Pre-operative iris fluorescein angiograms show age-related pupillary margin leakage. After surgery dye only leaks in the pupillary part.*

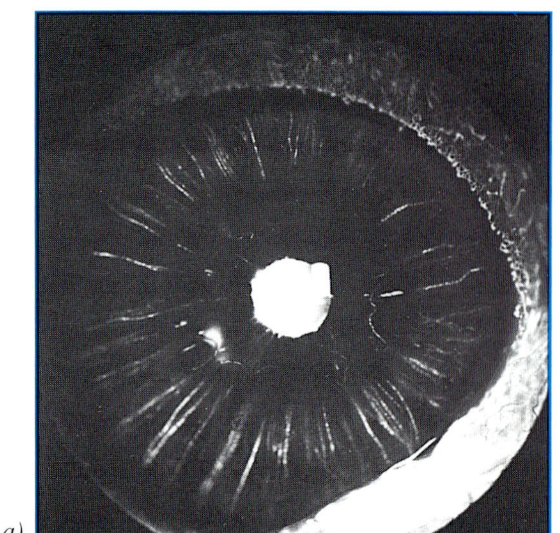

a)

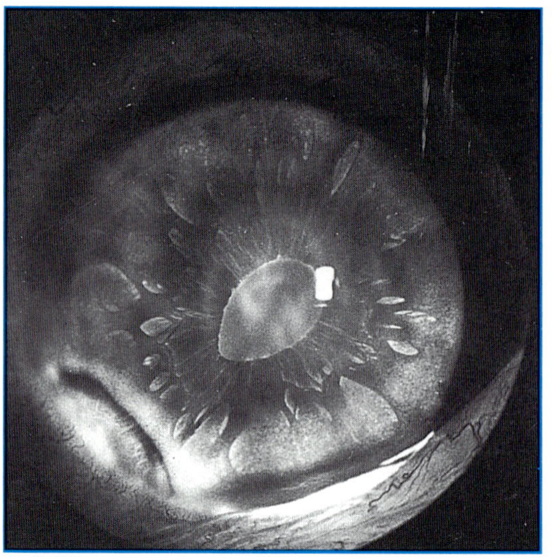

b)

*Fig. **4.9**,26 - Another case before (a) and after (b) cataract extraction with implantation of a posterior chamber intraocular lens. Pupillary deformation and diffuse breakdown of the blood-iris barrier can be seen. An irido-corneal synechia is visible at the 7-8 o' clock position.*

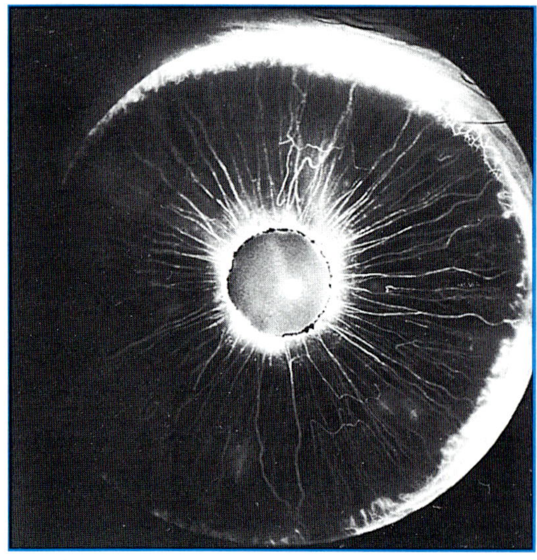

a)

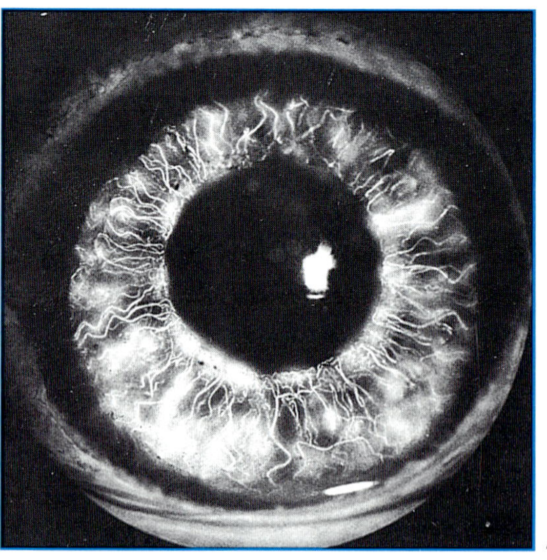

b)

*Fig. **4.9**,27 - Iris fluorescein angiography in an eye which had had anterior uveitis, that regressed in response to treatment. Dye leakage is visible only from the pupillary margin (a). Cataract extraction with implantation of an intraocular lens caused a recurrence of the uveitis. Congested vessels can be seen, with diffuse dye leakage over the whole iris surface (b).*

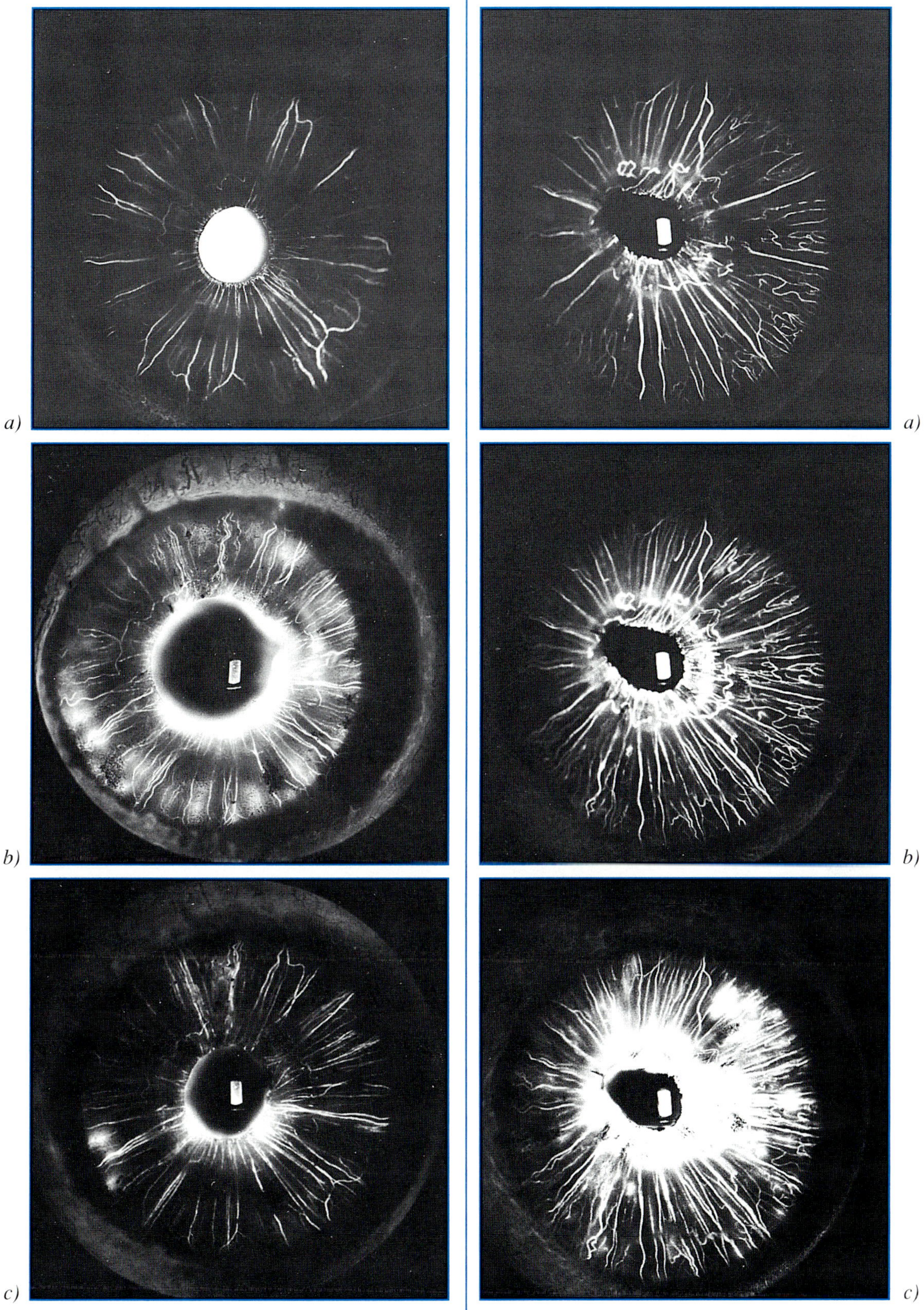

*Fig. **4.9**,28 - Same case before (a), one month (b) and four months (c) after cataract extraction with implantation of a posterior chamber lens. Iris fluorescein angiography before surgery showed no noteworthy abnormalities. Post-operative follow-up served to assess the iris vascular reaction to surgery (b) and its progress (c).*

*Fig. **4.9**,29 - Pseudophakic eye with a deformed pupil and rupture of the sphincter two months after surgery (iris fluorescein angiographic phases: a,b,c). Congestion is marked in the pupillary vessels, and dye leaks from most of the radial vessels in the later phases (c).*

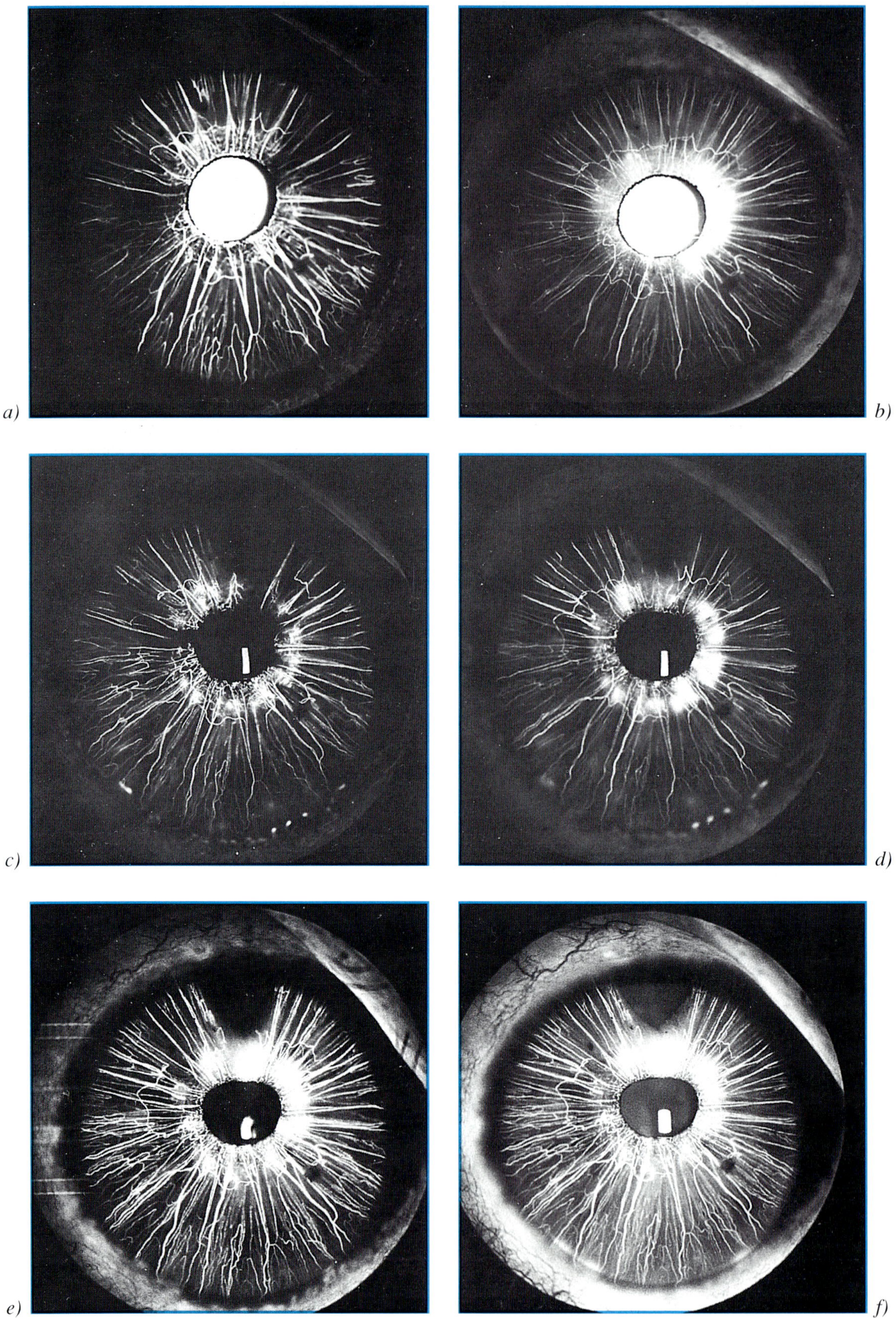

*Fig. **4.9**,30 - Pseudophakic eye before (a,b), one month (c,d) and two years (e,f) after cataract extraction with lens implantation in the capsular bag. The permeability of vessels in the pupillary part was already abnormal preoperatively.*

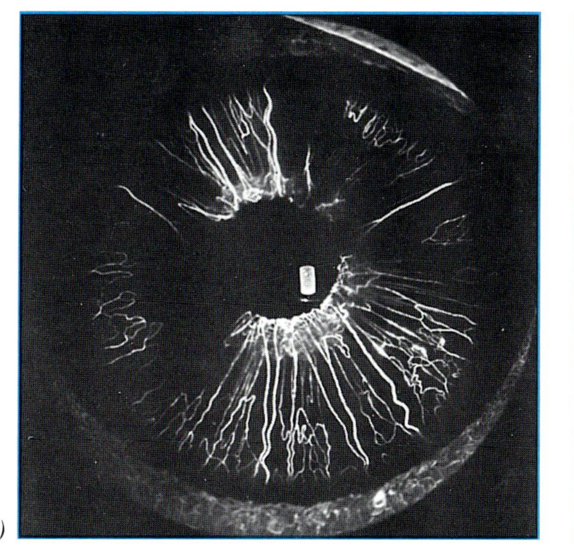
a)

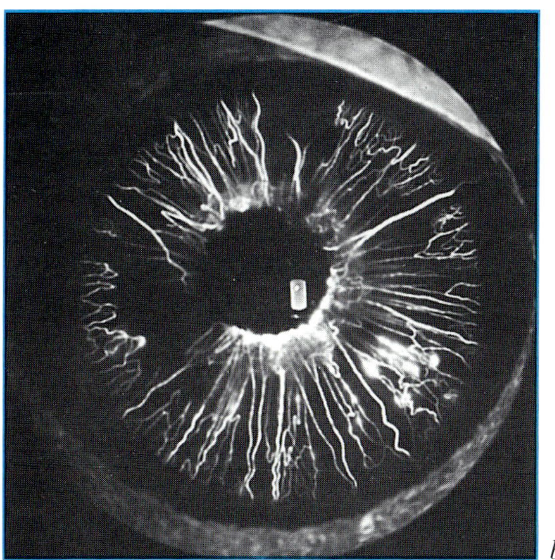
b)

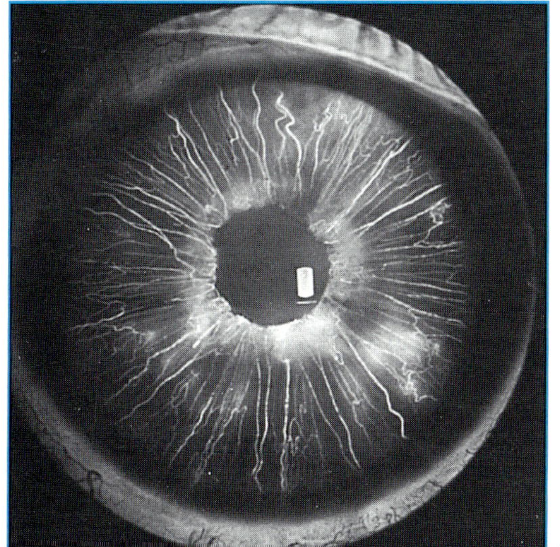
c)

*Fig. **4.9**,31 - Iris fluorescein angiographic phases (a,b,c) two months after cataract extraction with lens implantation in the ciliary sulcus. Findings include filling delays, well-visualized recurrent vessels, some radial vessels filling retrogradely and others with abnormal caliber, sac-like dilatations and increased permeability. Dye leakage can be seen from the pupillary border.*

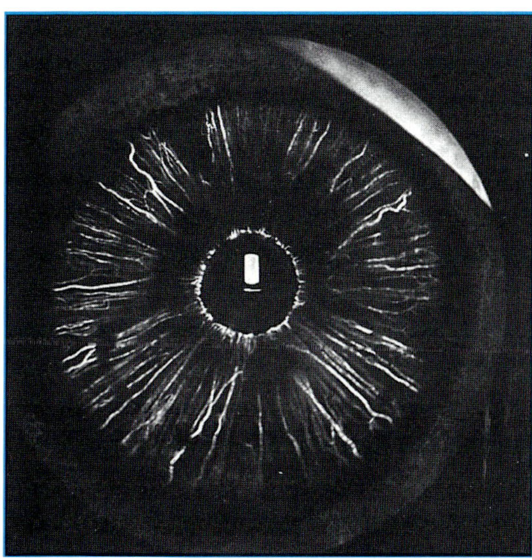

*Fig. **4.9**,32 - Two months after extracapsular cataract extraction with implantation of a Hydrogel posterior chamber intraocular lens this eye shows no iris fluorescein angiographic signs of edematous iridopathy.*

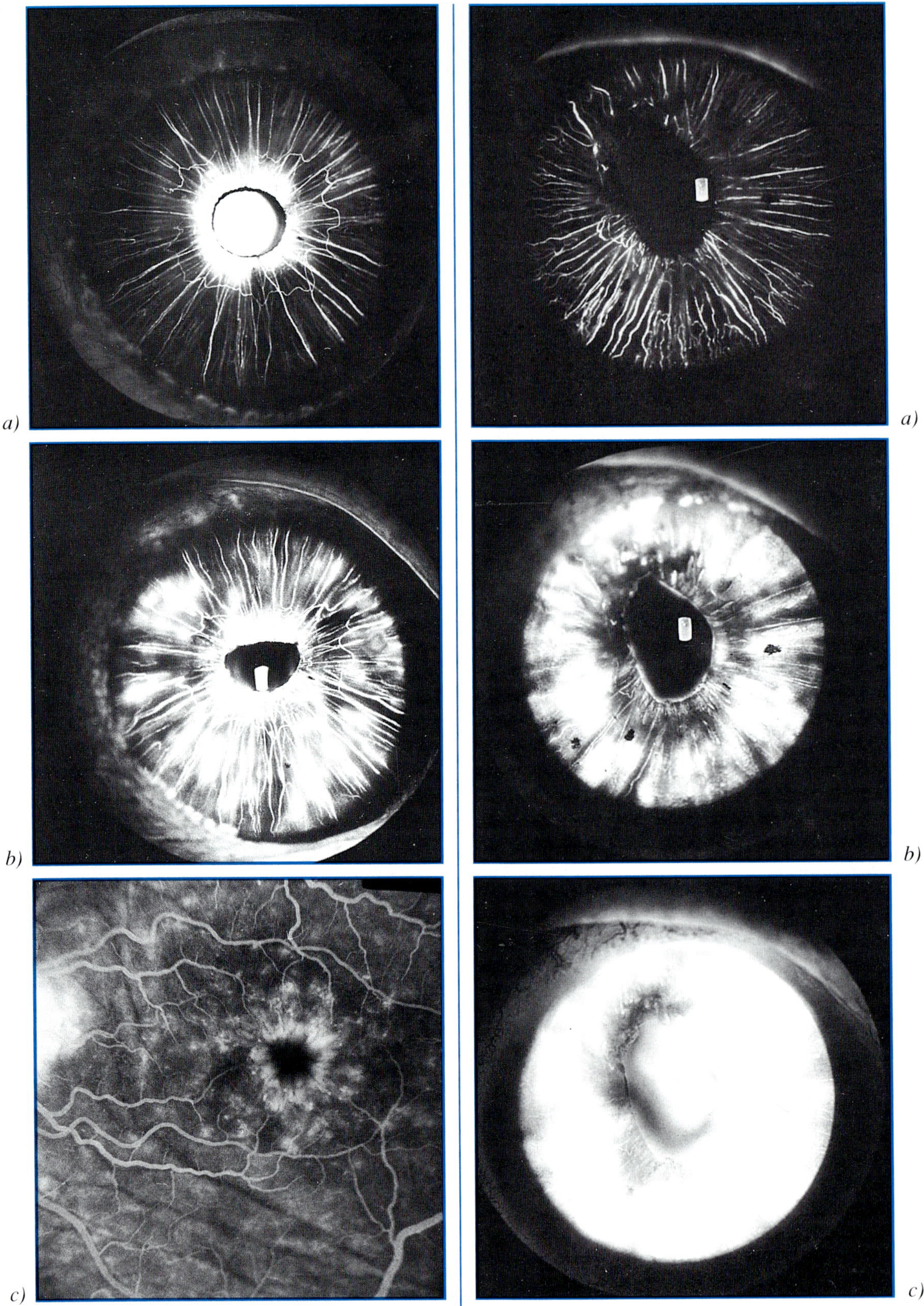

*Fig. **4.9**,33 - Iris fluorescein angiography before (a) and after (b) cataract extraction. The preoperative view is within the limits of normal. Dye leakage from the pupillary margin is age-related (a). Two months post-operatively (b) vascular permeability throughout the iris is increased. The associated cystoid macular edema (c: retinal fluorescein angiogram) leads to a diagnosis of Irvine-Gass syndrome.*

*Fig. **4.9**,34 - Another case with Irvine-Gass syndrome one month after surgery. Iris fluorescein angiography (phases a,b,c) shows massive edematous iridopathy causing dye leakage, increasing in subsequent angiographic phases until in the late phase (c) it masks the whole iris surface.*

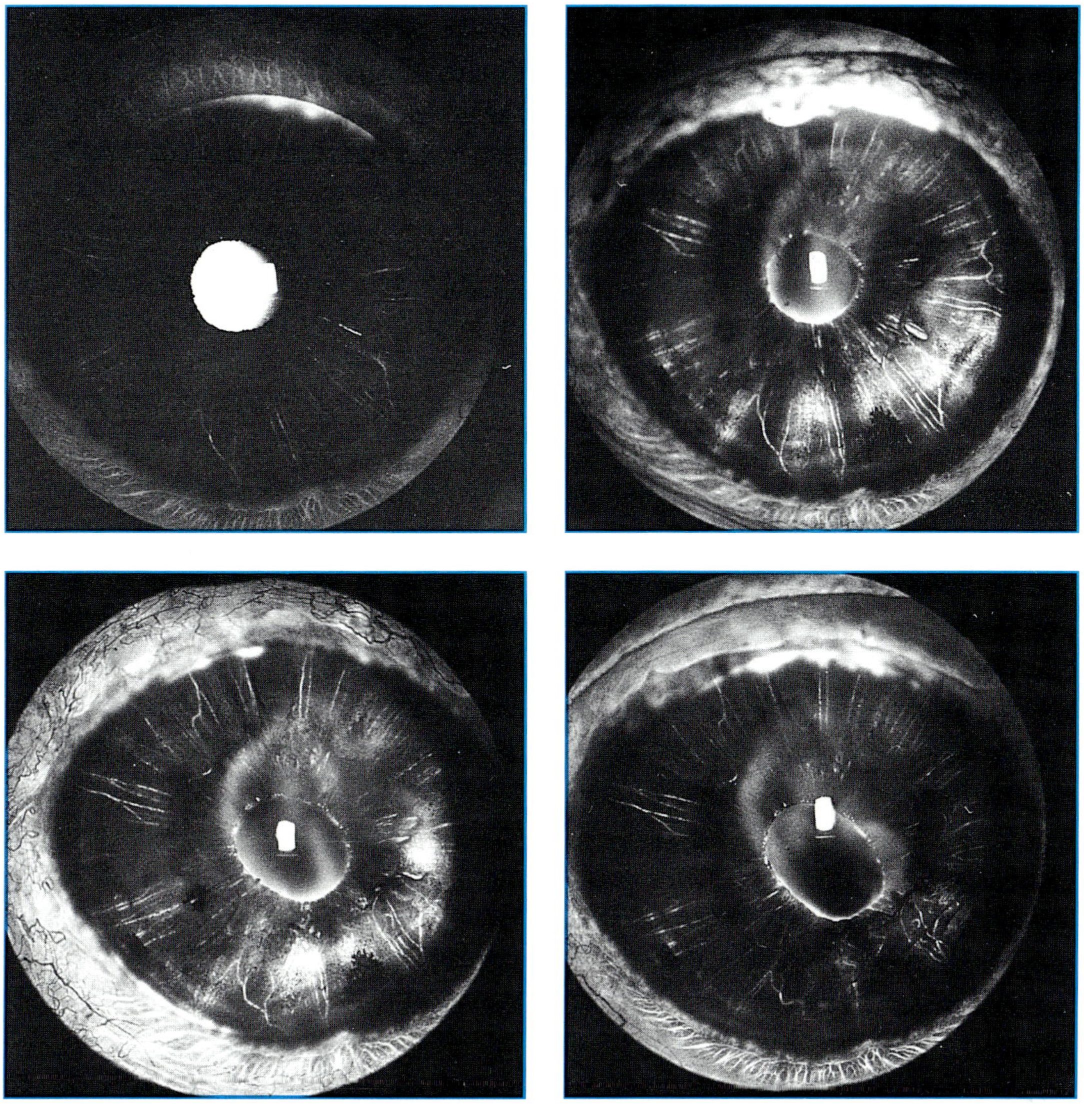

a) b)

c) d)

*Fig. **4.9**,35 - Iris fluorescein angiographic findings in another patient with Irvine-Gass syndrome before (a), one month (b), three months (c) and one year (d) after cataract extraction. Only the last examination showed a reduction in the damage to the blood-iris barrier, in response to anti-inflammatory therapy.*

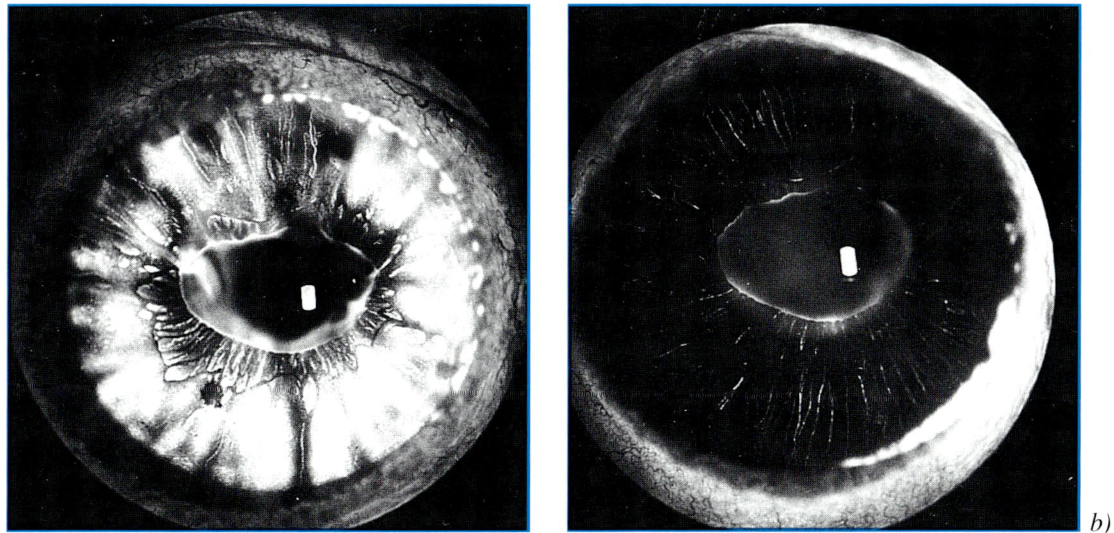

a) b)

*Fig. **4.9**,36 - Another case of Irvine-Gass syndrome in which iris fluorescein angiography served to follow the damage to the blood-iris barrier (a) as it regressed (b) in response to anti-inflammatory therapy.*

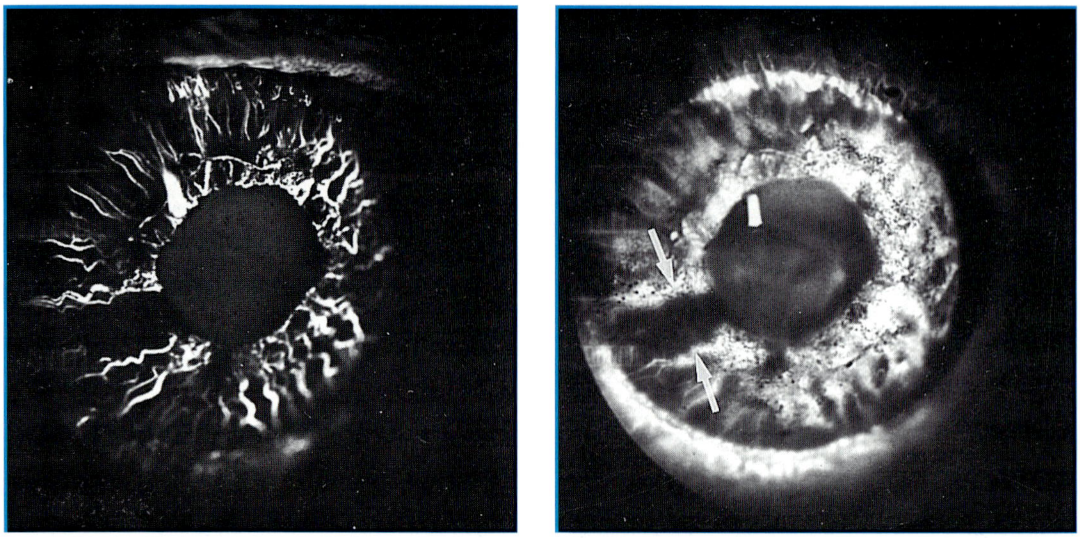

a) b)

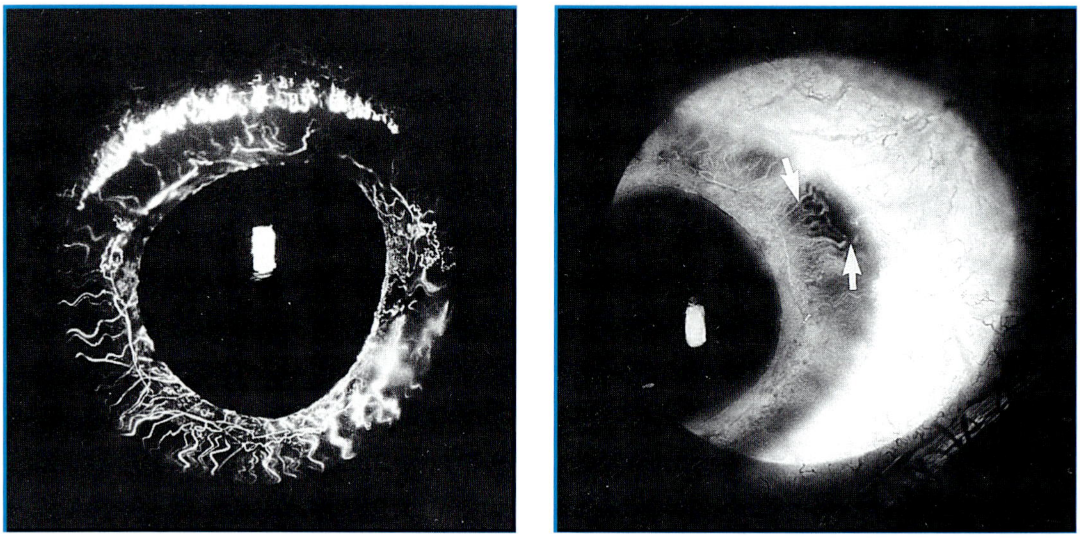

a) b)

Figs. ***4.9****,37,38 - Two cases of anterior segment ischemia after surgery for retinal detachment (a,b: iris fluorescein angiographic phases). The pupil is dilated and deformed and shows filling defects; perfused radial vessels are distorted, congested and abnormally permeable. In late phases of the examination (b) a veil of fluorescence covers the surface of the iris, with the hypofluorescent areas of ischemia standing out (arrows).*

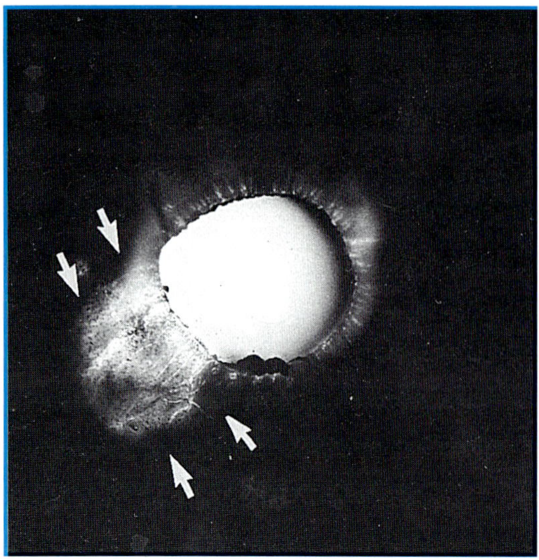

Fig. ***4.9****,39 - Iris fluorescein angiographic view of anterior segment ischemia in an eye with a brown iris, after surgery for retinal detachment. Ischemia has led to marked alterations in one sector of the iris stroma, which has become atrophic (arrows). Pigment thinning in that sector means that the abnormally permeable residual vascular network can be seen.*

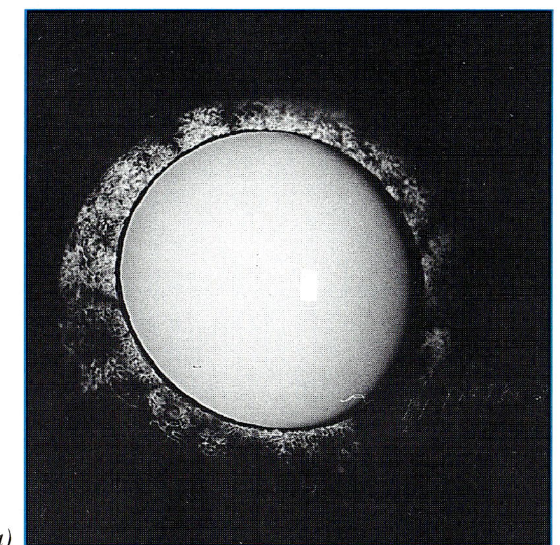
a)

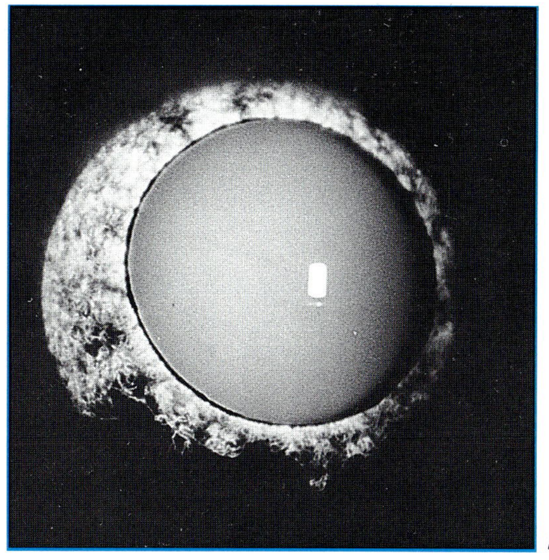
b)

*Fig. **4.9**,40 - Iris fluorescein angiographic phases (a,b) in a case of anterior segment ischemia after encircling buckle for retinal detachment. Filling delays and defects can be seen, loss of radial vascular architecture and diffuse, marked leakage from the anomalous vessels.*

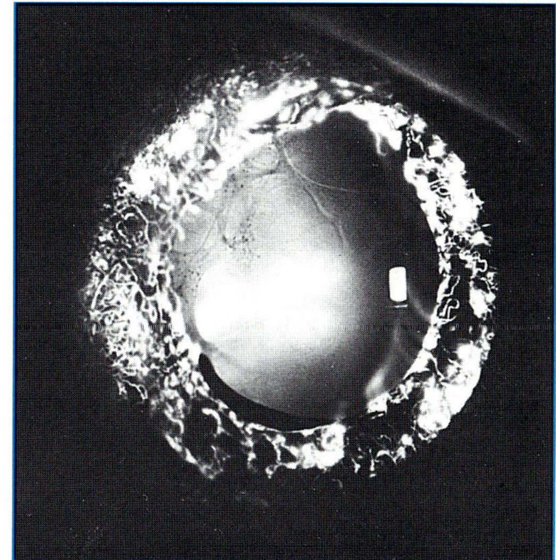

*Fig. **4.9**,41 - Anterior segment ischemic syndrome in an eye operated for retinal detachment. The nonperfused areas are associated with iris neovascularization and the vascular architecture is virtually lost (iris fluorescein angiographic view).*

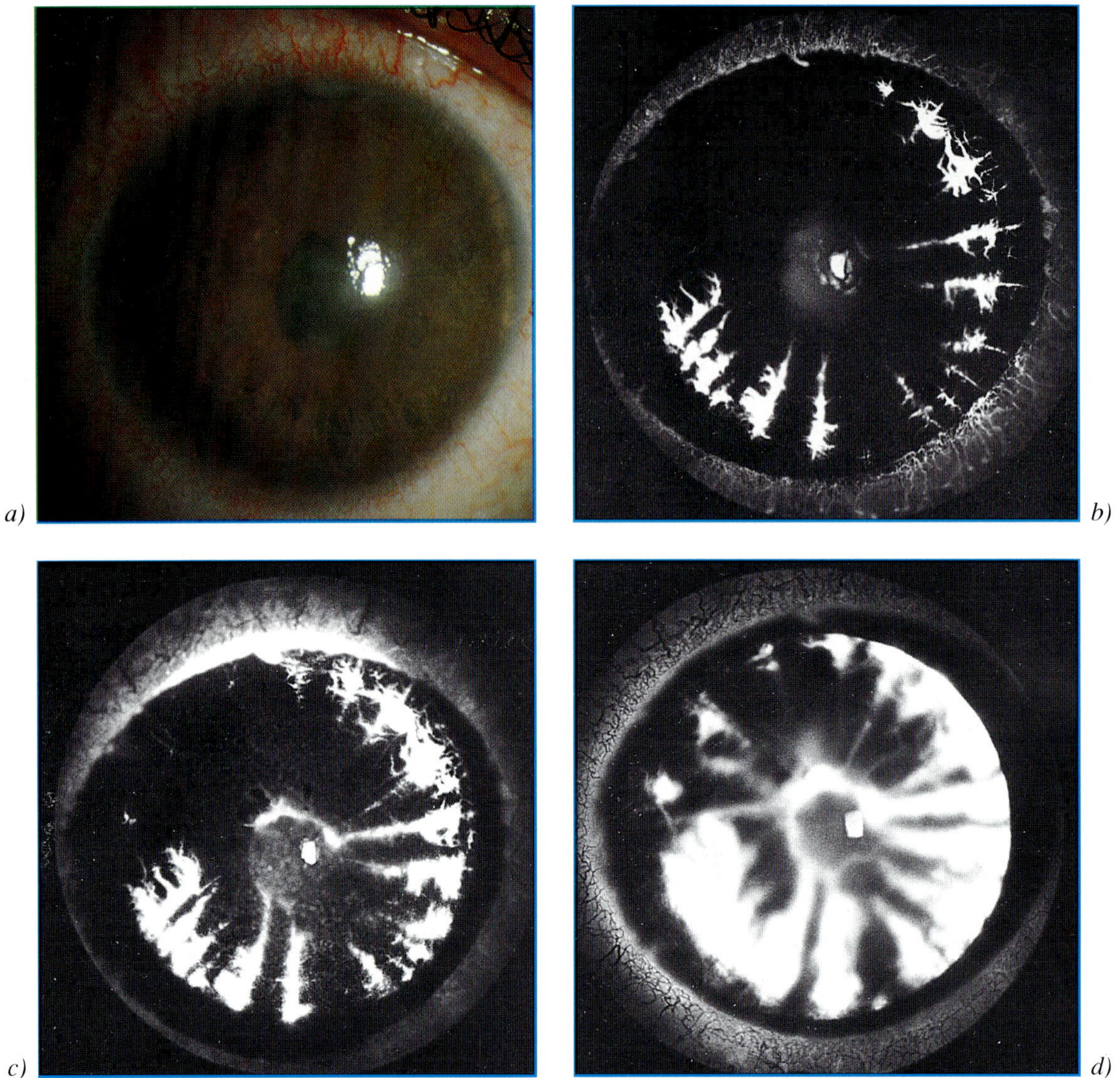

*Fig. **4.9**,42 - Massive corneal opacity, observed with the biomicroscope (a), makes it hard to visualize the iris surface. Iris fluorescein angiographic phases (b,c,d) in this eye with severe anterior segment ischemia after surgery for retinal detachment show the ischemic areas; perfused radial vessels are congested and there is heavy early dye leakage along their path (b), increasing in subsequent phases of the examination (c,d).*

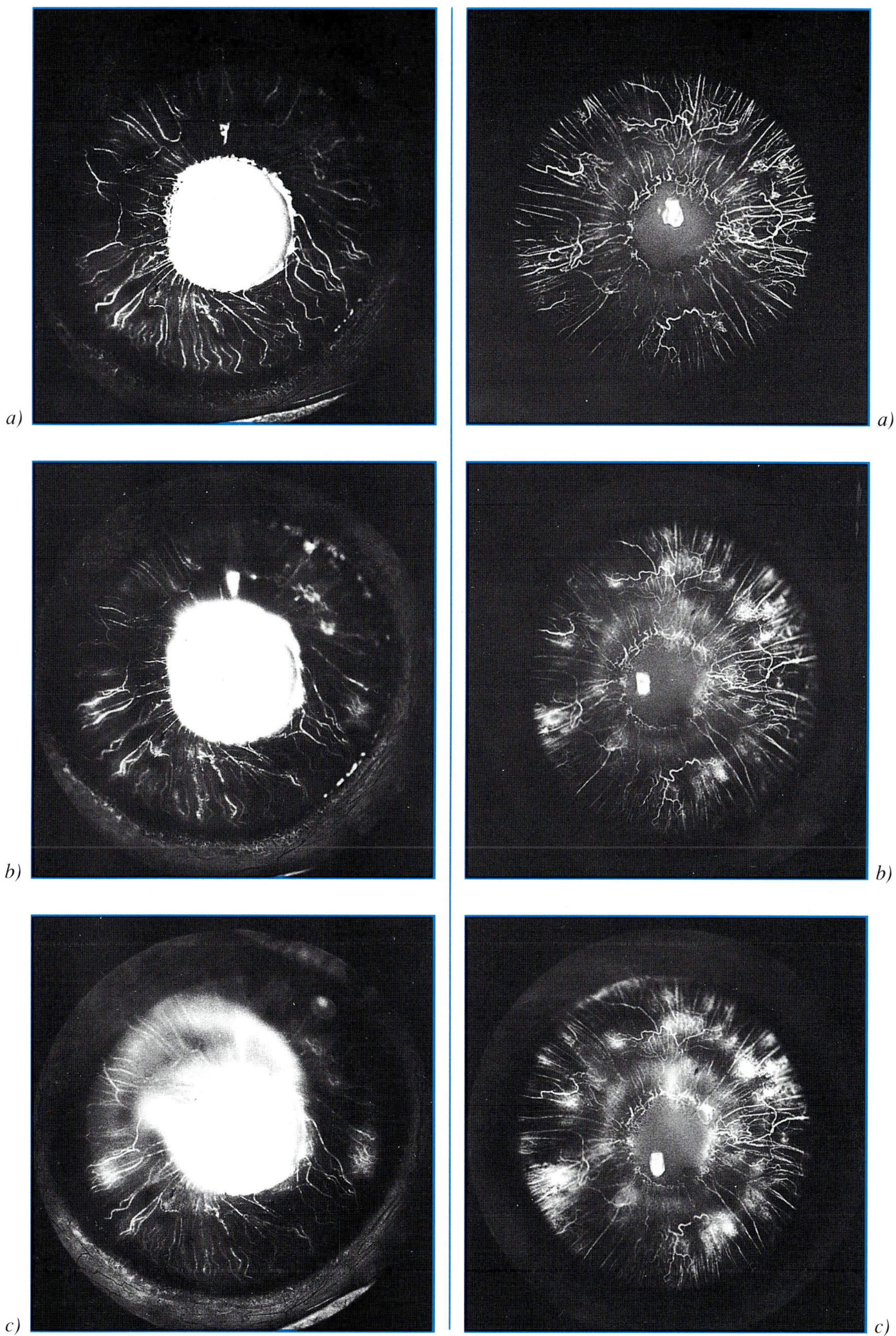

*Figs. **4.9**,43,44 - Iris fluorescein angiographic views (phases a,b,c) in eyes after buckling for retinal detachment. Fig. **4.9**,43 shows slight torsion of the iris stroma and initial neovascularization at the pupillary margin and in circumscribed areas in the pars ciliaris. In Fig. **4.9**,44 the vascular network is definitely distorted. Anomalous vessels with increased permeability can be seen over the whole surface of the iris and in the pupillary field.*

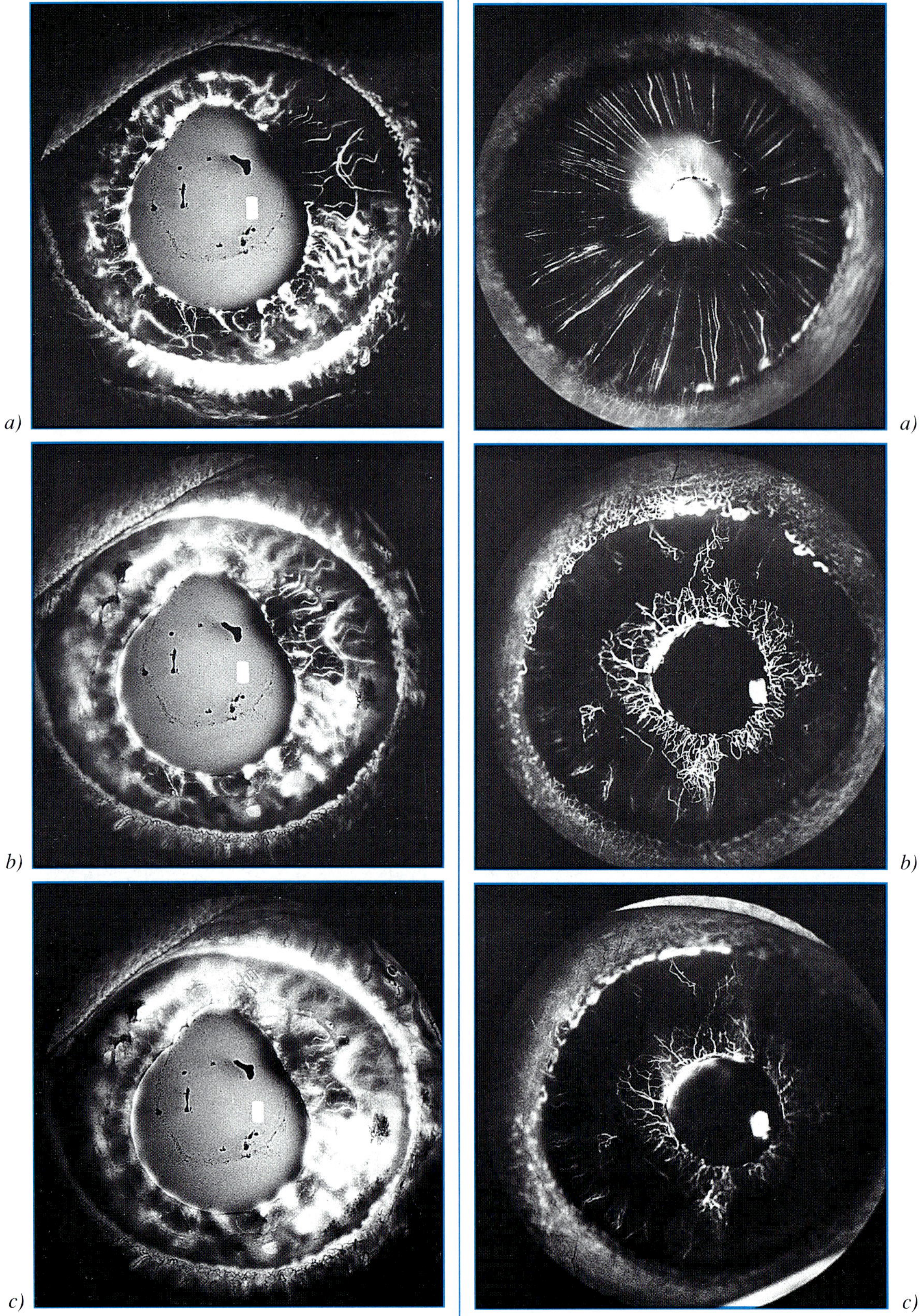

*Fig. **4.9**,45 - Imposing inflammatory reaction in an eye after vitrectomy for tractional retinal detachment (iris fluorescein angiographic phases a,b,c). Pigment dispersion can be seen on the anterior lens, with filling defects and delays, vascular congestion and diffuse breakdown of the blood-iris barrier.*

*Fig. **4.9**,46 - Iris fluorescein angiography before (a) and after (b,c) vitrectomy in a diabetic patient. Preoperatively the eye presented initial neovascularization at the pupillary margin; after surgery the pupillary part in particular showed a dense network of anarchic vessels (b) which leak dye slightly in later phases (c).*

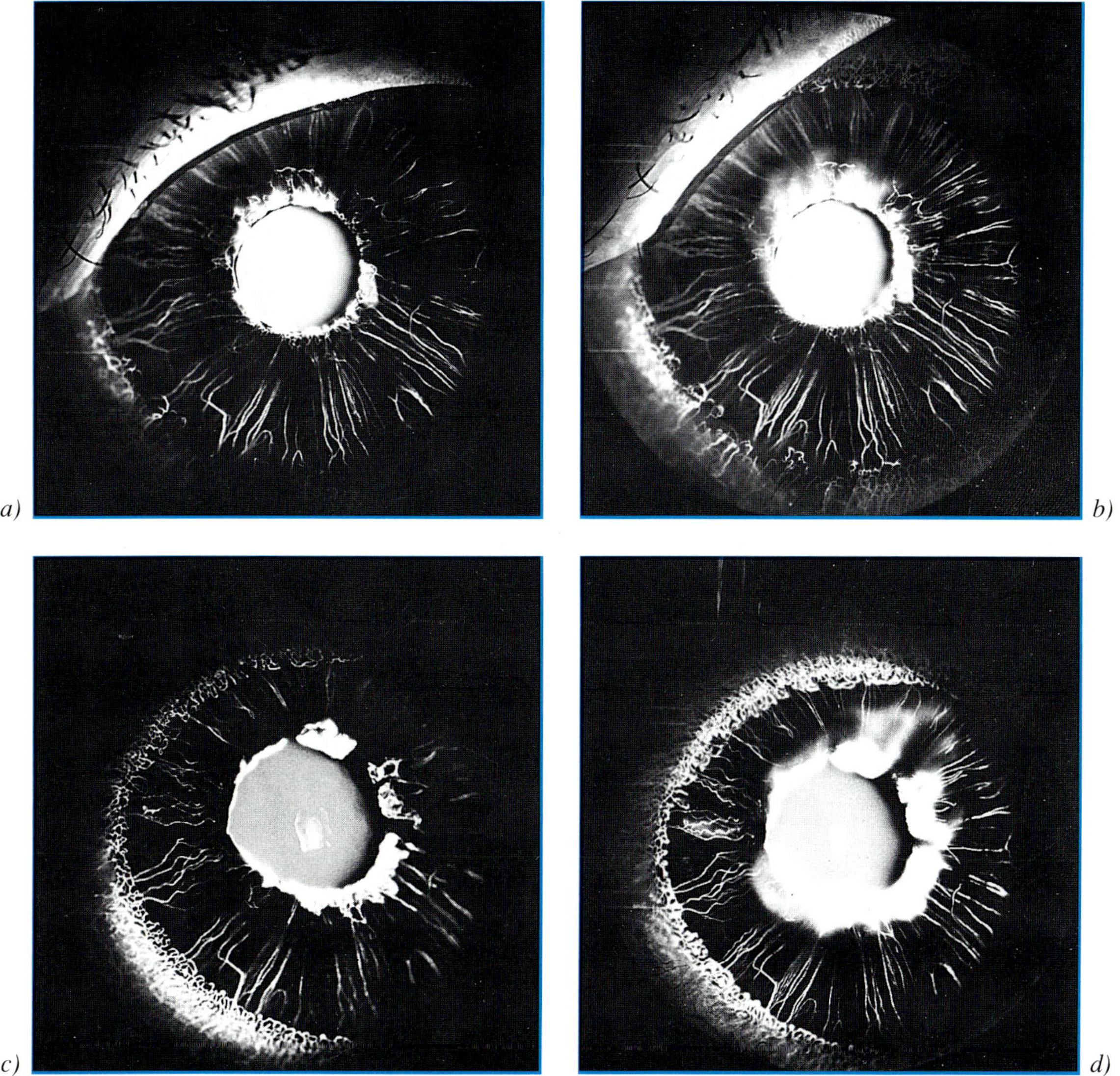

*Fig. **4.9**,47 - In this case of diabetic proliferative retinopathy complicated by tractional retinal detachment, the proliferative iridopathy already present before vitrectomy (a,b) is progressive but after surgery it still remains circumscribed to the pars pupillaris (c,d).*

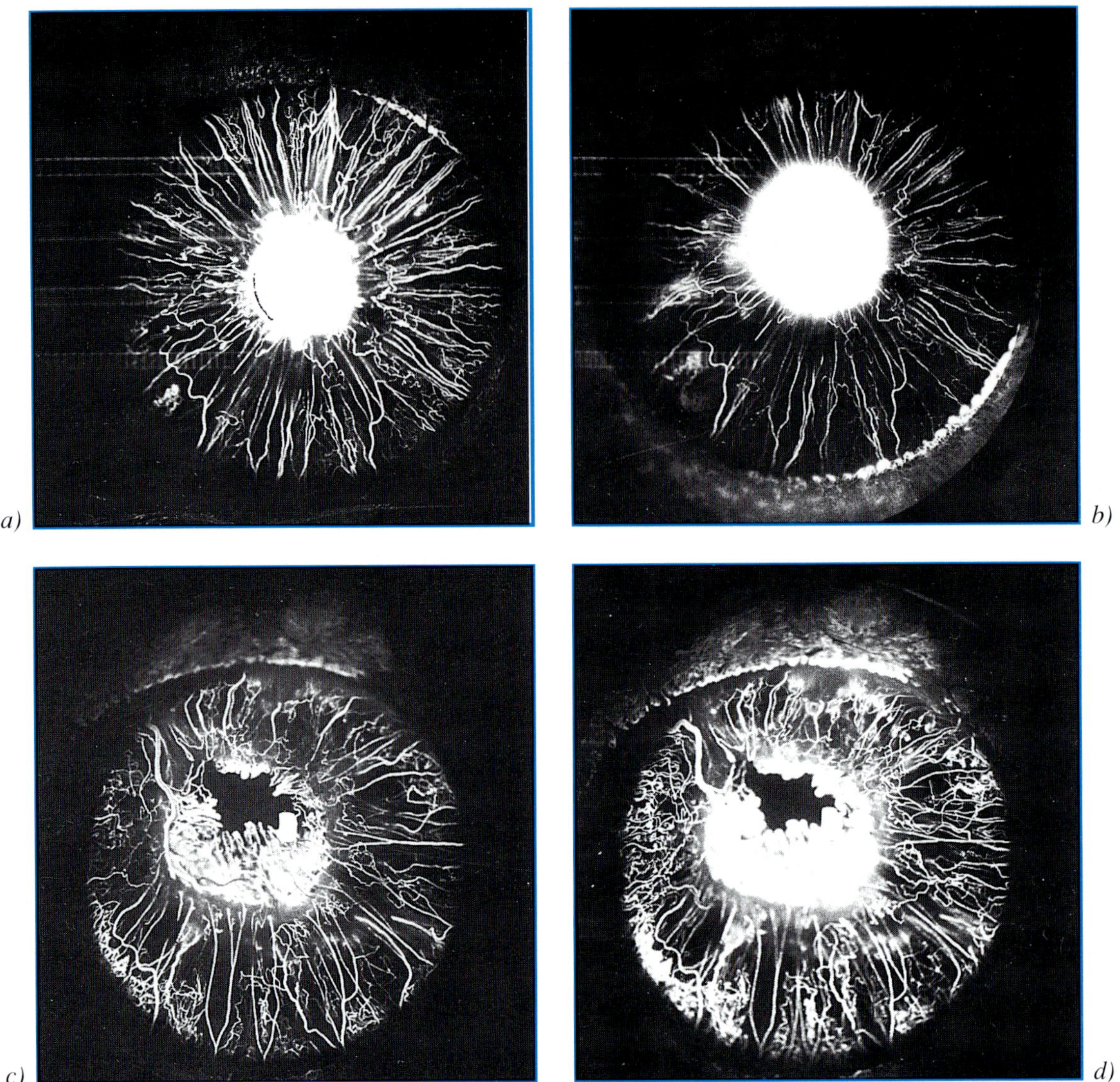

Fig. ***4.9****,48 - Neovascular glaucoma after vitrectomy and cataract extraction (c,d) in an eye with proliferative diabetic retinopathy and secondary retinal detachment. The preoperative picture showed new vessels at the pupillary border and in the stroma (a,b). The irreversible progression of the iridopathy is due to the failure to ensure photocoagulative ablation of the ischemic retina during or after surgery.*

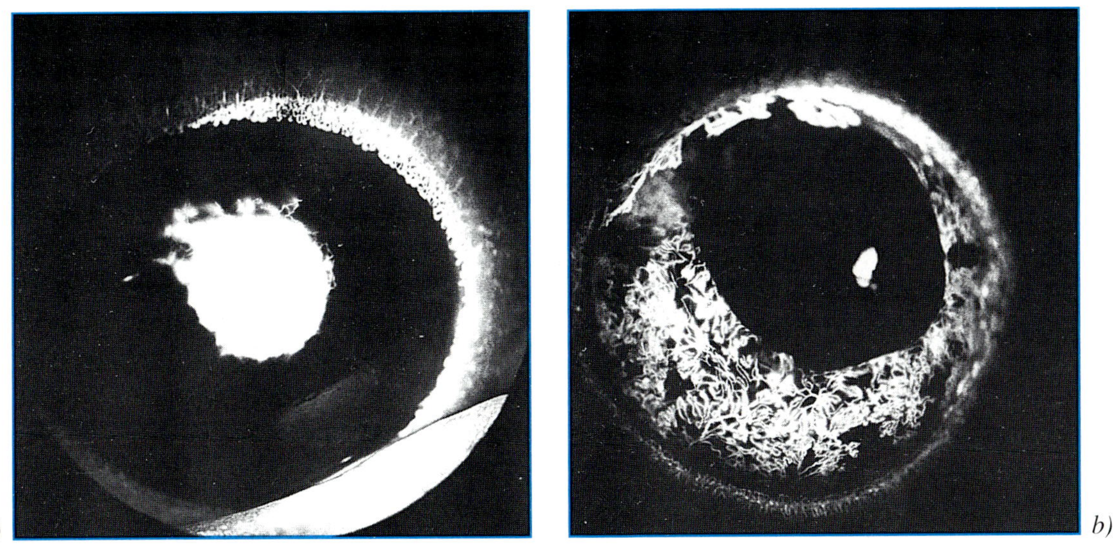

*Fig. **4.9**,49 - A case of diabetic iridopathy circumscribed to the pupillary margin preoperatively (a). After vitrectomy and cataract extraction, not followed by photocoagulation of the ischemic retina, neovascular glaucoma was visible (b).*

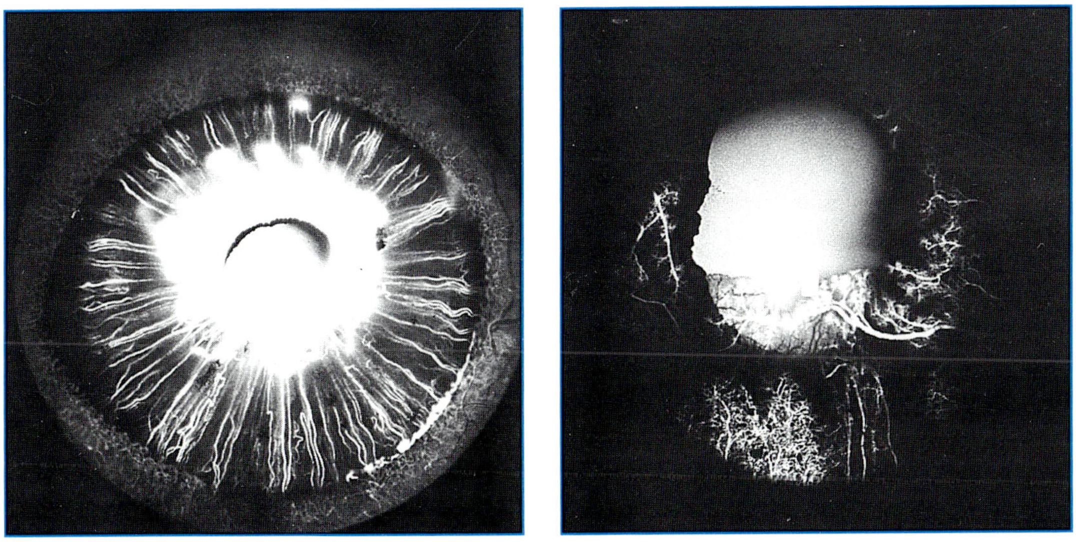

*Fig. **4.9**,50 - A case similar to the previous one, before (a) and after (b,c) vitrectomy.*

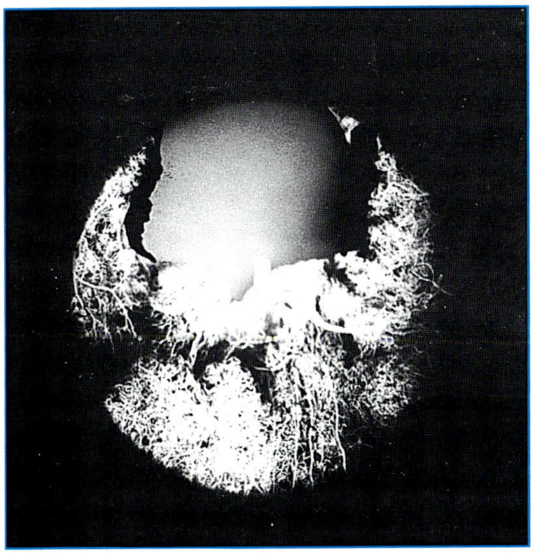

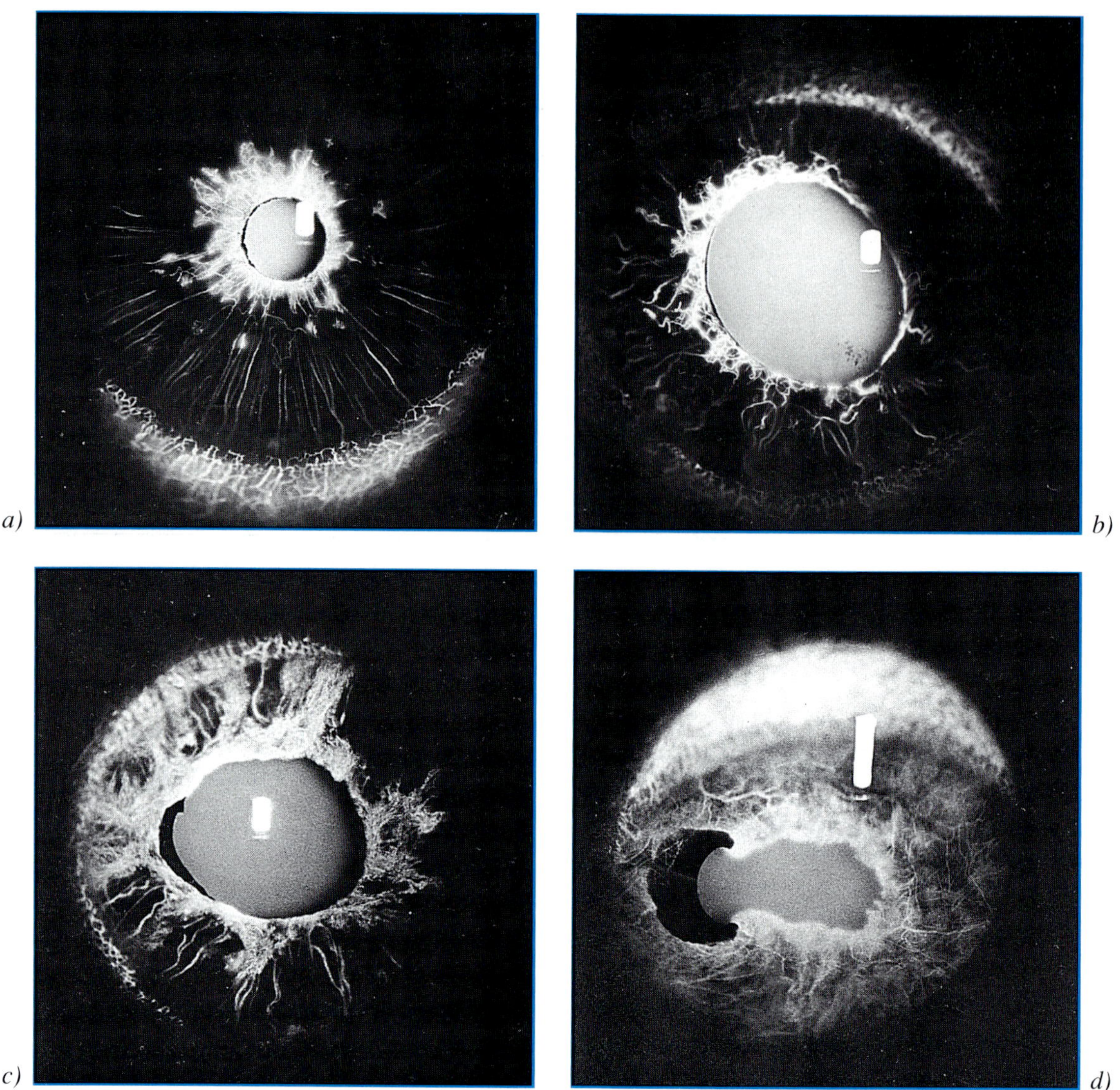

*Fig. **4.9**,51 - Iris fluorescein angiographic findings before (a), one month (b), four months (c) and one year (d) after vitrectomy for tractional retinal detachment in proliferative diabetic retinopathy. The proliferative iridopathy can be followed as it progresses to neovascular glaucoma.*

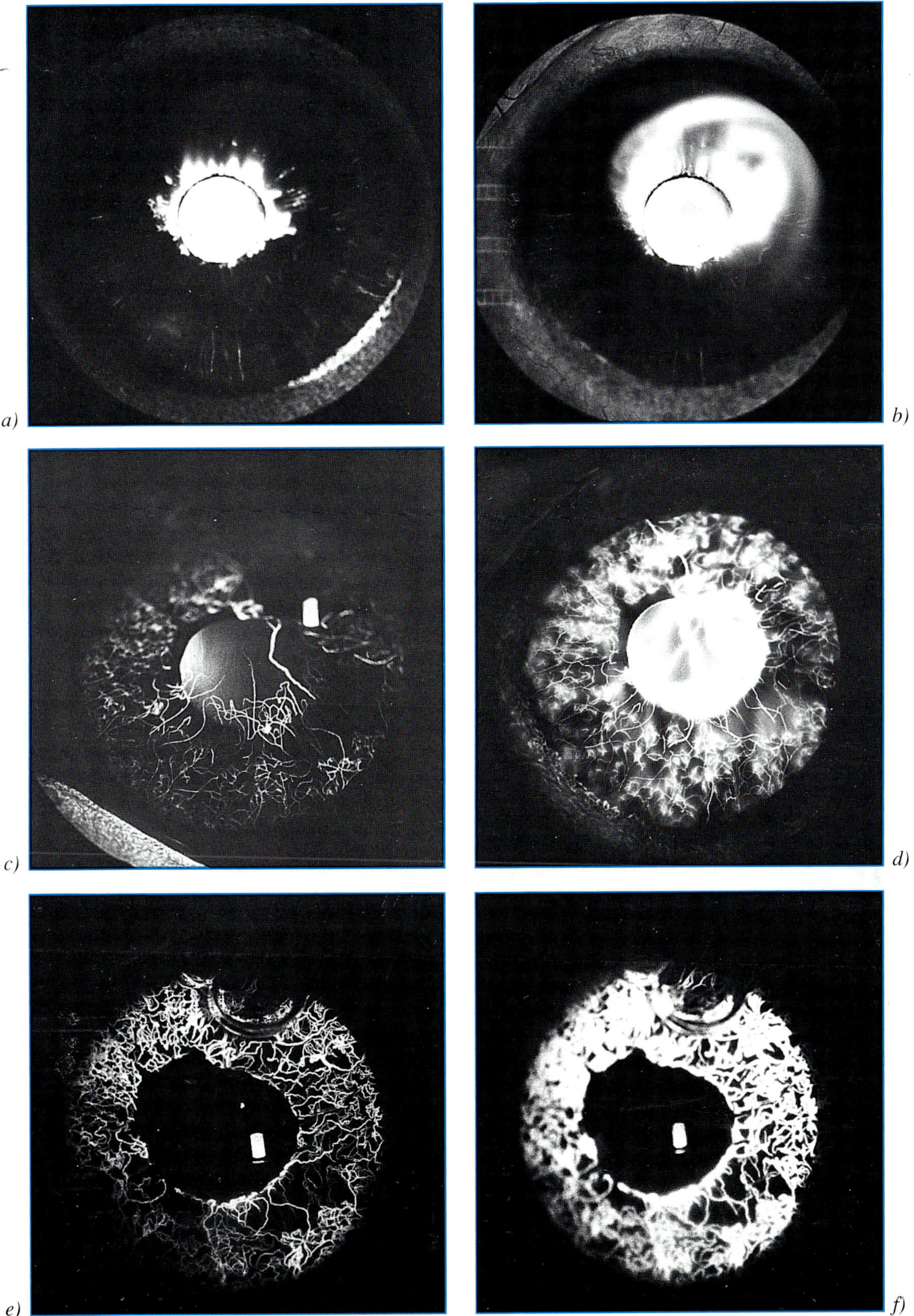

*Fig. **4.9**,52 - An eye of a diabetic patient with neovascularization at the pupillary border before (a,b) and after cataract extraction (c,d). Proliferative iridopathy has progressed severely. Despite the new vessels over the whole surface of the iris and in the pupillary field, vitrectomy was subsequently done to deal with serious proliferative retinopathy and tractional retinal detachment. Postoperatively (e,f) iris new vessels appear more florid, congested and leak more dye - a situation of neovascular glaucoma. A silicone bubble can be seen at the 12-1 o'clock position.*

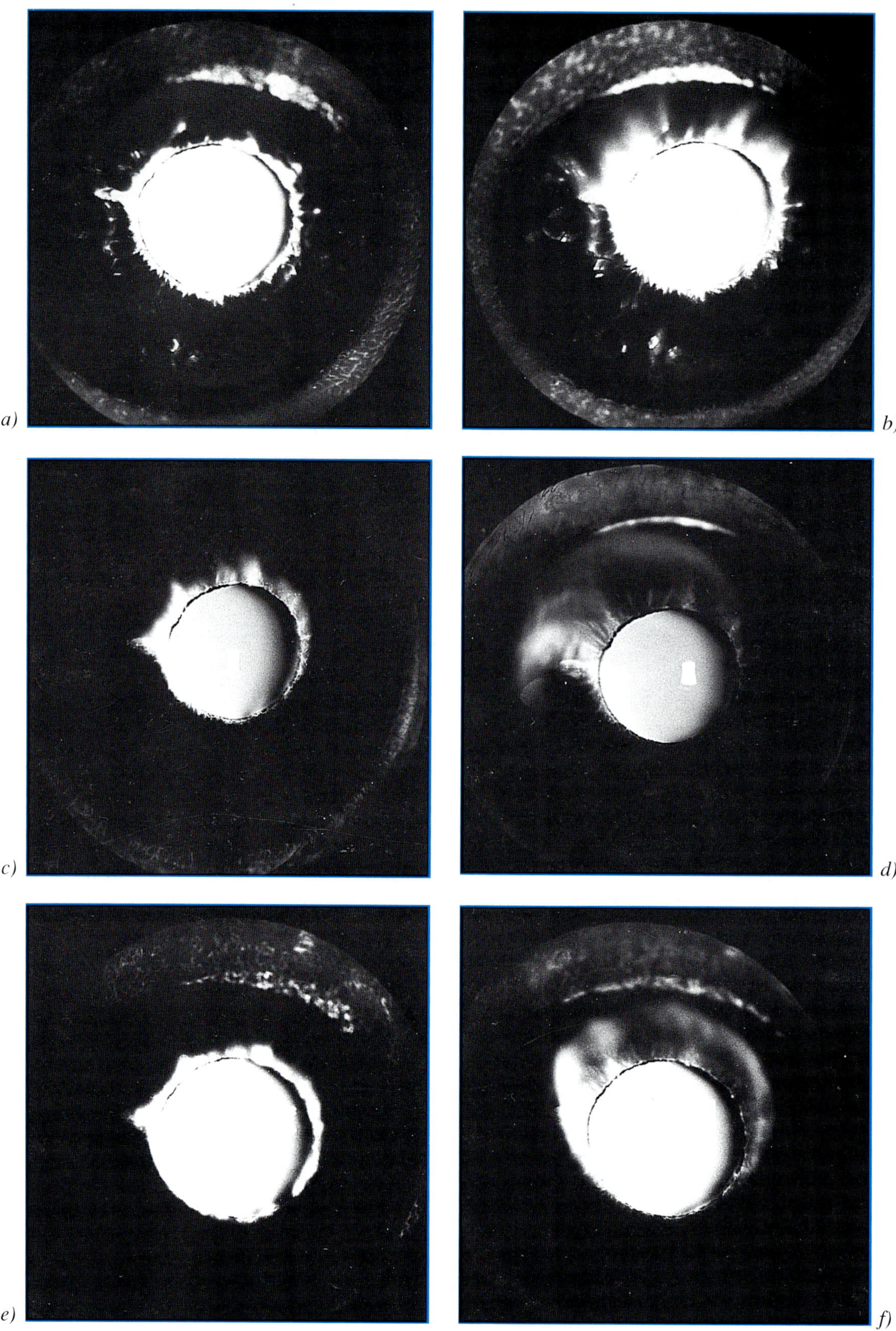
a)
b)
c)
d)
e)
f)

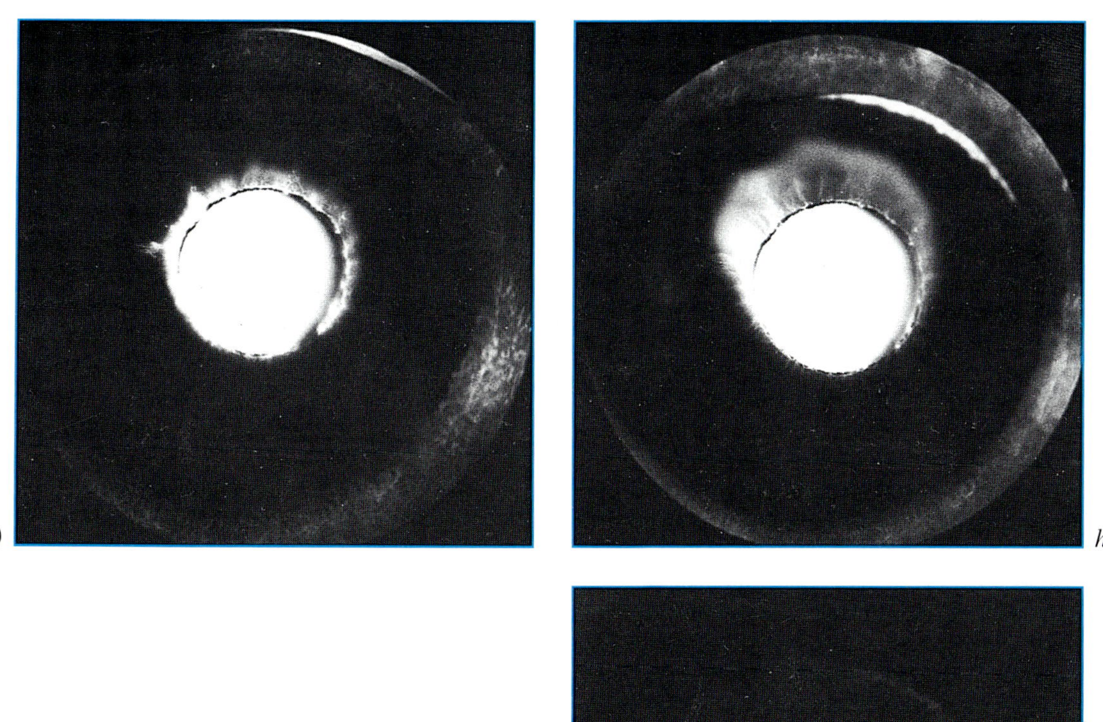

g) h)

i)

Fig. ***4.9***,*53 - Serious bilateral proliferative diabetic vitreo-retinopathy. Iris fluorescein angiography in the right eye before (a,b) and after (c,d) retinal cryocoagulation shows a reduction in the iris new vessels. The patient was then operated for vitrectomy and endophotocoagulation. Immediately postoperatively new vessels at the pupillary border increased slightly (e,f). Ablation of the ischemic retina was then completed by transpupillary photocoagulation and the new vessels diminished (g,h) and eventually disappeared (i).*

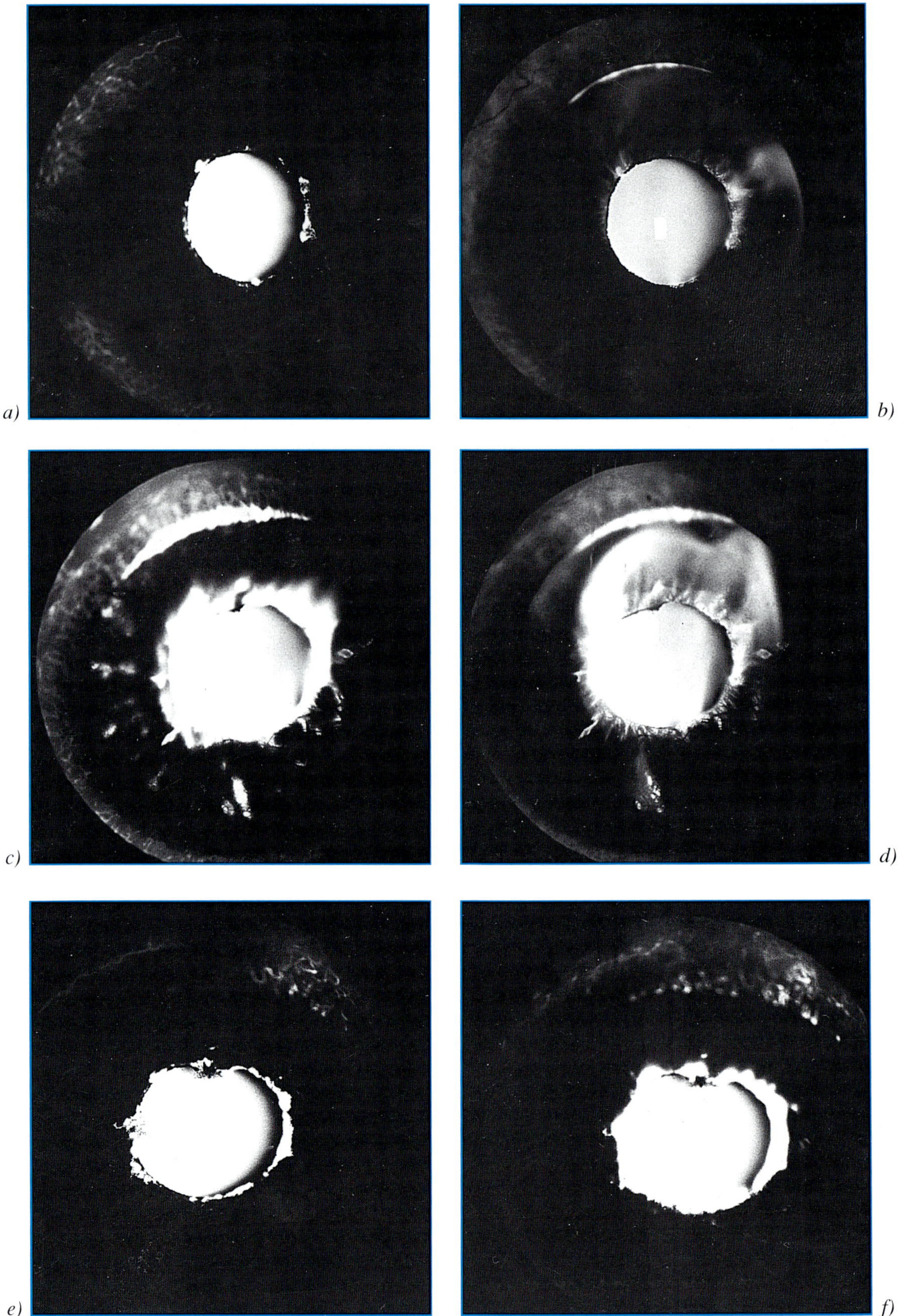

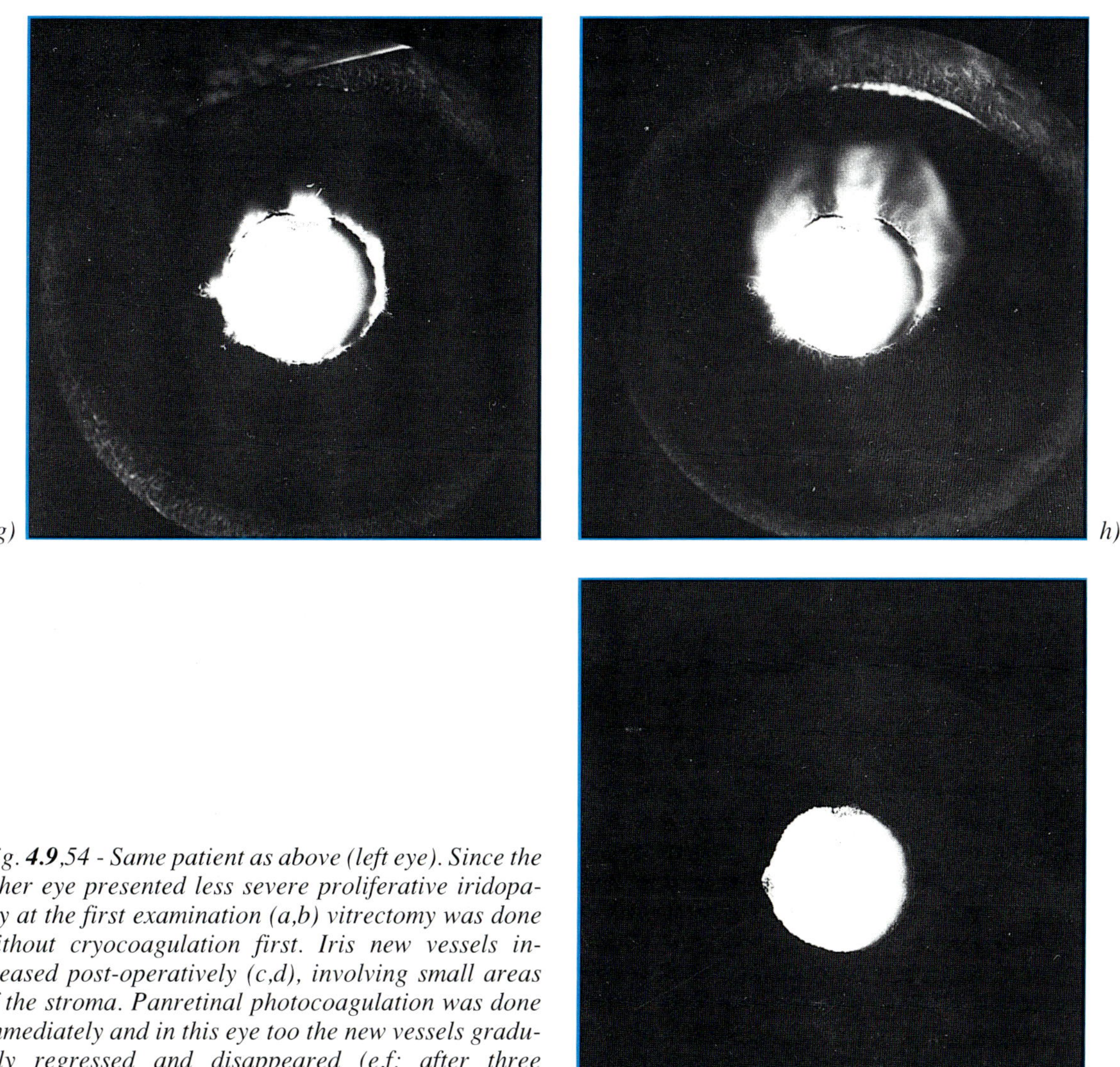

*Fig. **4.9**,54 - Same patient as above (left eye). Since the other eye presented less severe proliferative iridopathy at the first examination (a,b) vitrectomy was done without cryocoagulation first. Iris new vessels increased post-operatively (c,d), involving small areas of the stroma. Panretinal photocoagulation was done immediately and in this eye too the new vessels gradually regressed and disappeared (e,f: after three months; g,h: after six months; i: one year after surgery).*

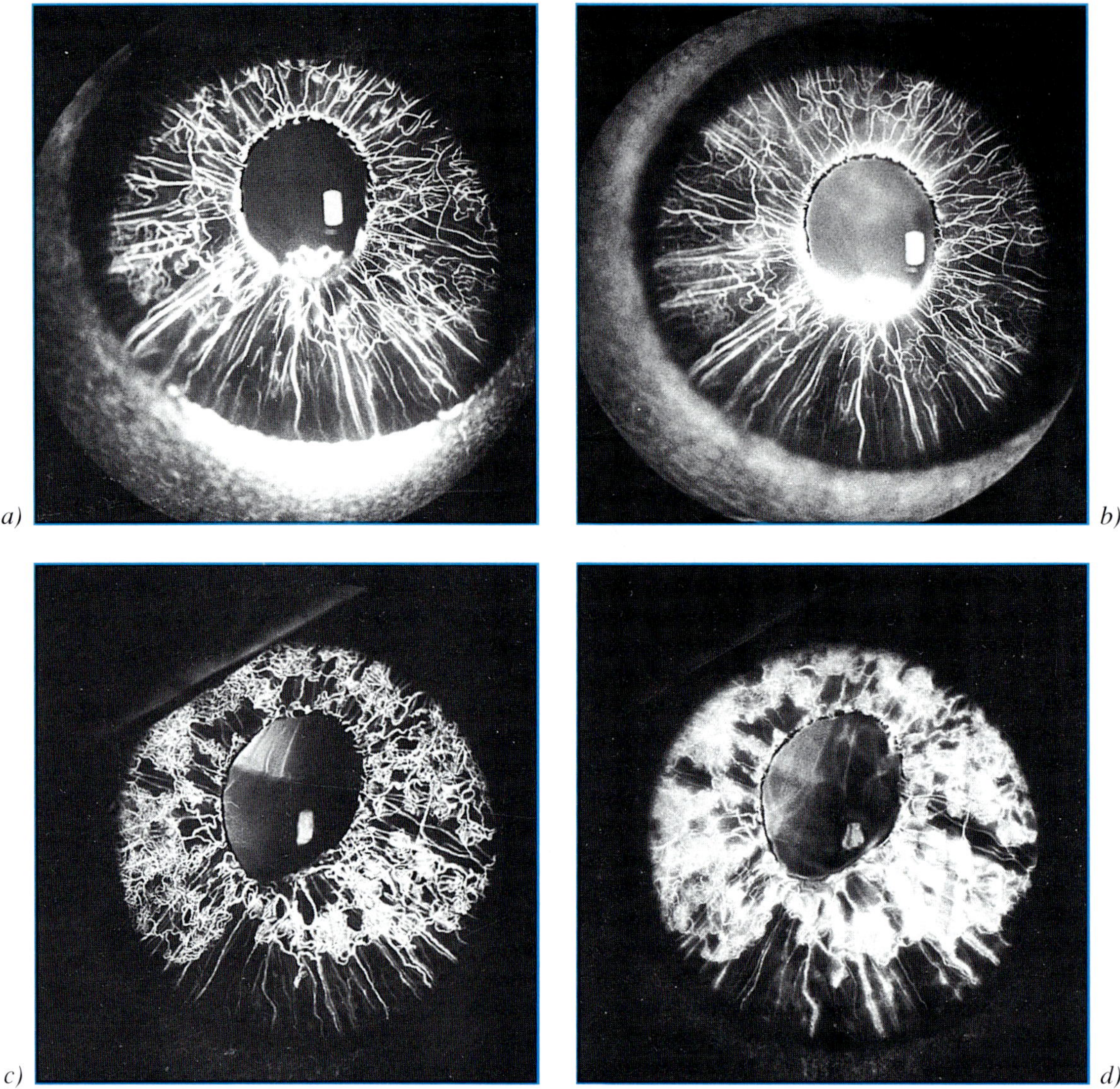

*Fig. **4.9**,55 - Proliferative iridopathy (iris angiographic phases: a,b) in a patient with retinal angiomatosis complicated by secondary retinal detachment. There was marked progression of iris new vessels after vitrectomy (c,d).*

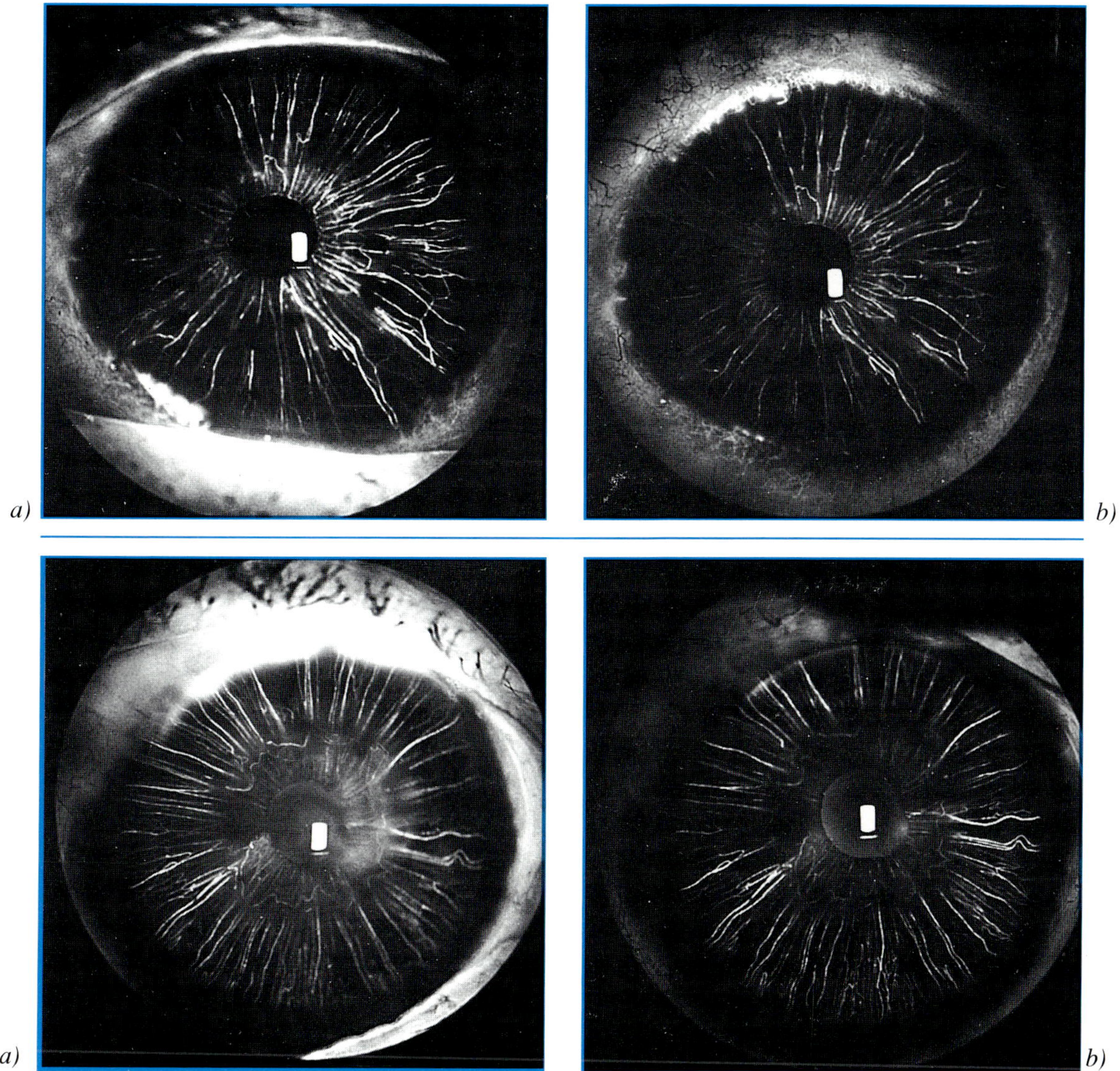

*Figs. **4.9**,56,57 - Iris fluorescein angiography in two aphakic eyes before (a) and after (b) capsulotomy with the Nd:YAG laser. Permeability of the blood-iris barrier appears unaffected.*

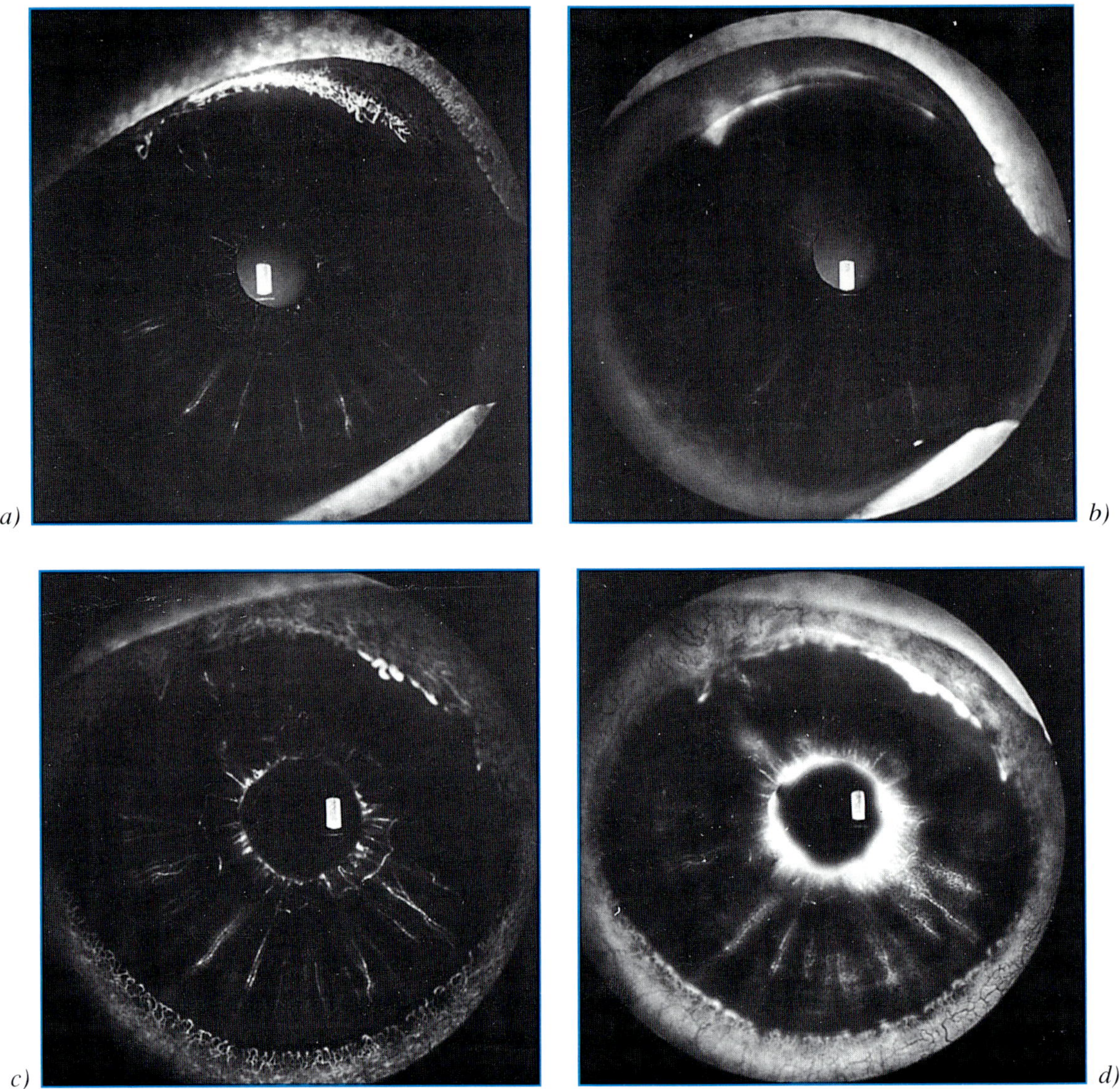

*Fig. **4.9**,58 - A case of aphakic eye with secondary cataract operated by capsulotomy with the Nd:YAG laser (iris fluorescein angiographic phases a,b: before; c,d: after). Dye leakage from the pupillary margin has increased.*

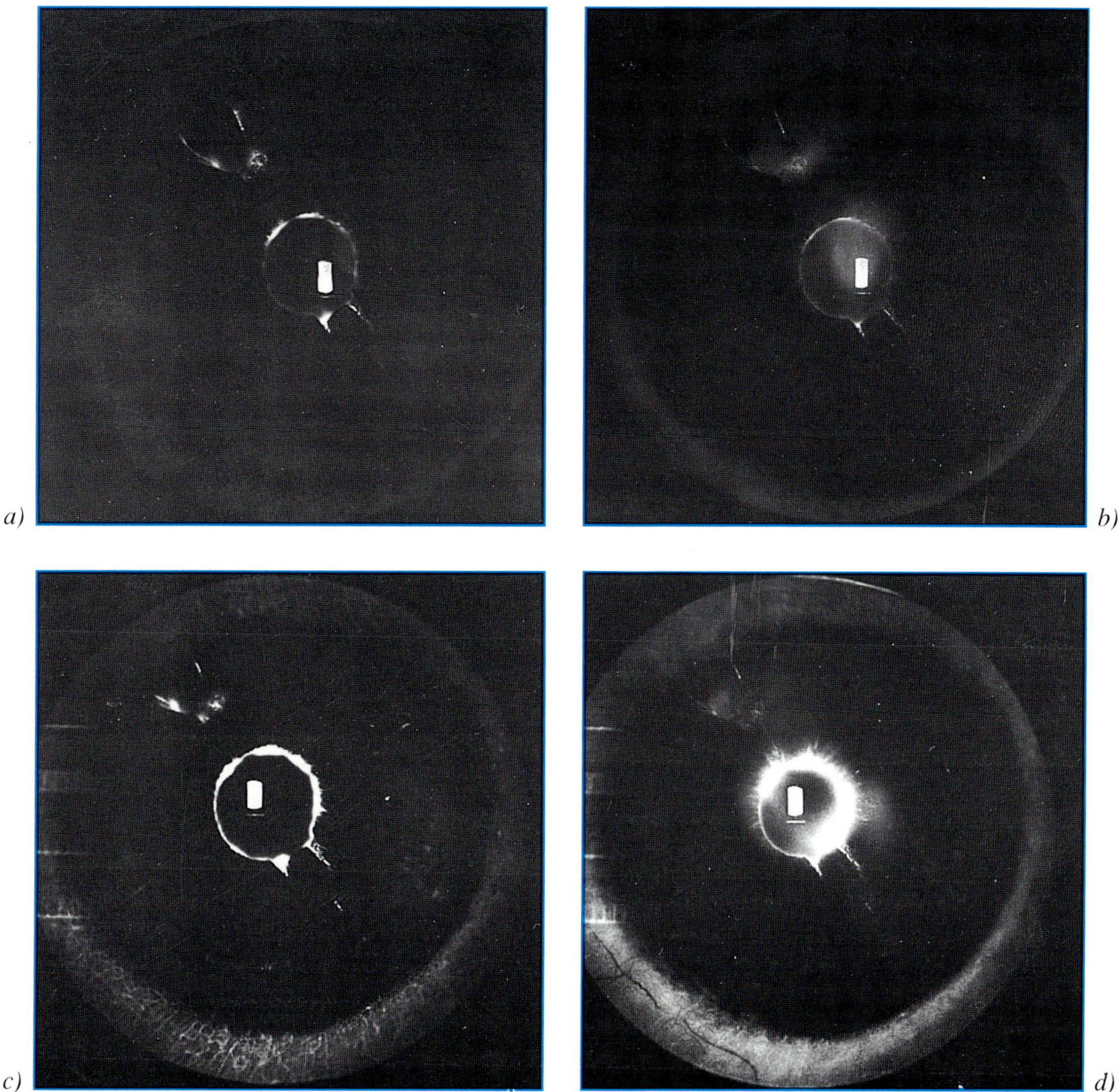

*Fig. **4.9**,59 - Similar case as in Fig. **4.9**,58 (a,b: before; c,d: after Nd: YAG capsulotomy).*

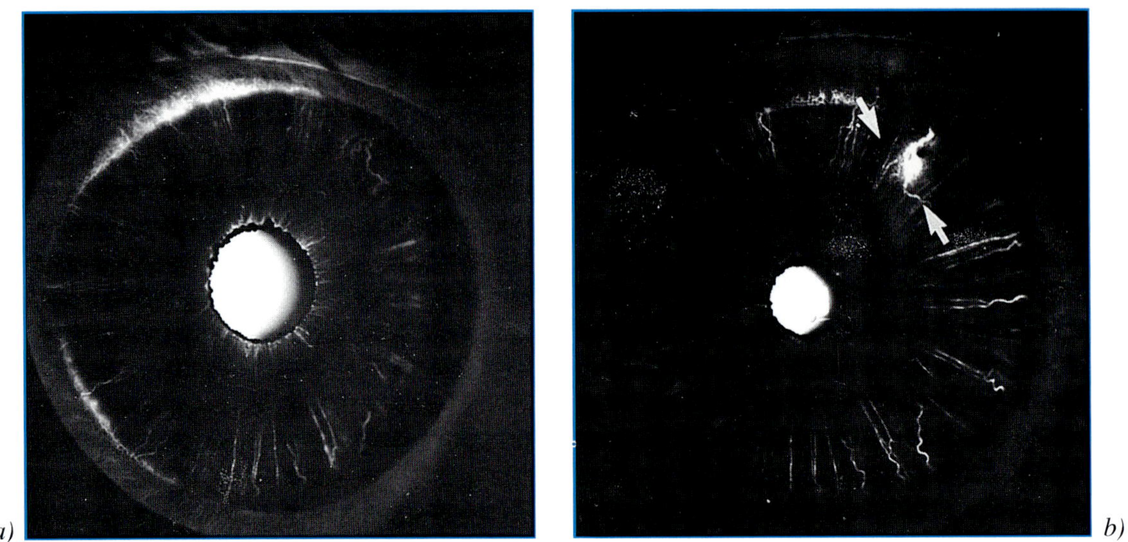

*Fig. **4.9**,60 - Iridography in an eye with chronic angle closure glaucoma before (a) and two hours after (b) iridotomy with the Nd:YAG laser. There is slight dye leakage from the vessels around the edges of the iridotomy (arrows). There appear to be no other breakages in the blood-iris barrier.*

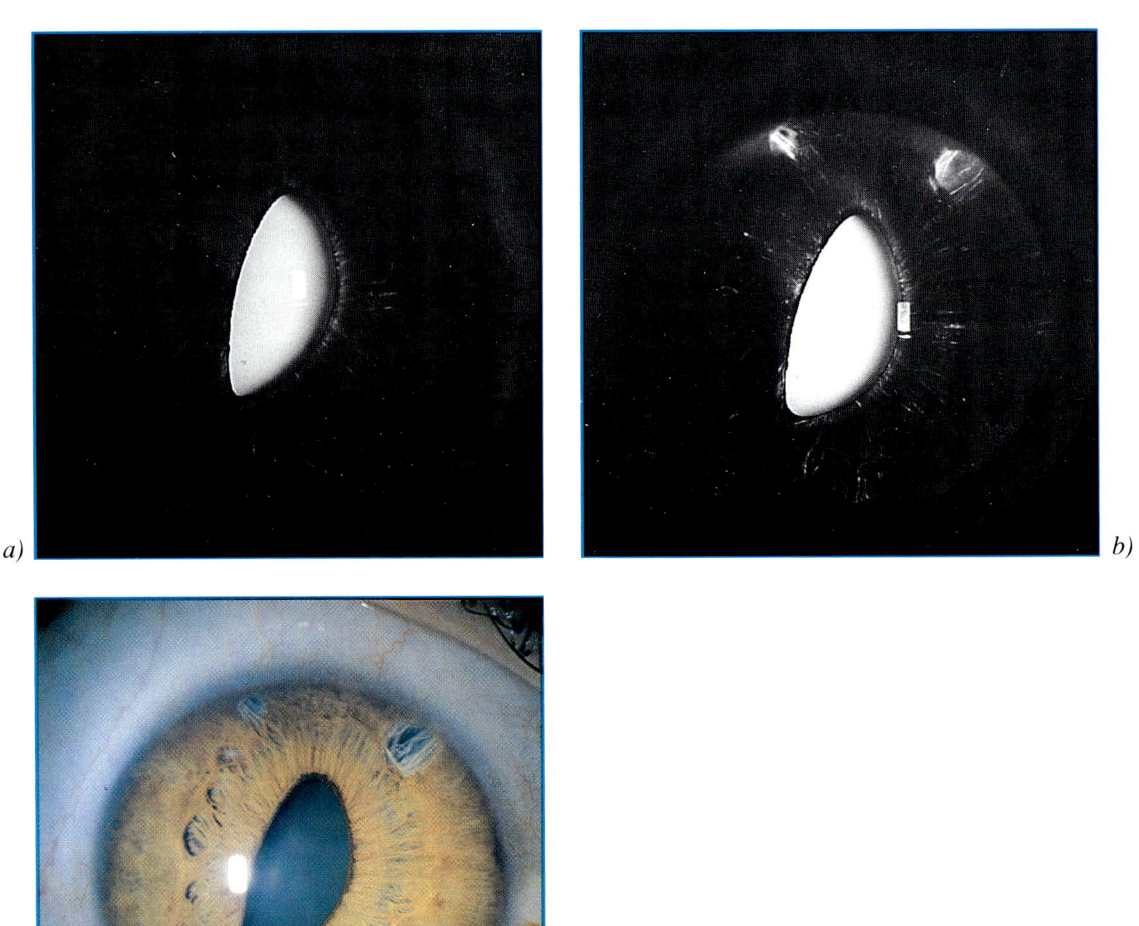

*Fig. **4.9**,61 - Iris fluorescein angiography before (a) and after (b) double iridotomy. Where the iris is perforated right through at the iridotomies, biomicroscopic examination (c) shows up radial vessels. Iris fluorescein angiography shows no damage to the iris outside the iridotomies (b).*

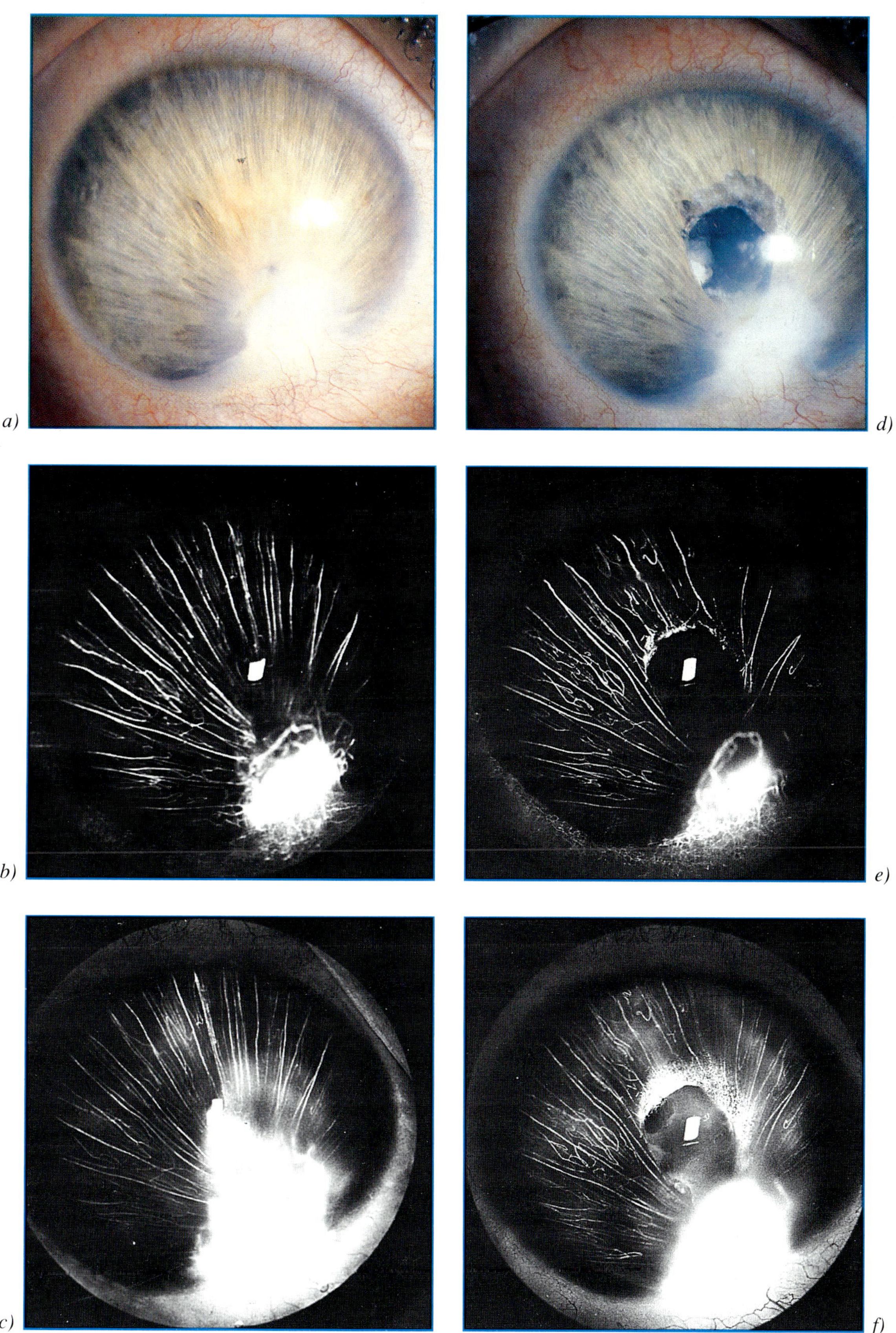

Fig. ***4.9****,62 - Same case of perforating trauma before (a,b,c) and after (d,e,f) Nd:YAG laser coreoplasty (a,d: biomicroscopy; b,c,e,f; iris fluorescein angiography). At the hole in the iris no gross alterations can be seen in the angiogram, except for dye leakage at the new-formed pupil.*

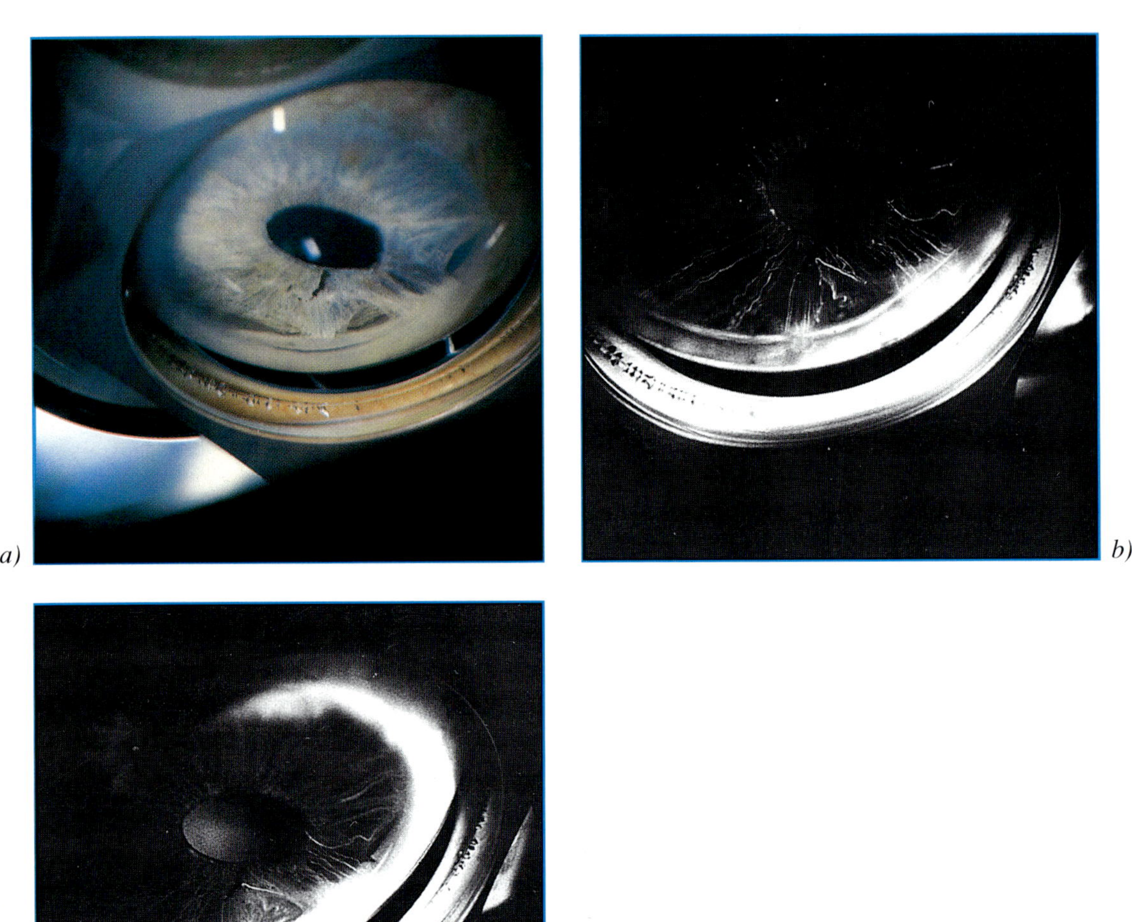

a)

b)

c)

*Fig. **4.9**,63 - Iridocorneal strands in an aphakic eye (a: gonioscopy). Iris fluorescein angiography (b,c) indicates they are avascular so Nd:YAG laser resection can be planned.*

R. Brancato, F. Bandello, R. Lattanzio
Atlas of Iris
Fluorescein Angiography
Kugler & Ghedini Publications 1995

Chapter 4.10

Iris masses

Space-occupying lesions of the iris give different fluorescein angiography patterns depending on their cytological and clinical features. Fluorescein angiography findings, despite the fact that sometimes they are difficult to interpret, are useful in most cases for early diagnosis and identification of the nature of the mass.

Space-occupying lesions of the iris can be very roughly grouped under two headings: *cysts* and *tumors*.

Iris cysts

Iris cysts may be congenital or acquired.

Congenital cysts are usually due to incomplete closure of the space between the two neuroectodermal layers of the optic vesicle, or to its reopening. They may also originate from the pigmented epithelium of the iris, or the conjunctive epithelium, from an ectopic lacrimal duct, from the unpigmented neuroepithelium or from the iris stroma.

Acquired cysts may be idiopathic, post-traumatic, post-surgical or cysts of the pupillary border. Generally idiopathic cysts are diagnosed in young or middle-aged subjects, and are more frequent among women (Figs **4.10**,1,2). They often shift the iris forward, causing thinning of the overlying iris stroma, inflammatory reactions and ocular hypertension.

Iris cysts may be pigmented (Fig. **4.10**,3) and it is often hard to make a differential diagnosis from melanoma (Fig. **4.10**,4). However, they are frequently mobile and - above all - are transparent to direct and indirect light from the slit lamp.[87]

Fluorescein angiographic findings with iris cysts tend to vary widely depending on the type and size of the lesion. Some forms present virtually no angiographic alterations (Fig. **4.10**,5)[15,39,58] while others seriously disrupt the iris vascular network (Fig. **4.10**,6,7).

Small congenital cysts rarely take up the dye and the surrounding vessels do not behave pathologically (Fig. **4.10**,8).[8] Around voluminous cysts, on the other hand, vascular anomalies may be seen, with dye leakage.

The fluorangiographic picture of acquired cysts depends largely on the pathogenesis of the cyst.[8] The cyst may be hypofluorescent and surrounded by dilated vessels from which no dye leaks (Fig. **4.10**,9).[58] In other cases there may be anomalous, tortuous, dilated iris vessels in the area of the cyst, generally, however, not letting the dye spread (Fig. **4.10**,10). Some leakage may be seen at the pupil or, more rarely, in adjacent areas.[58] In some cases dye may accumulate in the cystic space. Apparent filling defects or asymmetries may be the result of the iris tilting because of the cyst.[57]

Iris tumors

Tumors of the iris may be *benign* or *malignant*, *primary* or *secondary*, *pigmented* or *non pigmented*.

The pigmented forms are by far the most common and their clinical aspects at presentation may differ.

Correct diagnosis of a tumor of the iris must be based on a careful biomicroscopic examination, gonioscopy, transillumination, ultrasound examination, 32P test,[89] and cytological examination of the aqueous humor. However, an analysis of its clinical behaviour, cytological examination of an excisional biopsy specimen and fluorescein iridography are essential for confirmation.

We classify iris tumors as follows:

Primary

Pigmented	Nonpigmented
Benign	
– Hyperplasia of the pigment epithelium	– Hemangiomas
	– Leiomyomas
– Iris freckles	– Neorilemmomas
– Nevi	– Schwannomas
– Melanocytosis	– Neurinomas
– Ota nevus	– Neurofibromas (often in von Recklinghausen's disease)
	– Adenomas of the pigmented epithelium of the iris
Malignant	
– Leiomyoblastomas	– Leiomyosarcomas
– Melanomas	– Rhabdomyosarcomas
	– Amelanotic melanomas

Secondary

- By direct propagation
- Metastatic

Pseudotumoral lesions

- Granulomatous pseudotumors
- Juvenile xanthogranulomas

Lesions arising in systemic diseases

- Leukemic nodules
- Pigmented masses (in siderosis and hemosiderosis)
- Granulomas arising in
  * syphilis
  * tuberculosis

Pigmented iris tumors

Iris freckles

These small flat coloured spots are, histologically, foci of stromal melanocyte proliferation full of pigment. They appear on the anterior surface of the iris, and show no potential for malignant change.[12]

Melanocytosis

This rare congenital form is unilateral, and is characterised by diffuse or segmentary hyperpigmentation of the episclera and uvea. In the iris there is a dense concentration of strongly pigmented melanocytes which may give rise to heterochromia (Figs. **4.10**,11-13).

Ota nevus or oculodermic melanocytosis

This nevus can be distinguished from melanocytosis because it is associated with marked pigmentation of the eyelids and surrounding skin and sometimes also of the nasal and oral mucous membranes. Epidemiological data[12] indicate that patients with Ota nevi develop malignant melanomas of the skin, iris, choroid, orbital, meninges and brain more frequently than unaffected subjects.

Nevi

Nevi of the iris appear as roundish or oval, brown or greyish masses, varying in size.

Histologically they consist of a clearly circumscribed mass of anomalous spindle-shaped or polygonal melanocytes. Electron microscopy shows that the lesion is made up of two cell types.[54] The first are polygonal cells, with a peripheral nucleus, ample cytoplasm with numerous large melanosomes. The second are smaller, spindle-shaped cells, with a fairly high nucleus-to-cytoplasm ratio. The cytoplasm contains small melanosomes, numerous mitochondria, abundant rough endoplasmic reticulum and an evident Golgi system.

Clinically nevi present as nodules tending to rise under the anterior leaflet of the iris and extending towards the stroma, not protruding more than 1 mm on the anterior face of the iris.[88] Generally they are small but some may occupy a whole sector or even the whole iris. It is hard to establish any firm classification based on the size of these nevi as a means of deciding whether they are benign or malignant, although published reports indicate that lesions smaller than 3 x 3 x 1 mm are usually benign, whereas larger ones are usually malignant.[88] Like melanomas, nevi are usually found in the lower part of the iris, especially in the infero-temporal quadrant.[12,17,106]

Although most nevi are not aggressive, they may nevertheless grow and affect adjacent structures in the eye. Malignant transformation is possible, but rare. The very possibility, though, makes it essential to plan careful follow-up when a sufficiently reliable clinical diagnosis is available. Should a nevus change its shape, get bigger, become vascularized, or change its colour, and should new pigmented spots appear in the iris, or evident clinical symptoms arise (such as ocular hypertension due to invasion of the angle of the anterior chamber), malignant degeration of the nevus must be suspected.[12,28]

A recent study found that only eight out of 175 pigmentary neoformations of the iris (4.6%), followed for an average of 4.7 years, showed a tendency to get bigger.[2] Factors associated with this tendency were medial localization of the mass, pigmentary dispersion of the surrounding iris and at the angle. The study found that tumor growth was not correlated with other factors such as the patient's age or sex, intraocular pressure, colour of the iris, size and vascularization of the mass, pupillary deformation, ectropion of the iris or sectorial cataract.

Iris nevus syndrome (Cogan-Reese's syndrome)

This is a diffuse nevus of the iris involving multiple unilaterial iris nodules, ectopia of the Descemet membrane and secondary glaucoma.

Melanomas

Uveal melanoma is the most frequent malignant eye tumor (71%) among the white population. However, such tumors amount to only 11% of all malignant melanomas.[21] They usually arise in the choroid (93%), being much more rare in the iris (3%) and ciliary body (4%).[53] Other studies assess the frequency of melanoma of the iris at between 3 and 12%.[48,49,71,78]

With today's possibilities for early diagnosis melanomas of the iris are now generally found in younger subjects (on average 10-20 years younger) than other melanomas of the posterior uveal tract. It is frequent to encounter these tumours in subjects aged 25-46 years[3,9,30,73,78] and the ratio of males to females is 6:4.[103]

There are certain acknowledged risk factors for malignant melanomas of the iris, such as a pale iris,[56,79] nevi or melanocytosis, exposure to sunlight,[45,71,83,89] or certain chemicals and some viral infections.

Clinically melanoma of the iris presents as a flat or slightly raised mass, varying in size, generally strongly pigmented. These melanomas are found with particular frequency in the lower half of the iris; they may have a clear-cut outline or may be diffuse with ragged edges, involving the whole thickness of the iris.

The tumoral infiltration may cause ectropion of the iris, and involvement of the irido-corneal angle may result in secondary glaucoma. Melanomas that become necrotic may show irregular nodularity at the angle as necrotic fragments are deposited (black hypopyon). Hyphema may occasionally be the presenting symptom, especially if the melanotic mass is richly vascularized.

Three morphological varieties of malignant melanoma of the iris are known:[81,88]
- *Diffuse melanoma* involving the whole surface of the iris, down to the angle. It presents as a diffuse pigmentation, often associated with glaucoma;[77]
- *Tapioca melanoma (Reese's melanoma):* this is characterized by an atypical growth of pale, transparent nodules, in single or multiple foci.[50,52,69,72,98,101] It used to be believed that this lesion was always benign, but in some cases spindle-cell or epithelioid melanomas have been detected, and in other metastases have been reported.[101] It has also been proposed that this is a variant of von Recklinghausen's disease;
- *Ring melanoma* is an intermediate form involving simultaneously the base of the iris, the irido-corneal angle and the anterior ciliary body. It runs in a ring around the perivascular space of the main arterial circle of the iris and along the base of the ciliary muscle.[3,52]

The finding that smaller uveal melanomas generally have a better prognosis than the larger ones has led to numerous studies aimed at establishing reliable prognostic criteria. Methods have been sought to define the site and size of the tumor with precision.[53,85] Other prognostic factors are the patient's age,[96] the extrascleral extension,[92] the cell type[12,67] and the mitotic activity. Elderly patients with larger tumors containing epithelioid cells which have been shown to extend beyond the sclera have a worse prognosis after enucleation.[88]

The main characteristic of tumor cells is that the cytoplasm of one cell may contain melanosomes at different stages of maturation, whereas in a normal melanocyte most of the melanosomes are at the same stage. The melanosomes may also vary in number and stage of maturity from one tumor to another and from one cell to another within the same tumor. However, generally there are more melanosomes in early stages of maturation than in the later stages.[64]

The vascular system too may vary widely. There may be large bloodless areas into whose thin walls the tumoral cells are inserted directly. Foci of necrosis are not rare.

Today we still consider essentially valid the histopathological classification of malignant uveal melanomas proposed by Callender in 1931, describing two basic types of cells, both of neuroectodermal origin:[12]
- *spindle cells*, dividable into subtypes A and B;
- *epithelioid cells*.

On the basis of their cytology, Callender identified six types of melanoma:
- *spindle A melanoma;*
- *spindle B melanoma;*
- *fascicular structured melanoma,* with bands of spindle A and B cells;
- *mixed melanoma,* with spindle and epithelioid cells (probably the spindle cells, which are relatively benign, can transform to highly malignant epithelioid cells);
- *necrotic melanoma,* in which the foci of necrosis are so large as to prevent any more precise classification;
- *epithelioid cell malanoma.*

Subsequently McLean[63] modified Callender's classification, in relation to the three cell types detectable (spindle subtypes A and B, and epithelioid cells). He divided melanomas into three classes with increasing malignity: if only spindle A cells are present the mass is considered a nevus; if it contains only spindle B cells, or subtypes A and B, it is considered a melanoma with low malignant potential; if it comprises spindle and epithelioid cells (mixed form) it is considered a highly malignant melanoma. The degree of pigmentation may also vary widely.

The importance of the histopathological subdivision of melanomas lies in the fact that it largely dictates their clinical course, prognosis being worse for the less differentiated cell types. Survival seems to be less for epithelioid cell melanomas (only 25% after five years) and better for patients with spindle cell melanomas (68% survival after five years).[32] The observation that survival varies so widely with malignant uveal melanomas has led to numerous investigations to identify the anatomoclinical parameters on which to base a reliable forecast of the clinical course of the tumor. Analysis of the time of onset of symptoms, tumor site, and patients' age and sex brought to light no significant indications for prognosis but the tumor size, cell type and mitotic activity have proved more useful.

It was largely considered in the past that melanomas of the iris, even those with evident infiltration, were only slightly metastatic and that mortality was lower than with tumors of the ciliary body and choroid.[18] One explanation was that tumors in the iris could be diagnosed and treated earlier.[55]

There are 38 published cases of metastastic deaths from primary melanomas of the iris.[10] Recent, documented caselists indicate that 2.4-4.8% of patients die of multiple metastases.[93] The frequency of metastasis is estimated at around 3%[42,44] and these are generally hepatic.[13,59,102] The mean interval to metastasis, on the basis of several studies, is 8.5 years.[2,30,55,71,78,93] Recently a case of hepatic metastasis was described as arising from a diffuse iris melanoma 17 years after enucleation;[90] in another case 30 years after enucleation hepatic and pulmonary metastases were reported with an orbital relapse of the iris melanoma.[95]

As they are slow-growing, iris melanomas rarely recur and when this happens it can usually be traced back to incomplete removal of the original mass.

Fluorescein angiographic patterns of pigmented iris tumors

It is not easy clinically to establish a reliable diagnosis of pigmented iris tumors. Iris fluorescein angiography may show up alterations characteristic of malignant forms and is therefore useful in achieving a correct diagnosis when faced with pigmented neoformations of the iris. Fluorescein angiography of the iris shows up the vascular network of the neoformation and the effects of its growth on surrounding tissues.

The fluorescein angiographic aspects of pigmented iris neoformations have been widely analysed, with often discordant conclusions. Summarized here are the three different classifications of these masses proposed by Demeler, Jakobiec and ourselves. We shall also analyse the iris fluorescein angiographic findings described in other studies.

Demeler[24,25] divided neoformations into three fluorescein angiographic classes:

1) tumors in which angiography shows no blood vessels and no fluorescein uptake and leakage. These tumors retain their clinical and angiographic characteristics unchanged over long periods. Demeler found that these tumors were benign and recommended follow-up every 6-12 months;
2) tumors with a well developed but irregular vascular system, filling in the very early angiographic phases. In the late phases they present mottled or diffuse staining. Demeler assessed tumors in this group as "potentially malignant" and recommends frequent angiographic follow-up (every 3 months);
3) tumors with their own stainable vascular system, or masses containing so much pigment that the vessels cannot be seen even in the late angiographic stage. A common feature of this third category is early dye leakage which becomes stronger in the later phases, particularly around the edges of the mass. Dye also spreads to the other stromal vessels. All tumors showing these angiographic features were dealt with surgically and histological examination showed malignancy. Demeler concluded that peripheral fluorescence is a sign of malignancy and may arise through two possible mechanisms:
   1) staining starts from the tumor vessels but it is only visible at the periphery because of the strong pigmentation;
   2) staining starts from the iris whose walls are damaged by stasis caused by the tumor obstructing venous return.

   Neoformations with these angiographic characteristics are, in Demeler's opinion, "definitely malignant" and should be excised.

Jakobiec[51] divides pigmented lesions of the iris into four categories, based on their fluoridographic patterns:

1) tumors with such dark pigmentation that no vasculature can be detected by fluorescein angiography. Biopsy was done in three cases (out of 11 examined) and showed various patterns of nevoid spindle-cell proliferations;
2) tumors with their own regular vascular network, almost geometrical, that fluoresces early and in synchrony with the rest of the radial vasculature of the iris. The tumor vessels have slightly larger caliber than the radial arteries and are often anastomosed. In the later phases dye often leaks into the tumor and stains a small amount of the neighbouring stroma. Histological examination of two lesions (out of seven examined) showed spindle cells with abundant cytoplasm that were interpreted as nevus cells;
3) tumors with a fine vascular network that takes up the dye early (with no late leakage), with alternating non-fluorescent areas. Histological examination of one specimen (out of three) showed nevoid spindle cells alternating with stromal tissue;
4) tumors with an irregular network of vessels of different calibers and orientation, in which fluorescein leaks early and tends to spread to neighbouring stroma. In the two biopsy specimens considered mixed-cell or spindle B-type melanomas were found.

Demeler's and Jakobiec's classifications, confirmed in some cases by biopsy findings, have the disadvantage of not taking account of changes in fluorescein diffusion over time, and do not consider the effects of the tumors on adjacent structures.

We have drawn up a four-section classification of the fluorescein angiography findings in iris tumors:[4]

1) pigmented masses that mask the normal vascular network of the iris and show no

fluorescein leakage at any stage of angiography. This iridographic pattern is characteristic of benign forms. Followed over time, the morphology and angiographic findings of these masses remain unchanged;

2) faintly or very faintly pigmented masses which show filling of the newly-formed vascular network in the early stages of angiography, and in which the dye diffuses to varying extents, with different degrees of uniformity, but never leaks from the mass itself. Neoformations with these features are assessed as "probably benign", and are most likely leiomyomas. In fact in the cases followed over some time the morphology and iris fluorescein angiographic findings remain unchanged;
3) pigmented formations showing fluorescein diffusion throughout the mass but only in the late angiographic stages, associated with slight distortion of the pupillary border (tending to become more evident with time) with or without ectropion uveae. These are very probably "potentially malignant" lesions, this potential being linked not only to the fact that dye diffusion in the mass increases at successive visits, but also to the progress of the pupillary border deformation and ectropion uveae over time;
4) pigmented masses that start to fluoresce from the initial angiographic phases, increasingly so in the later stages, with marked pupillary distortion and varying degrees of ectropion uveae, which also tends to become more marked with time. We consider these neoformations as "definitely malignant", or at the very least highly suspect. Histological examination of three enucleated eyes confirmed malignant melanoma in all cases.

Many other authors have analysed the fluorescein angiographic aspects of iris neoformations and most of them agree that a pigmented lesion that masks fluorescence (angiographic silence) and shows no tendency to diffusion of the dye can be considered benign.(9,15,22,24,51,58) This is the case in 44% of benign tumors.(22) Pigmented benign neoformations, iris freckles and foci of hyperplasia in the pigmented epithelium block fluorescence in the underlying vascular meshwork and generally show no angiographic anomalies (Figs. **4.10**,14-22).(58)

Pigmented neoformations of the iris with fluorescein angiographic features comparable to nevi, but causing deformation of the pupil and ectropion uveae can be regarded as mid-way between the benign and malignant forms (Figs. **4.10**,23-25). The presence of a geometrical, regular pattern of vessels within a mass is usually considered a sign of a benign formation.(9,51) Some, however, view it as a sign of potential malignancy,(24) and yet others maintain it can be found in all tumor types.(22)

Early hyperfluorescence in an irregular, disorganized vascular network (Figs. **4.10**,26,27) which alters the radial structure of the iris (Figs. **4.10**,28-31) is considered to indicate a malignant tumor.(16,51,58,62) Some authors maintain that dye diffusion(15) especially if marked(9,24,51) is a sign of a malignant tumor; this leakage may mask the tumor's disorderly vascular system (early hyperfluorescence) and the surrounding stroma.(15) This fluorescence tends to become more intense from the early to late angiographic phases, and may cause diffuse staining lasting 30-40 minutes.(9)

Thus, whenever early hyperfluorescence, dilated and tortuous vessels altering the radial vascular network, and delayed dye leakage are observed, the tumor should be considered suspect for malignancy.(16,62)

There is still much debate on the significance of dye leakage in or around tumor. However, it has been shown that the vessels within a tumor are lined with anamalous endothelial cells(58) or tumor cells without a basement membrane,(100) which would explain the dye leakage (Figs. **4.10**,32,33).

In a very densely pigmented tumor fluorescence may be blocked and the vascular network will not be visible (Figs. **4.10**,34-36).(24) A fluorescent ring around a hypofluorescent area in a tumor should arouse suspicion of malignancy (Fig. **4.10**,37).[24] Two mechanisms can produce this peripheral fluorescence:

1) fluorescence diffuses from the tumor vessels but can only be seen at the periphery because of dense pigmentation;
2) fluorescence diffuses from the iris vessels whose walls are damaged by venous stasis due to compression by the tumor mass.

In any event, the angiographic picture may vary widely in different conditions, for example:

- no dye leakage from the tumor vessels because of sclerosis or hyalinization of their walls;[24]
- dye diffusion from radial vessels around the tumor, whose caliber and path is usually altered (Fig. **4.10**,38);[16]
- dye leakage from the iris vessels themselves because of the damage caused by stasis resulting from compression by the tumor;[24]
- areas of leakage some distance from the tumor or at the pupillary margins (Figs. **4.10**,39,40);[24,51]
- the pupillary border may be distorted and when the eye presents ectropion uveae fluorescence may appear limited on account of excess pigment in that particular district (Figs. **4.10**,41,42);
- the tumor fills with dye at different phases of the angiographic examination.[22]

The classification of pigmented iris tumors remains, however, a difficult clinical problem.

The grading system we used is based on color photographs and fluorescein angiographic patterns.[5] This method of classification was employed for the retrospective assessment of 44 pigmented iris tumors observed during the last 12 years in our Department. Of these 44 neoformations, 25 (56.5%) had a biomicroscopic and fluorescein angiographic follow-up (mean: 29.6 months ±26.6).

The *parameters* considered in *color photographs* were as follows:

1) thickening of the iris, scored 2 for thickened and 0 for flat neoplasms;
2) pupillary distortion and/or ectropion uveae, with a score from 0-2;
3) uneven pigment density. This was graded 0 for even and 2 for an uneven pattern.

The *iris fluorangiographic parameters* considered were:

1) early visibility of an anomalous tumor vascular network (scored from 0-2);
2) hyperfluorescence inside or around the tumor (scored from 0-2);
3) dye leakage at sites remote from the tumor (scored from 0-2).

In order to assess whether the method could in fact single out active tumors, out of the 44 cases we considered only:

- cases surveyed for at least one year;
- eyes examined histologically;
- patients who had died from metastases.

The results did highlight the active tumors. We took as active tumors all cases showing changes in the parameters (worsening) during a follow-up of at least one year, all cases with histological diagnosis of melanoma and those who died from metastases. Inactive tumors were taken as all cases that showed no change over a follow-up of at least one year. This method gave a sensitivity of 73% and specificity of 100%. The positive predictive value was 100% and the negative was 73%. The method can thus recognise benign tumors much more reliably than potentially active ones.

Uneven pigment density and early visibility of an anomalous network were the only parameters employed in this biomicroscopic-iris fluorescein angiographic classification system that distinguished significantly ($p < 0.01$) between active and inactive tumors.

The translucent nodules of *tapioca melanoma* of the iris[69,98] give a special fluorescein angiographic picture. The angiogram promptly shows up the tumor outline, and later phases reveal injection of an irregular vascular network within the tumor mass. The late-phase angiogram shows diffuse leakage of fluorescein from the tumor vessels but no leakage to the rest of the iris.[69]

In *melanocytoma* the excess of pigment blocks early-phase visualization, but in the later phases there is evident fluorescence.[47]

The angiographic pattern of a *mucus-secreting adenoma* of the iris has been reported,[11] apparently derived from the pigmented epithelium. In the early angiographic phases a fine, irregular capillary network was visible within the non-pigmented tumor which filled with dye before the normal vessels of the iris. In later angiographic phases the whole area became diffusely fluorescent but no dye passed into the aqueous humor. The rest of the iris appeared angiographically normal.

Melanomas of the cilary body

Fluorescein angiography examination of melanomas of the ciliary body must be done with the eye midriatic, so as to visualise the neoformation behind the iris to the best possible extent (Figs. **4.10**,43,44). If the tumor has shifted the iris, angiography can be done directly, in the normal way (Figs. **4.10**,45,46). When the tumor is at the angle a gonioscopic lens will be needed during the examination (Fig. **4.10**,47).

The fluorescein angiographic findings in these cases are similar to those for iris tumors.[97]

Non pigmented iris tumors

Hemangiomas

The literature provides numerous descriptions of iris angiomas, but only a few have been confirmed histologically. This is in fact a rare finding, frequently accompanied by the facial angioma of the Sturge-Weber or von Hippel-Lindau syndromes. Angiomas of the iris are so rare that their existence has even been questioned.[56]

Gross diagnosis is not always straightforward as the angioma may be confused with a juvenile xanthogranuloma or simply with granulation tissue.[1] The less vascular forms may simulate small melanomas (fibrangiomas, Fig. **4.10**,48), as do the pigmented forms because of repeated hemorrhage.

Generally the biomicroscope shows the mass as rich in new vessels, limited to one sector of the iris. The tissue in a clearly circumscribed zone appears to be replaced by new, thin-walled vessels lined with normally shaped endothelial cells; the thin walls explain the extravasations of blood into the iris or the anterior chamber.

Glaucoma may be seen, resulting from angle blockage by the tumor or from blood congestion in the trabecular structures.

Only one published iris fluorescein angiography study of angioma provided histological confirmation; in this case there was no hyperfluorescence, particularly at the lesion and this finding was interpreted as ruling out inflammatory or malignant formations.[1] Fluorescein angiography thus appears to be useful for establishing the therapeutic approach to these iris angiomas, which require conservative surgical management consisting of sector iridectomy followed by histological examination.[1]

Numerous descriptions have appeared of vascular tufts near the pupillary margin, interpreted as microhemangiomas.[6,18,19,68,80] These limited saccular ectasias of the iris vessels can cause spontaneous hyphema. The angiographic patterns produced by these microhemangiomas are described in the chapter dealing with vascular abnormalities of the iris. The same chapter deals with the iris fluorescein angiographic picture of cirsoid aneurysm of the iris (Fig. **4.10**,49).

Leiomyomas

Leiomyomas are benign, non-pigmentary tumors, frequently encountered in the iris. These tumors of the sphincter and iris dilating muscles, despite the neuroectodermal origin of the iris muscles, can be considered typical leiomyomas; histologically they are identical to smooth muscle tumors in different localizations, of mesodermic origin. Leiomyomas are high vascular, with scant pigment, and consist of spindle cells which tend to be arrayed in palisades. The presence of myofibrils is diagnostic.

Clinically leiomyomas are nodules of various sizes, red-brown or grey-yellow, with a uniform appearance, generally found in the pupillary area or lower part of the iris. Advanced tumors of this type cause localized ectropion uveae, unilateral or sector cataract, hyphema and irregular astigmatism caused by the growing tumor itself. The course is always benign.

Those that show an invasive tendency are classified as leiomyosarcomas and respond well to local excision.

The fluorescein angiogram of leiomyoma gives a typical picture from which the tumor's exact extension can be judged and its vascularization assessed.[84] The tumoral mass contains a knotty mass of vessels (green leaf veins)[9] which fills early (in the arterial phase) and shows early and substantial fluorescein leakage. The resulting fluorescent area extends a few millimeters beyond the limits of the clinically affected part. Dye leakage extends into the immediately adjacent iris but there is a clear cut-off from non-involved tissue (Figs. **4.10**,50,51).[20,69,84] The fluorescence tends to disappear fairly promptly.[69] No dye leakage is seen into the rest of the iris. These are therefore well-formed neovessels that remain circumscribed. Radial adjacent vessels show no change in caliber and path, indicating the absence of deformation or retraction (Fig. **4.10**,52).

Neurofibromas, schwannomas and neurinomas

These tumors are a proliferation of the Schwann cells around peripheral nerves. They are very rare but are often associated with neurofibromatosis in von Recklinghausen's disease. They appear as small fibrotic nodules, often multiple, almost always without pigment, in a heterochromic iris.[99] They may become bigger until they produce a spot visible to the naked eye (Fig. **4.10**,53). Generally they are spindle cells with fibrous strands, with a very limited vascular component. They often cause considerable thickening of the iris, with consequent intraocular hypertension.

Rubeosis and neovascular glaucoma have been described together with this tumor.[41]

Amelanotic melanomas

These tumors have the same features as pigmented melanomas, differing only in the absence of melanin; this means that the vascular network can be viewed simply by biomicroscopy.

In these cases fluorescein angiography gives an even more precise picture of the vessels as there is none of the typical masking effect of pigmented tumors (Figs. **4.10**,54,55).

Secondary tumors

Metastases to the eyes are fairly rare. Nevertheless, in some cases they may point to a primary tumor in some other site, not yet causing any clinical signs or symptoms.[7,36]
The iris and ciliary body may be involved in two ways:
1) by direct propagation of epibulbar or intraocular tumors;
2) through the blood, by neoplastic emboli crossing the long posterior ciliary arteries.

Tumors that most frequently metastasize to the eyes are breast (60-70%), lung (10-15%), gastrointestinal tract (7%), renal, prostatic, ovarian, testicular, uterine cancers and skin melanomas (8-20%).

Iris metastases are usually multiple, gelatinous, translucent nodules, with an irregular surface, highly vascularized and tending to invade surrounding tissue.

Iris fluorescein angiography produces early hyperfluorescence, resulting from the fact that the vascular network is richer than can be clinically detected. Dye subsequently leaks out later especially at the edges of these nodules, whose margins are not generally clear-cut.[38] Leakage may even occur on zones of the iris beyond the actual metastic nodules themselves.[69] As they expand iris metastases may cause changes in the pupillary margin, revealed by fluorescein leakage points. Sometimes the tumors cause atrophy in the iris which shows up angiographically as ischemic areas.[38]

A variety of clinical pictures may be seen with metastases of the iris: inflammation which may simulate iridocyclitis, intraocular hypertension, hypopion, recurrent hyphema or rubeosis of the iris.[38] Fluorescein angiographic findings therefore vary in relation to the clinical picture (Figs. **4.10**,56,57). The miliary form presents as small whitish flakes.[32,81,83,88]

Pseudotumoral lesions

In patients with *iris masses of inflammatory origin* (reactions to foreign bodies, tuberculoma, adherent leucoma, etc.) iris fluorescein angiography shows up anamalous vessels and marked dye leakage often not limited to the involved area but spreading throughout surrounding tissue.[58] The intensity and extension of the dye diffusion area are always greater than reported for tumoral lesions.[58]

Granulomatous iritis is an inflammatory disorder in which iris nodules are found. Angiography shows extensive vascular dilatation and dye leakage,[69] not just in the affected part of the iris.

Granulomatous pseudotumor (iris abscess) may clinically simulate malignant melanoma[41] but generally its iris angiogram is typical. In the early phases the dye marks out a rich capillary network within the pseudotumoral mass, but the fluorescence subsequently leaks out copiously. In the later phases the granuloma presents diffuse staining with blurred edges.[9,57] The rest of the iris also contains multiple foci of dilated capillaries with marked dye uptake; these indicate diffuse mild inflammation that is hard to assess clinically.[57]

Juvenile xanthogranuloma (nevoxanthoendothelioma)

This is typically found in infants, and is considered congenital even if it appears after a few months of life. The child presents ocular and skin lesions, rarely also visceral. Yellow-brown nodules are distributed mainly in the periorbital areas, conjunctiva and soft tissues of the orbit. Inside the eye the iris and ciliary body are mainly affected.

Biomicroscopy shows a yellowish mass, localized, highly vascular and with little pigment; often corneal edema is caused by contact between the tumor and the Descemet membrane. Recurrent spontaneous hemorrhage in the anterior chamber is frequent. More rarely the child suffers photophobia, lacrimation and blepharospasm. Intraocular hypertension often results from blockage of the angle by inflammatory goniosynechiae and from the extent of histiocyte proliferation.[104,105] Histologically, in fact, the lesion is seen to consist of vigorously proliferating histiocyte elements with a foamy appearance; among them are multinucleate giant cells and a few inflammatory cells.

This is currently considered to be a granulomatous, non-neoplastic lesion and it has been suggested that it is a thwarted form of Hand-Schuller-Christian disease.

The iridographic pattern in juvenile xanthogranuloma is similar to that of an iris abscess. However, the patient's age, the scant pigmentation, rich vascularization and fast growth of the mass, and the presence of blood in the angle of the anterior chamber permit a differential diagnosis. Atypical forms of iris xanthogranuloma have been described in which dye leaked profusely even in unaffected areas of the iris.[65]

Iris lesions in systemic diseases

Leukemic nodules in the iris are bilateral and present together with systemic disease. The iris appears diffusely invaded, pale and sometimes micronodules are found. Iris fluorescein angiography shows hyperfluorescent spots with blurred outlines over the nodules, from which dye tends to leak in the later phases.

In *hemosiderosis* (and *siderosis* when a metal foreign body enters the eye) pigment masses are found in the iris, the resulting colour change sometimes simulating melanoma ("hyperchromic heterochromia") because of recurrent hemorrhage in the anterior chamber.[32,81,83,88] Iris fluorescein angiography shows hyperfluorescent spots over these pigment masses because they mask the underlying vascular network.

Differential diagnosis of iris neoformations

At this stage it is clear how hard it is to diagnose malignant tumor of the iris clinically. Numerous neoformations have similar characteristics and some melanomas may present an atypical appearance.

In 1965 Ferry[34] already noted that 35% of eyes enucleated for melanoma of the iris were found histologically to have been misdiagnosed. In another study of 200 iris neoformations presumed to be melanomas, only 24% actually were.[86] The other cases that simulated malignant neoformations proved to be cysts (38%), nevi (31%), essential atrophy of the iris (5.7%), foreign bodies (4.5%), anterior peripheral synechiae (2.5%), iris metastases (2.5%) and, in the remainder, leiomyomas, melanocytomas, luymphjoid reactive hyperplasia, adenoma of the pigment epithelium, iridoschisis, congenital heterochromia. Some of these 200 cases had been differentially diagnosed on a clinical basis, the others on the basis of histology. It was concluded that the following clinical factors point the way to a correct diagnosis of melanoma: diameter more than 3 mm and thickness 1 mm, marked vascularization, ectropion iris, cataract and glaucoma secondary to gradual growth.

There is a large range of investigational methods for reaching a correct diagnosis of iris neoformations. Anterior segment fluorescein angiography is one of these. In differential diagnosis of iris lesions, however, this technique has aroused controversy in the recent literature, since there is still no agreement on the pictures for the different neoformations that can be considered as characteristic, let alone pathognomonic.

The table **4.10**,I summarizes the iris fluorescein angiographic findings described in various studies in relation to different iris neoformations.

Table 4.10,I: Angiographic findings described in different neoformations.

FLUORESCEIN ANGIOGRAPHIC CHARACTERISTICS	Cyst																
	congenital	acquired	Nevus	Melanocytoma	Melanoma	Tapioca melanoma	Amelanotic melanoma	Hemangioma	Neurofibroma	Leiomyoma	Metastases	Inflammatory mass	Granulomatous iritis	Granulomatous pseudotumor	Juvenile xanthogranuloma	Leukemic Nodules	Hemosiderosis Nodules
Normal angiogram	+								+								
Masking effect		+		+			–										+
– complete (angiographic silence)			++														
– partial					+					+							
– and/or ectropion uveae					+						+				+		+
– and/or blood extravasation										+	+			+	+		
Own vascular network														+	+		
– regular						+	++	+	+								
– irregular					++					++	+						
Filling time																	
– early (in relation to iris filling)			+		+			+	+	+	+	+	++			+	
– simultaneous (in relation to iris filling)																	
– late (in relation to iris filling)																	
– incomplete					+												
Pooling		+															
Early injection of tumor edges						+											
Late fluorescent peritumoral ring					+												
Dye diffusion																	
– in tumor - early				–	+					++		++		+			
- late			±	++	++	+	++		+	+	+	++	+	++		+	
– surrounding stroma		+	±		+						+	++		+			
– distant stroma					+	–				–	+	+		+			
– pupillary margin		+			+			+	+	–	+	+		+			
– extended				+	+						+	+++	++	+			
Anomalies of radial vessels													+	+			
– dilated and tortuous ("sentinel")	+	+	+		++					–				+			
– peripariental diffusion	+				+					–				+			
– disorderly pattern					+												
New vessels																	
– margin									+		+						
– stroma									+		+						
– neovascular glaucoma									+		+						
Atrophy or iris ischemia					+						+						

The most typical features of a malignant tumor are thus: early injection of an anarchic vascular network and late dye leakage; fluorescent peritumoral ring, dye spread at the pupillary margin and surrounding stroma; anomalies of adjacent radial vessels, disorder of the radial structure, ectropion uveae.

Despite these apparently clear indications, in clinical practice one still meets tumors presenting features common to the benign and malignant types. In other cases masses presenting all the typical characteristics of malignant forms remain unchanged over time. In such cases, iris fluorescein angiography - although not decisive - is extremely useful. If nothing else it provides objective findings that can be compared over time, and permits direct visualization of the morphology of the tumor vascular network and of the effects of its growth on surrounding tissues.

References

1 Amasio E, Vitale Brovarone F, Musso M: Angioma of the iris. Ophthalmologica (Basel) 180: 15, 1980.

2 Arentsen JJ, Green WR: Melanoma of the iris: report of 72 cases treated surgically. Ophthalmic Surg 6: 23, 1975.

3 Ashton N: Primary tumors of the iris. Br J Ophthalmol 48: 650, 1964.

4 Bandello F, Brancato R, Lattanzio R et al: Fluoreszenzangiographische diagnostik bei iristumoren. Akt Augenheilkd 19: 10, 1994.

5 Bandello F, Brancato R, Lattanzio R et al: Biomicroscopy and fluorescein angiography of pigmented iris tumors: a retrospective study on 44 cases. Int Ophthalmol 18:61, 1994.

6 Blanksma LJ, Hooijmans JMM: Vascular tufts of the pupillary border causing a spontaneous hyphaema. Ophthalmologica (Basel) 178: 297, 1979.

7 Block RS, Gartner S: The incidence of ocular metastatic carcinoma. Arch Ophthalmol 85: 673, 1971.

8 Brancato R, Menchini U, Carnevalini A: Atlante di iridografia a fluorescenza. C.I.C. Edizioni Internazionali Gruppo Ed. Medico, Roma, 1981.

9 Brovkina AF, Chichua AG: Value of fluorescein iridography in diagnosis of tumors of the iridociliary zone. Br J Ophthalmol 63: 157, 1979.

10 Brown D, Boniuk M, Font RL: Diffuse malignant melanoma of iris with metastates. Surv Ophthalmol 34: 357, 1990.

11 Bujara K, Domarus DV, Demeler U: Adenoma of the iris pigment epithelium. Ophthalmologica (Basel) 177: 336, 1978.

12 Callender GR: Malignant melanotic tumors of the eye: a study of histologic types in 111 cases. Surv Ophthalmol 34: 357, 1990.

13 Char DH: Anterior uveal tumors. In Char DH: Clinical ocular oncology. Churchill Livingstone, New York, 1989.

14 Charteris DG: Progression of an iris melanoma over 41 years. Br J Ophthalmol 74: 566, 1990.

15 Cheng H, Bron AJ, Easty D: A study of the iris masses by fluorescein angiography. Trans Ophthalmol Soc UK 91: 199, 1971.

16 Christiansen JM, Wetzig PC, Thatcher DB et al: Diagnosis and management of anterior uveal tumors. Ophthalmic Surg 10: 81, 1979.

17 Cleasby GW: Malignant melanoma of the iris. Arch Ophthalmol 60: 403, 1958.

18 Cobb B: Vascular tufts at the pupillary margin. A preliminary report on 44 patients. Trans Ophthalmol Soc UK 88: 211, 1968.

19 Coleman ST, Green WR, Patz A: Vascular tufts of pupillary margin of the iris. Am J Ophthalmol 83: 881, 1977.

20 Cornand G, Brisore B, Cozette P et al: Un cas de leiomyoma irien. Arch Ophtalmol (Paris) 35: 245, 1975.

21 Cutler SJ, Joung JL: Third National Cancer Survey: Incidence data. Dhew Publication, National Cancer Institute, Bethesda, 1975.

22 Dart JK, Marsh RJ, Garner A et al: Fluorescein angiography of anterior uveal melanocytic tumors. Br J Ophthalmol 72: 326, 1988.

23 Davidorf F: The melanoma controversy. A comparison of choroidal, cutaneus and iris melanoma. Surv Ophthalmol 25: 373, 1980.

24 Demeler U: Fluorescence angiographical studies in the diagnosis and follow-up of tumors of the iris and ciliary body. Adv Ophthalmol 42: 1, 1981.

25 Demeler U: Verlaufskontrollen von iristumoren mit hilfe der fluoreszenzangiographie. Adv Ophthalmol (Karger-Basel) 35: 167, 1978.

26 Demeler U: Irisangiographische besonderheiten bei malignen melanomen der aderhaut. Ophthalmologica (Basel) 177: 70, 1978.

27 Demeler U: Klinik fluoreszenzangiographie und eines ringmelanom der iris. Klin Monatsbl Augenheilkd 168: 387, 1976.

28 Dhermy P: Les tumours de l'iris et du corps ciliarie. J Fr Ophtalmol 2: 501, 1979.

29 Dorn HF, Cutler SJ: Morbidity from cancer in the United States. Public Health Monograph N.56, VS Government Printing Office, Washington, 1959.

30 Duke JR, Dunn SN: Primary tumors of the iris. Arch Ophthalmol 59: 204, 1958.

31 Editorial: Melanoma of the iris. Br J Ophthalmol 73: 586, 1989.

32 Fabris G, Mazzola A, Ravalli I: Anatomia patologica dei tumori del bulbo oculare e dell'orbita. In Rossi A: Clinica dei tumori dell'occhio e dell'orbita. S.A.T.E., Ferrara, 1981.

33 Felberg WT, Mione T, Shields JA et al: In vitro characteristics of uveal malignant melanomas. Arch Ophthalmol 100: 987, 1982.

34 Ferry AP: Lesions mistaken for malignant melanoma of the iris. Arch Ophthalmol 74: 9, 1965.

35 Ferry AP: Hemangiomas of the iris and ciliary body. Do they exist? A search for a histologically proved case. Int Ophthalmol Clin 12: 177, 1971.

36 Ferry AP, Font RL: Carcinoma metastatic to the eye and orbit. Arch Ophthalmol 92: 276, 1974.

37 Foulds WS: Management of intraocular melanoma (Mini review). Br J Ophthalmol 74: 559, 1990.

38 Freeman TR, Friedman AH: Metastatic carcinoma of the iris. Am J Ophthalmol 80: 947, 1975.

39 Friedburg D, Schultheiss K, Wigger H: Differential diagnose von neubildungen im bereich der iris mit hilfe der irisangiographie. Verr Rhein-Westf Augenartz 126: 13, 1973.

40 Fries PD, Char DH: Fluorescein angiography in ciliary body melanomas. Ophthalmologica 201: 57, 1990.

41 Gass DM: Iris abscess simulating malignant melanoma. Arch Ophthalmol 90: 300, 1973.

42 Geisse LJ, Robertson DM: Iris melanomas. Am J Ophthalmol 99: 639, 1985.

43 Gilman JP, Maio M: Documentation of iris tumors: slit-lamp biomicrography, goniophotography and anterior segment angiography. J Ophthalmic Photography 13: 25, 1991.

44 Green WR: Uveal tract. In Spencer WH: Ophthalmic pathology. An atlas and textbook. Saunders WB, Philadelphia, 1986.

45 Hakulinen T, Teppo L, Saxen E: Cancer of the eye. A review of trends and differentials. World Health Stat Q 31: 143, 1978.

46 Heath P: Tumors of the iris: classification and clinical follow-up. Trans Am Ophthalmol Soc 62: 52, 1965.

47 Hodes BL, Gildenhar M, Chromokos E: Fluorescein angiography in pigmented iris tumors. Arch Ophthalmol 97: 1086, 1979.

48 Hogan MJ, Zimmerman LE: Ophthalmic pathology: an atlas and textbook. Saunders WB, Philadelphia, 1962.

49 Holland G: Zurklinik und pathologie der pigmenttumoren der iris. Klin Monatsbl Augenheilkd J 150: 359, 1967.

50 Iwamoto T, Reese AB, Mund M: Tapioca melanoma of the iris. II. Electron microscopy of the melanoma cells compared with normal iris melanocytes. Am J Ophthalmol 100: 1288, 1982.

51 Jakobiec FA, Depot MJ, Henkind P et al: Fluorescein angiography pattern of iris melanocytic tumors. Arch Ophthalmol 100: 1288, 1982.

52 Jakobiec FA, Silbert G: Are most iris melanomas "really naevi"? Arch Ophthalmol 99: 2117, 1981.

53 Jensen DA: Malignant melanomas of the uvea in Denmark: 1943-1952. Acta Ophthalmol 75 (Suppl): 57, 1963.

54 Juarez CP, Tso MOM: An ultrastructural study of melanocytoma of the optic disk and uvea. Am J Ophthalmol 90: 48, 1980.

55 Kersten RC, Tse DT, Anderson R: Iris melanoma. Nevus or malignancy? Surv Ophthalmol 29: 423, 1985.

56 Kliman GH, Augsburger JJ, Shields JA: Association between iris color and iris melanocytic lesions. Am J Ophthalmol 100: 547, 1985.

57 Kottow MH: Anterior segment fluorescein angiography. William & Wilkins, Baltimore, 1979.

58 Kottow MH: Fluorescein angiographic behaviour of iris masses. Ophthalmologica (Basel) 174: 217, 1977.

59 Margo CE, Groden LR: Iris melanoma with extensive corneal invasion and metastases. Am J Ophthalmol 104: 543, 1987.

60 Makley TA Jr: Management of melanomas of the anterior segment. Surv Ophthalmol 19: 135, 1974.

61 Makley TA, Kapetansky FM: Iris nevus syndrome. Ann Ophthalmol 20: 311, 1988.

62 Mc Gallard JN, Johnstone PB: A study of iris melanoma in Northern Ireland. Br J Ophthalmol 73: 591, 1989.

63 Mc Lean IW, Foster WD, Zimmerman LE et al: Inferred natural history of uveal melanomata. Invest Ophthalmol Vis Sci 19: 760, 1980.

64 Mincione GP, Campana G, Vannelli G: Observations sur l'ultrastructure des melanomes malins de l'uveé. J Fr Ophtalmol 10: 531, 1979.

65 Naumann G, Ruprecht KW: Xanthom der iris: ein klinisch pathologischer befundberich. Ophthalmologica 164: 293, 1972.

66 Nordman J, Brini A: Von Recklingausen's disease and melanoma of the uvea. Br J Ophthalmol 54: 641, 1970.

67 Paul EV, Parnell BC, Fraker M: Prognosis of malignant melanoma of the choroid and ciliary body. Int Ophthalmol Clin 2: 387, 1962.

68 Podolsky MM, Srinivasan BD: Spontaneous hyphaema secondary to vascular tuft of pupillary margin of the iris. Arch Ophthalmol 97: 301, 1979.

69 Price MJ, Bell RA, Willis WE et al: Tapioca melanoma of the iris: clinico-pathological correlation with results of fluorescein angiography. Can J Ophthalmol 16: 195, 1981.

70 Racz J, Shabo J: Two cases of neurilemmoma of the anterior uvea. Klin Monatsbl Augenheilkd 163: 605, 1973.

71 Raivio I: Uveal melanoma in Finland: an epidemiologic, clinical, histological and prognostic study. Acta Ophthalmol 133 (Suppl): 3, 1977.

72 Reese AB, Mund M, Iwamoto T: Tapioca melanoma of the iris: clinical and light microscopy studies. Am J Ophthalmol 74: 840, 1972.

73 Reese AB: Tumors of the eye. Harper & Row Publishers, New York, 1976.

74 Riffenburgh RS: Recurrent spontaneous iris arterial hemorrhage. Am J Ophthalmol 53: 319, 1965.

75 Rydberg M: Svenska Ogonlakarforeningens Sammanträde. Nord Med 72: 1488, 1964.

76 Rohrbach JM, Roggendorf W, Thanos S et al: Simultaneous bilateral diffuse melanocytic uveal hyperplasia. Am J Ophthalmol 110: 49, 1990.

77 Rones B, Zimmerman LE: The production of heterochromia and glaucoma by diffuse malignant melanoma of the iris. Trans Am Acad Ophthalmol Otolaryngol 61: 447, 1957.

78 Rones B, Zimmerman LE: The prognosis of primary tumors of the iris treated by iridectomy. Arch Ophthalmol 60: 193, 1958.

79 Rootman J, Gallangher RP: Color as a risk factor in iris melanoma. Am J Ophthalmol 98: 558, 1984.

80 Rosen E, Lyons D: Microhemangiomas at the pupillary border. Am J Ophthalmol 67: 846, 1969.

81 Rossi A: Clinica dei tumori dell'occhio e dell'orbita. S.A.T.E., Ferrara, 1981.

82 Schwartz LK, O'Connor GR: Secondary syphilis with iris papules. Am J Ophthalmol 90: 380, 1980.

83 Scotto J : Melanoma of the eye and other non cutaneous sites epidemiologic aspects. J Nat Cancer Inst 56: 489, 1976.

84 Sevel D, Tobias B: The value of fluorescein iridography with leiomyoma of the iris. Am J Ophthalmol 9: 475, 1972.

85 Shammas HF, Blodi FC: Orbital extension of choroidal and ciliary body melanomas. Arch Ophthalmol 93: 63, 1977.

86 Shields JA, Sanborn GE, Augsburger JJ: The differential diagnosis of malignant melanoma of the iris: a clinical study of 200 patients. Ophthalmology 90: 716, 1983.

87 Shields CL, Shields JA, Cook GR et al: Differentiation of adenoma of the iris pigment epithelium from iris cyst and melanoma. Am J Ophthalmol 100: 678, 1985.

88 Shields JA: Diagnosis and management of intraocular tumors. CV Mosby, St Louis, 1983.

89 Shields JA, Packer S: Radioactive phosphorus uptake test for the diagnosis of malignant melanoma of the choroid. Seminars in Nuclear Medicine XVI: 1, 1984.

90 Shields JA, Shields CL: Hepatic metastases of diffuse iris melanoma 17 years after enucleation. Am J Ophthalmol 106: 749, 1988.

91 Sihota R, Tiwari HK, Azad RV et al: Photocoagulation of large iris cysts. Ann Ophthalmol 20: 470, 1988.

92 Starr HJ, Zimmerman LE: Extrascleral extension and recurrence of malignant melanoma of the choroid and ciliary body. Int Ophthalmol Clin 2: 369, 1962.

93 Sunba MSN, Rahi AHS, Morgan G: Tumors of the anterior uvea. I. Metastasizing malignant melanoma of the iris. Arch Ophthalmol 98: 82, 1980.

94 Sunba MSN, Rahi AHS, Morgan G et al: Prognostic parameters in malignant melanoma of the iris. In Lommatzch PK, Blodi FC: Intraocular tumors. Springer, Berlin, 1983.

95 Territo C, Shields CL, Shields JA et al: Natural course of melanocytic tumors of the iris. Ophthalmology 95: 1251, 1988.

96 Westervel-Brandon ER, Zeeman WPC: The prognosis of melanoblastoma of the choroid. Ophthalmologica 134: 20, 1958.

97 Wilensky JT, Holland MG: A pigmented tumor of the ciliary body. Arch Ophthalmol 92: 219, 1974.

98 Wilson RS, Fraunfelder FT, Hanna C: Recurrent tapioca melanoma of the iris and ciliary body treated by the argon laser. Am J Ophthalmol 82: 213, 1976.

99 Wolter JR, Butler RG: Pigment spots of the iris and ectropion uveal with glaucoma in neurofibromatosis. Am J Ophthalmol 56: 964, 1963.

100 Yanko L: An angiographic and histologic study of the vasculature of choroidal malignant melanoma. Acta Ophthalmol 51: 12, 1973.

101 Zakka KA, Foos RY, Sulit H: Metastatic tapioca melanoma. Br J Ophthalmol 63: 744, 1979.

102 Zakka KA, Foos RY, Omphroy CA et al: Malignant melanoma: analysis of an autopsy population. Ophthalmology 87: 549, 1980.

103 Zimmerman LE: Clinical pathology of iris tumors. The Ward Burdick Award Contribution. Am J Clin Pathol 39: 214, 1963.

104 Zimmerman LE: Ocular lesions of juvenile xanthogranuloma (nevoxanthoendothelioma). Trans Am Acad Ophthalmol Otolaryngol 69: 412, 1965.

105 Zimmerman LE: Ocular lesions of juvenile xanthogranuloma: nevoxanthoendothelioma. Am J Ophthalmol 60: 1011, 1965.

106 Zimmerman LE: Histopathologic considerations in the management of tumors of the iris and ciliary body. Ann Inst Barraquer 10: 27, 1972.

107 Zimmerman LE, Mc Lean IW, Foster WD: Statistical analysis of follow-up data concerning uveal melanomas and the influence of enucleation. Ophthalmology 87: 557, 1980.

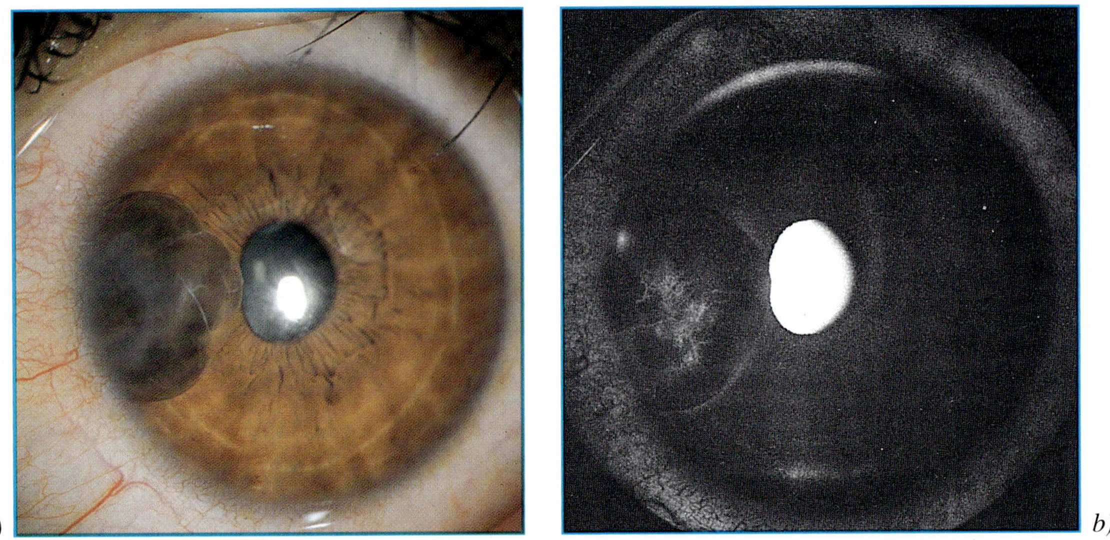

*Fig. **4.10**,1 - Biomicroscopic appearance of an idiopathic serous cyst of the anterior layer of the iris (a); in iris fluorescein angiography (b) injection of a fine superficial vascular network from which dye leakages, can be seen.*

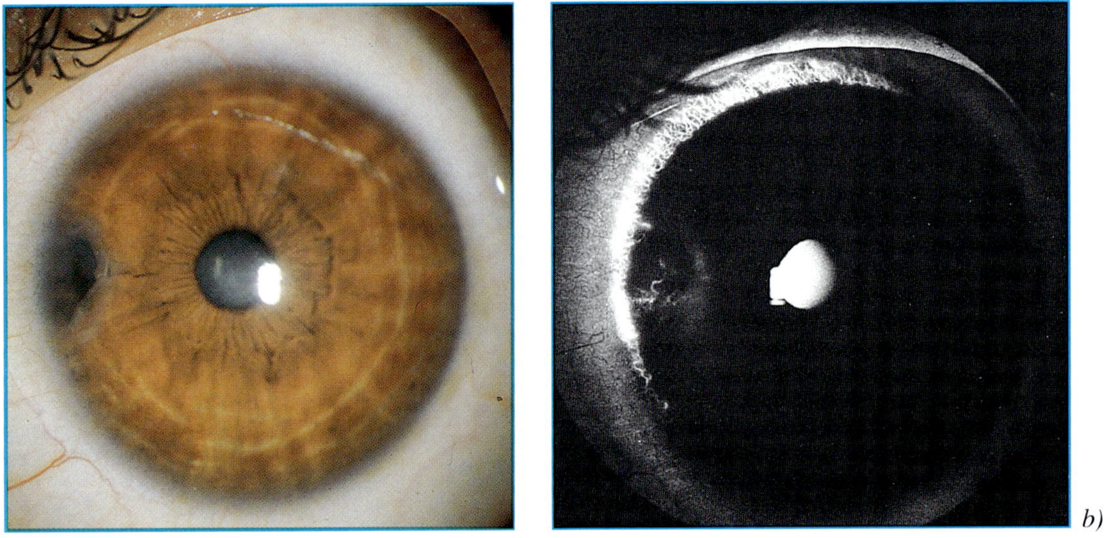

*Fig. **4.10**,2 - Same case as Fig. **4.10**,1 after Nd:YAG laser treatment: (a) color photo; (b) iris fluorescein angiography.*

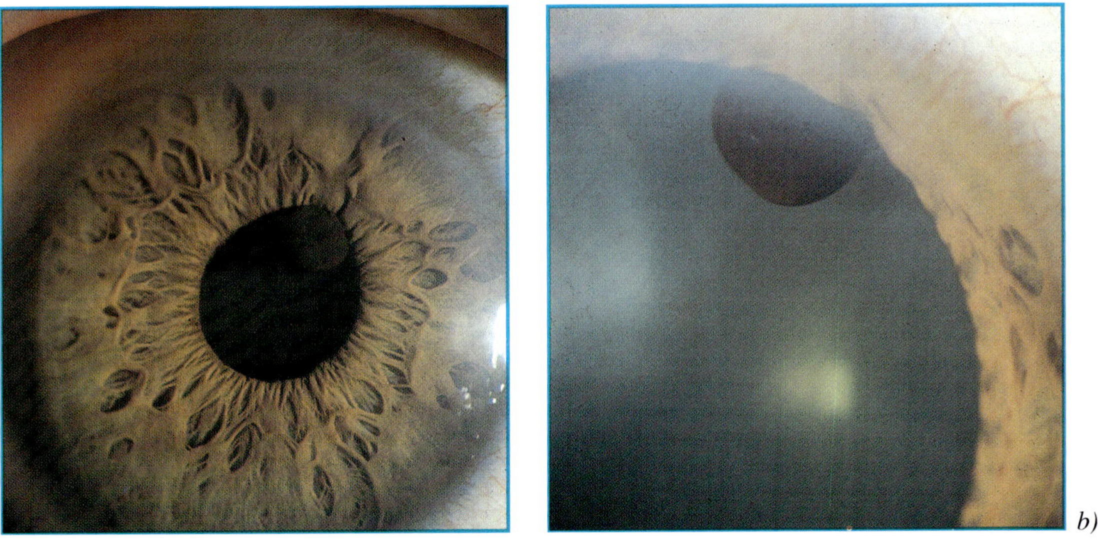

*Fig. **4.10**,3 - When the cyst is located posteriorly (a) pharmacological midriasis must be induced to visualize it better (b).*

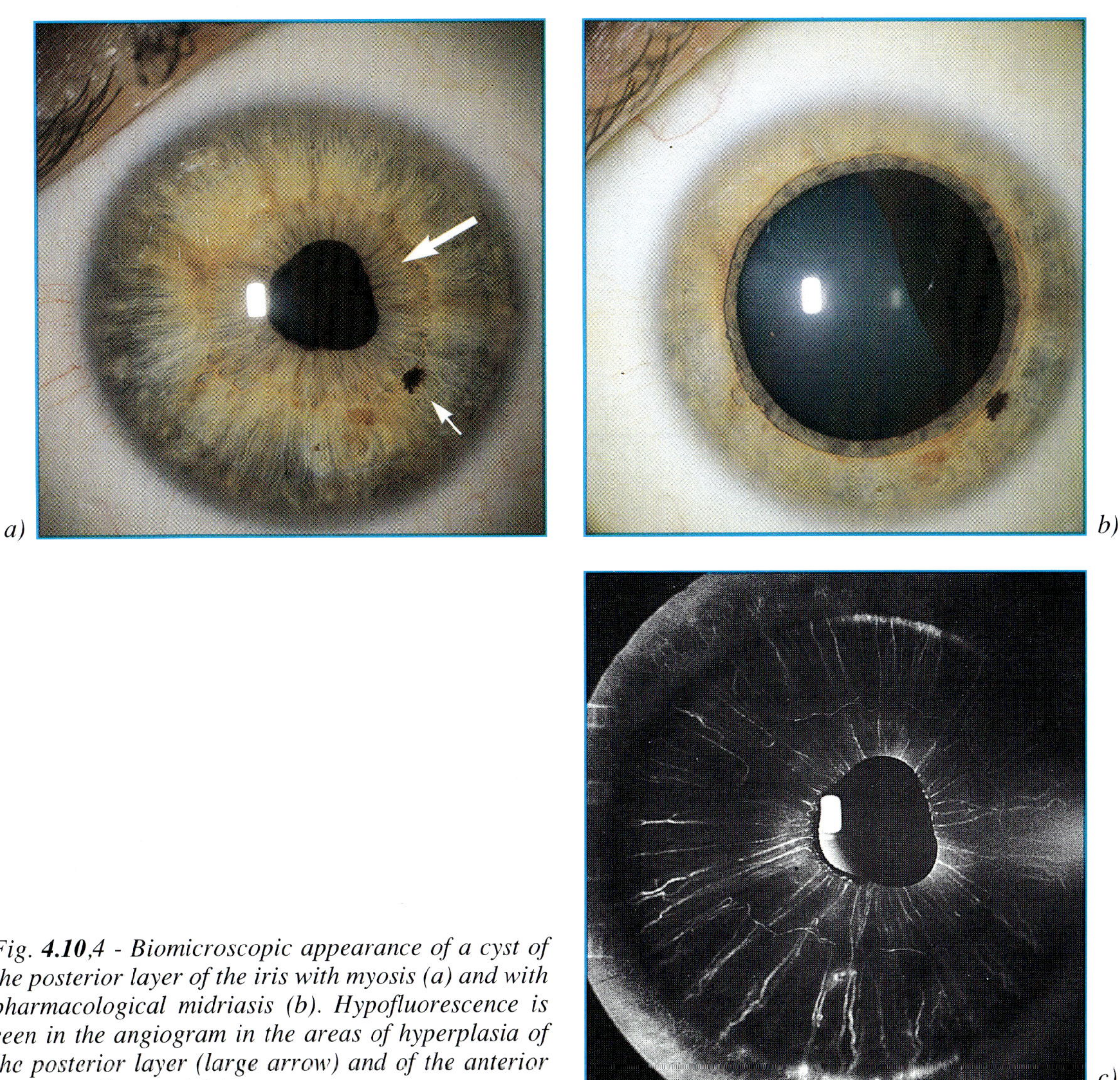

a) b) c)

*Fig. **4.10**,4 - Biomicroscopic appearance of a cyst of the posterior layer of the iris with myosis (a) and with pharmacological midriasis (b). Hypofluorescence is seen in the angiogram in the areas of hyperplasia of the posterior layer (large arrow) and of the anterior layer (small arrow) (c).*

a) b)

*Fig. **4.10**,5 - In cases of iris cysts (a: see arrow) fluorescein angiography may give a normal picture (b).*

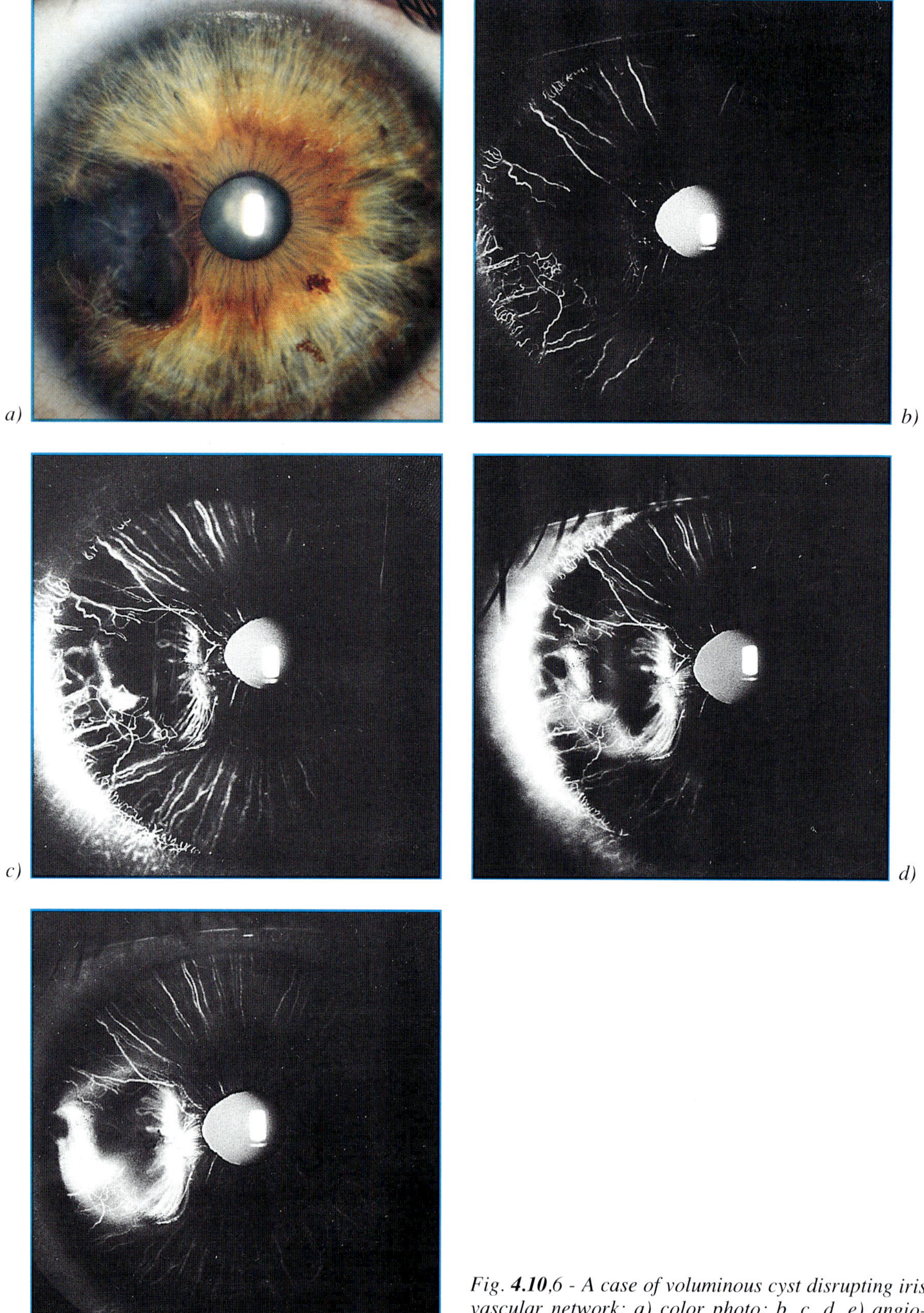

*Fig. **4.10**,6 - A case of voluminous cyst disrupting iris vascular network: a) color photo; b, c, d, e) angiographic phases.*

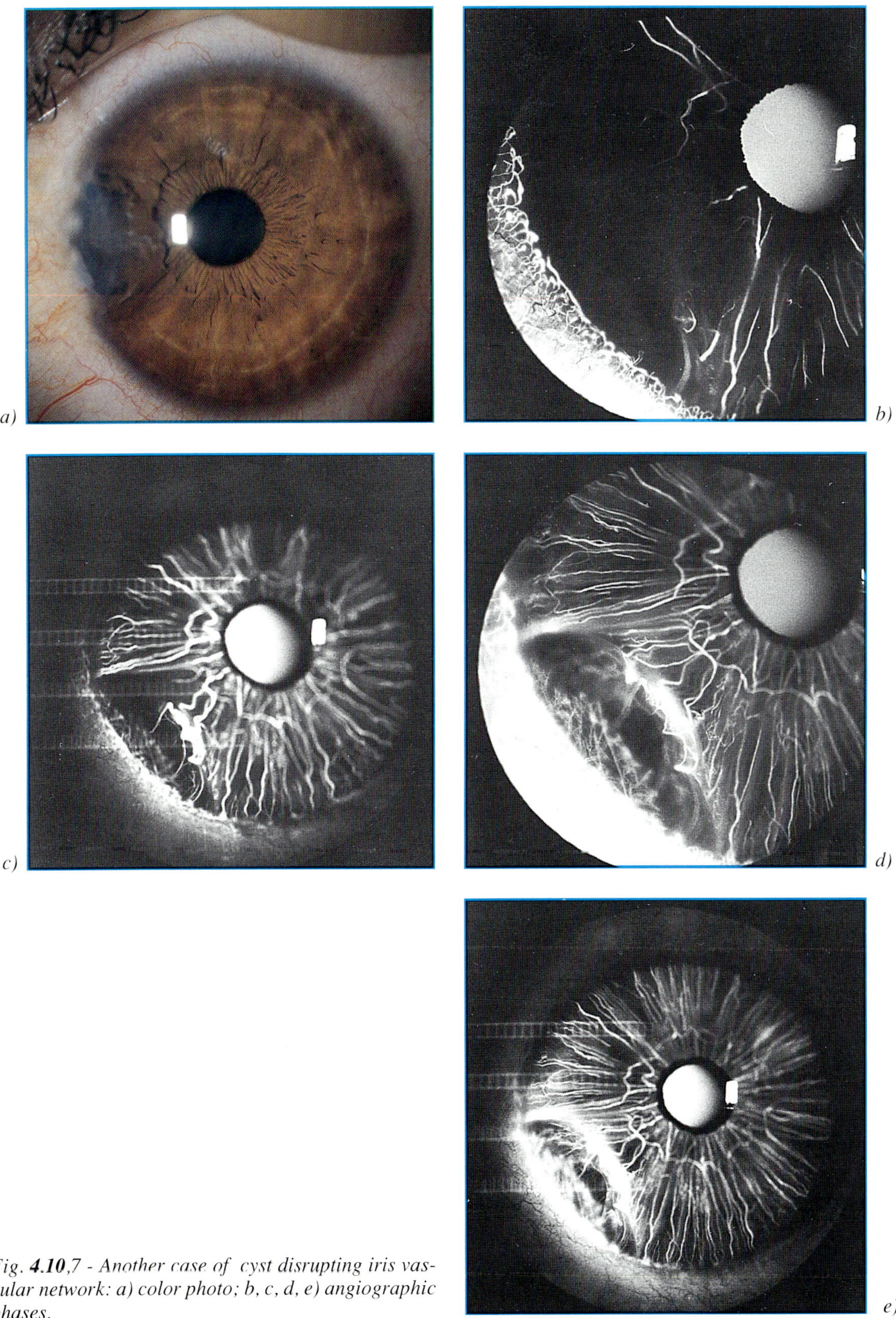

Fig. ***4.10****,7 - Another case of cyst disrupting iris vascular network: a) color photo; b, c, d, e) angiographic phases.*

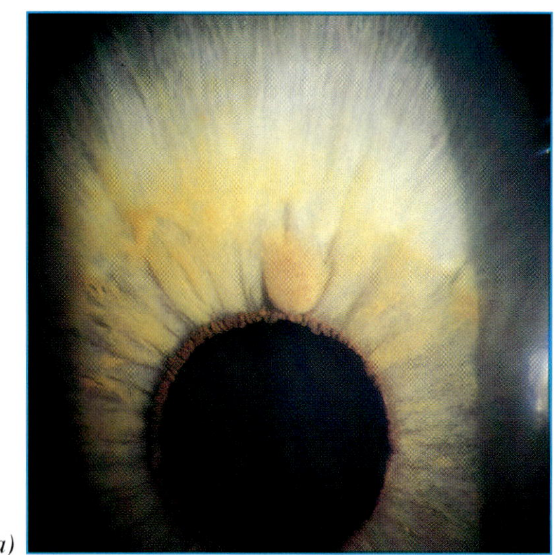
a)

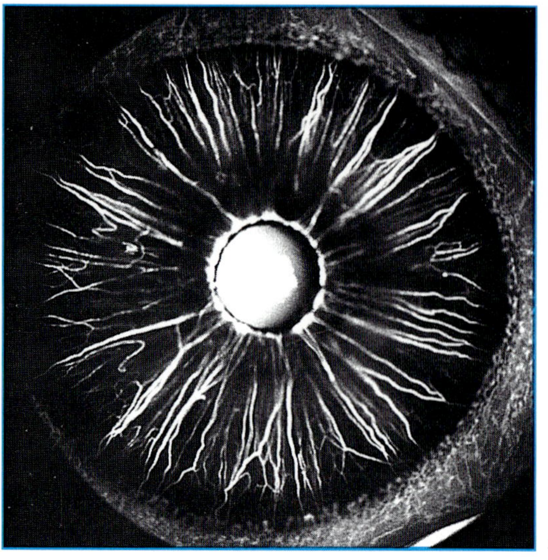
b)

*Fig. **4.10**,8 - Small congenital iris cysts (a), examined by iris fluorescein angiography (b) generally do not take up the dye and their surrounding vessels show no noteworthy changes.*

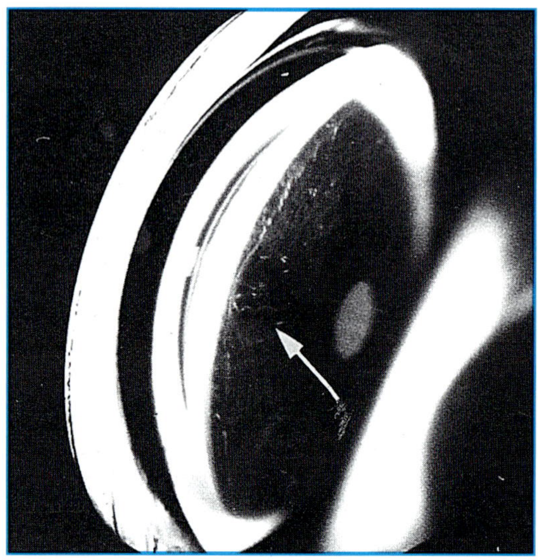

*Fig. **4.10**,9 - The area of the cyst (arrow) in this case shows low fluorescence in the angiogram. Overlying and surrounding radial vessels appear dilated but there is no dye leakage.*

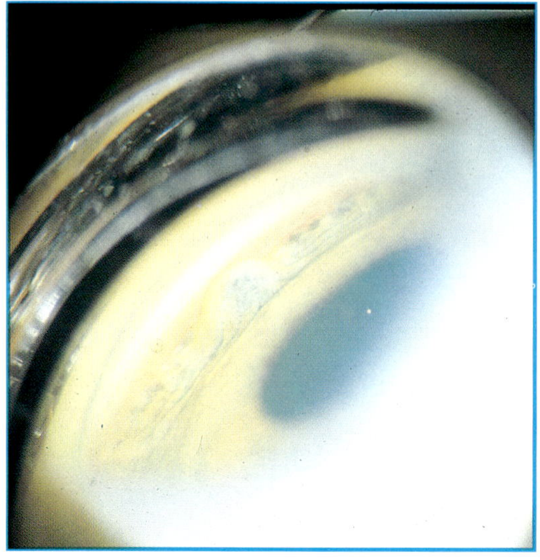
a)

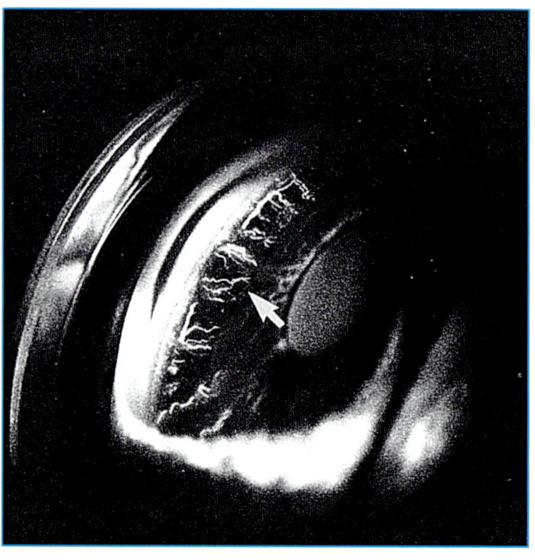
b)

*Fig. **4.10**,10 - Biomicroscopic picture (a) and fluorescein angiogram (b) of a stromal cyst of the iris (arrow) which appears overlaid by anomalous, tortuous iris vessels.*

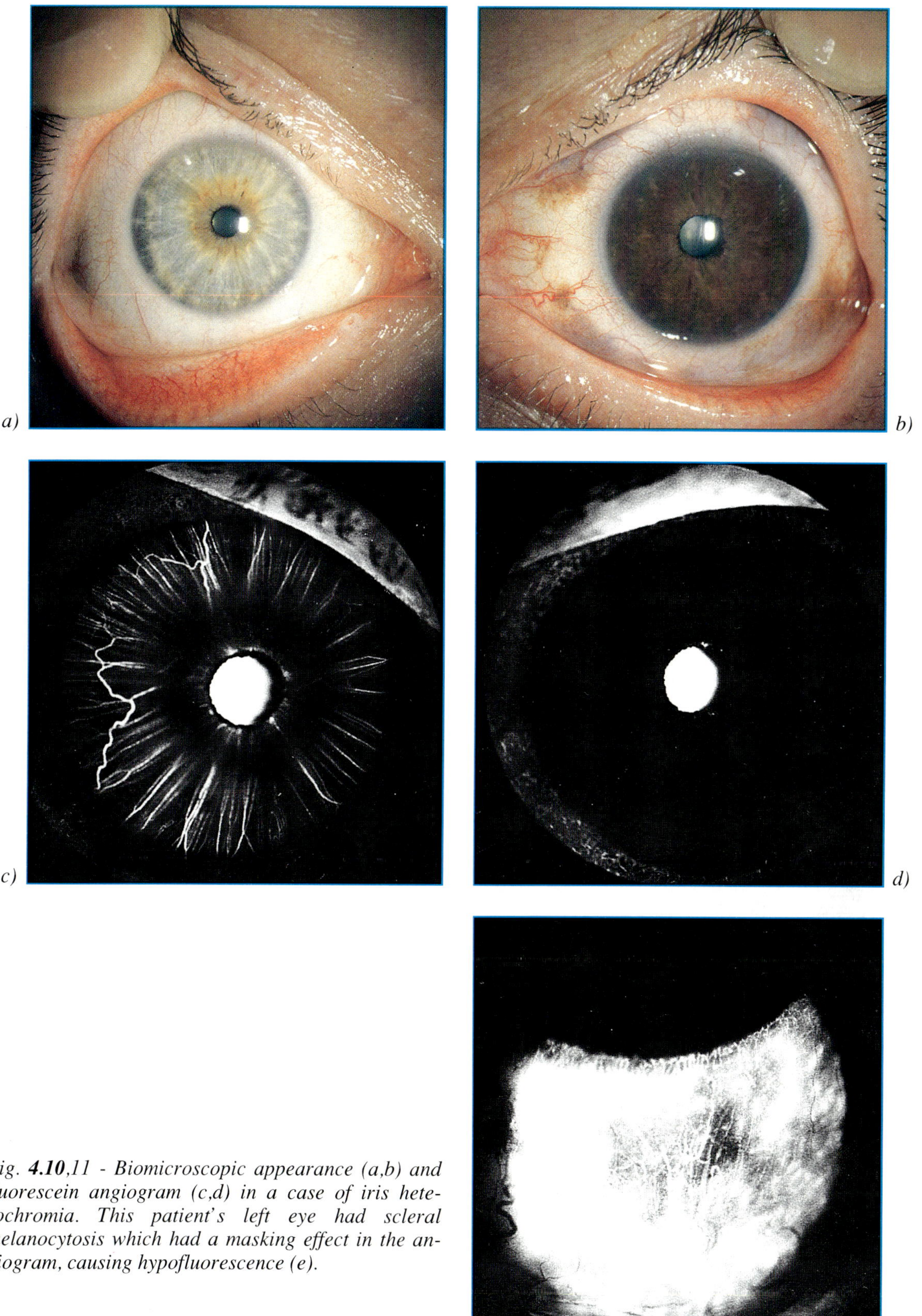

*Fig. **4.10**,11 - Biomicroscopic appearance (a,b) and fluorescein angiogram (c,d) in a case of iris heterochromia. This patient's left eye had scleral melanocytosis which had a masking effect in the angiogram, causing hypofluorescence (e).*

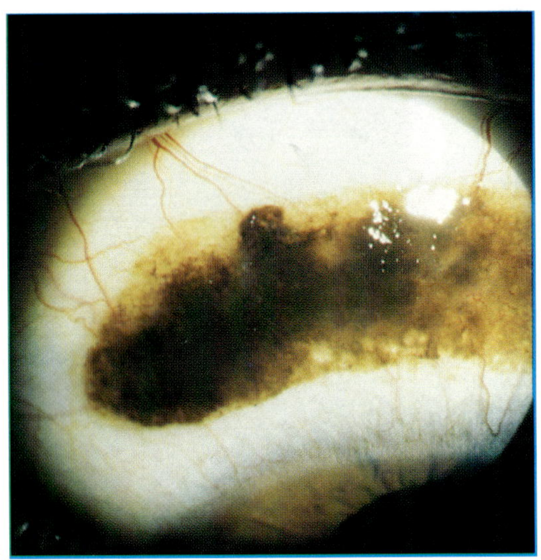
a)

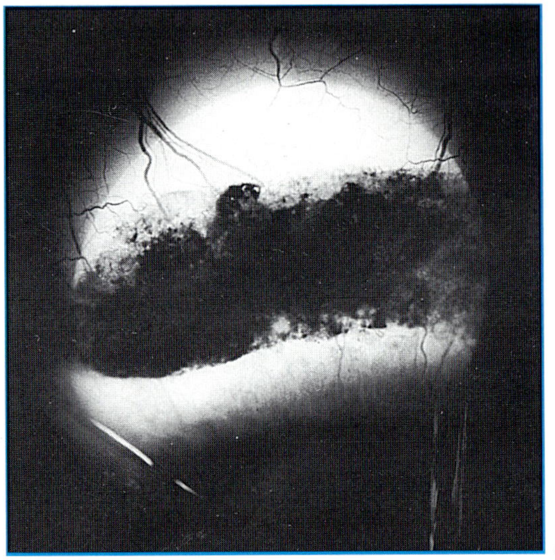
b)

*Fig. **4.10**,12 - Melanocytosis : a) color photo, b) fluorangiographic pattern.*

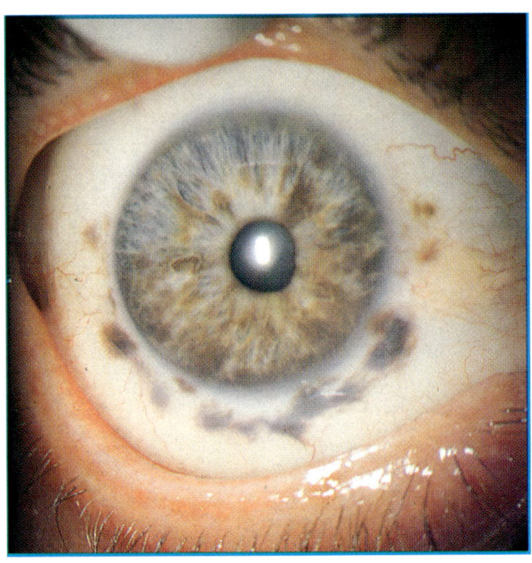

*Fig. **4.10**,13 - Pigment accumulation in the sclera may indicate tissue invasion by a choroidal melanoma, as in this instance. It can be distinguished from simple melanocytosis by the fact that there is a malignant melanoma in the posterior segment of the eye, by its progressive growth, and by its focal, not diffuse, proliferation.*

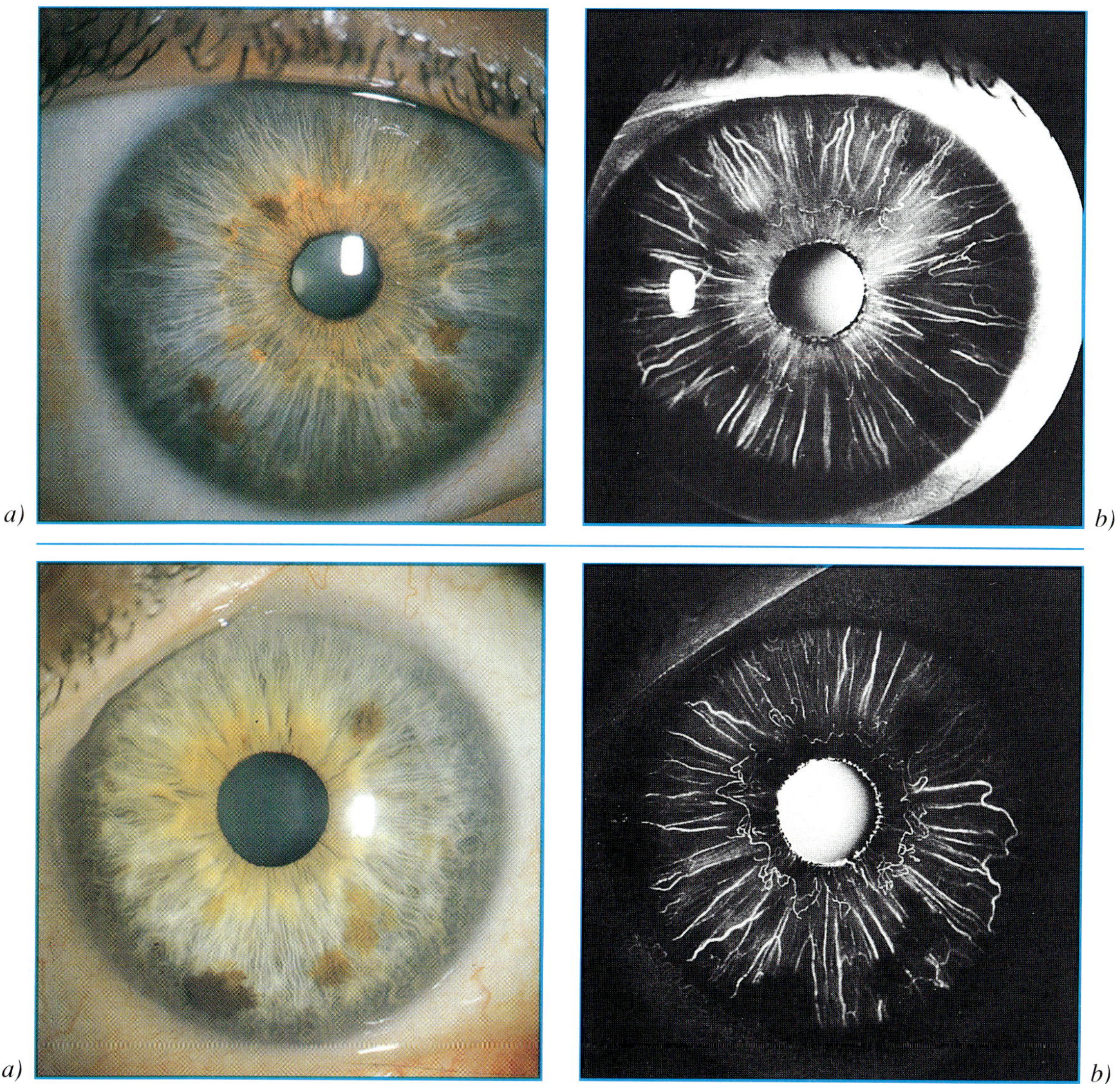

*Figs. **4.10**,14,15 - The masking effect causes hypofluorescent areas in the angiogram (b) corresponding with the hyperpigmented foci in the iris, visible biomicroscopically (a).*

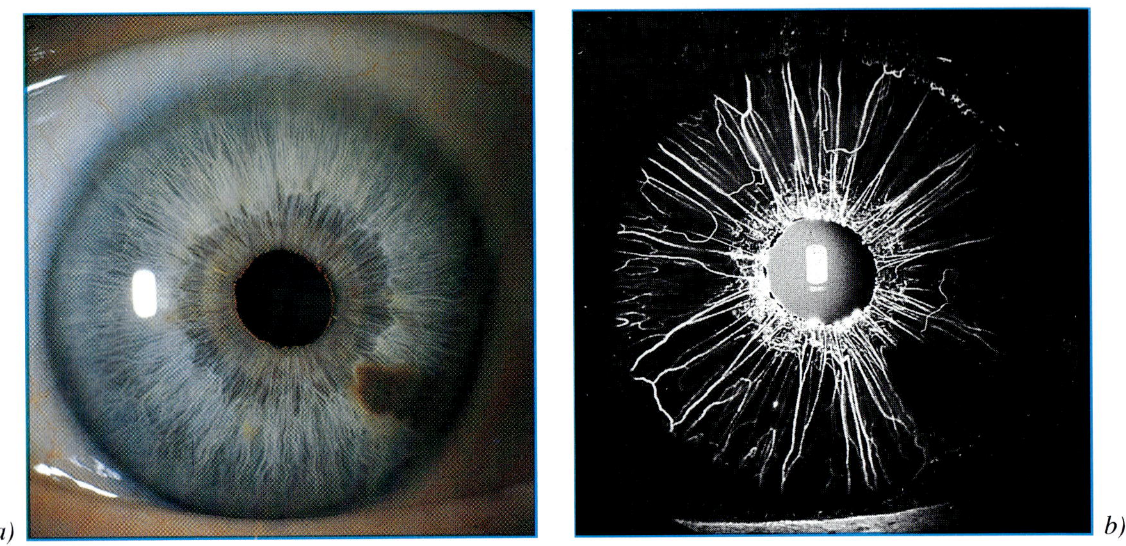

a) b)

Fig. ***4.10****,16 - The nevus visible in the color photo (a) masks the iris vascularization (angiographic silence) in the angiogram (b).*

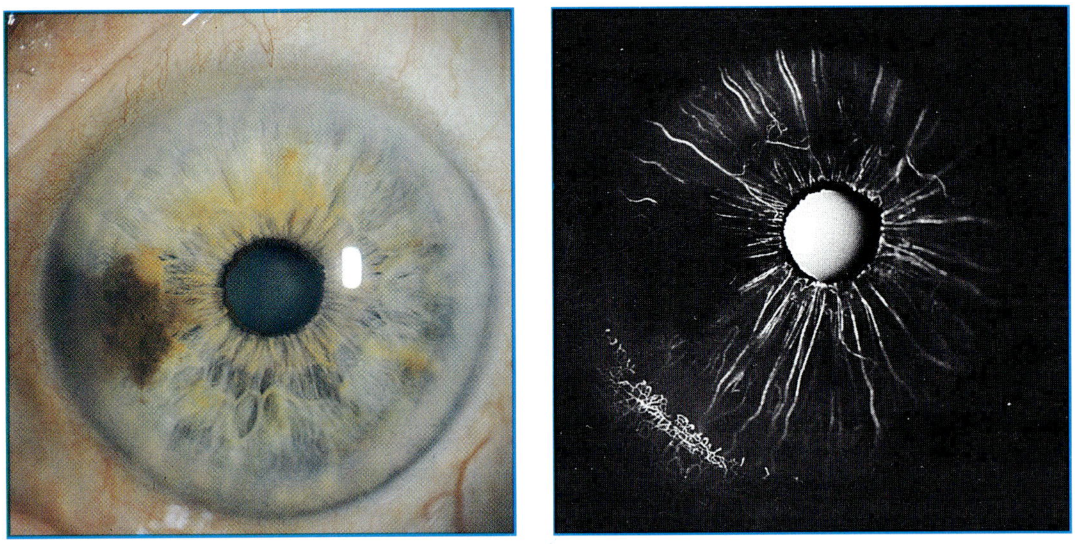

a) b)

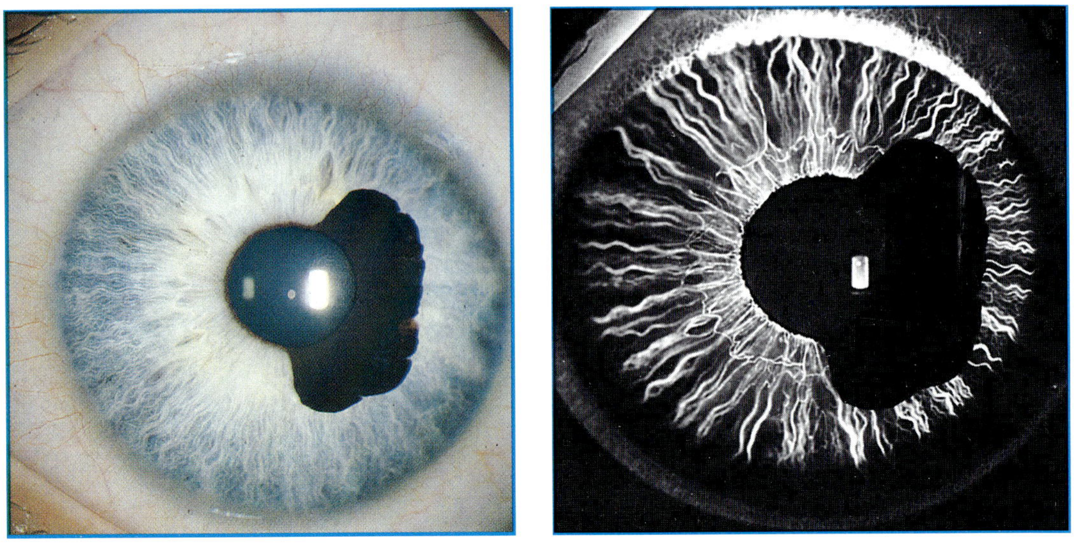

a) b)

Figs. ***4.10****,17,18 - Two cases similar to that in Fig.* ***4.10****,16.*

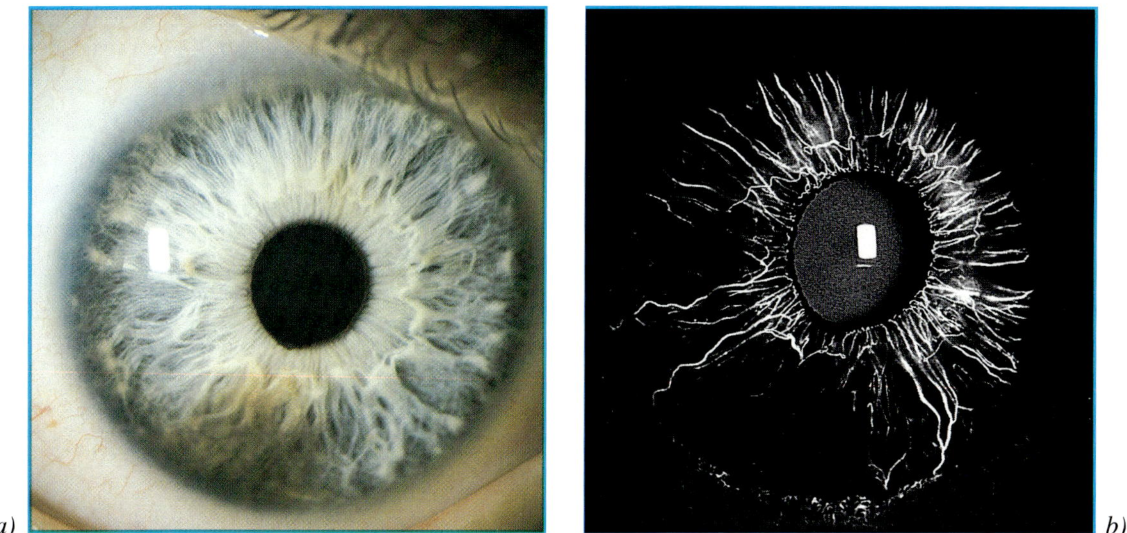

a) b)

Fig. ***4.10****,19 - The excess of pigment in the nevus, visible biomicroscopically (a), in this case partially masks the vascular network of the iris in the angiogram (b).*

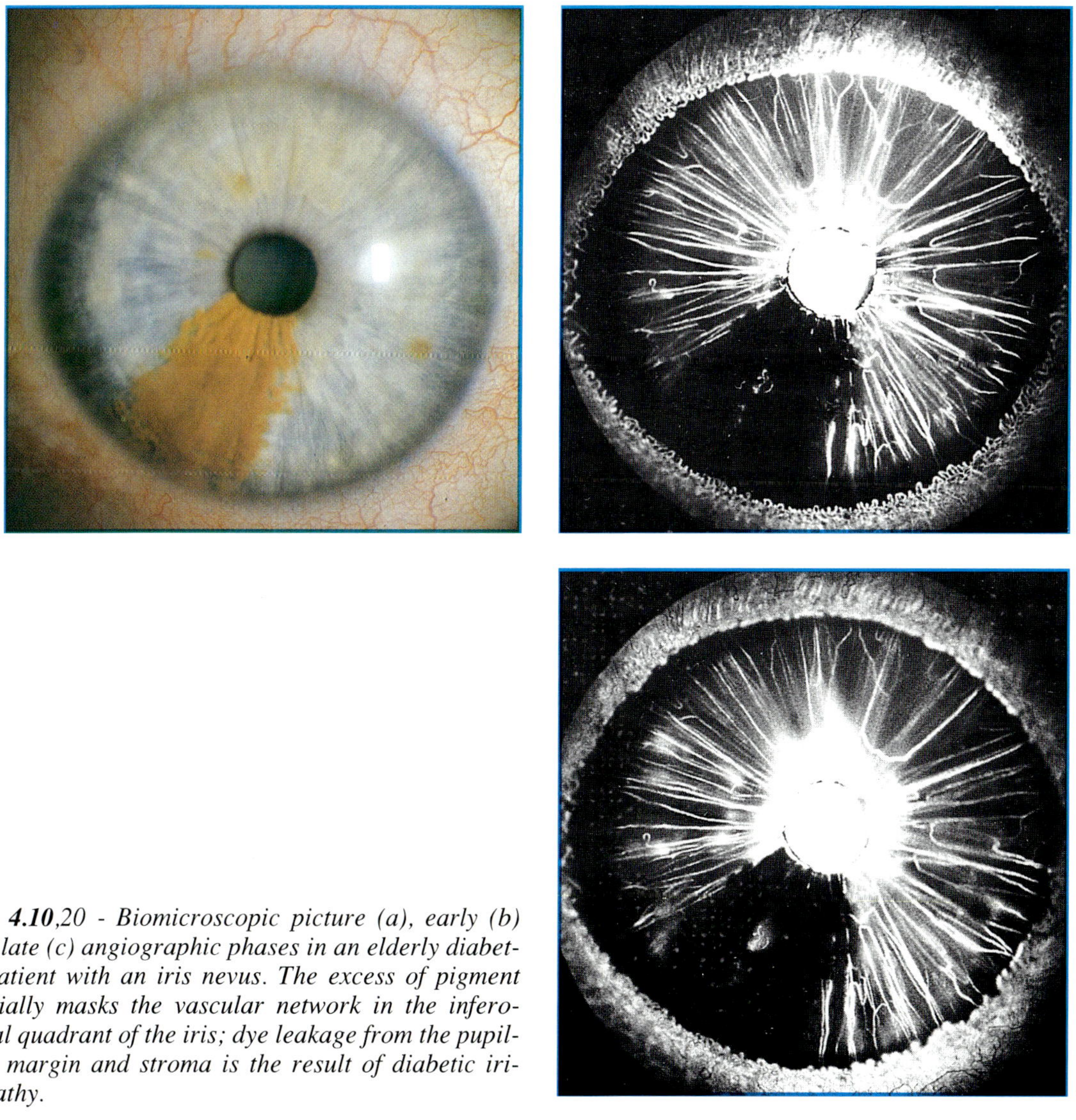

a) b)

c)

Fig. ***4.10****,20 - Biomicroscopic picture (a), early (b) and late (c) angiographic phases in an elderly diabetic patient with an iris nevus. The excess of pigment partially masks the vascular network in the inferonasal quadrant of the iris; dye leakage from the pupillary margin and stroma is the result of diabetic iridopathy.*

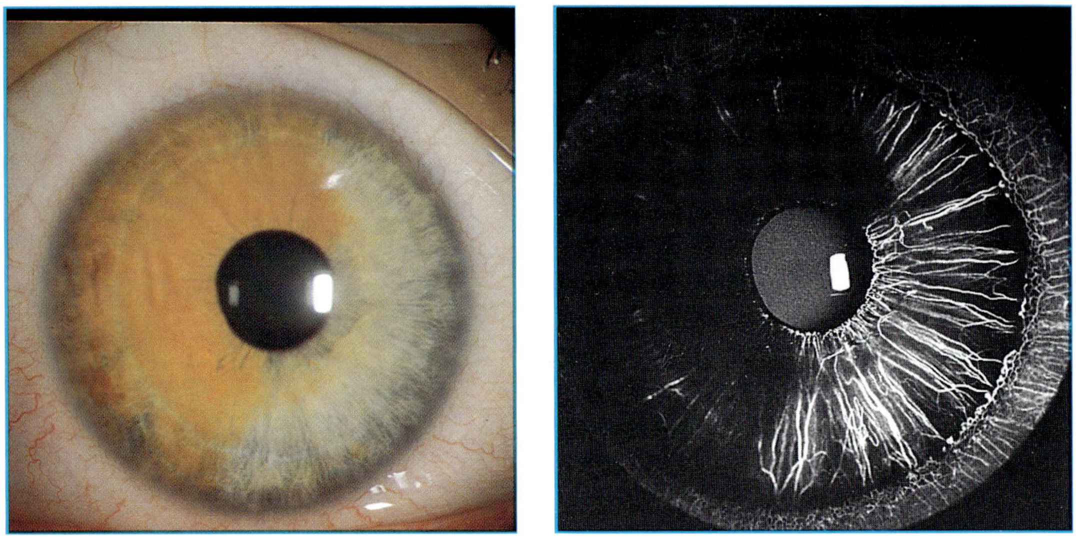

Figs. ***4.10****,21,22 - Hyperpigmentation of the iris in these cases involves whole sectors (a); the absence of noteworthy fluorescein angiographic anomalies (b) indicates the lesions are probably benign.*

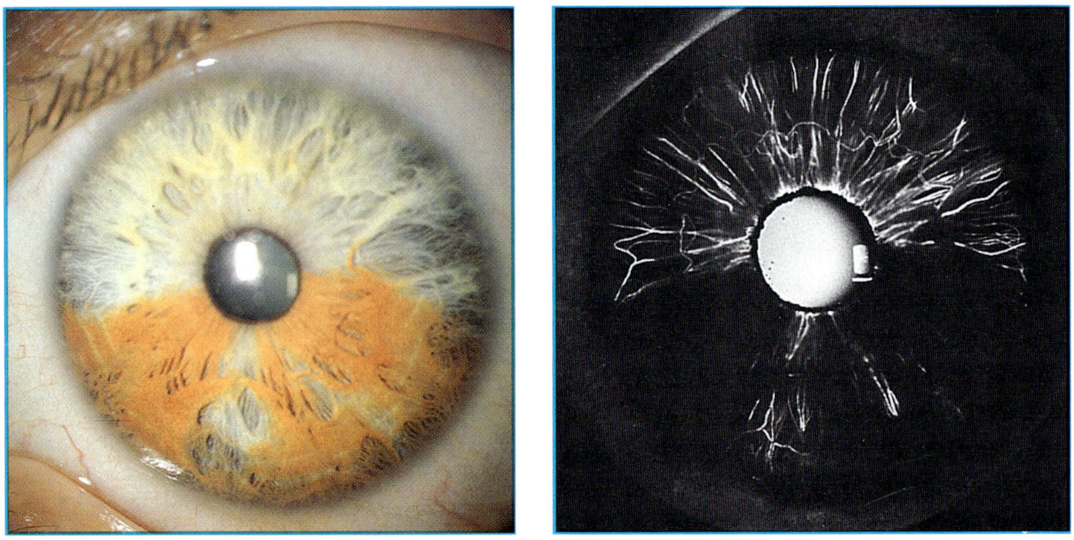

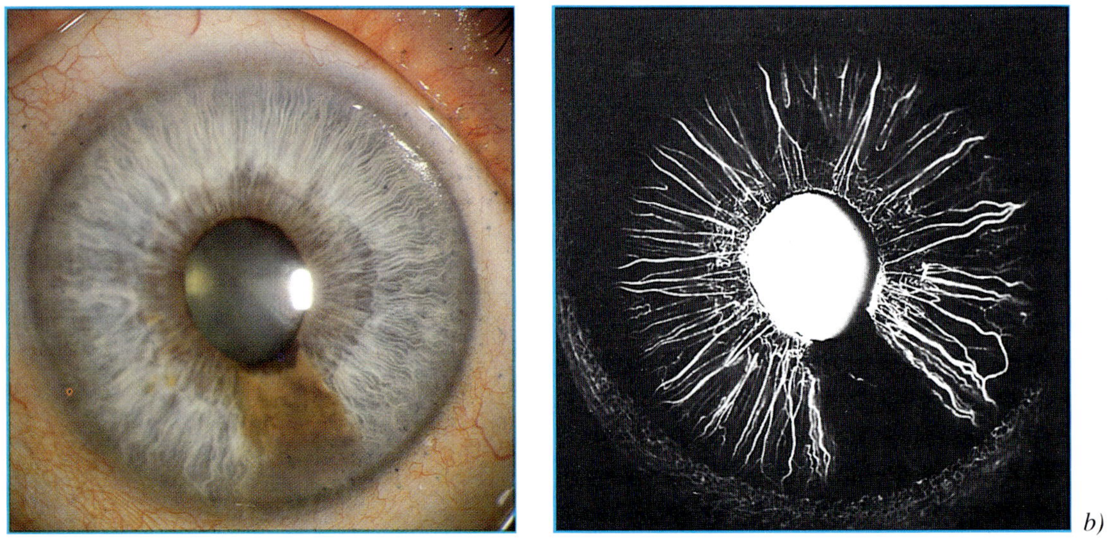

Fig. ***4.10****,23 - The area of low fluorescence in the angiogram (b) corresponds to the hyperpigmented area in the color photo (a). In this case the pupillary margin is deformed in the affected sector and the hypofluorescence caused by the ectropion uveae is hard to distinguish from the hypofluorescence of the nevus itself.*

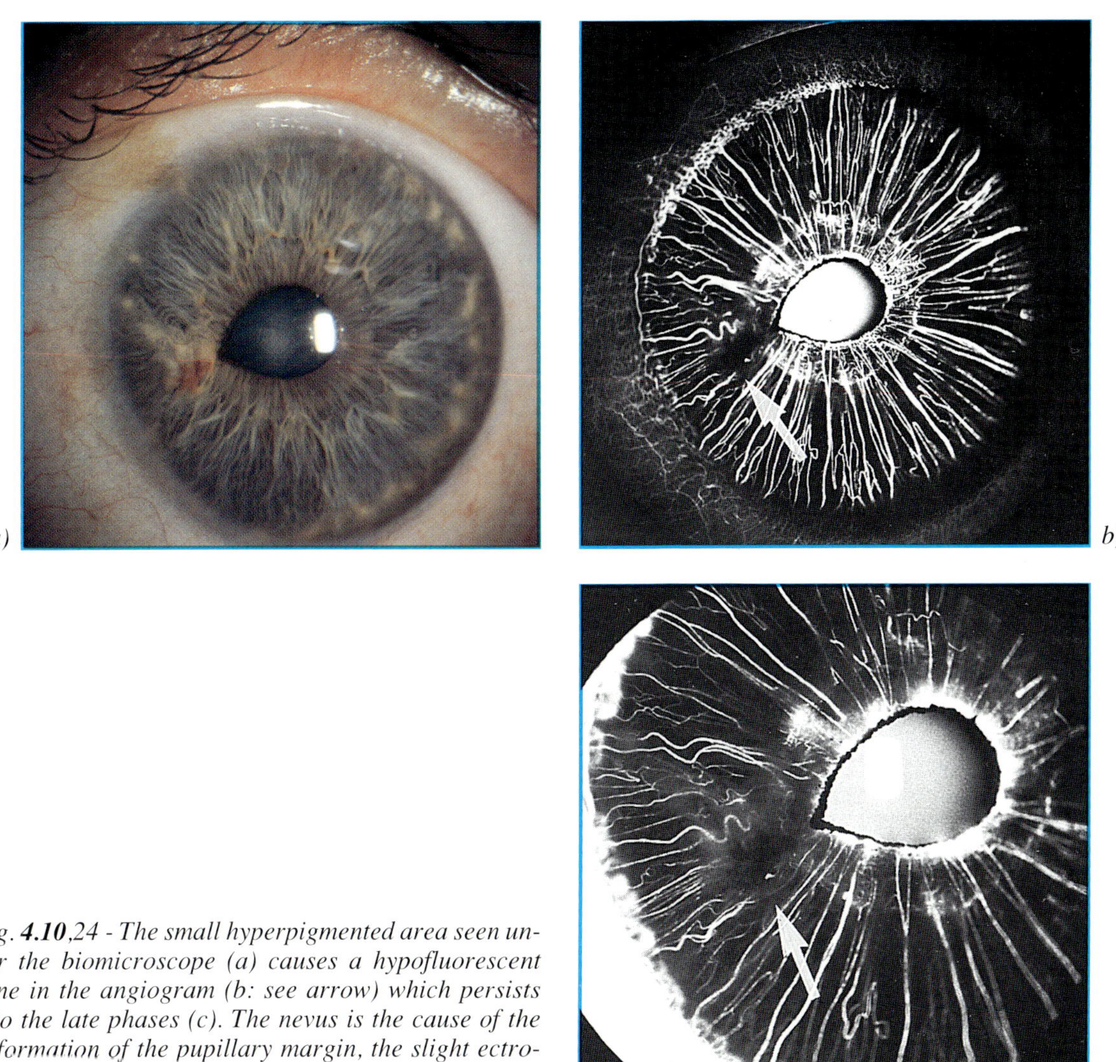

*Fig. **4.10**,24 - The small hyperpigmented area seen under the biomicroscope (a) causes a hypofluorescent zone in the angiogram (b: see arrow) which persists into the late phases (c). The nevus is the cause of the deformation of the pupillary margin, the slight ectropion uveae and the anomalies in the surrounding radial vessels.*

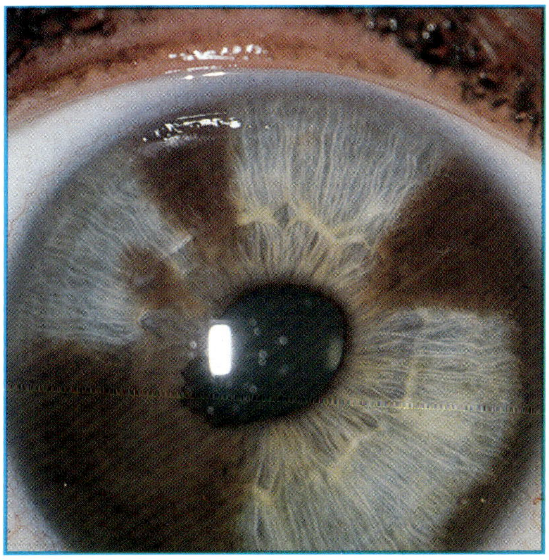

a) 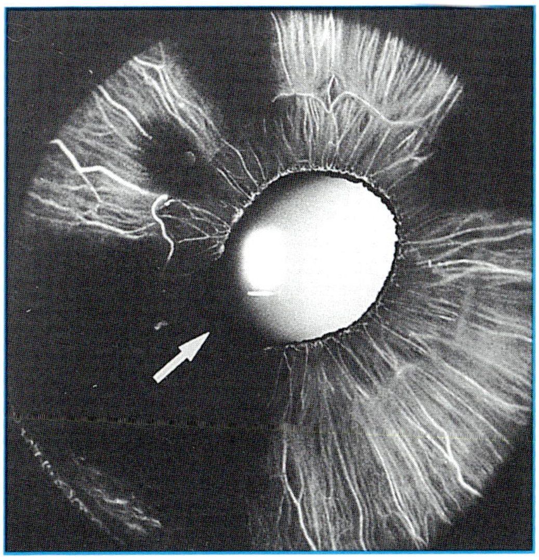 b)

*Fig. **4.10**,25- In this case there is pigment accumulation in various sectors of the iris (a); these present low fluorescence in the angiogram (b). The area with more hypofluorescence at the pupillary margin (arrow) is the ectropion uveae.*

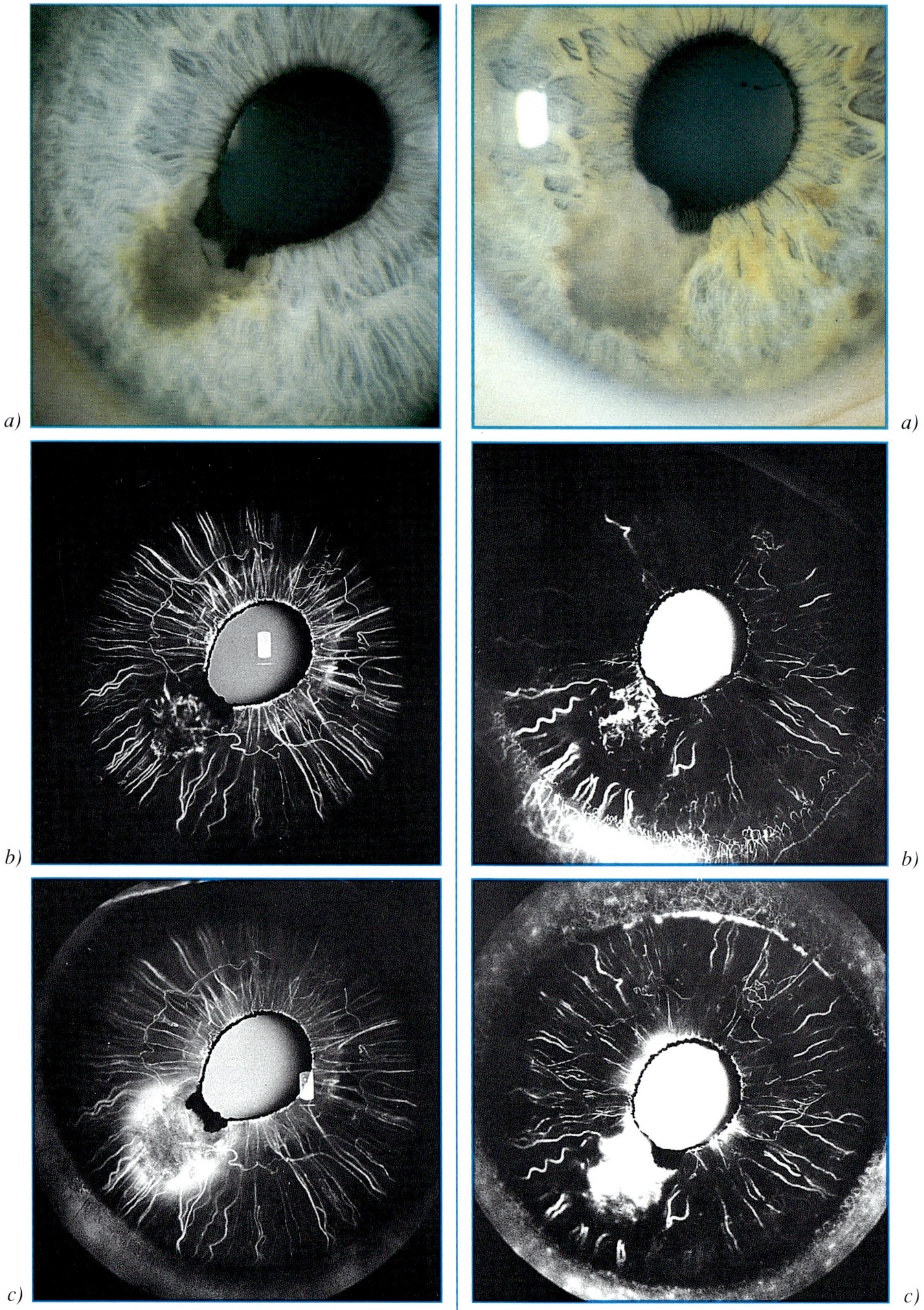

*Fig. **4.10**,26 - Color photo of a pigmented neoformation of the iris (a); angiography shows early fluorescence in the tumor, irregular vascular network (b) and a tendency for dye to leak late (c). The tumor causes deformation of the pupillary margin and ectropion uveae.*

*Fig. **4.10**,27 - Neoformation with biomicroscopic (a) and fluorescein angiographic (b,c) features similar to the previous case: in the late phases (c) hyperfluorescence of the mass covers the anarchic vascular network of the tumor, which showed early hyperfluorescence (b).*

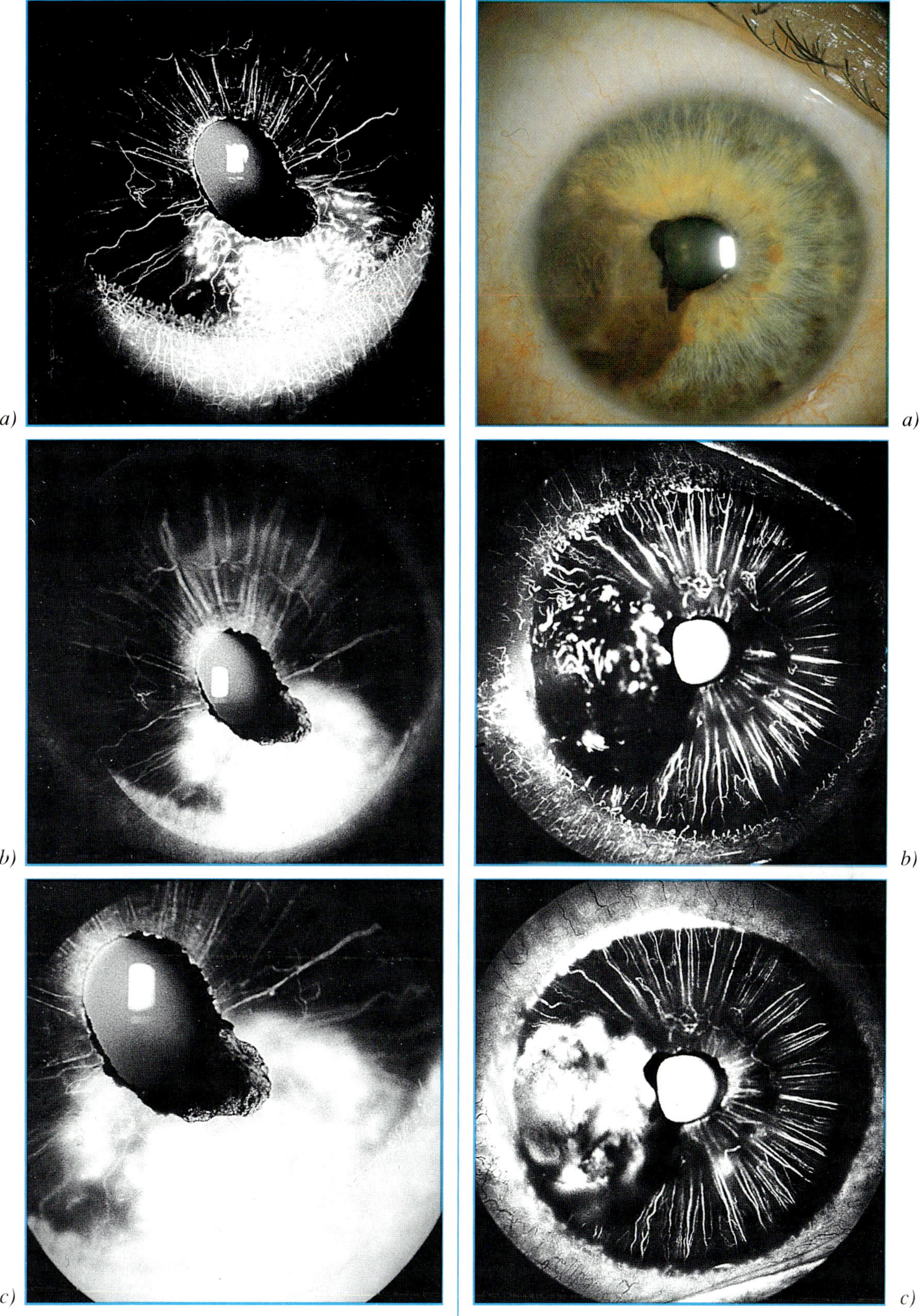

*Fig. **4.10**,28 - The tumor's intricate vascular network shows hyperfluorescence early (a) and dye leaks out in the later phases of the examination (b,c). Hypofluorescence at the pupillary margin is a result of ectropion uveae caused by the traction of the mass which also deforms the pupillary margin.*

*Fig. **4.10**,29 - Early injection of dye into the tumor's anarchic vascular network (b) is followed in the later phases of the examination (c) by diffuse hyperfluorescence in the mass. a) Biomicroscopy.*

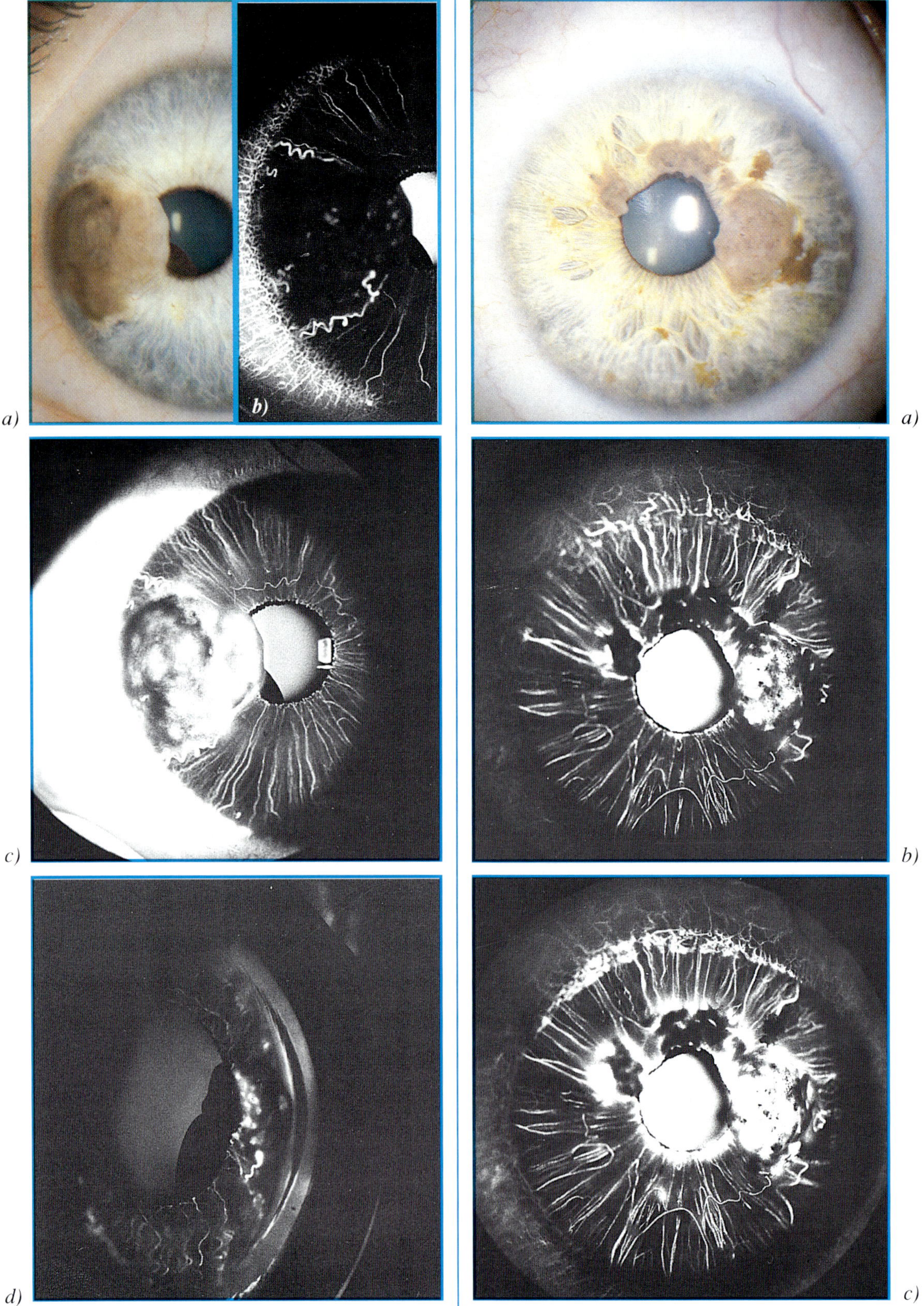

*Fig. **4.10**,30 - Biomicroscopic (a) and fluorescein angiographic (b,c) pictures of another iris melanoma. The radial vessels of the iris around the tumor are dilated and tortuous as a result of the stasis caused by the mass ("sentinel" vessels). Fluorescein angiography under pharmacological midriasis (d) shows up better the details behind the iris.*

*Fig. **4.10**,31 - When the iris melanoma is extensive (a) the fluorescein angiographic pictures (b,c) are more complex, with alternating low- and high-fluorescence areas.*

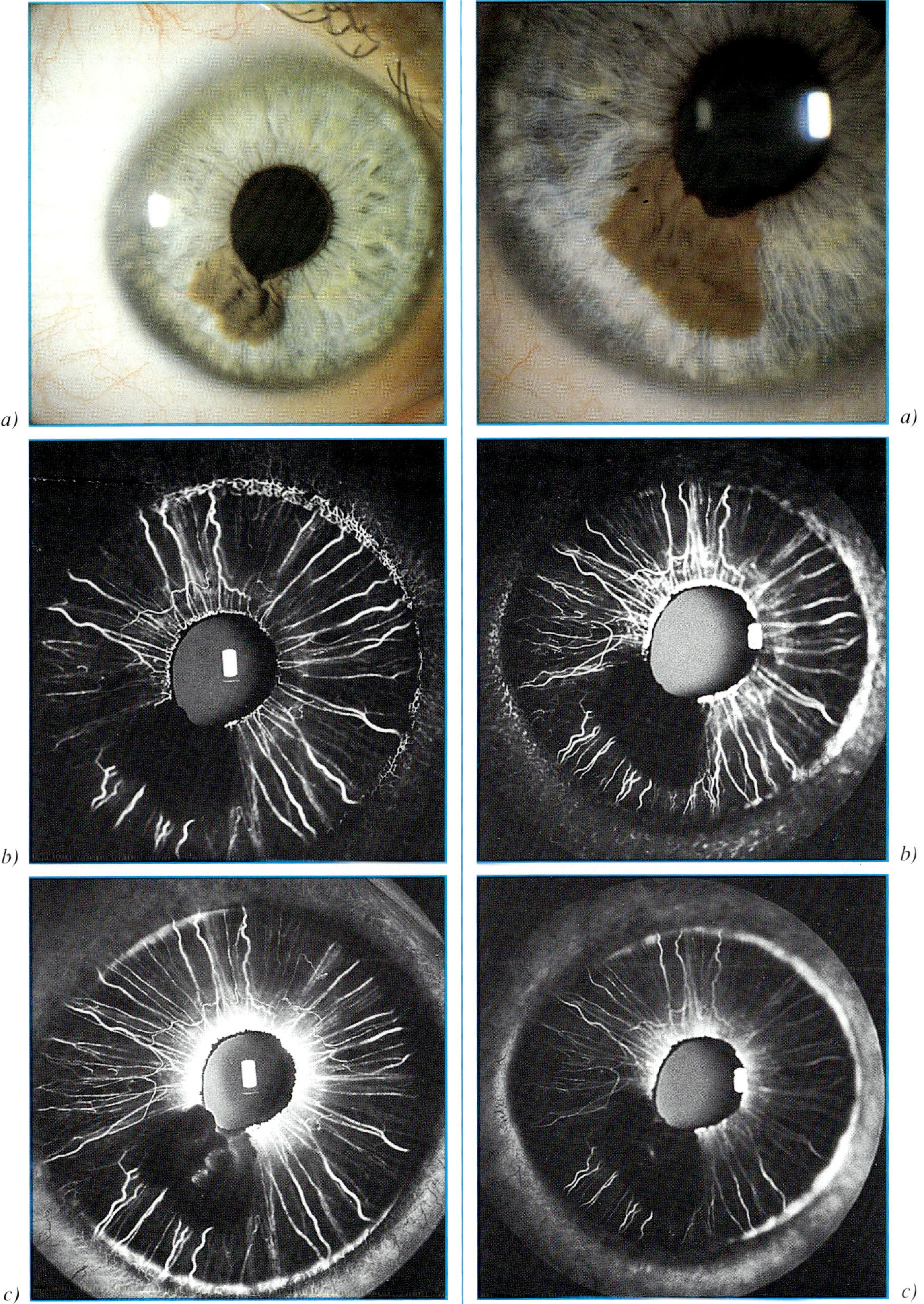

*Fig. **4.10**,32 - The excess of pigment in the mass itself (a) totally masks the tumor vascular network in the early fluorangiographic phase (b) and partially still masks it in the later phase (c). The pupillary opening is deformed and there is dye leakage at the margin.*

*Fig. **4.10**,33 - Same case as in Fig. **4.10**,32 six years later. The hyperpigmented area (a) appears bigger but its fluorescein angiographic characteristics (b,c) are still the same.*

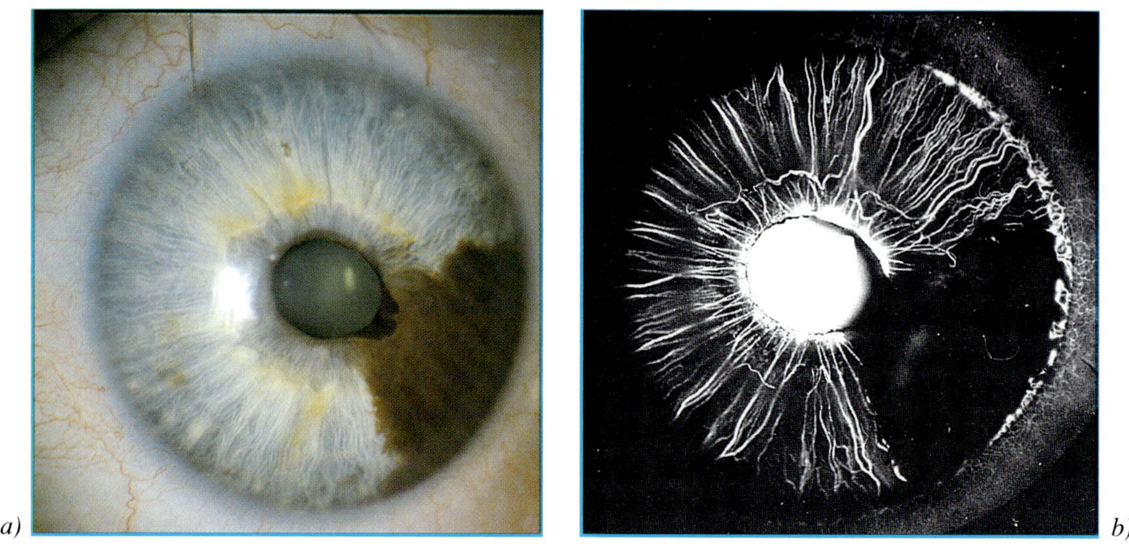

Fig. ***4.10****,34 - Pigmented neoformation of the iris (a) which on fluorescein angiographic examination (b) blocked the fluorescence. There was however late dye diffusion in the mass, which itself caused deformation of the pupillary opening and ectropion uveae.*

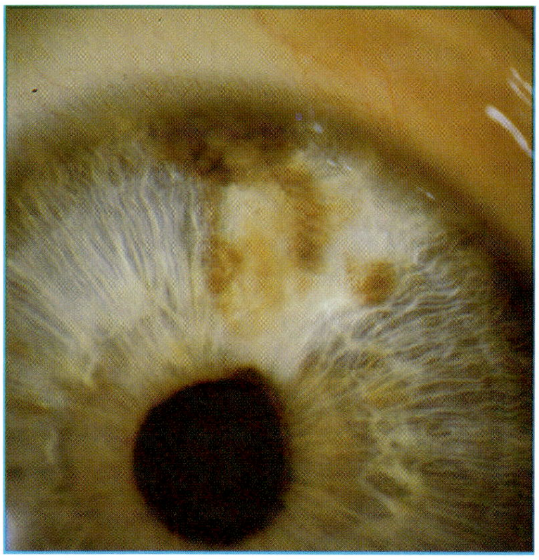

a)

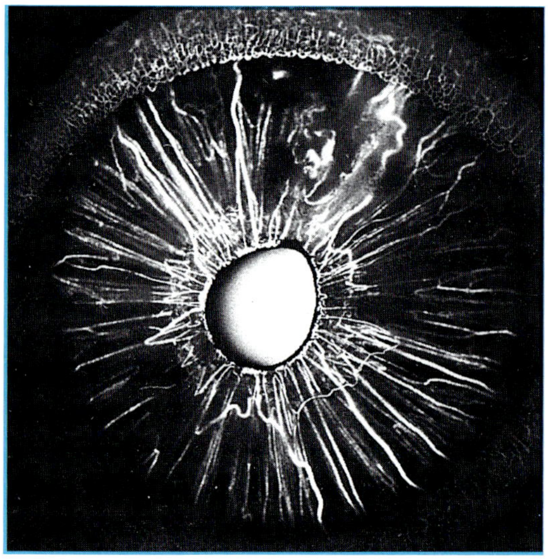

b)

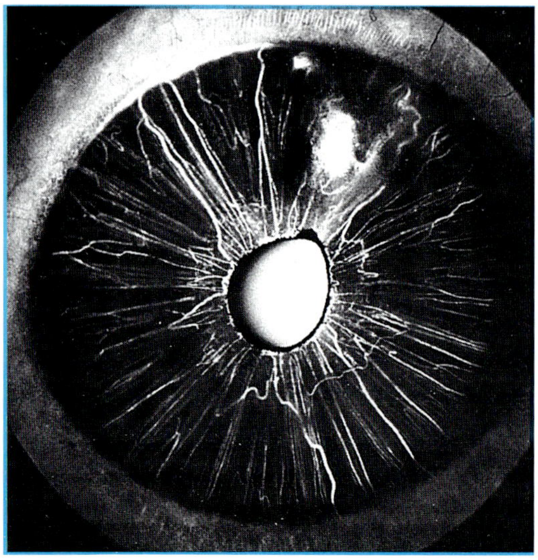

c)

Fig. ***4.10****,35 - The uneven distribution of pigment in the neoformation (a) masks the tumor fluorescence in some areas of the angiogram (b,c).*

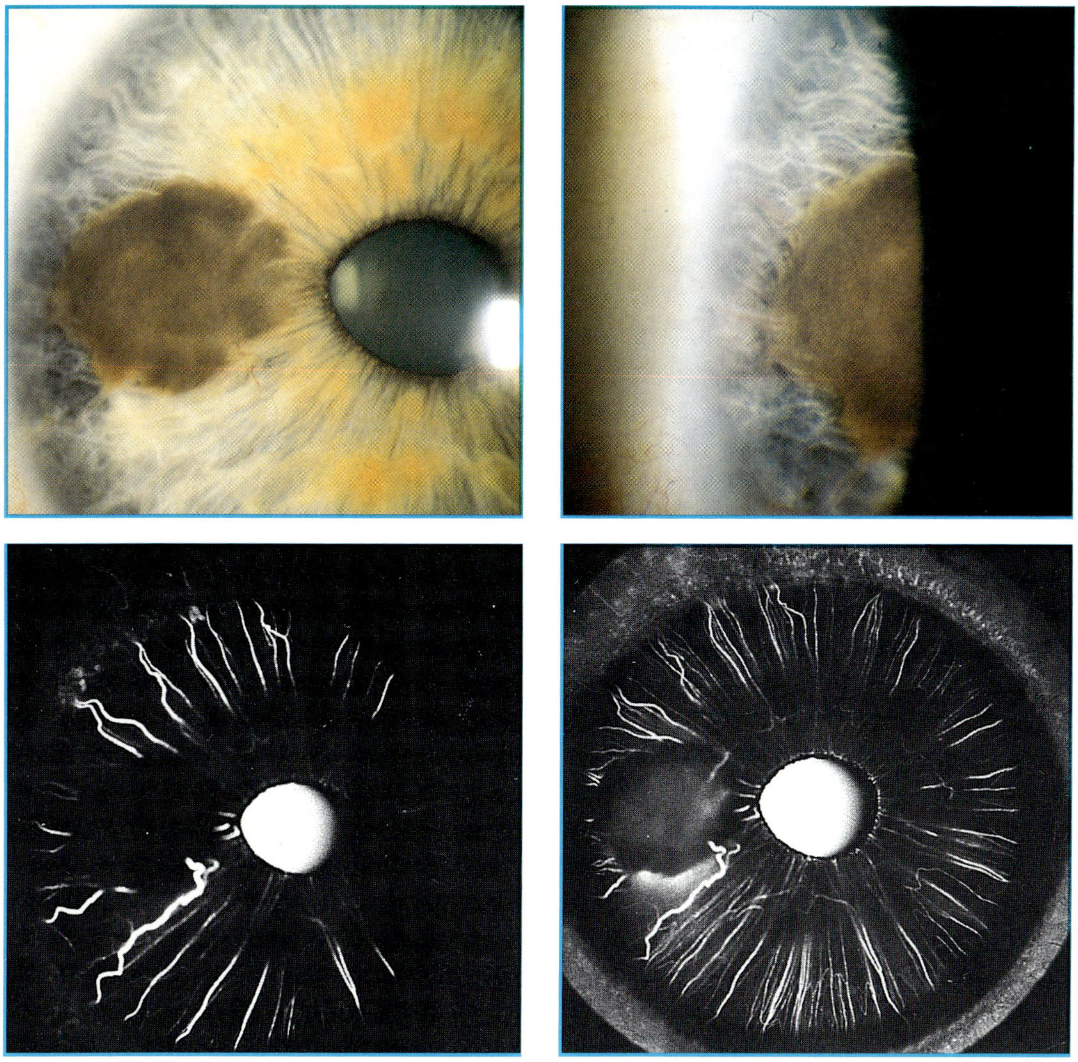

a) b)

c) d)

Fig. ***4.10****,36 - On account of the excess of pigment in the mass fluorescence is mainly visible at the periphery of the tumor and in the late phases of the angiographic examination (d). Iridography shows up the physiological nature of the peritumoral vessels which are tortuous and congested but nevertheless have the same path as the radial vessels and do not leak the dye (c,d). a,b) Color photographs.*

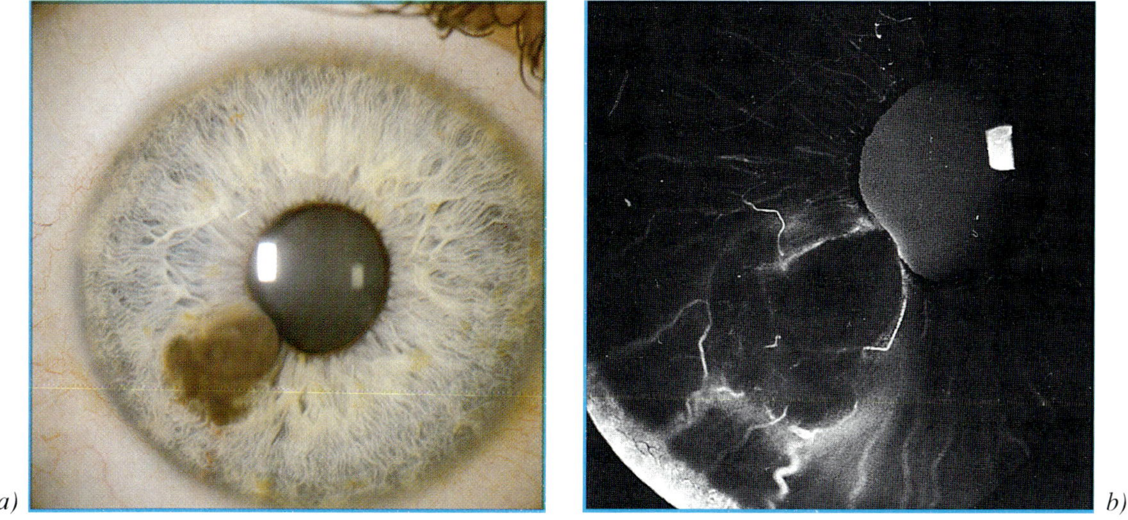

a) b)

Fig. ***4.10****,37 - In this case the excess of pigment in the neoformation (a) blocks fluorescence in the angiogram (b) and prevents the vascular network being seen. However, the fact this case presented a fluorescent ring around the hypofluorescent area points to probable malignancy. Peritumoral radial vessels appeared dilated and tortuous.*

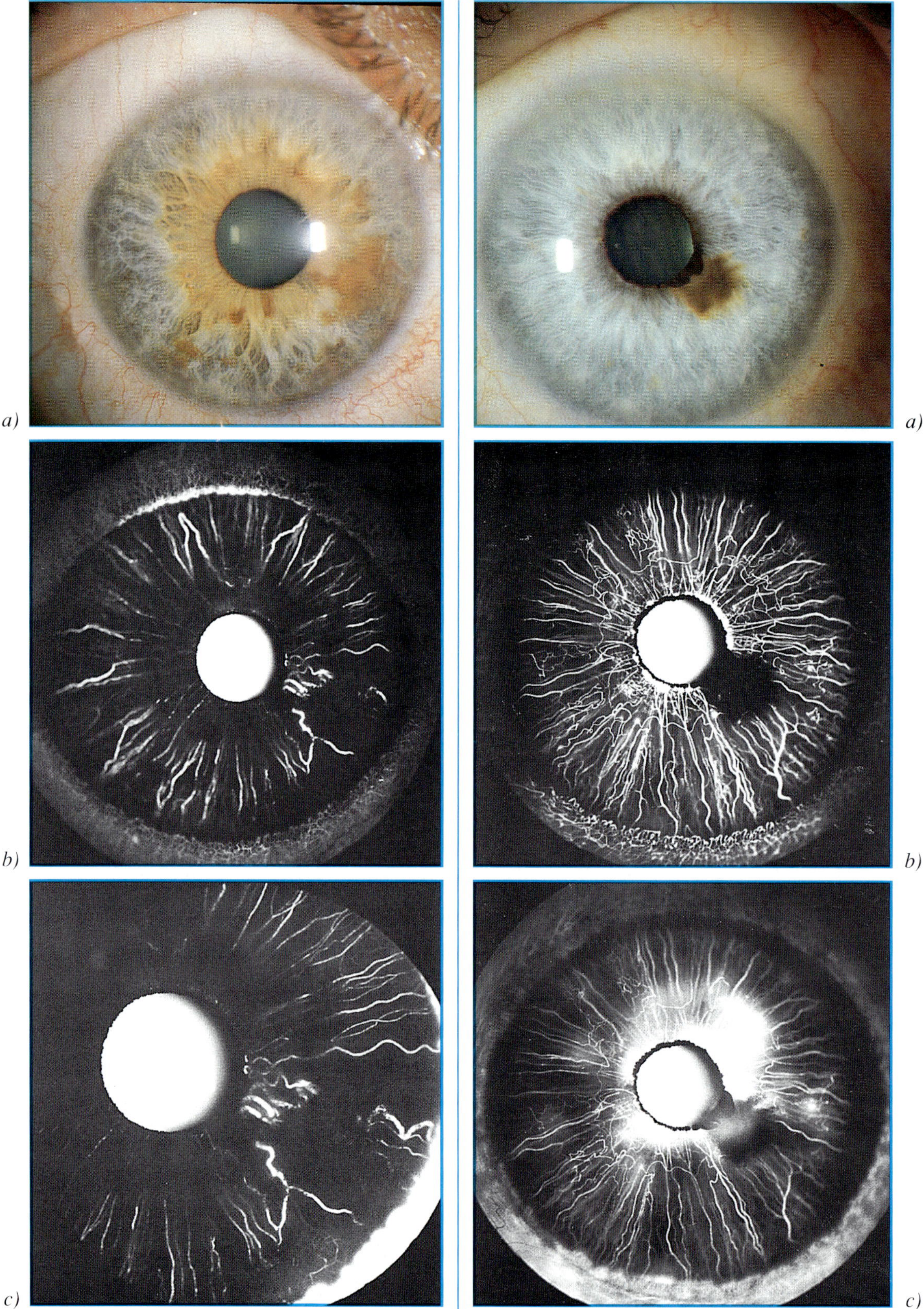

*Fig. **4.10**,38 - In this case too the iris vessels at the edges of the hypofluorescent mass (b,c) show alterations in caliber and path, and in the late phases (c) there is some dye leakage due to damage to the vessel walls resulting from the stasis induced by the tumor. a) Color photograph.*

*Fig. **4.10**,39 - Here again large amounts of pigment, visible biomicroscopically (a), block the fluorescence (b,c). Other angiographic findings are the more marked hypofluorescence at the ectropion uveae and the marked dye leakage at the pupillary margins and in the stroma, more visible in the later phases of the examination (c).*

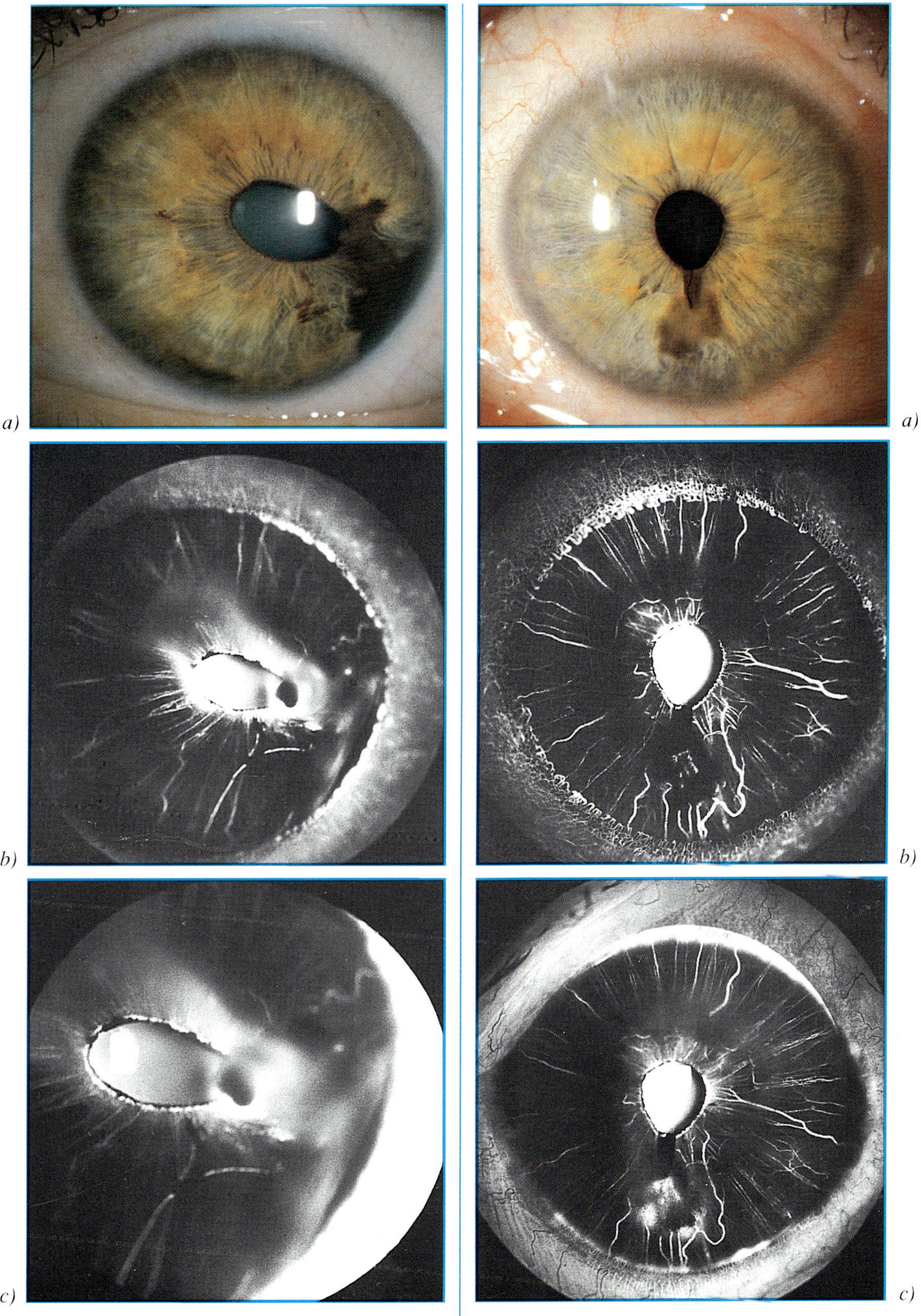

*Fig. **4.10**,40 - In this right eye the architecture of the infero-nasal quadrant of the iris is upset by the presence of the mass, best seen biomicroscopically (a). Fluorescein angiography (b, c) shows dye diffusion from the superficial vessels of the neoformation, despite the huge amount of pigment, and from vessels in the pupillary microcirculation.*

*Fig. **4.10**,41 - Biomicroscopic (a) and fluorescein angiographic pictures (b,c) of a pigmented iris neoformation, which caused ectropion uveae and damage to the surrounding vessels in the iris.*

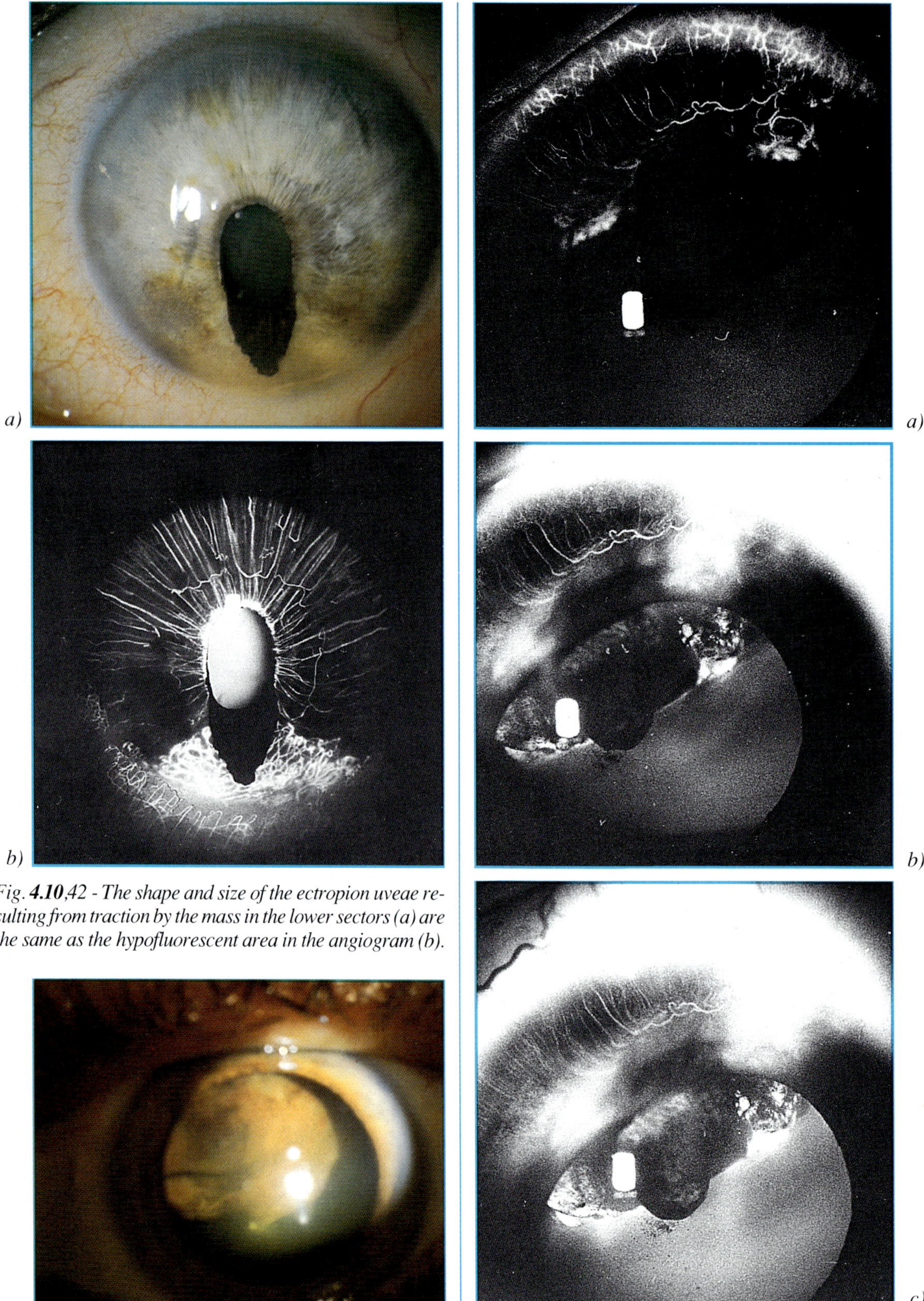

a)

b)

*Fig. **4.10**,42 - The shape and size of the ectropion uveae resulting from traction by the mass in the lower sectors (a) are the same as the hypofluorescent area in the angiogram (b).*

*Fig.**4.10**, 43 - In this case of melanoma of the ciliary body, examination under pharmacological midriasis permits better visualization.*

a)

b)

c)

*Fig. **4.10**,44 - Melanoma of the ciliary body: in the early fluorescein angiographic phase (a) dye can be seen injecting the neoformed iris vessels and the tumor vascular network from which the fluorescence leaks in the later phases (b,c).*

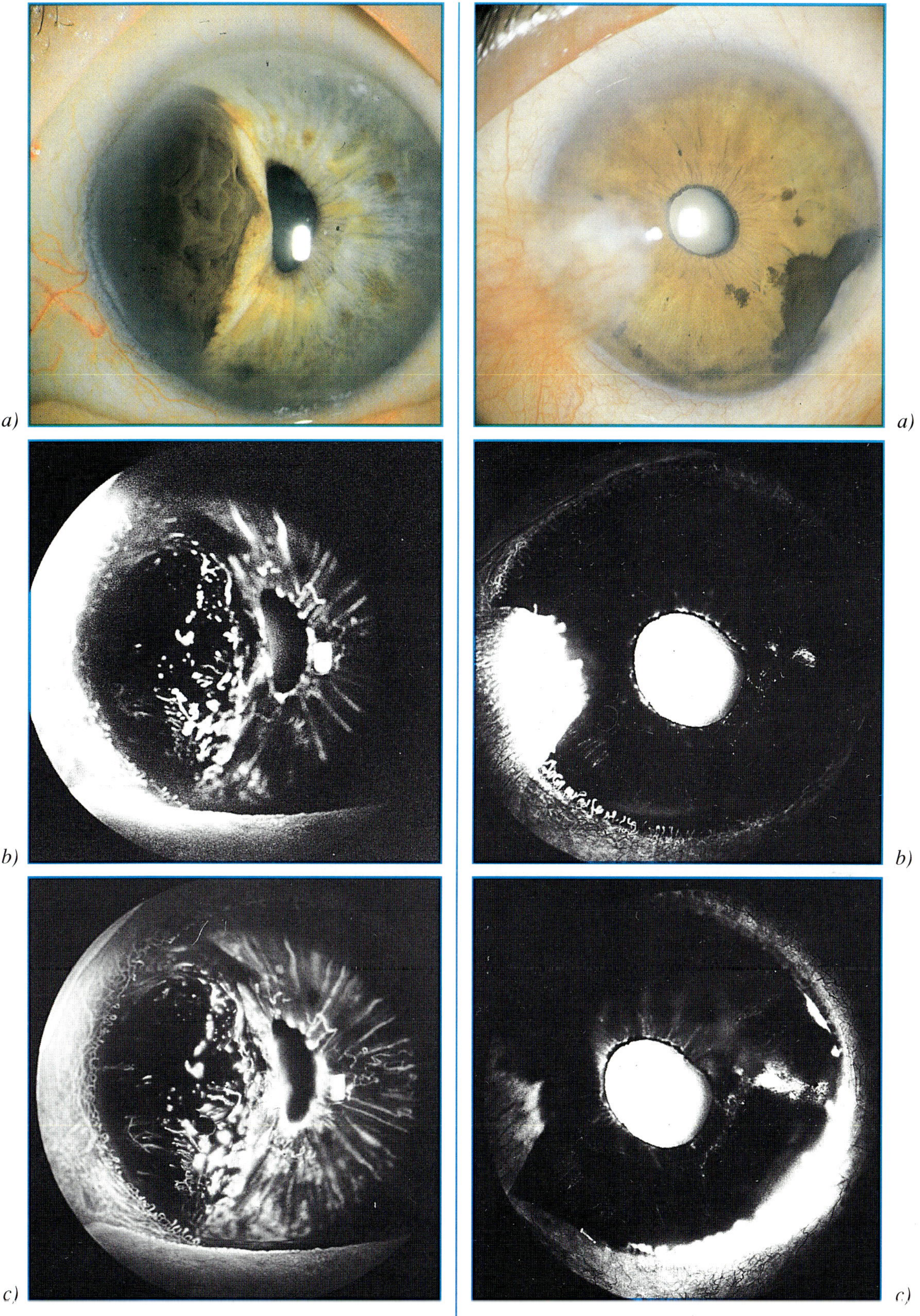

*Fig. **4.10**,45 - Fluorescein angiography (b,c) in a case of melanoma of the ciliary body going beyond the angle and invading the anterior chamber. There is early fluorescence of the tumor vessels (b), the dye leaking out later in the examination (c), with complete upheaval of the iris structure. a) Color photograph.*

*Fig. **4.10**,46 - In this case the neoformation, starting at the angle, detaches the iris and tends to invade the stroma (a). The excess of pigment masks the tumor fluorescence which is only visible at the upper edges of the mass (b,c). At the pterygium - detectable biomicroscopically (a) - there is early hyperfluorescence (b).*

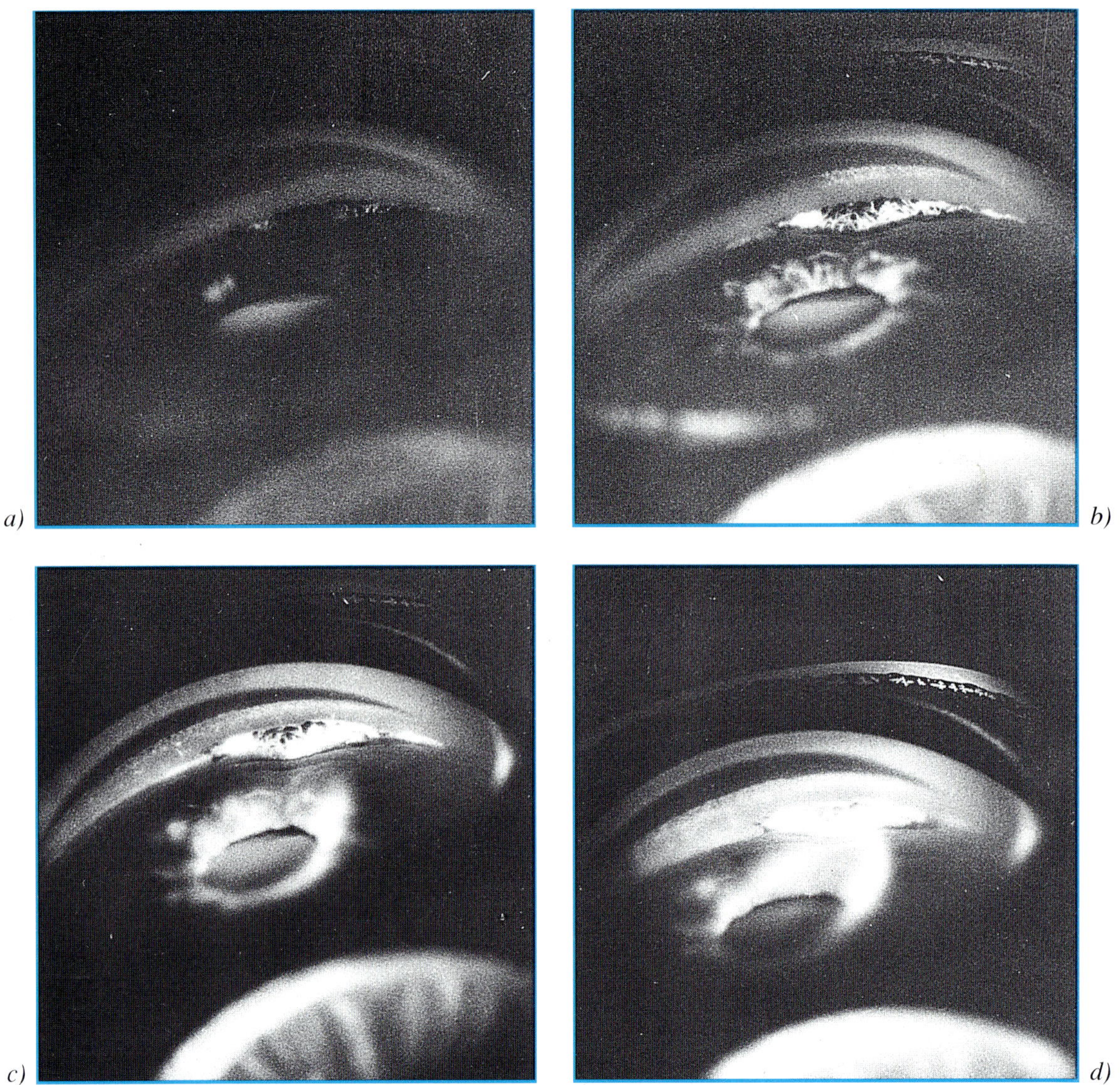

*Fig. **4.10**,47 - Fluorescein angiography done using a Goldman three-mirror lens to examine a neoformation at the angle. a, b, c, d) The various phases of the examination.*

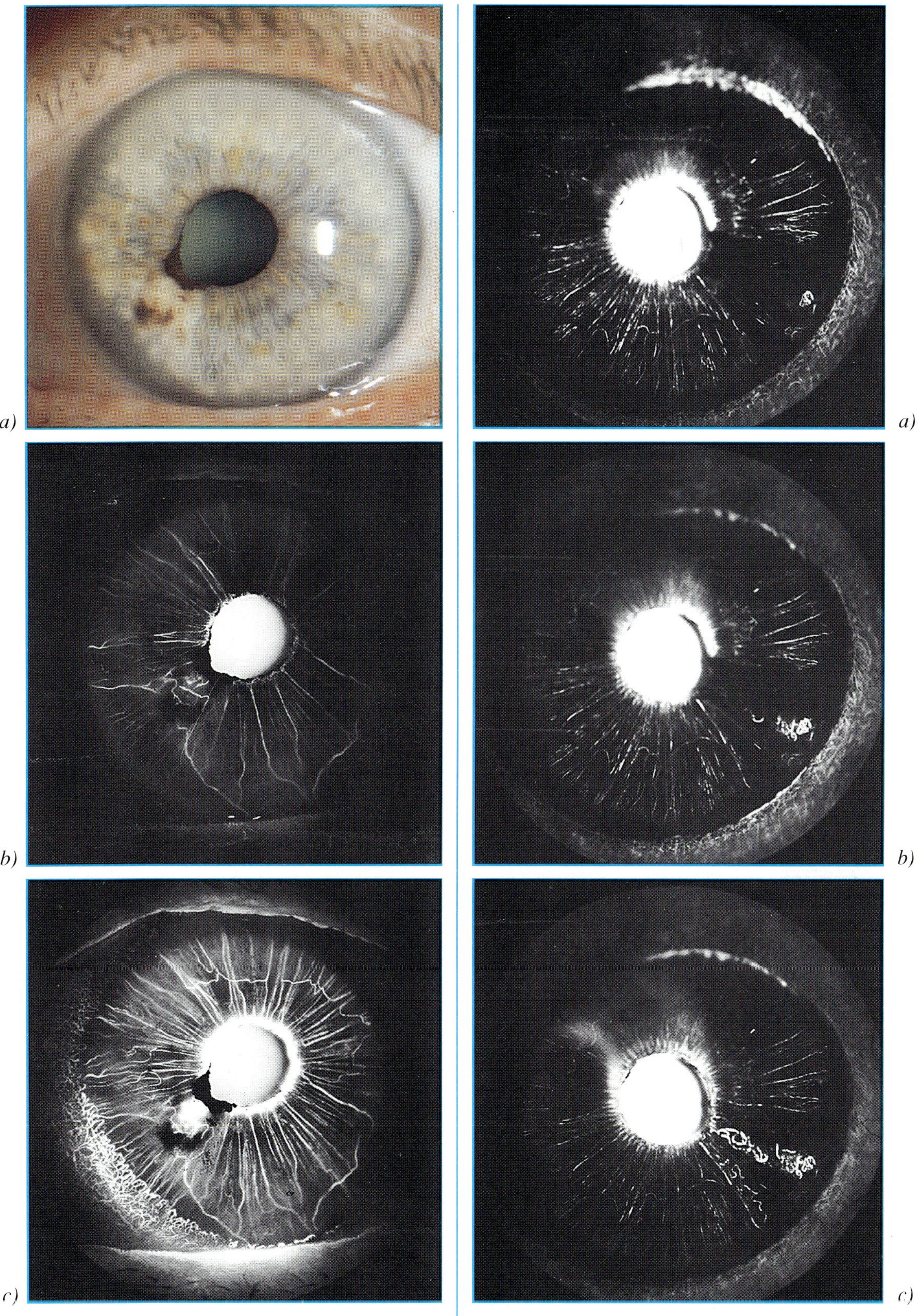

*Fig. **4.10**,48 - Biomicroscopic (a) and fluorescein angiographic (b,c) findings in a case of angiofibroma of the iris.*

*Fig. **4.10**,49 - In cases of artero-venous anastomosis a dilated, tortuous vascular trunk picks up dye in the later phases of the examination (a,b) because of slow circulation and excess of pigment; no dye leakage is seen even in the very late phases (c).*

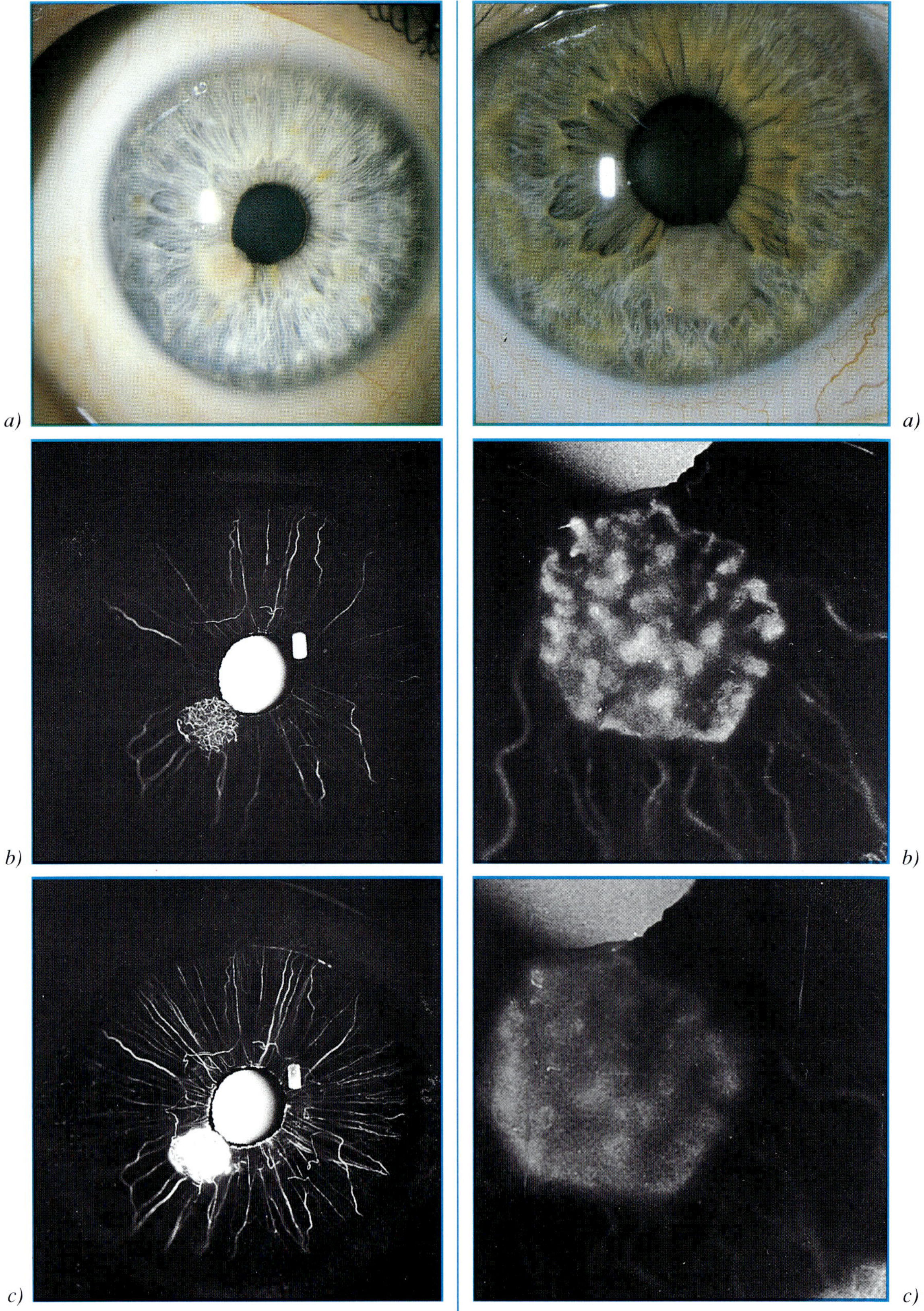

Fig. ***4.10****,50 - Typical iris leiomyoma (a) which on fluorescein angiographic examination takes up dye early in an intricate vascular network (b), followed immediately by intense dye diffusion (c).*

Fig. ***4.10****,51 - Biomicroscopic picture (a) and fluorescein angiogram (b,c) in another case of iris leiomyoma.*

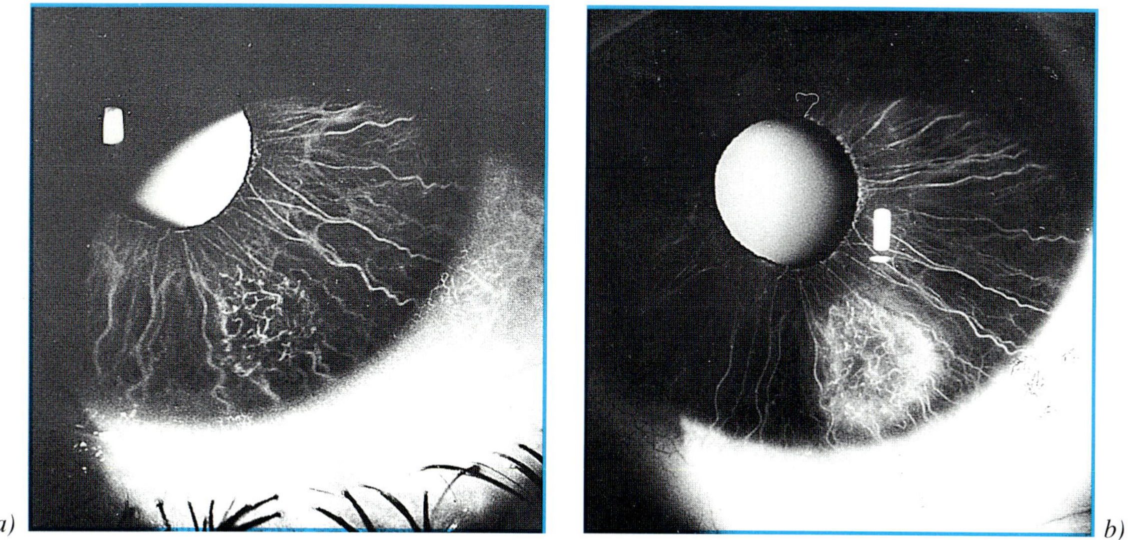

*Fig. **4.10**,52 - Neoformation of the iris with fluorescein angiographic features comparable to a leiomyoma (a,b).*

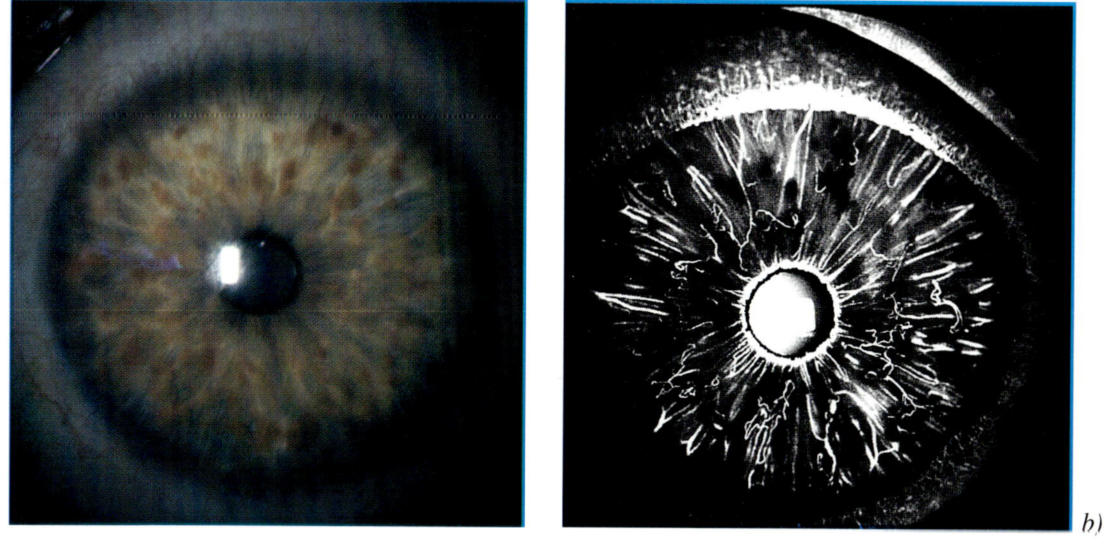

*Fig. **4.10**,53 - Biomicroscopic picture (a) and fluorescein angiogram (b) in von Recklinghausen's disease.*

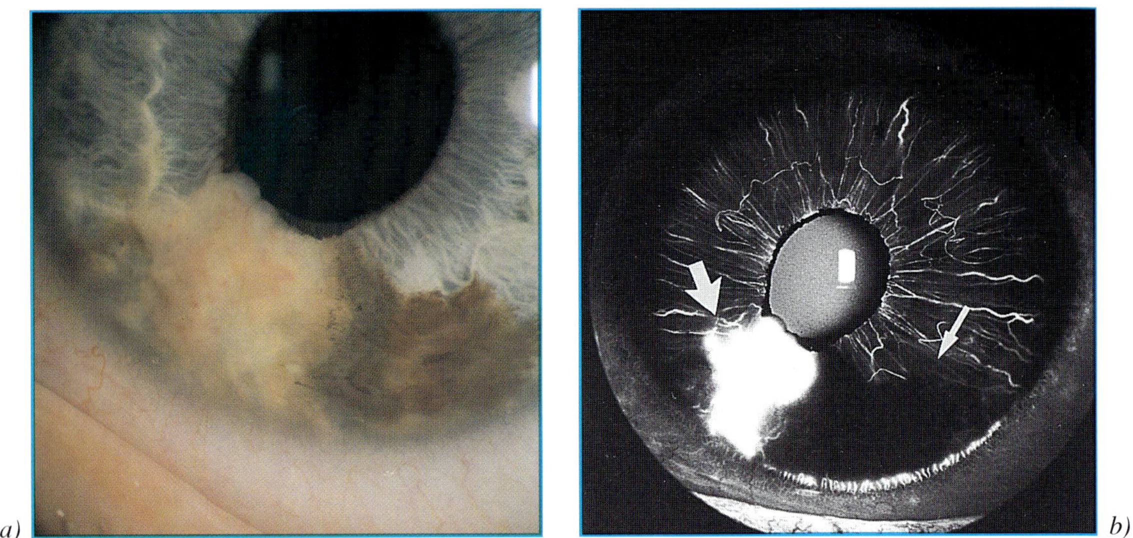

a) *b)*

Fig. ***4.10**,54 - In this case there are two neoformations with different biomicroscopic (a) and fluorescein angiographic (b) characteristics. They can be interpreted as an amelanotic mass (large arrow) and a nevus (small arrow).*

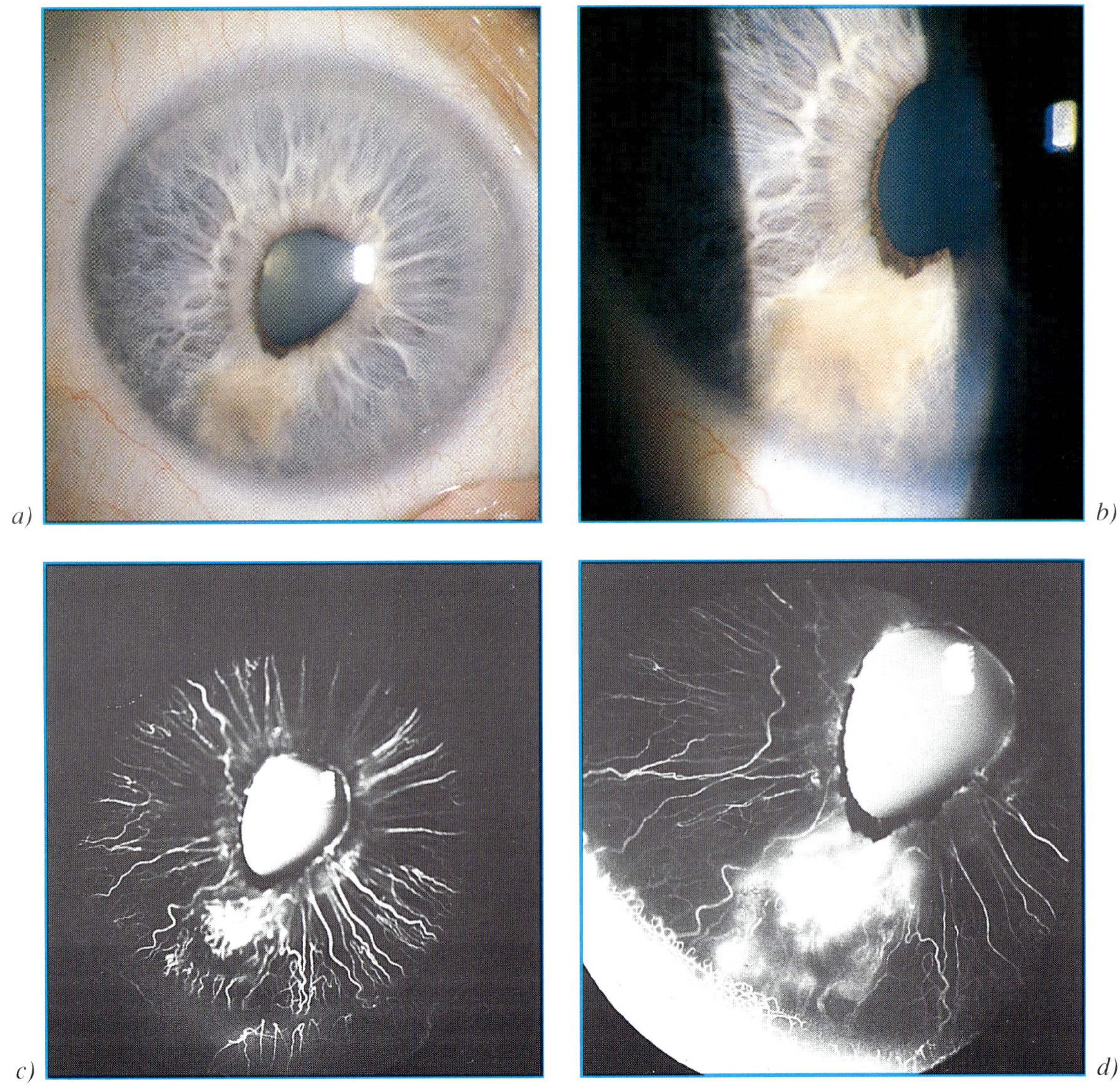

a) *b)*

c) *d)*

Fig. ***4.10**,55 - In this case of amelanotic melanoma (a,b) the lack of melanin permits a clear fluorescein angiographic view of the vascular network of the tumor, which perfuses rapidly (c) and leaks dye in the later phases (d).*

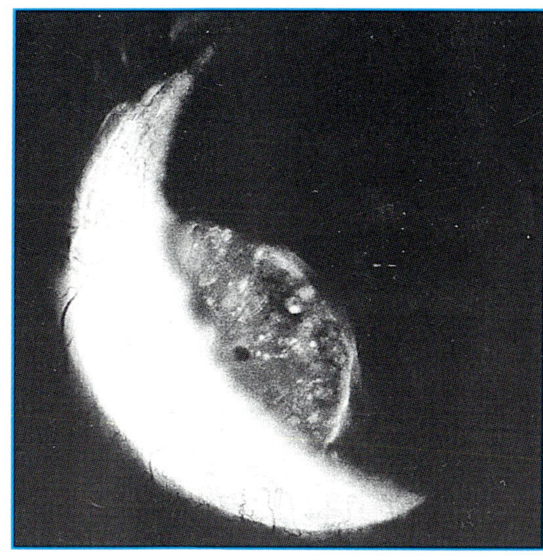

Fig. ***4.10****,56 - Metastatic adenocarcinoma of the ciliary body: iris fluorescein angiographic findings.*

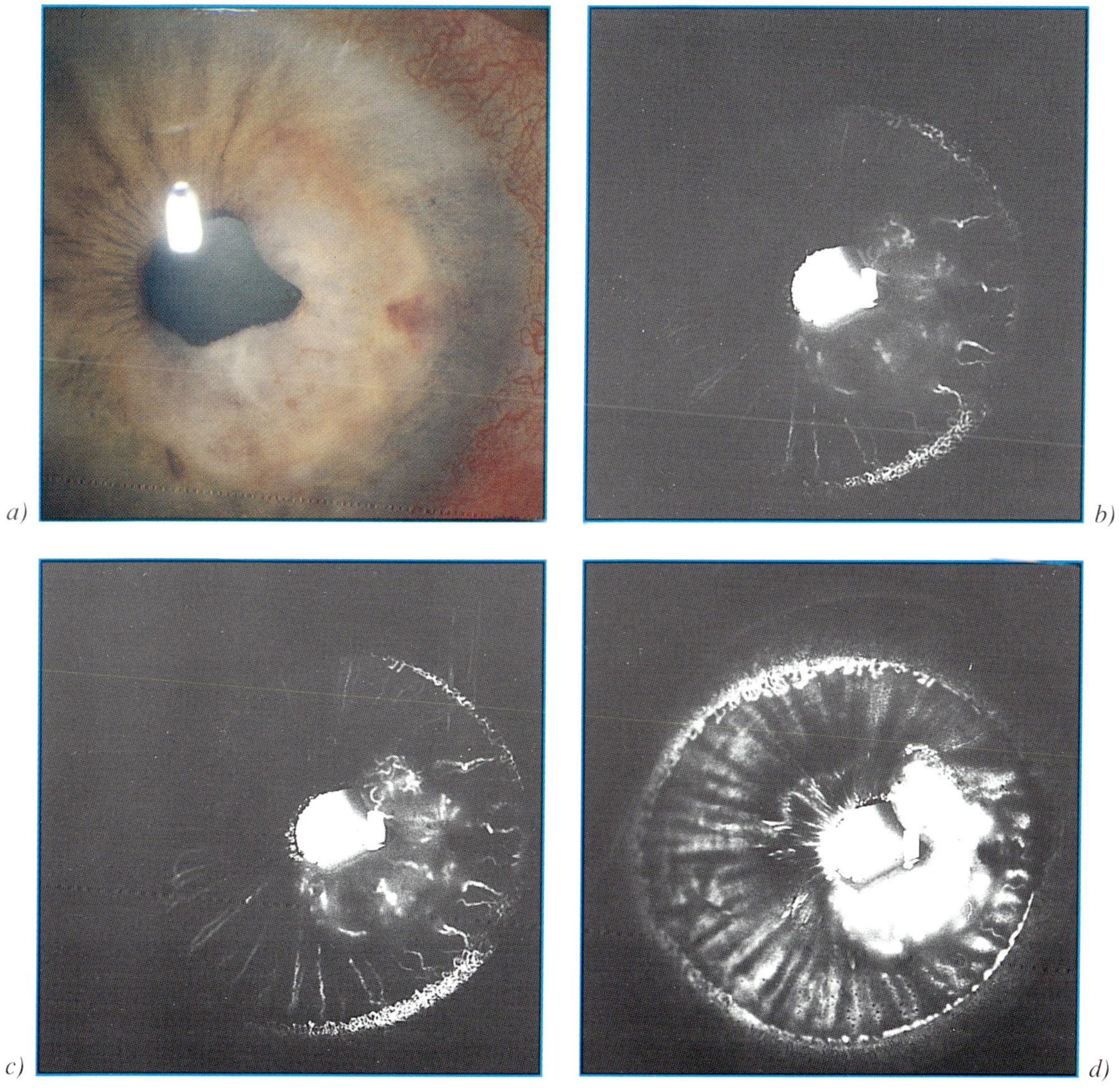

a) *b)*

c) *d)*

Fig. ***4.10****,57 - Iris mass metastatized from a primary pulmonary cancer. Biomicroscopic (a) and fluorangiographic patterns (b,c,d).*

R. Brancato, F. Bandello, R. Lattanzio
Atlas of Iris
Fluorescein Angiography
Kugler & Ghedini Publications 1995

Chapter 4.11

Traumas

The iris is one of the parts of the eye that is most frequently damaged as a consequence of bulbar lesions. The damage may be related to *blunt* or *perforating* traumas. Even minor trauma may involve the iris directly or indirectly with major effects on the dynamics and permeability of iris vessels.

Fluorescein angiography is once again useful for studying vascular damage to the iris caused by trauma.[1,2,5,6,7] Biomicroscopy alone cannot in fact always show up these alterations objectively, or follow their progress.

The wide variety of possible iris lesions depends on the type and severity of the trauma, the therapy provided and whether or not intraocular hypertension was associated. These lesions include, among others, alterations to the dynamics and site of the pupil, pupillary margin or sphincter rupture, iris rupture or lacerations, and - in the most severe cases - actual splitting of the iris, known as iridodialysis (Figs. **4.11**,1,2). Various other ocular lesions may cause indirect damage to the iris: partial or total dislocation of the lens, melting cataract secondary to laceration of the lens capsule, and blood effusion into the anterior chamber (primary or secondary traumatic hyphema).

A foreign body remaining inside the globe after a perforating lesion may cause severe problems, and the prognosis depends on the nature of the intruding article. Some become encysted and remain silent throughout the patient's lifetime; others, after some time, may give rise to inflammation; others - like ferrochrome - dissolve and the resulting metal salts infiltrate all the ocular membranes (Fig. **4.11**,3).

In relation to the time elapsed between the actual trauma and its effects, post-traumatic lesions are classified as recent and old. Iris fluorescein angiographic findings of recent traumas are not always straightforward to interpret, as there may be corneal opacity or blood in the anterior chamber (Figs. **4.11**,4,5). However, they all present dye leakage from the pupillary microvessels and from stromal vessels. The severity and extension of damage to the blood-iris barrier is generally directly proportional to the gravity of the trauma itself. This is probably a reflection of the release of substances such as prostaglandins which give rise to inflammation, causing an increase in vascular permeability. How long the blood-iris barrier is ruptured also depends on the severity of the trauma. Hyperpermeability may last a few hours or several days. There must be no permanent anatomical damage if the blood-iris barrier is to heal.

More serious contusive trauma may cause alterations to the dynamics of the iris circulation, detected as filling delays, mainly in the upper parts of the iris. There may occasionally be areas of actual nonperfusion, where the vascular damage is serious enough to have broken off the circulation.

A perforating trauma to the iris may cause a variety of damage: dialysis, pupillary displacement, synechiae with the corneal endothelium, the lens or at the angle. Iris fluorescein angiographic findings in such cases, when the damage is recent, are normally dominated by signs of inflammation: there is widespread rupture of the blood-iris barrier with dye leakage from radial vessels and from the pupillary border. In cases with iridodialysis the circulation is always interrupted at some point. Generally such cases present filling delays in the sectors below the split and, in later phases, some hyperfluorescence around it (Fig. **4.11**,6).

In patients with old wounds from blunt trauma iris fluorescein angiography may be useful to check whether the blood-iris barrier is still broken, and whether there are zones in the iris where vascular filling is delayed or lacking. In cases presenting intraocular hypertension secondary to the trauma, these angiographic signs may be more marked (Figs.**4.11**,7,8).

In old perforating trauma cases with pupillary ectopia and breakage of the iris, the normal vascular lay-out becomes distorted, taking a different pattern depending on the new morphology of the iris. In certain cases the changes in circulation needed to adapt to the new situation may be clear: some stromal vessels which, judging from their position, should certainly be considered arteries, fill retrogradely and take longer than normal to do so. In other cases the blood-iris barrier is still broken, indicating that the globe is still in an unbalanced state. Sometimes there may be areas of nonperfusion and neovascularization (Figs. **4.11**,9-20).

Another important point in these cases is the likelihood of sympathetic ophthalmia (see chapter on Uveitis). Iris fluorescein angiography is useful in such cases as it shows up any problems in the undamaged eye early. There may be varying degrees of rupture of the blood-iris barrier and sometimes inflammation may persist in the originally healthy eye even after enucleation of the injured one. Fluorescein angiography is therefore useful not just for assessing the state of healing of the traumatized eye - it is also a means of monitoring the uninjured eye, giving prompter and more detailed information than biomicroscopic examination.

In our experience, the iris fluorescein angiographic examination gives extremely useful information for scheduling surgery and deciding on the best approach to deal with traumas. The angiograms provide a basis for assessing the inflammation, the state of balance achieved, the patency of vessels in the membrane, adhesions, and scars that the trauma may have left.

References

1 Bechetoille A, Chabanais JL, Jallet G: Contusion et permeabilité de la barriere hematoaqueuse à la fluorescéine. J Fr Ophtalmol 1: 129, 1978.

2 Brancato R, Menchini U, Carnevalini A: Atlante di iridografia a fluorescenza. C.I.C. Ed Int Gruppo Ed Medico, Roma, 1981.

3 Chan CC, Benezra D, Hsu SM: Granulomas in sympathetic ophthalmia and sarcoidosis. Immunohistochemical study. Arch Ophthalmol 103: 198, 1985.

4 Font RL, Fine BS, Messmer E: Light and electron microscopic study of Dalen-Fuchs nodules in sympathetic ophthalmia. Ophthalmology 90: 66, 1983.

5 Kottow MH: Anterior segment fluorescein angiography. William & Wilkins, Baltimore, 1978.

6 Menchini U, Carnevalini A, Scialdone A et al: Aspetti fluoroiridografici dei traumi bulbari. Clin Oc 4: 310, 1984.

7 Musso M, Brovia P, Coggi G: Fluorangiografia dell'iride negli oftalmocontusi. Atti LX Congresso Società Italiana Oftalmologia, Roma. Cappelli Ed, Bologna, 1980.

8 Rao NA, Marak GE: Sympathetic ophthalmia simulating Vogt-Kojanagi-Harada's disease: a clinicopathologic study of four cases. Jpn J Ophthalmol 27: 506, 1983.

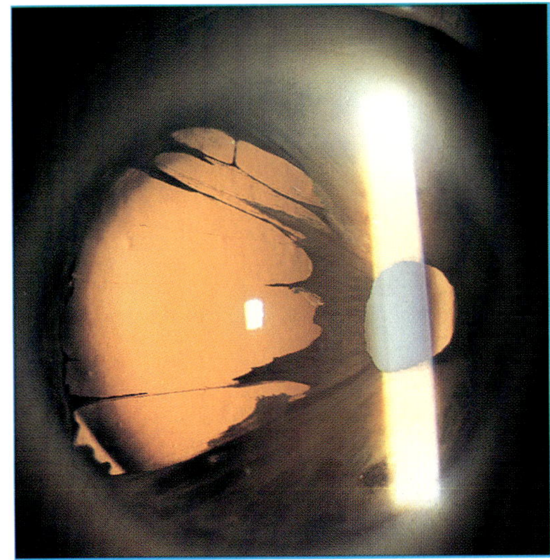

*Fig. **4.11**,1 - Biomicroscopy with retroillumination in a case of massive post-traumatic iridodialysis. In the areas of separation the iris is lacerated and retracted; a few fine strands of iris are stretched across the gap.*

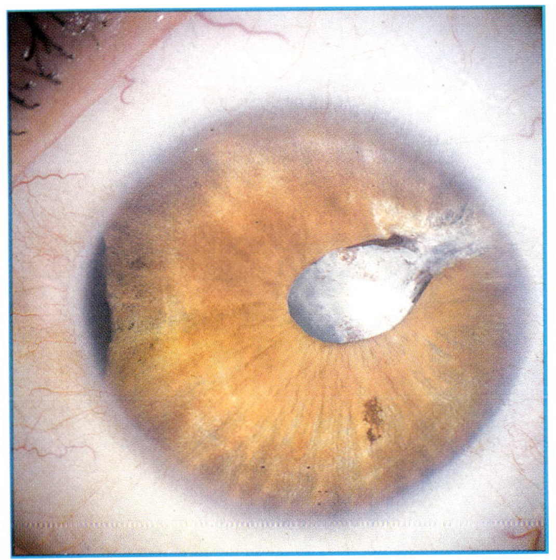

a)

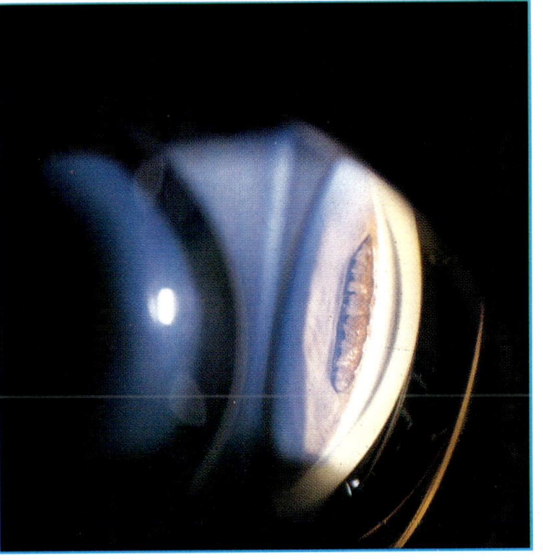

b)

*Fig. **4.11**,2 - Biomicroscopy (a) in a case of old trauma. The traumatic cataract can be seen with an iridocorneal strand at 2 o'clock and a corresponding ample area of atrophy on the iris, pupillary deformation and iridodialysis at the 9 o'clock position. Gonioscopy (b) shows up the ciliary bodies through the separated portion of the iris.*

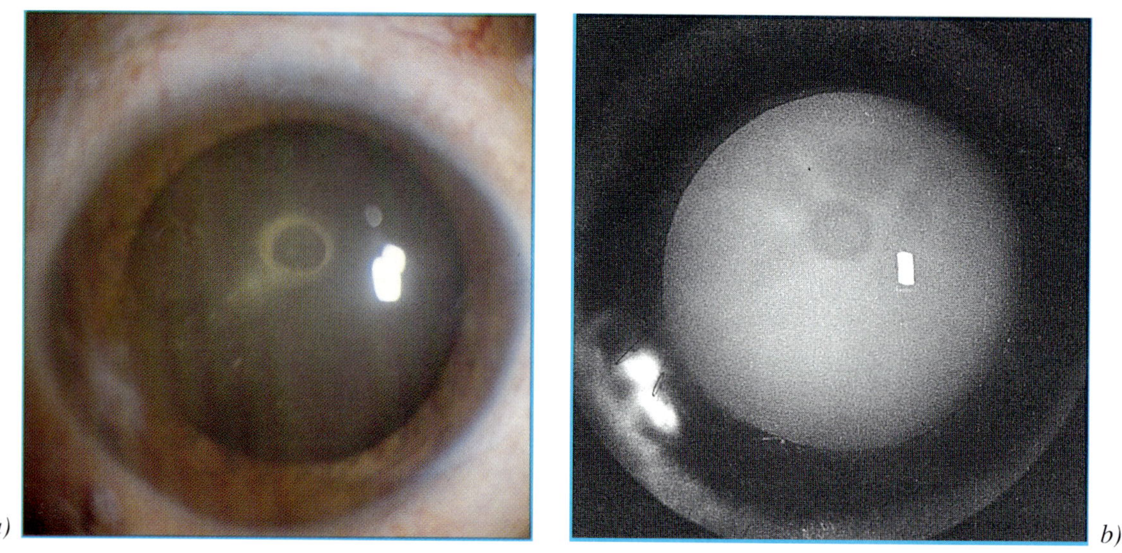

*Fig. **4.11**,3 - Biomicroscopy in mydriasis (a) in a case of perforating trauma with a retained intraocular foreign body (iron rifle shot). Fluorescein angiography (b) shows hyperfluorescence in the 8 o'clock position around the scar. Permeability of the iris vessels looks virtually normal.*

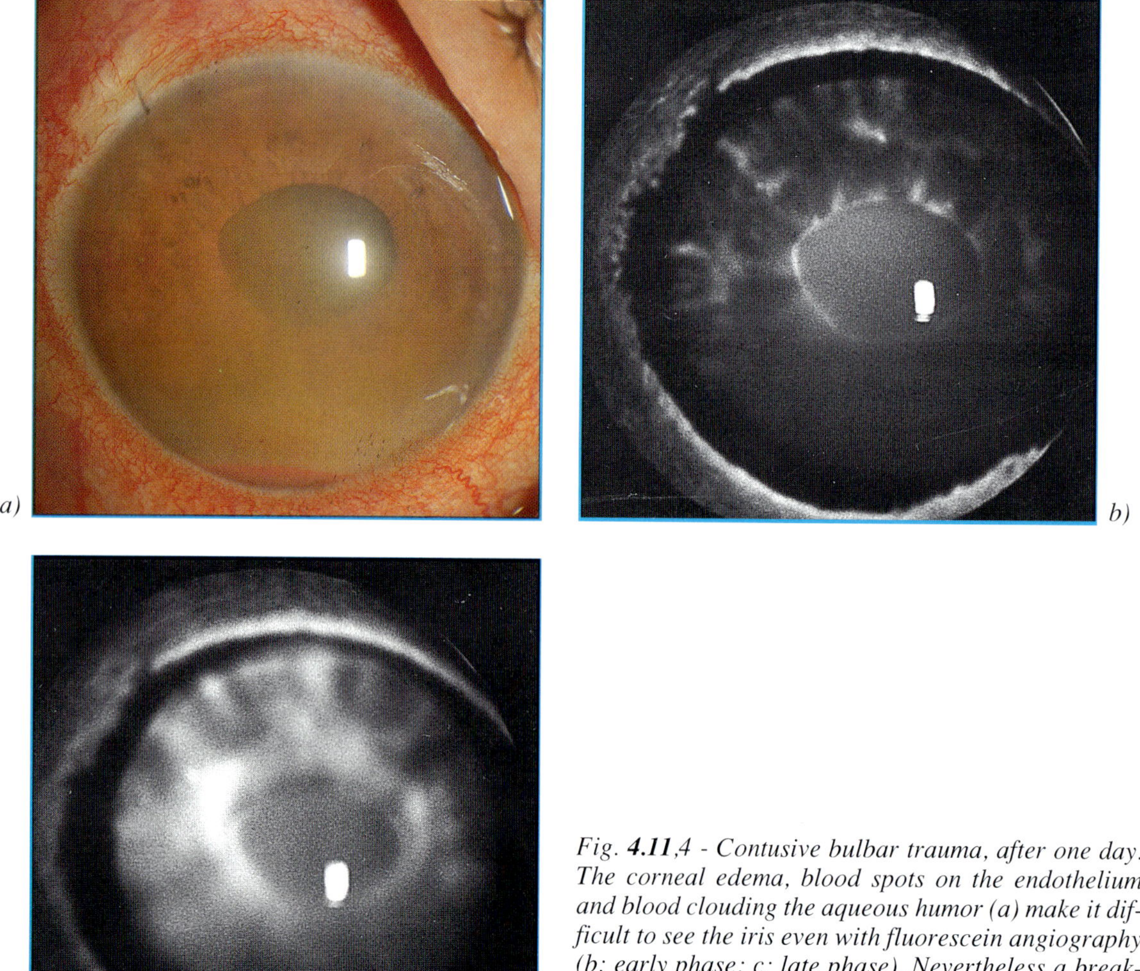

*Fig. **4.11**,4 - Contusive bulbar trauma, after one day. The corneal edema, blood spots on the endothelium and blood clouding the aqueous humor (a) make it difficult to see the iris even with fluorescein angiography (b: early phase; c: late phase). Nevertheless a breakdown can be seen in the blood-iris barrier, involving stromal vessels as well, and giving rise to diffuse paravascular leakage which becomes more marked in later phases.*

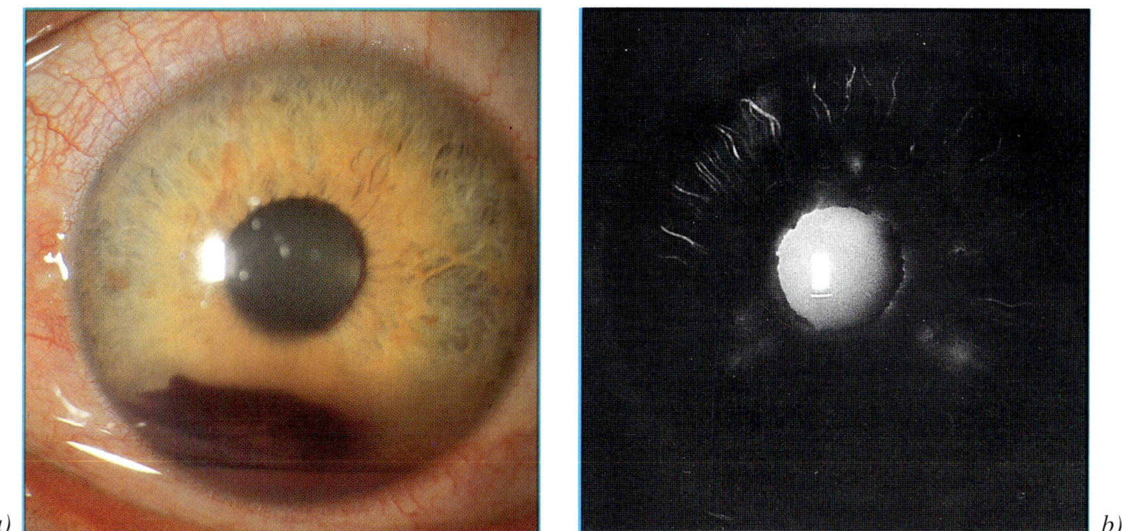

Fig. ***4.11****,5 - Post-traumatic hyphemà visible with the biomicroscope (a) makes it impossible with fluorescein angiography (b) to see the radial vessels in the lower sectors of the iris. Hyperfluorescent spots are visible in the sectors not covered by blood, indicating localized areas of increased vascular permeability.*

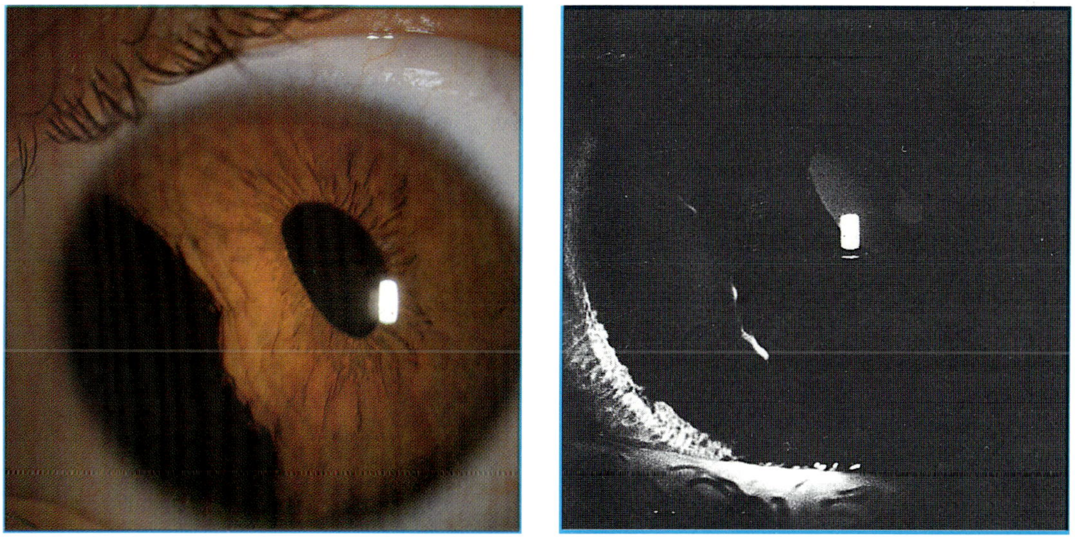

a) b)

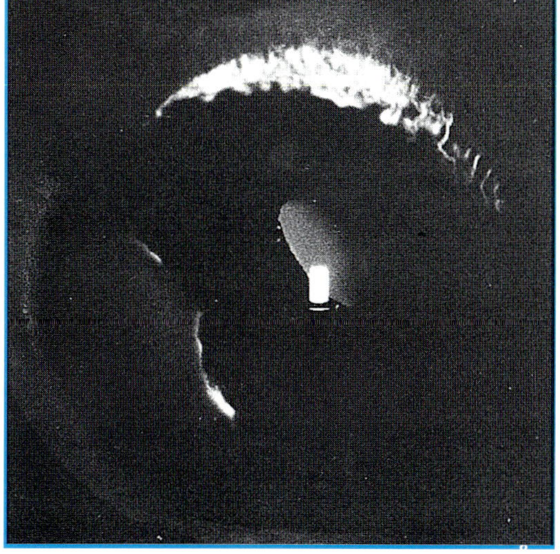

c)

Fig. ***4.11****,6 - Post-traumatic iridodialysis (a). Fluorescein angiography (b,c) shows that permeability of the iris vessels is within normal limits (globe quiescent). There is slight hyperfluorescence along the edges of the split.*

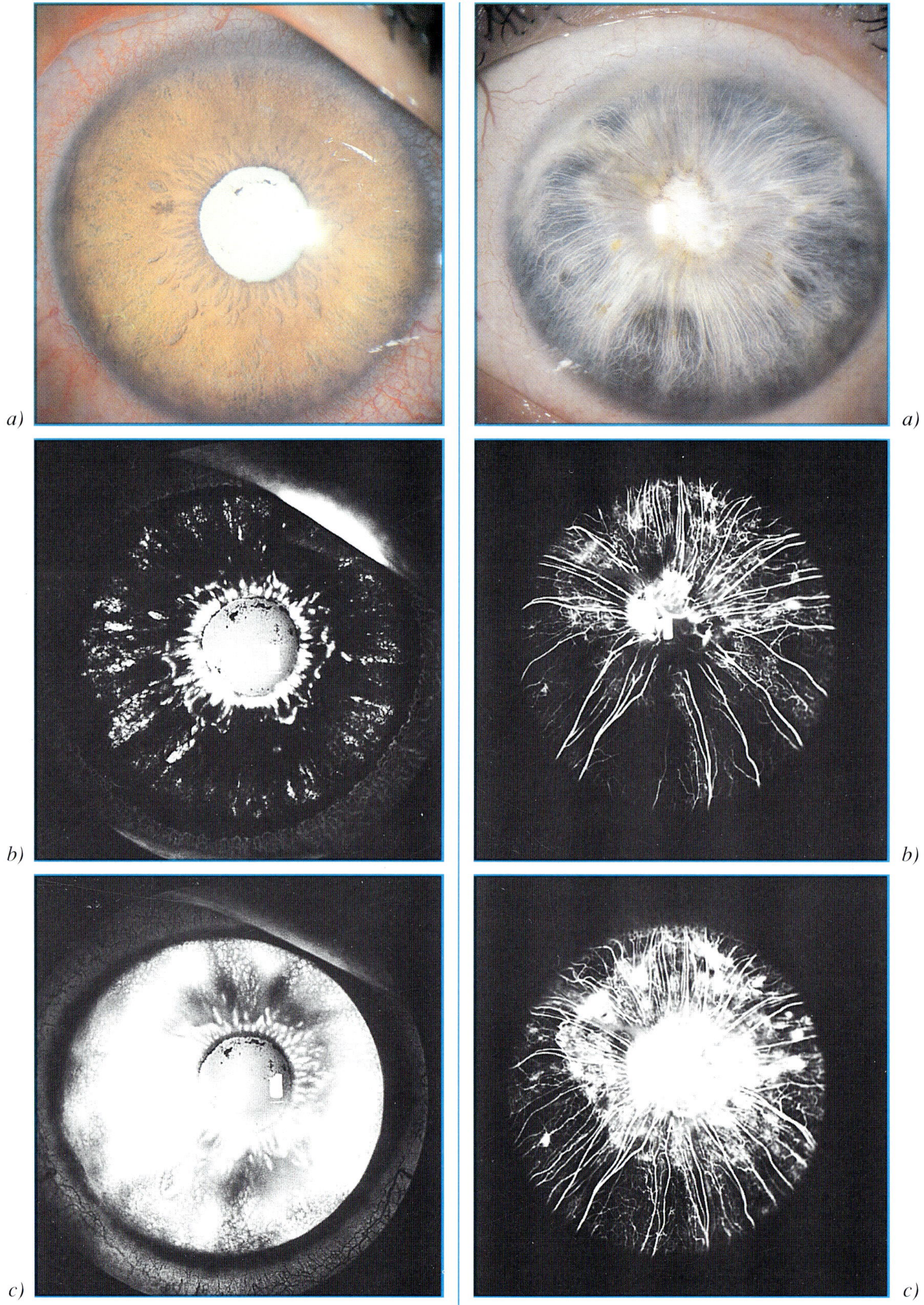

*Fig. **4.11**,7 - Cataract due to old contusive trauma: biomicroscopic picture (a). The concomitant ocular hypertension explains why, even after so much time, there is still marked rupture of the blood-iris barrier in the pupillary and ciliary vessels (b,c).*

*Fig. **4.11**,8 - Post-traumatic cataract and pupillary occlusion (a: biomicroscopy). Iris angiography phases (b,c) show details of the new-formed iris vessels even in the pupil area.*

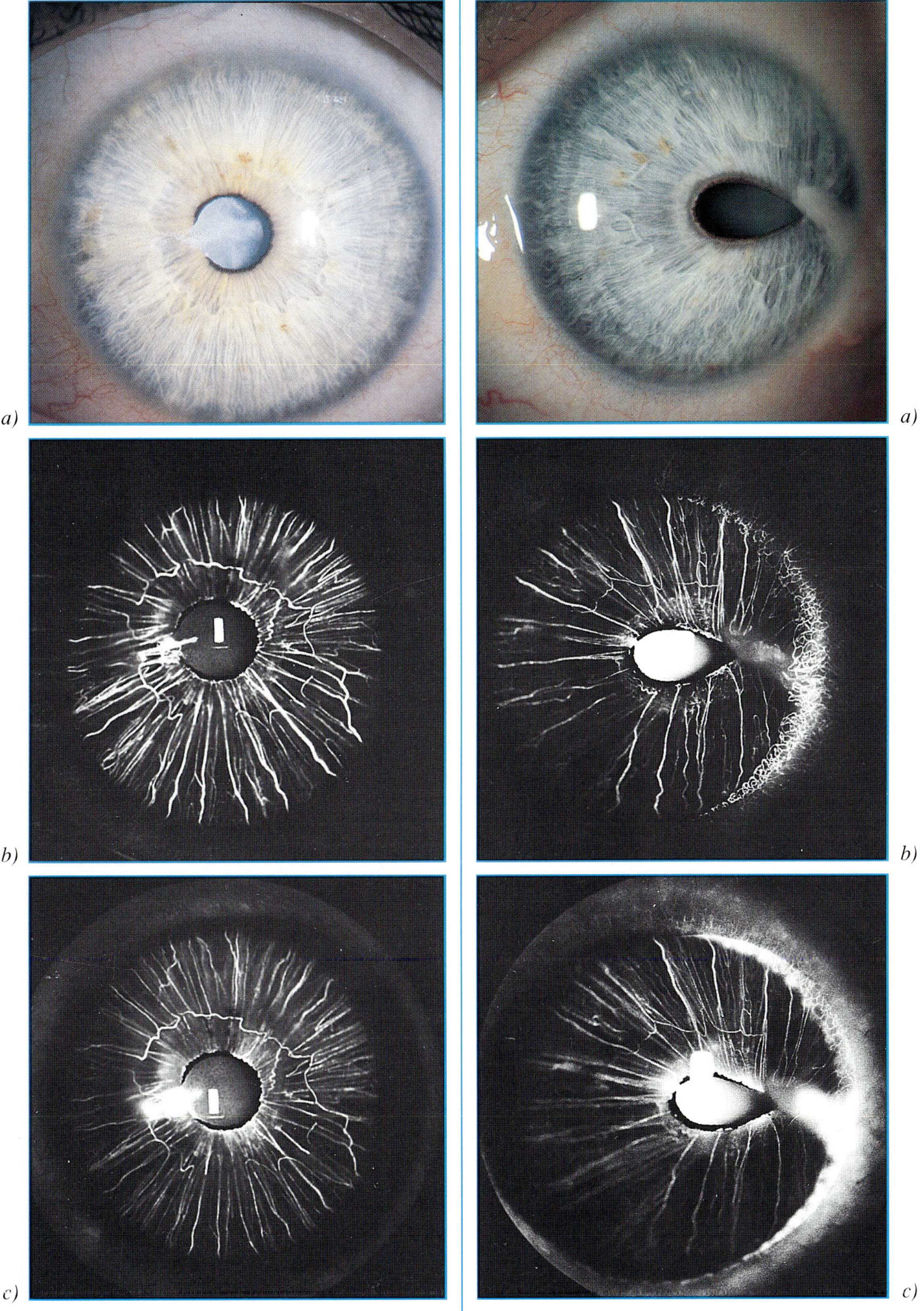

Fig. ***4.11****,9 - Traumatic cataract with scarring involving the cornea, iris and lens: biomicroscopy (a). Iris angiography (b,c) shows that vascular permeability is within normal limits. Dye leakage, increasing with subsequent phases, corresponds to the area of scarring.*

Fig. ***4.11****,10 - Post-traumatic iridocorneal adhesions causing stretching and pupillary ectopia (a: biomicroscopy). Fluorescein angiography (b,c) shows dye accumulating and leaking from the strand. Vascular permeability is increased, especially in the pupillary portion.*

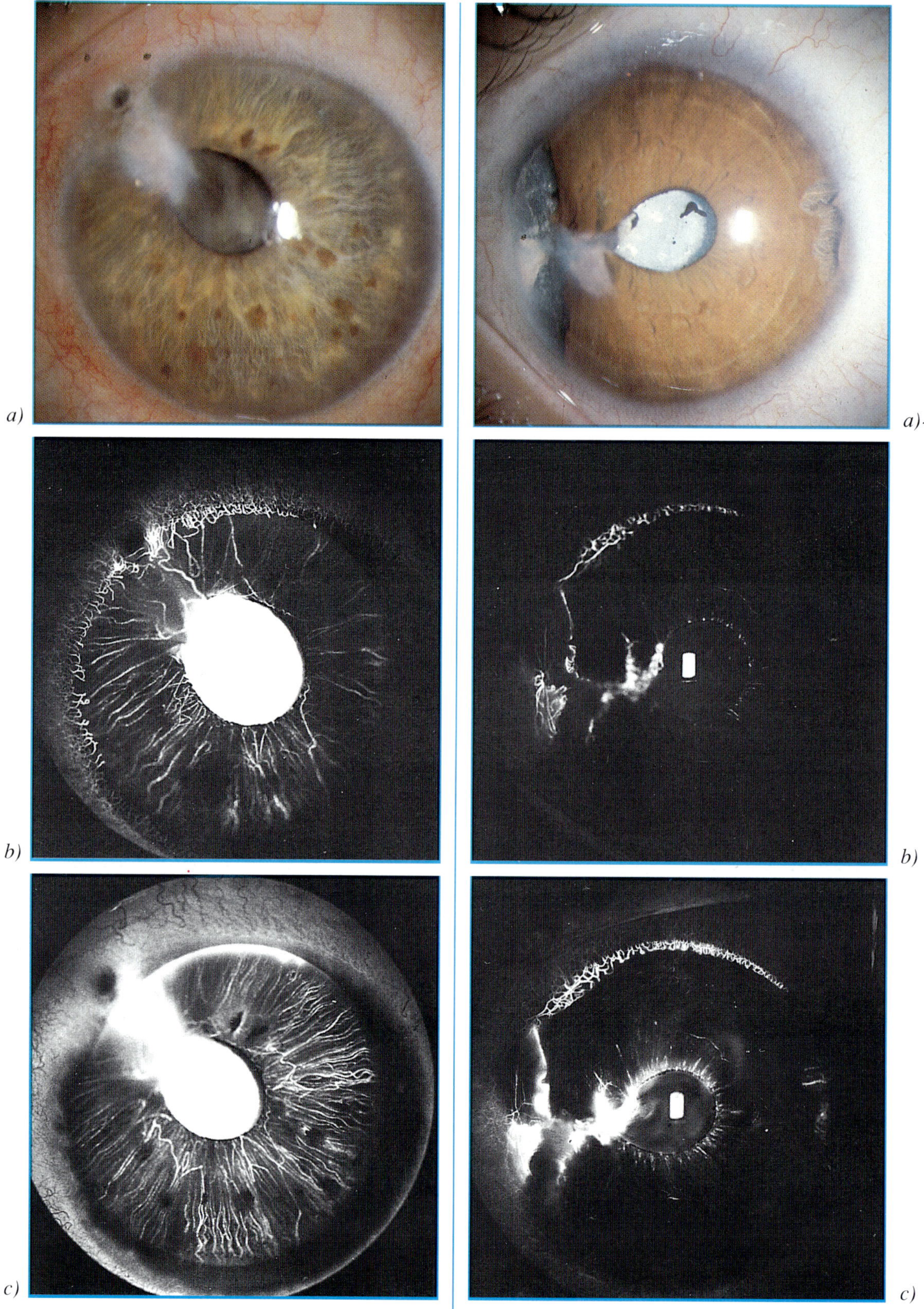

Fig. ***4.11****,11 - Biomicroscopy (a) in another case of perforating trauma. The hole where the foreign body entered the eye can be seen in the 11 o'clock position. The position, path, diameter and permeability of vessels in the corresponding sector of the iris can all be seen to be altered on fluorescein angiographic examination (b,c). Dye accumulates at the iridocorneal fibrous strand.*

Fig. ***4.11****,12 - Biomicroscopy (a) and early (b) and late (c) fluorescein angiography. In this case the trauma has produced corneal scarring, iridodialysis, iridocorneal and iridolenticular adhesions, pupillary deformation and cataract. Hyperfluorescence, increasing in subsequent phases of the examination, can be seen around the scar, the retracted iris and at the edges of the iridodialysis.*

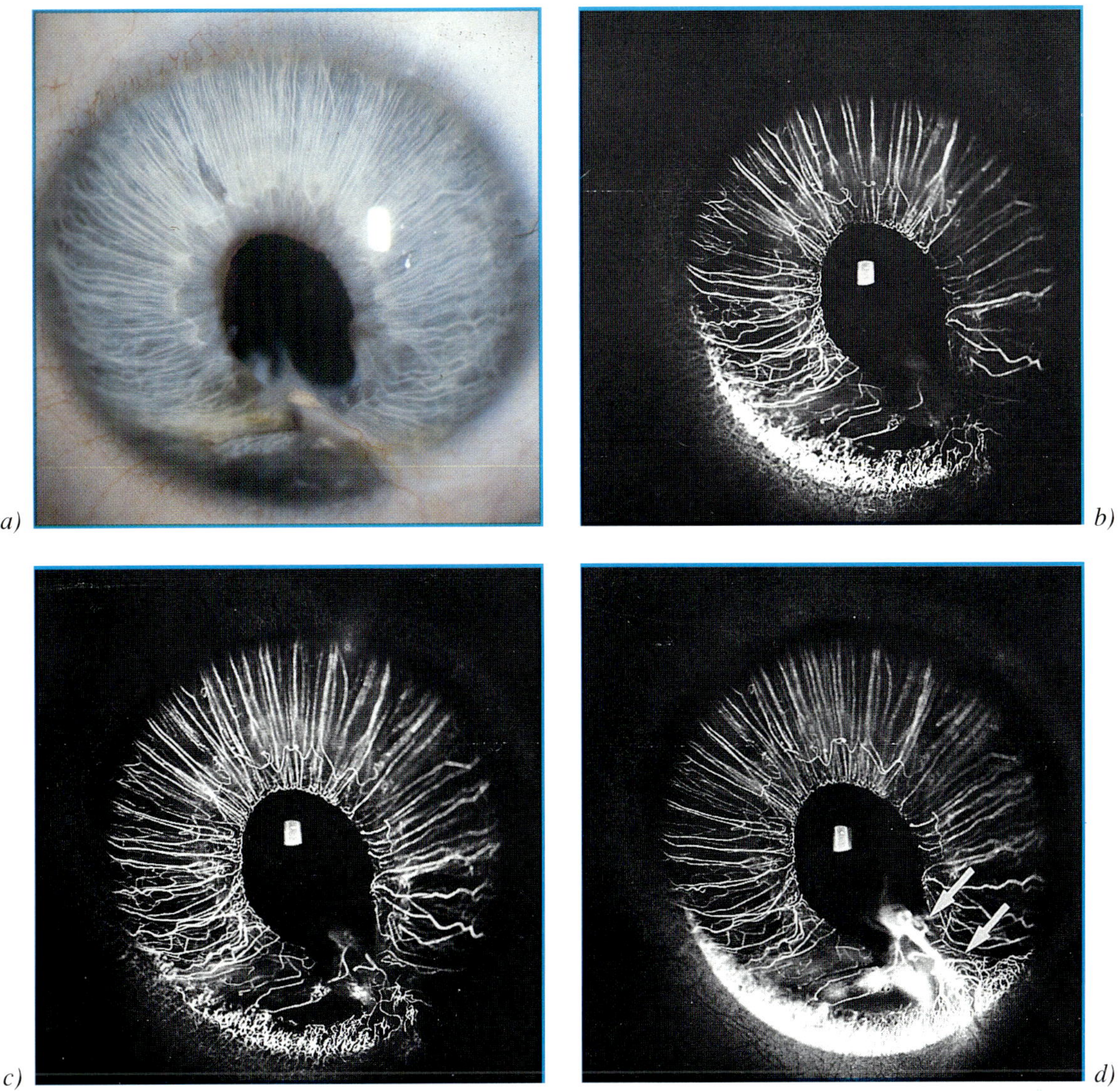

*Fig. **4.11**,13 - In this case the lower sectors of the iris appear stretched and delaminated and present synechiae with adjacent structures (a: biomicroscopy; b,c,d: fluorescein angiographic phases). The evident hyperfluorescence in the later phases (d) (see arrows) starts mainly from a corneal new vessel in the scar.*

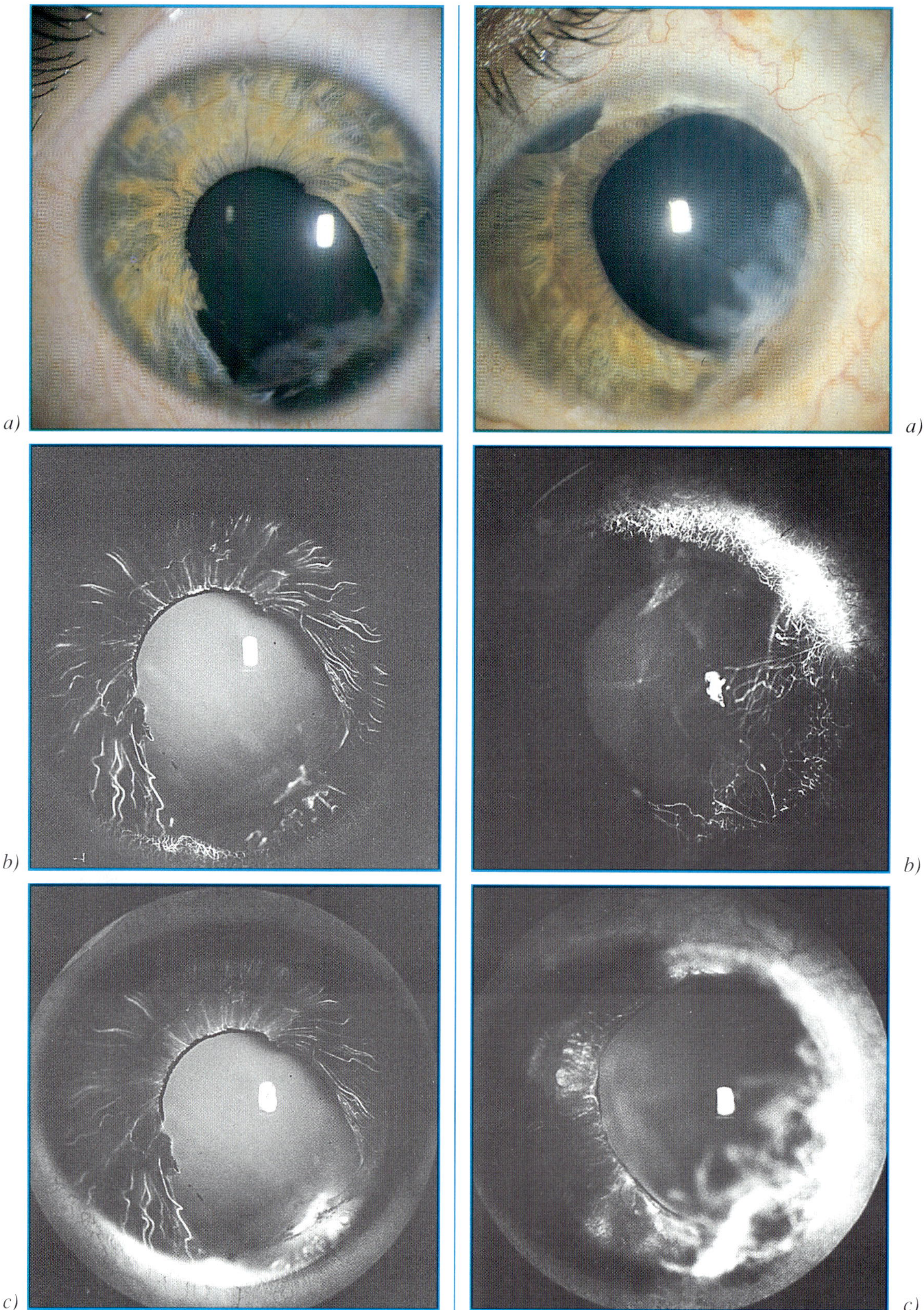

*Fig. **4.11**,14 - Old perforating wound with enlargement of the pupil because of massive laceration of the lower hemi-iris (a: biomicroscopy; b,c: fluorescein angiographic phases).*

*Fig. **4.11**,15 - Vascularized corneal scar after a perforating trauma. Biomicroscopic view (a). The fluorescein angiographic picture is dominated by early hyperfluorescence from the corneal new vessels (b), becoming more marked in later phases (c). There is clearly breakage of the blood-iris barrier, also in the stromal vessels.*

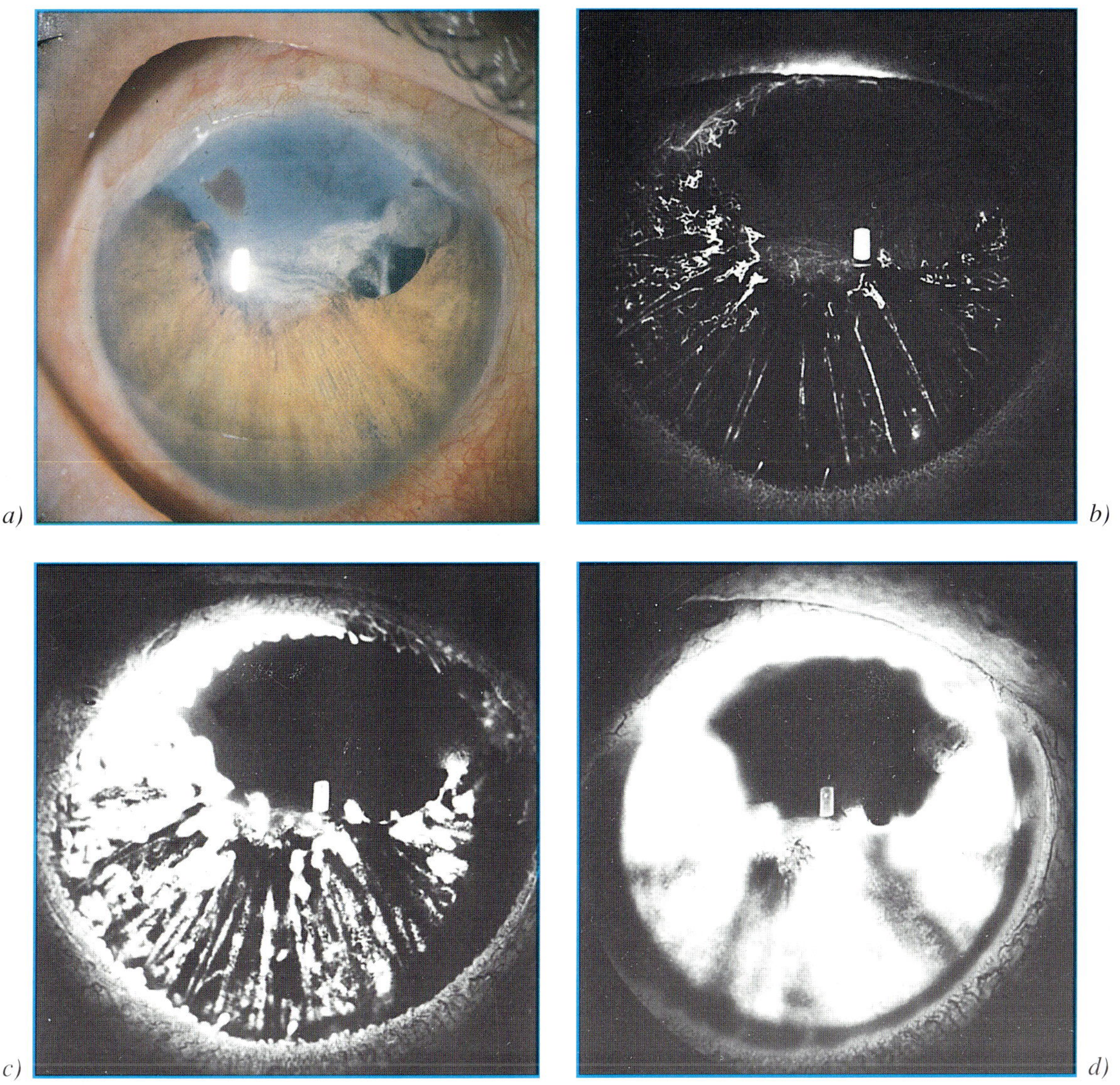

*Fig. **4.11**,16 - Biomicroscopy (a) in a case of severe post-traumatic distortion of the iris. Iris fluorescein angiography (b,c,d) shows marked congestion of the remnant radial vessels, areas of nonperfusion and neovascular tufts. The marked hyperfluorescence in the later phases (c,d) is due to the increased permeability of the stromal vessels and also to dye leakage from new-formed vessels.*

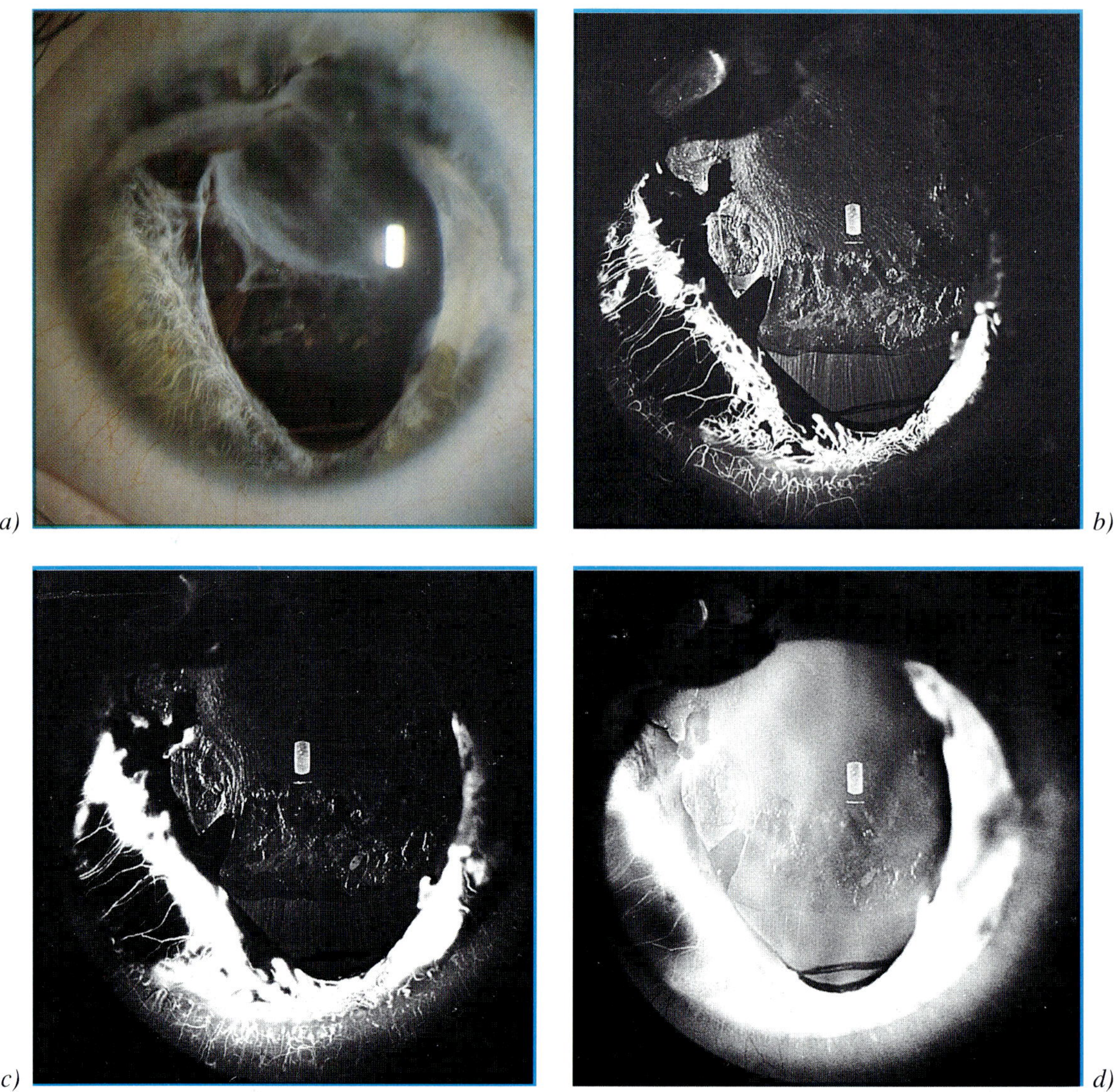

Fig. ***4.11****,17 - Biomicroscopy (a) in another ocular trauma case. The fluorescein angiographic picture (b,c,d) is dominated by ischemia and neovascularization in the remnants of the lacerated iris. Strands of posterior iris structures are joined by synechiae to the lenticular masses.*

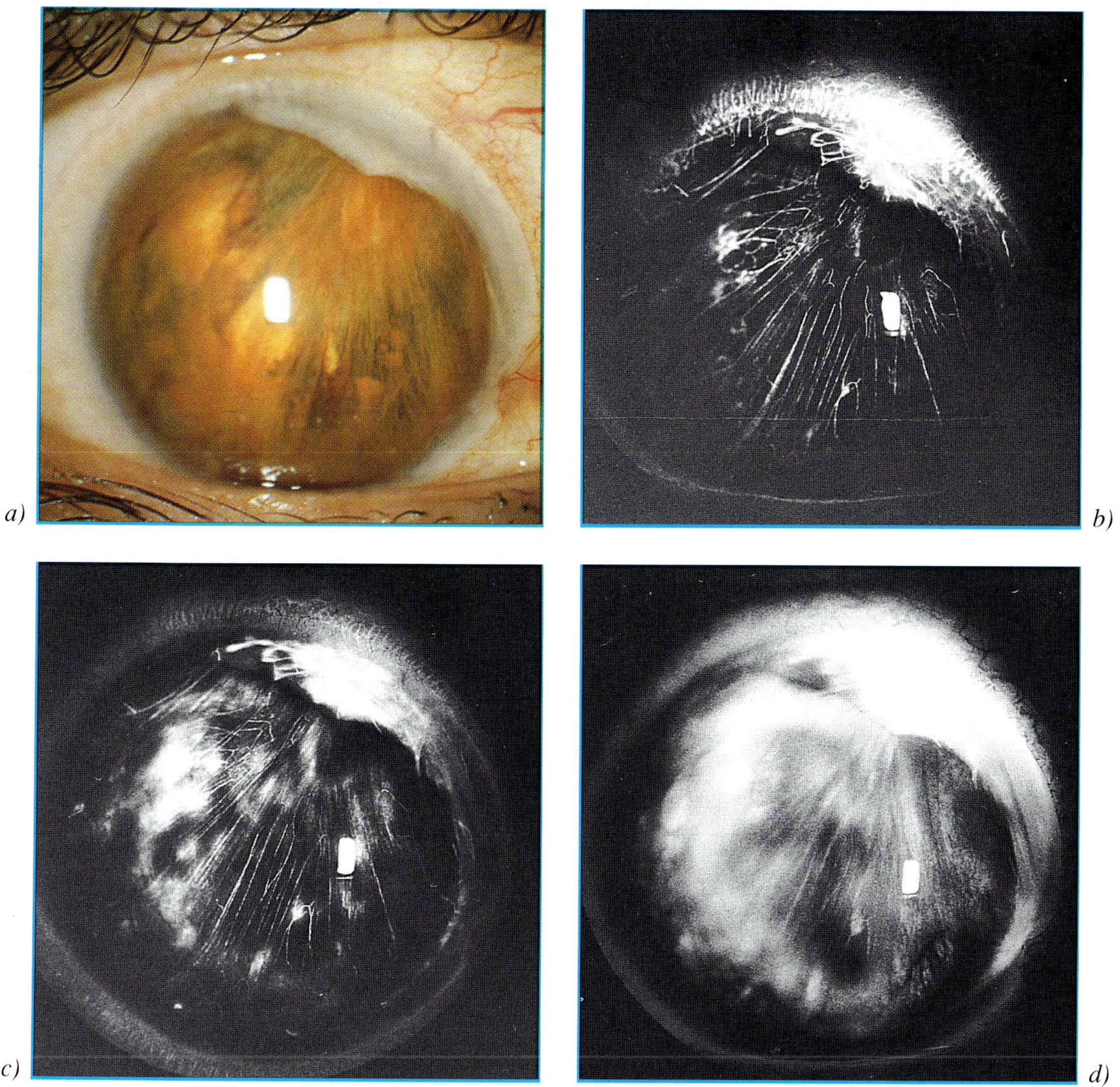

*Fig. **4.11**,18 - Biomicroscopy (a) in a case of old trauma in which the pupil has risen and become obliterated. In this case the persistent rupture of the blood-iris barrier and the fact that there are some new vessels indicates that the globe has not yet reached a state of balance (b,c,d: angiographic phases).*

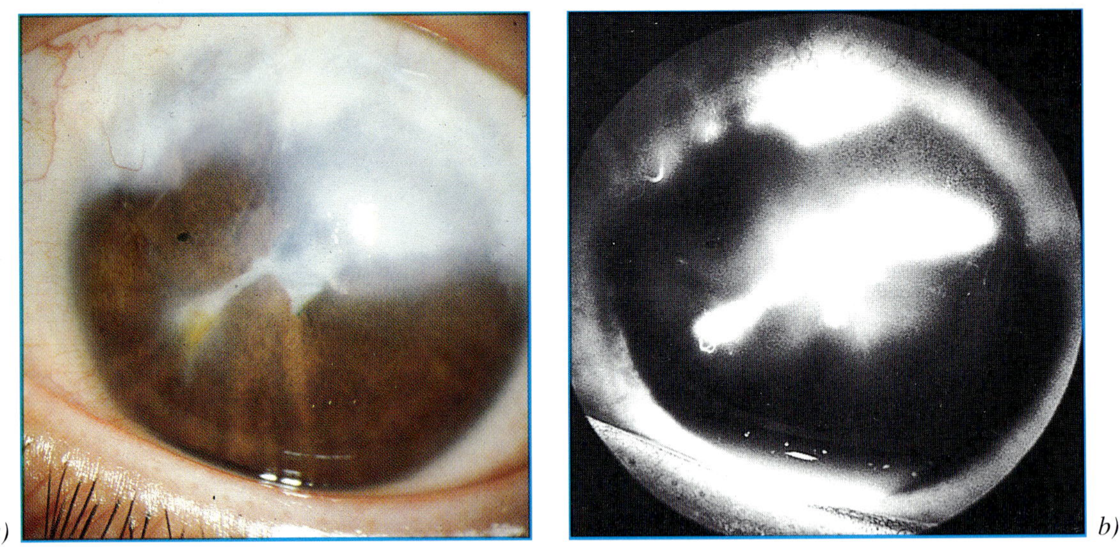

Fig. ***4.11****,19 - Old perforating trauma with a scantily vascularized leukoma in the upper sectors of the cornea, cataract and fibrotic irido-corneal-lenticular bands. Biomicroscopy (a) and fluorescein angiography (b).*

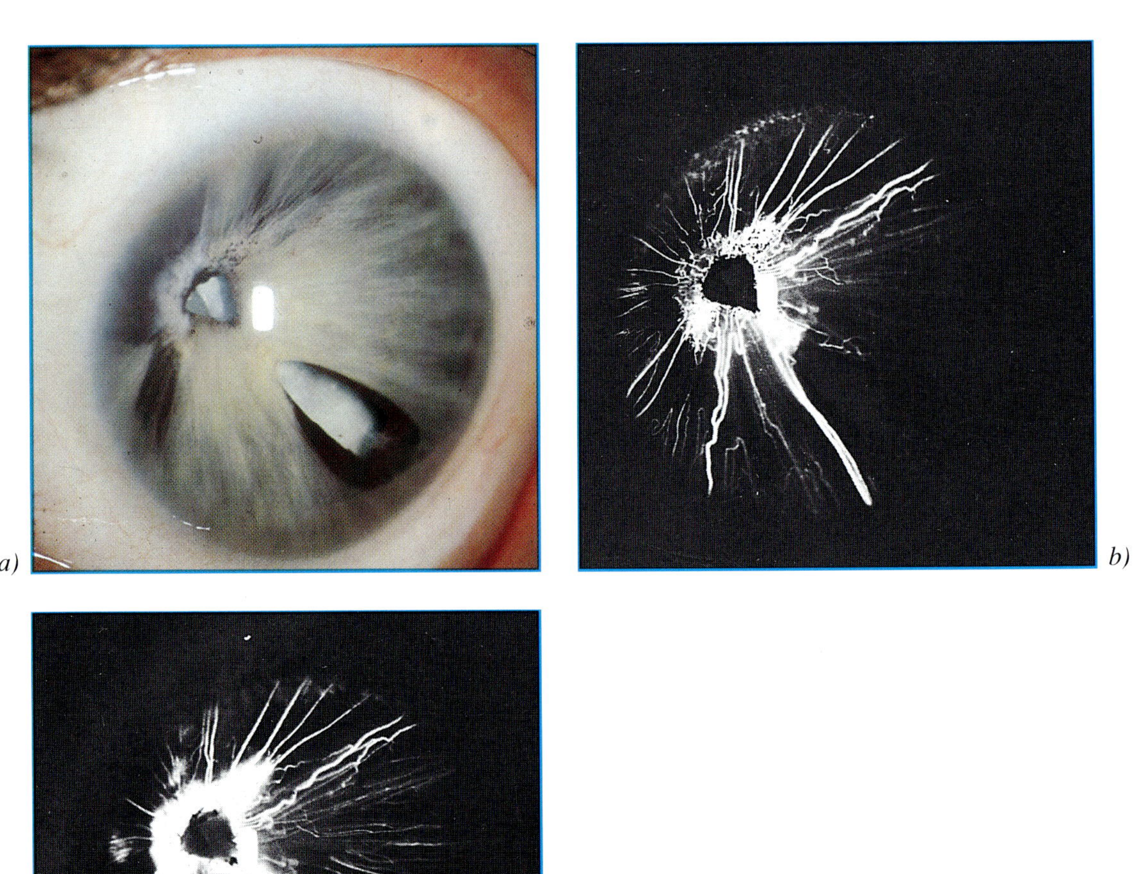

Fig. ***4.11****,20 - Pupillary ectopia, holes in the iris, opacity and subluxation of the lens in an old trauma (a: biomicroscopy). Iris angiography shows the iris vessels (b,c) have taken an abnormal path to adapt to the new conditions, though vascular permeability is normal. New vessels can be seen in the peripupillary portion.*

Analytical index of pictures